Diagnostic Ultrasound

Text and Cases

Diagnostic Ultrasound
Text and Cases

Edited by

Dennis A. Sarti, M.D.
Department of Radiology
University of California at Los Angeles
Center for the Health Sciences
Los Angeles, California

W. Frederick Sample, M.D.
Department of Radiology
University of California at Los Angeles
Center for the Health Sciences
Los Angeles, California

G. K. Hall Medical Publishers
70 Lincoln Street
Boston, Massachusetts 02111

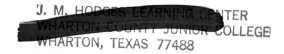

G. K. Hall Medical Publishers
70 Lincoln Street
Boston, Massachusetts 02111

83   84   /   10   9   8

Sarti, Dennis A.

Diagnostic Ultrasound

Includes index.
1. Diagnosis, Ultrasonic. 2. Diagnosis, Ultrasonic—Cases, clinical reports, statistics. I. Sample, William Frederick, joint author. II. Title.
RC78.7.U4S27   616.07'54

Library of Congress Catalog No. 79-184

ISBN 0-8161-2110-9

The authors and publisher have worked to ensure that all information in this book concerning drug dosages, schedules, and routes of administration is accurate at the time of publication. As medical research and practice advance, however, therapeutic standards may change. For this reason, and because human and mechanical errors will sometimes occur, we recommend that our readers consult the *PDR* or a manufacturer's product information sheet prior to prescribing or administering any drug discussed in this volume.

To Sunny
and to
Marc, Jennifer, and Jeffrey
    Dennis A. Sarti

To my family, which has
provided so much support
for so long.
    W. Frederick Sample

In Memoriam

W. FREDERICK SAMPLE, M.D.,

*for his many contributions
to diagnostic ultrasound*

Contents

Foreword

The concept of writing a textbook enters your thoughts fleetingly at first and gradually builds. You discuss the project with others who have accomplished the task and hear, "It was very rewarding, but I'll never do it again." You become cautious but optimistic, for the others all survived. Naively, you make a decision to undertake the project. The mental commitment occurs early on. You have no idea of the time commitment necessary until you are too far along to turn back. It is only at this point that you can decide intelligently whether or not to undertake the project. Alas, it is too late.

Diagnostic ultrasound has undergone numerous recent advances that have consistently and often dramatically improved image quality. This has created difficulties in textbook writing. The time frame necessary from when a case is scanned initially to when it appears in print can be as long as two to three years. This presents a dilemma for the practicing ultrasonographer whose current images are of much better quality and are more informative than those in the textbooks. Information becomes outdated by the time it reaches those for whom it was intended.

However, there has been little change in B-scan image quality since the development of the gray scale. Recent research has been oriented toward a digital scan converter and real-time image improvement. Although the digital scan converter has increased system stability, it has not improved image quality dramatically, if at all. Realtime images presently do not compare with high quality B-scan images. Therefore, the time appears right for an extensive, well-illustrated text in the field.

When developing the groundwork or format for a textbook, an author tries to orient his or her material toward a specific audience. Those who are in most need at the present time for such a book are the practicing ultrasonographers and radiologists who have had no formal training in this specific area. Also, the expanding field of radiology will shortly confront its residents with ultrasonography at the board examinations. It is toward these two groups that this text is specifically oriented with the hope that others, such as medical students, technologists, and referring physicians, may also benefit from it.

Much of the design format for this text came from the suggestions of practicing radiologists who visited the UCLA Ultrasound Laboratory for one- to two-week intervals to acquire further training. While visiting, they often asked to peruse a teaching file or some other organized form of case material. With these requests in mind, we decided to develop this text as an ultrasound teaching file.

The textbook chapters are divided according to organ systems. Each chapter contains two major sections: written text and case material. The written text describes technique, normal anatomy, and pathological states. The initial section of each chapter is primarily the work of the various outstanding contributors, with minor changes by the editors.

The second section of each chapter is comprised of case material compiled and discussed by the editors. Most of the images were obtained from the diagnostic laboratory of the UCLA School of Medicine in Westwood, California, with some from the Harbor General Hospital Campus in Torrance, California. A few of the images were obtained from outside laboratories and will be so noted in the text.

Since diagnostic ultrasound is a visual field, the case material section has been given great attention. The editors have maintained strict control of, and responsibility for, this section for two reasons: (1) the teaching file approach necessitates a uniform presentation; and (2) image quality and extensive labeling are, therefore, more consistent.

Each of the 1192 figures in the text is abundantly labeled. The decision to maintain extensive labeling was both intentional and time-consuming and was accomplished because we felt that the beginning and intermediate ultrasonographer can learn a great deal of anatomy from these images, through the labeling, in addition to the obvious pathology for which each case was presented.

As a project such as this reaches completion, it becomes obvious that the efforts and energies of many individuals are responsible for the end result. Most of the images in this text were performed by, or with the assistance of, technologists who are intelligent, highly motivated, and extremely independent. The excellent technical skills of the following individuals were invaluable in compiling the cases: Gerta Awender, Bob Clark, Fred Gardner, Rosemary Glenny, Janel Parker, Pamela Scarlett, and Kathleen Weber.

Since the text contains a large number of images, photography plays an extremely important role. We have been fortunate to have the assistance of Kim Willis who worked long hours under adverse conditions to accomplish what at many times must have seemed an insurmountable task. Lastly and most importantly, we wish to express a special thanks to Jean Slater who provided the secretarial assistance necessary in this endeavor. In addition to her other duties, which are burdensome, she found the time and energy to complete this project; and she was there to give encouragement at the numerous low points along the way.

Dennis A. Sarti
W. Frederick Sample

Contributors

Catherine Cole-Beuglet, M.D.
Associate Professor of Radiology
Jefferson Medical College
Thomas Jefferson University
Philadelphia, Pennsylvania

Peter Cooperberg, M.D.
Assistant Professor of Radiology
University of British Columbia
Chief, Section of Ultrasound
Department of Diagnostic Radiology
Vancouver General Hospital
Vancouver, British Columbia, Canada

Ken Erikson
Rohe Scientific Corporation
Santa Ana, California

Harvey M. Goldstein, M.D.
Radiologist
S. W. Texas Methodist Hospital
Clinical Professor of Radiology
University of Texas Health Science Center
San Antonio, Texas

Barry Green, M.D.
Assistant Professor and Co-Director of Diagnostic
  Ultrasound
Departments of Diagnostic Radiology and Pediatrics
The University of Texas System Cancer Center
M. D. Anderson Hospital and Tumor Institute
Houston, Texas

Anthony A. Mancuso, M.D.
Assistant Professor
Ultrasound/CT Section
Department of Radiology
University of California School of Medicine
Los Angeles, California

Michael M. Raskin, M.D.
Clinical Assistant Professor of Radiology
University of Miami School of Medicine
Director of Nuclear Medicine and Ultrasound
St. Francis Hospital
Associate Director of Radiology
St. Francis Hospital
Miami Beach, Florida
Florida Medical Center
Lauderdale Lakes, Florida

W. Frederick Sample, M.D.
Associate Professor
Ultrasound/CT Section
Department of Radiology
University of California School of Medicine
Los Angeles, California

Dennis A. Sarti, M.D.
Assistant Professor
Ultrasound/CT Section
Department of Radiology
University of California School of Medicine
Los Angeles, California

Michael S. Shaub, M.D.
Staff Radiologist
Centinela Valley and Daniel Freeman Hospitals
Assistant Clinical Professor of Radiology
University of California School of Medicine
Los Angeles, California

Diagnostic Ultrasound

Text and Cases

1.
Basic Principles of Diagnostic Ultrasound

W. Frederick Sample, M.D.
Kenneth Erikson

Sound Wave Characteristics

Mechanical Waves

Unlike the electromagnetic waves responsible for most imaging systems, sound waves are mechanical phenomena that require an elastic, deformable medium for their propagation. Sound can be envisioned as a displacement or pressure wave with the particles of the medium oscillating about their average positions. This vibration produces localized changes in the density of the medium (fig. 1.1). Increases in density above that of the undisturbed medium are termed condensations and are regions of increased pressure. Density or pressure decreases are called rarefactions. Mechanical energy propagates through the medium without actual "flow" of the molecules of the medium since they vibrate about the same position.

Sound waves are longitudinal or transverse vibrations, or they are combinations of both. In water and soft biological tissue, pure longitudinal waves predominate, with particle motion along the direction of propagation. In such solids as bone, transverse or shear waves also may be generated and have a particle motion normal (90°) to the wave propagation.

Wave Parameters

In a continuous-sound field the simplest wave is a plane wave in which the condensations and rarefactions travel in parallel, equally spaced planes in the direction of energy flow. If we freeze the wave at one instant of time, as in figure 1.1, a wavelength (λ) is defined as the distance between planes in the medium where the pressure, density, and, therefore, the displacement amplitudes are equal. Unfreezing the wave, successive planes of maximum pressure pass a given point in a regular sequence. The wave period (P) is the time required for the wave to move forward through a distance of one wavelength in the medium. The frequency (f) of the wave is equal to the number of cycles that pass a given point in the medium in one second ($P = \frac{1}{f}$). The unit of vibrational frequency is the Hertz (Hz) and equals one cycle per second (1 kHz = 10^3 cps and 1 MHz = 10^6 cps). Sound waves are further categorized, according to frequency, as infrasonic (less than 20 Hz); audible (20 Hz to 20 kHz); and ultrasonic (greater than 20 kHz).

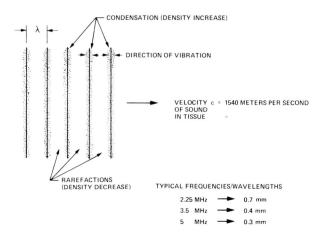

Fig. 1.1

Velocity of Sound

The velocity (c) of sound waves is a constant of a medium and is dependent upon the inertial (density, ρ) and elastic (bulk modulus of elasticity, E) characteristics of the medium. The units of the velocity of sound are meters per second (m/sec).

$$c = \sqrt{\frac{E}{\rho}}\, m/sec \quad (1)$$

For living, soft biological tissues in which the propagation of sound is longitudinal, there is essentially no dependence of the velocity of sound on frequency, at least not in the frequency ranges normally used in diagnostic ultrasound. Since elastic characteristics are temperature-dependent, velocity is temperature-dependent; however, over the temperature variations encountered in living biological materials, the effect on velocity is minimal.

The propagation velocity of a number of common biological materials is summarized in table 1.1. With the exception of air, bone, fat, water, and the lens of the eye, the velocity of sound is very similar in most biological tissues, averaging 1540 meters per second (m/sec). The relationship among velocity, frequency, and wavelength is given as follows.

$$\lambda = \frac{c}{f} \quad (2)$$

Typical wavelengths for commonly used sound frequencies in medical imaging are shown in figure 1.1. In reality, the small changes in the velocity of sound as a

sound wave of given frequency passes through different biological materials, produce important tissue interaction phenomena to be described later.

Table 1.1
Velocity of Sound in Some Common Biological Materials

Biological Material	Velocity of Sound (m/sec)
Air	330
Fat	1450
Water	1480
Human soft tissues (average)	1540
Brain	1540
Liver	1550
Kidney	1560
Blood	1570
Muscle	1580
Lens of eye	1620
Skull bone	4080

Acoustic Intensity

The intensity (I) of a sound beam represents the average rate of energy flowing through a unit area and is usually expressed in watts per cm². The intensity of a plane wave can be related to pressure amplitude, particle displacement amplitude, the velocity of sound, and the undisturbed density of the medium by various formulas. The intensity of a sound beam can also be related to the voltage applied to the transducer generating the sound energy. Sound intensities are difficult to measure directly.

Since the sound intensities encountered in medical imaging may vary over a range of at least a million to one, the decibel (dB) system is convenient for expressing ratios of intensities in a logarithmic form, with one level taken as a reference.

$$\text{Intensity Ratio} = 10 \log_{10} \frac{I_1}{I_0}\, dB \quad (3)$$

where I_1 is the measured intensity and I_0 is the reference intensity.

Therefore, if the relative intensities are 2/1, 10/1, or 1000/1, the decibel notation would be 3, 10, and 30 dB respectively. The decibel system is frequently used to express the relative amplitude of sound reflections or amplifier gains. Since amplitudes and intensities are related as ($I = A^2$), equation 3 becomes:

$$\text{Amplitude Ratio} = 20 \log_{10} \frac{\text{Amplitude}_1}{\text{Amplitude}_2} \, dB \quad (4)$$

Generation of Sound Waves

Piezoelectricity

Piezoelectricity is the physical phenomenon by which the sound waves used in medical imaging are generated. "Piézein" is a Greek word meaning "to squeeze." Piezoelectricity is only possible in materials, usually crystals or composites of crystals, which are anisotropic, with properties that are different in different directions. When a voltage is applied to a piezoelectric element, it will either expand or compress, according to the polarity of the voltage. If the element is in contact with a material, a sound wave will be generated. Conversely, when the element is mechanically compressed or expanded, as when a sound wave strikes it, a voltage will be produced. The same element can therefore generate and receive sound waves.

Some naturally occuring piezoelectric materials used to generate sound are quartz, lithium sulphate, and Rochelle salt. Although quartz is often still used above 20 MHz, most piezoelectric elements used for medical diagnosis (1–10 MHz frequencies) are synthetic ceramics. Mixtures of metallic oxides are fused at very high temperatures (1500°C) and shaped into elements. The most commonly used ceramic is lead zirconate titanate, often referred to by the trade name, PZT. To create the piezoelectric characteristic, the ceramic is reheated to a temperature (193°C for PZT) called its Curie point and then cooled down, with a high-DC voltage applied, which aligns the anisotropic molecules in the direction of the "poling" electric field. Once poled in this fashion, the ceramic cannot be reheated to the Curie point because it will be de-poled, and the piezoelectric characteristic will be lost.

Piezoelectric ceramic elements can be designed to vibrate in a variety of modes including length, thickness, and radial modes. In medical applications, we are primarily concerned with the thickness mode, and the elements are usually in the shape of a disk. Figure 1.2 shows such an element in a typical transducer sending a sound wave into a water tank. The element also generates an unwanted wave in the opposite direction. This

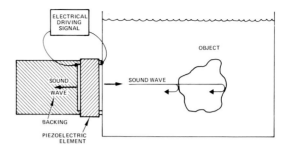

Fig. 1.2

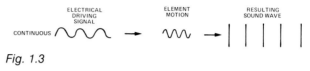

Fig. 1.3

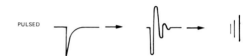

Fig. 1.4

must be absorbed in the backing, or spurious signals will result.

The sound wave is depicted striking an object in the water tank, with a portion reflected back toward the transducer. Some of the sound energy enters the object, where it is again reflected. If a continuous sinusoidal voltage (fig. 1.3) is applied to the element, a sound wave is established in the tank, but it is difficult to distinguish the reflected waves from the front and rear of the object. If the transducer is excited by a short electric pulse (fig. 1.4), however, separate echoes from the front and back surface will be received. This pulse-echo mode is essential for ultrasonic medical imaging as it is practiced today.

Frequency Characteristics

A piezoelectric element has a dominant or resonant frequency, much like that of a pendulum. When constructed to vibrate predominately in the thickness mode, the resonant frequency is determined by the thickness. The intensity of the sound emitted is maximum at the resonant frequency. If a sinusoidal voltage is applied to a piezoelectric element, it can be caused to vibrate at frequencies other than the resonant frequency, but a lower intensity will be achieved. As the driving frequency approaches the resonant frequency, the intensity will increase until internal damping factors, such as friction and heat loss, restrict the amplitude of the vibration.

When a short electric pulse is applied to a piezoelectric element, it will ring at its resonant frequency, much like a bell that is sharply struck. The magnitude of the vibration gradually decays to zero over a period of time, depending upon the mechanical losses or damping. To enhance the ability to distinguish or resolve closely spaced objects, a short pulse of ultrasound is desired. This cannot be achieved simply by making a shorter electric pulse, because the natural frequency of the transducer dominates, producing the slowly damped "tail" of the pulse (fig. 1.4). This can be minimized through proper transducer design. Another solution for better resolution would be to use a higher-frequency transducer. As discussed later, there are other considerations which limit the usefulness of this idea.

The waveform, or element motion, in the pulse case actually contains a continuum of many different frequencies dominated by the resonant frequency. The range of these frequencies is called the bandwidth of the transducer. For example, a typical 3.5-MHz transducer designed for pulse operation has substantial energy in a continuous range of frequencies from 2.5 to 4.5 MHz.

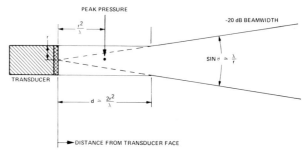

Fig. 1.5

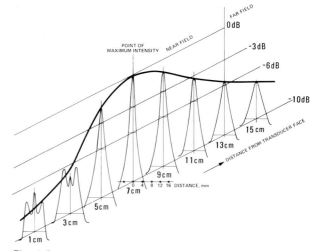

Fig. 1.6

Sound Beam Characteristics

The sound beam emitted by a planar, disk-shaped (unfocused) piezoelectric element is divided into two regions. In the near field, or Fresnel region, the beamwidth is relatively constant in diameter. In the far field, or Fraunhofer region, the beam diverges. The transition of the near and far fields (d) is determined by the radius of the element (r) and the wavelength (λ) (fig. 1.5). If the radius is reduced, the near field beamwidth is reduced, the distance to the near field–far field transition is shortened, and the angle of divergence in the far field is increased. Usually the element diameter is 10 to 20 times the wavelength in order to be adequately collimated. If the wavelength is shortened (i.e., the frequency is increased), the beamwidth in the near field is unchanged, the distance to the near field–far field transition is lengthened, and the angle of divergence in the far field is reduced. These are all desirable characteristics.

Although the general configuration of an unfocused sound beam is relatively simple, the energy distribution throughout the beam is complex. As the wave pro-

gresses outward from the source, there are maxima and minima of sound intensity (fig. 1.6). These peaks and valleys of intensity are the result of the superposition of the sound field, from the various vibrating regions of the element, that results in areas of addition or cancellation of the sound intensity. This effect is most significant in a narrow bandwidth transducer and becomes less pronounced as the bandwidth is increased. A last maximum occurs before the near field–far field transition, beyond which the sound intensity decreases as 1/(distance)^2 which is called the inverse square law.

Even though the near field sound beam of an unfocused transducer has a nondivergent, approximately cylindrical shape, the intensity is usually greatest along the central axis of the beam and falls off toward the edge. In addition, there may be side lobes of increased intensity (fig. 1.6).

Focused Sound Beams

A sound beam can be focused by means of an acoustic lens, mirror, or appropriate change in the shape of the

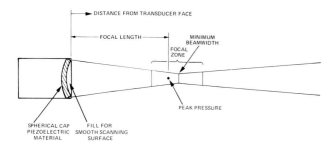

Fig. 1.7

Table 1.2
Specific Acoustic Impedance Values for Common Materials

Material	Z (Rayls) (10^6 kg/sec m^2)
Air	0.0004
Fat	1.38
Water	1.48
Kidney	1.62
Mean (soft tissues)	1.63
Liver	1.65
Plastic	3.20
Skull bone	7.80
Steel	40.00

piezoelectric element itself (fig. 1.7). The diameter of the sound beam at the focal point depends on the focal length and the diameter-to-wavelength ratio of the element. A larger element for a given frequency and focal length results in a smaller focal area. The length of the region of improved diameter or focal zone also is variable. It is shorter for more highly focused beams. The focal length of a transducer cannot be made longer than the distance of peak pressure (r^2/λ) of an unfocused transducer of similar diameter and frequency. Beyond that point, far field spreading dominates no matter what focusing is attempted.

The Interaction of Sound with Tissue

Sound energy interacts with tissue and targets by means of transmission, reflection, refraction, diffraction, scattering, and absorption. The type of interaction which occurs depends upon the characteristics of the material, the frequency of the sound, the wavelength relative to the size of the object, the orientation of acoustic interfaces, and the acoustic impedance.

Acoustic Impedance

The acoustic impedance (Z) of a substance is the product of its density (ρ) and the velocity of sound (c).

$$Z = \rho c \quad (5)$$

If equation (1) is substituted into (5) it can be shown that, in fact, acoustic impedance depends on the density and elasticity of a substance.

$$Z = \sqrt{\rho E} \quad (6)$$

Values of specific acoustical impedance for various materials are given in table 1.2, expressed in units of rayls or kilograms per m^2 per second. In general, the acoustic impedances of solids are higher than liquids, which, in turn, are higher than gases.

Reflection

When a sound beam encounters an interface between two substances, the type of reflection and the strength of the reflection depend upon many factors. When the sound beam strikes the interface perpendicularly, the fraction of energy that is reflected (R) versus the fraction that is transmitted (T) depends upon the acoustical impedances Z_1 and Z_2 of the two substances:

$$R = \frac{Z_1 - Z_2}{Z_1 + Z_2} \quad (7)$$

$$T = 1 - R \quad (8)$$

Figure 1.8 depicts the reflection and transmission of a plane sound wave through several common interfaces. For example, if a sound pulse is launched in water (Z_0) and then encounters bone (Z_1), 68% of the energy will be reflected with only 32% left to propagate through the bone. At the back of the bone, 68% of that remaining is again reflected, leaving only 10% (0.32 × 0.32) continuing into the water (Z_2). The 68% reflected at the Z_1–Z_2 interface returns toward the transducer, but it encounters the Z_0–Z_1 interface where 68% is reflected.

Thus, 14% (0.68 × 0.32 × 0.68) returns to the transducer from the back interface. This multiple reflection phenomenon continues as shown in figure 1.8 until the

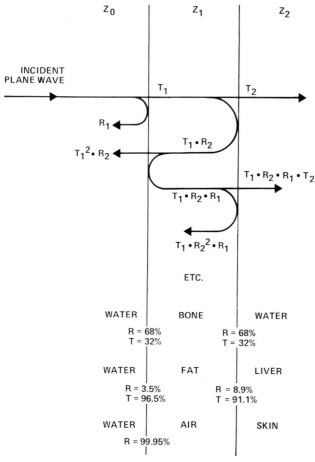

Fig. 1.8

normal to the axis of the transducer, a maximum amount of sound is returned to the transducer (left side of figure 1.9). As the interface is tilted (right side) even slightly, the reflected sound received decreases rapidly until it completely misses the transducer. The angle between the sound beam and the perpendicular to the interface (angle of incidence) is equal to the corresponding angle for the reflected beam (angle of reflection).

Refraction

When a sound beam strikes a large smooth acoustic interface at an angle off the perpendicular, and the velocity of the sound changes at the interface, a deviation of the transmitted beam occurs. This is called refraction (fig. 1.9, right side). Bending of the beam occurs because a portion of the wavefront travels at a different velocity in the second material than in the first. The amount of deviation changes with the angle of incidence. Fortunately, refraction is generally not much of a problem because the velocity of sound in soft tissue is relatively constant.

sound escapes or is absorbed in layer Z_1. Fortunately, soft tissues do not present the same problem. In the second example in figure 1.8 a water–fat liver interface shows that only 3.5% is reflected from the first interface, leaving 96.5% available for further use. In this case, weak signals are generated because the reflection coefficient is low. Thus, many interfaces can be traversed before the sound level is too small to be detected. In the third example, a water–air interface shows the necessity of using a coupling gel and excluding any air bubbles when scanning because the reflection coefficient when air is present is virtually 100%, preventing the sound from entering the body.

Specular Reflection

Specular reflection occurs when the sound beam strikes a large smooth interface (fig. 1.9). When the interface is

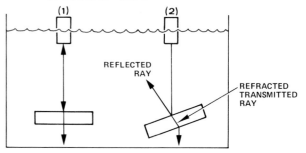

Fig. 1.9

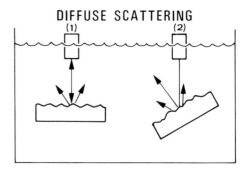

Fig. 1.10

Critical Angle Reflection

When a sound beam strikes a smooth acoustical interface at angles other than the perpendicular, more of the energy is reflected, and less is transmitted. An angle will eventually be reached, depending upon the velocity change across the interface, where the refracted sound travels along the interface. Beyond this critical angle, the sound is completely reflected, and none is transmitted. Clinically, this becomes extremely important when evaluating acoustic shadowing.

Diffuse Scattering

When a "rough" surface intercepts a sound beam, the sound is scattered in many directions in a random fashion (fig. 1.10). The designation, rough, refers to a surface texture of many wavelengths so that a few millimeters of roughness are needed at diagnostic frequencies. Although the signal amplitude is generally greatest when the interface is normal to the beam, it is much smaller than with the smooth reflector because energy is scattered away from the transducer. Unlike the smooth reflector, this interface returns energy to the transducer over a much wider range of inclinations. Specular reflectors are, therefore, harder to scan than diffuse ones, because a signal is only received within a limited range, and then it is likely to be an overloading signal. Anyone who has caught a momentarily blinding flash of bright sun from a piece of chrome on an automobile is familiar with this phenomenon of specular reflection.

Rayleigh Scattering

Rayleigh scattering is caused by particles smaller than a wavelength. Such objects are not resolved but merely send back a signal whose intensity varies as (d^6/λ^4), where d is the particle size. This has an interesting consequence for gray scale ultrasonography. Tissue can be thought of as resolvable structures, such as major vessels, and a huge collection of nonresolvable objects, such as minor vessels and other structures down to the microscopic cellular level. The fourth power relationship encourages us to go to higher frequencies so that signal levels from these nonresolvable structures are larger. For example, an increase in frequency from 2.25 MHz

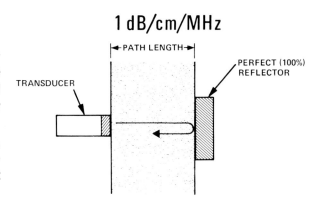

1 dB/cm/MHz

ATTENUATION = PATH LENGTH x FREQUENCY x 1 dB/cm/MHz

Fig. 1.11

to 3.5 MHz will lead to a sixfold increase in these signal levels. Unfortunately, absorption limits our ability to go as high in frequency as we wish.

Absorption

All of the interactions of sound in biological tissues considered to this point preserve the sound wave energy in its original form, although it may be directed differently. Absorption, however, results in the dissipation of sound into heat. The absorption process is poorly understood in tissue, although it has been studied extensively in blood where it is related to relaxation phenomena in the protein constituents of the blood. The resulting decrease in beam intensity is exponential and increases with frequency. In most biological soft tissues, the absorption is approximately proportional to frequency, whereas in bone it is a function of the frequency squared. Absorption is the most important determinant of the depth of penetration of the sound beam into the body.

Total Attenuation of Sound in Tissue

The reduction of the intensity of a sound beam as it passes through biological tissues, the result of scattering and absorption, is known as attenuation. Attenuation is conveniently expressed as a rate of decrease of intensity in decibels per centimeter depth of tissue and is found to increase linearly with frequency in most tissues (fig. 1.11). A crude rule of thumb is that attenuation is about 1 dB/cm/MHz where the one-way path-length is used for the total distance. The reference intensity of this decibel scale is taken to be the intensity at the front surface of the biological specimen examined.

Half-value Layer

A term used to express the role of attenuation of sound in tissue is the half-value layer, which is defined as the thickness of tissue, in centimeters, required to reduce the intensity of the beam by half, i.e., -3dB. The half-value layers for several tissues at three different frequencies are summarized in table 1.3. It should be noted that not all tissues are isotropic in their attenuation. For example, attenuation in muscle may be different by a factor of 2.5. This depends upon whether the sound beam passes along or across its fibers. In general, the echoes arriving back at the emitting transducer are substantially smaller than the initially transmitted pulse because of the low reflection coefficients and high attenuation.

Table 1.3
Half-value Thickness for Various Tissues
at Three Different Frequencies - cm

	Frequency (MHz)		
	2.25	*3.5*	*5.0*
Fat (cm)	3.0	1.92	1.34
Liver	1.55	1.0	0.7
Muscle	0.77	0.5	0.35

Instrumentation

In the design of any medical imaging system, the main goal is to maximize diagnostically useful information and to suppress artifact. One of the most important parameters is resolution. In ultrasound systems, resolution must be considered in two planes. Axial or depth resolution is defined as the ability of the system to separate objects in depth along the axis of the sound beam. Lateral or azimuthal resolution is defined as the ability to distinguish two objects laterally placed at the same depth, i.e., spatial resolution perpendicular to the sound beam. Axial resolution is determined by the pulse length which in turn has a minimum length determined by the

transducer frequency. Lateral resolution depends on the beamwidth which is primarily a function of transducer size, focal length, and frequency.

Both axial and lateral resolution may be improved by using higher frequency transducers. Unfortunately, absorption increases at higher frequencies, so less penetration or high input power levels must be accepted. Less penetration is acceptable for scanning regions close to the skin, but higher power levels may be inadvisable, especially in obstetrics, where biological effects are not well understood.

Another approach to improving penetration is to improve system sensitivity. Sensitivity is defined as the ability to detect weak signals and is normally limited by thermal noise in the amplifiers used. Fortunately, most modern ultrasound systems are operating near this thermal noise limit. This means, however, that increasing power levels is one of the few ways of improving penetration at higher frequencies.

A generalized block diagram of a modern gray scale ultrasound system is shown in figure 1.12. The basic elements can be implemented in many different ways, but in general, any ultrasound system must have them. The inclusion of the subject and the viewer are meant to remind us of the importance of patient variability and the training of the viewer in a successful diagnostic application.

In this section each component of a modern gray scale ultrasound B-scan system will be discussed in terms of its influence on system performance, including the variables under the operator's control. Techniques available to the operator for calibrating and standardizing the function of each component are provided in the references to this chapter.

Coupling Medium

The coupling medium between the patient and the transducer is an important part of the diagnostic system. In practice, one of the most common causes of decreased sensitivity and poor results is insufficient coupling material. An adequate amount of coupling medium eliminates an air gap or air bubbles which have a reflection coefficient approaching 100%, thus decreasing the transmitted sound to practically zero.

Either mineral oil or water-soluble gels are used as coupling agents for contact B-scan systems. Both mate-

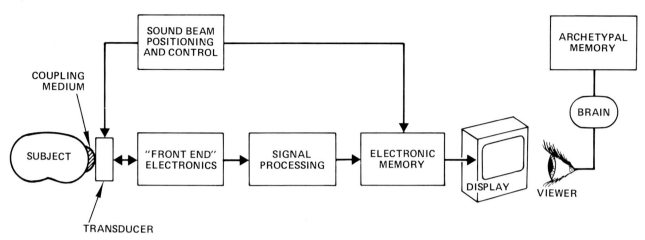

Fig. 1.12

rials have good acoustic properties. A single application of a water soluble gel tends to last longer but is more expensive.

Confined water can also serve as a coupler between the transducer and the patient. In fact, water-path systems can use larger aperture transducers which are more sensitive and which have better focused beam profiles. In the future, water coupled systems may become more common, although the requirement for mechanical movement of the bulkier transducer with attendant cost and complexity may limit their widespread application.

Transducer

Many of the factors limiting sensitivity and resolution are determined by the transducer. Generally, higher frequency transducers have better axial resolution, since the wavelengths are shorter. Realistic values of axial resolution in tissue are 2 mm for 2.5 MHz, 1 mm for 5 MHz, and 0.6 mm for 7.5 MHz center frequency transducers.

The lateral resolution of an ultrasound system is determined by the transducer beamwidth characteristics. Most transducers in use today are focused at a fixed distance. As a result, the best lateral resolution occurs in a focal zone over a limited depth around the focal length. It is important to select a transducer focused for the depth of interest. Larger diameter transducers generate better lateral resolution, but over a more limited range. Contact scanning becomes cumbersome with transducers of diameter above about 25 mm.

The beam profile characteristics of the transducer being used should be known by the ultrasonographer. These can be requested from the manufacturer or can be determined using relatively simple phantoms or acoustical probes.

The displayed beamwidth of a transducer depends strongly on the subsequent signal processing. Figure 1.13 illustrates this with a simulated B-scan of a group of rods. At low gain the targets are somewhat smeared horizontally by the beamwidth, while at higher gain they are greatly exaggerated. With a perfect gray scale system, the peak portion of this scan could be distinguished. In a practical system, however, strong echoes are compressed into one or two shades of gray. Thus, the beamwidth appears to be worse on the display.

The sensitivity and resolution of a given transducer

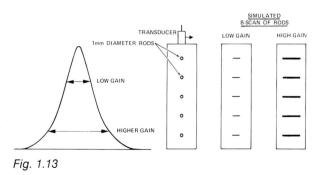

Fig. 1.13

are fixed and can only be altered by changing transducers. As will be discussed later, however, other components in the system can affect resolution and must be considered.

In the future, electronically variable focused transducers may replace existing fixed focused transducers. By means of complex signal processing, the beam can be effectively focused over a long range, thus improving overall scan quality. Real-time scanning systems using sequenced linear arrays and phased arrays are becoming common; however, discussion of these systems is beyond the scope of this book. The interested reader may refer to the work of Carson (1976; 1977) for more information.

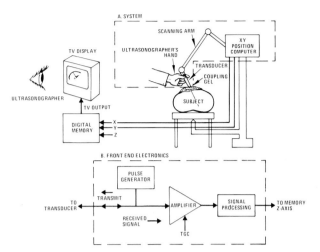

Fig. 1.14

Scanning Arm

A more detailed diagram of a manually operated contact B-scanner is shown in figure 1.14. The beam positioning information is generated by an articulated scanning arm. The transducer is attached by this arm to a support which in turn is attached to a mobile base on the floor next to the patient. The scanning arm serves two critical functions: (1) it determines the spatial orientation of the sound beam, so that the origin of a reflection from within the patient is correctly placed into the electronic memory; and (2) it constrains the scanning to a plane, so that a meaningful "cut" can be made. The X and Y coordinates of the sound beam are determined by the angles at the joints of the arm which are measured by potentiometers or optical digital encoders. If the scanning arm is not functioning properly, the spatial information is improperly registered. This function should be checked routinely with one of the various versions of the AIUM test object that are available.

Transmitter

The transmitter generates the electrical pulses which excite the transducer. Since a single transducer serves as the transmitter and the receiver, echoes must be received from the deepest structures before another pulse is transmitted. This sets an upper limit on the pulse repetition rate. In most systems, the pulse repetition rate is not under operator control and is fixed at about 1000 pulses per second. Since each pulse is about one

microsecond long, the system is capable of receiving 99.9% of the time between pulses.

The transmitter output control affects the amplitude of the emitted pulses and is often an operator variable control calibrated in decibels. A reduction of 6 dB would therefore reduce the amplitude of the pulses by one-half.

Receiver

At the transducer, sound energy is converted to an electrical signal which contains amplitude and phase information. In most present ultrasound scanning systems, amplitude information alone is used.

The electrical signal generated by piezoelectric elements from a typical weak echo is extremely small and must be amplified, often by a factor of 100,000 (100 dB) or more. The bandwidth characteristics of the amplifier must be closely matched to those of the transducer if the signal-to-noise ratio is to be kept high and if amplitude information is to be optimally preserved. The design of the amplifier is one of the most important and difficult tasks in a modern ultrasound system.

This tremendous signal range is illustrated in figure 1.15 in which signal levels from typical targets are displayed as a function of depth for different frequencies. The signal levels are referenced to a perfect (100%) reflector which corresponds to 0 dB. A strongly reflecting tissue interface with a 1% reflection (−40 dB) at the skin represents the largest signal.

Signal levels are rapidly reduced due to attenuation;

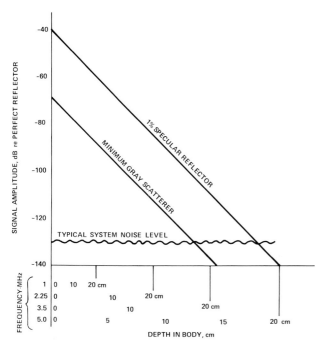

Fig. 1.15

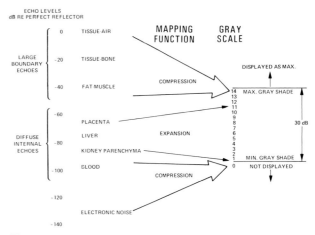

Fig. 1.16

and by using the rule of thumb, 1 dB/cm/MHz, at a depth of 20 cm in the body, the sound energy from this 1% specular interface is reduced by 20 dB at 1 MHz, up to 100 dB at 5 MHz. Thus, if only these interfaces were to be reproduced, scanning at 5 MHz could easily be accomplished to a depth of almost 20 cm before the system noise level overwhelmed the echoes.

In a gray scale system, however, much smaller echoes from small structures are of interest. For purposes of this example, suppose the weakest target of interest is 30 dB lower (32 times) than the specular interface at 2.25 MHz. Then from figure 1.15 this target could easily be detected, well beyond 20 cm at 2.25 MHz, but only to about 18 cm at 3.5 MHz and 12 cm at 5 MHz.

Signal Processing

The large signal dynamic range has additional implications for an ultrasound system. First, most displays are high quality television monitors with a dynamic range of 30 dB at best. Furthermore, since the human eye can only separately distinguish 8–10 shades of gray on a television display, each gray shade should be made to convey the most clinical information possible to the operator. Fitting a wide range of echoes into the dy-

namic range of the TV requires a special mapping or compression function (fig. 1.16). High-amplitude reflections are generally produced by specular reflection at organ boundaries and represent important spatial information. Intensity variations in these boundaries, however, have not been found clinically significant. The intensity of weak reflections produced by diffuse reflectors within tissue parenchyma has been found to convey important information concerning the nature of the tissue and certain disease processes. Therefore, in the compression scheme, the weaker echoes should be displayed through a disproportionately large part of the restricted dynamic range and assigned as many separate shades of gray as possible. Conversely, the stronger specular reflectors should be maximally compressed into a few separately detectible shades of gray. The lowest level signals, such as those from blood, are purposely blanked out to provide luscent structures on the display.

Time Gain Compensation

Another system requirement is to display the same structure at the same gray level regardless of depth in the body. This is accomplished by changing the amplification or gain as a function of depth (or echo return time) to compensate for attenuation in the body and is called time gain compensation or TGC. Depth gain compensation and swept gain are also terms sometimes used. The TGC function is illustrated in figure 1.17 where interfaces separate different attenuating materials.

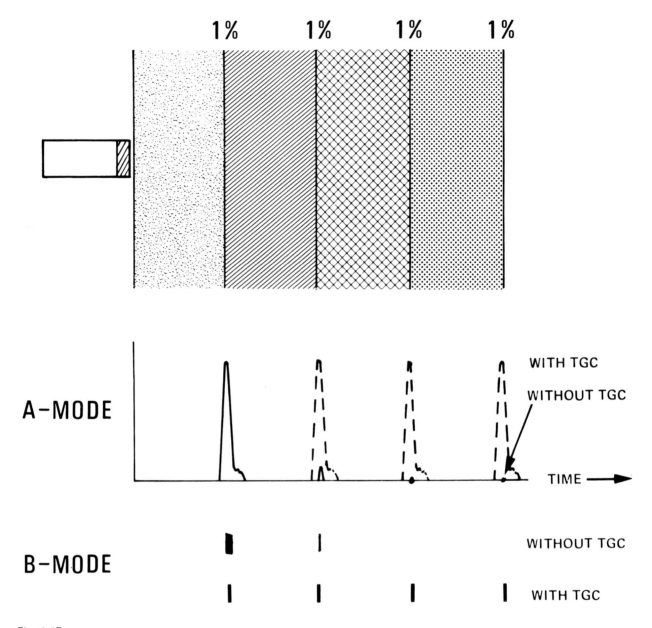

Fig. 1.17

Without TGC, the signals from the interfaces decrease rapidly and in the B-mode display only the first few would be displayed because of the dynamic range of the display. The proper amount of TGC provides a uniform display. TGC is basically an exponential function with depth, but considerable flexibility is available to the operator to compensate for patient variables. A near gain setting (fig. 1.18) separately controls the first few centimeters of amplification and is used primarily to attenuate large-amplitude echoes from skin–fat interfaces near the transducer. A delay or slope-start setting con-

trols when the time gain compensation function actually begins. The slope setting alters the rate of time gain compensation which is measured in decibels of gain increase per centimeter of depth. Some instruments also allow the operator to control the rate of change of the slope as well as provide additional amplification at any depth. Finally, a far gain setting independently controls the enhancement or suppression of distant reflections. Far gain is usually used only in echocardiology.

More sophisticated systems also attempt to correct for known variations in beam intensity throughout the

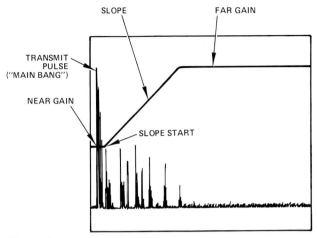

Fig. 1.18

field. Even for an unfocused transducer, the variations in signal amplitude related to attenuation and beam intensity variation are complex and different for specular and diffuse reflectors (fig. 1.19). This correction is not under the operator's control.

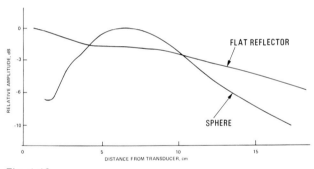

Fig. 1.19

Electronic Memory

There are two types of electronic memory in use today. The analog scan converter, in use since 1972, was responsible for making gray scale ultrasound a practical reality. The digital scan converter, recently introduced, promises to replace the analog systems, primarily because of its greater stability.

The analog scan converter (ASC) is an electron tube with an electron gun at one end and a matrix target at the other end. The electron beam can be deflected left and right, and up and down, by the X and Y axis signals generated by the position sensors in the scanning arm. The output of the amplifier carrying the ultrasound amplitude information modulates the electron beam. The electron beam impinges on the target, storing charges

at the X and Y locations in proportion to the signal amplitude. At a later time, the stored charge on the target is interrogated nondestructively by the same electron beam to make a standard television raster scan which is displayed on a television monitor.

A digital scan converter (DSC) performs the same function by converting amplitude information to binary numbers which are stored in a memory similar to a computer memory. The memory is organized in a three-dimensional matrix, typically $512 \times 512 \times 4$ or 5 bits. The X and Y information from the scanning arm is used to generate addresses for echo location in the 512×512 plane. The amplitude information is stored in the 4- or 5-bit direction (16 or 32 levels of gray respectively). This matrix is read out in a raster into a television monitor as in the ASC.

In an ASC, the operator has a number of available controls which must be clearly understood if high-quality images are to be obtained. The enhance, or read level, control varies the reading beam current to the scan convertor target being displayed. Scans tend to have increased contrast and deteriorate more rapidly as the read level voltage is increased. A zoom control allows magnification of any portion of the image after it has been written. Like all postprocessing magnification techniques, there is no real improvement in resolution, just a size increase. It is better to rescan the area of interest at a smaller field size to gain a real improvement in resolution. One of the major drawbacks to analog scan converters is drift which causes the gray scale assignment and the focus to vary, leading to deterioration of the image. Furthermore, variation of the gray scale mapping makes comparative studies difficult. Fortunately, phantoms to check the stability of the gray scale mapping are now in the developmental stages. Learning to recognize faulty analog scan converter performance without such a phantom takes considerable experience. Visualizing the gray scale test patterns that are electronically generated by an instrument gives some clue to the stability and allows us to learn how the various controls affect the gray scale map. These internally generated patterns often test only a portion of the complete system.

DSCs have no controls related to the storage function itself and are inherently more stable, since discrete numbers, rather than an analog charge, are stored for each point. In addition, they have a writing speed which is much greater than that of an ASC. This allows so-called "flicker-free" scanning in which new information is stored without disturbing the TV display. Thus, a scan can be done with minimal interference.

Both types of scan converters receive information from the Z axis signal processing described previously. In most systems, the greatest amplitude signal within a picture element is stored (peak detection). If this picture element is scanned over again, a new amplitude will be stored only if it is greater than that previously stored. This prevents overwriting with consequent loss of detail and contrast in the scan. DSCs are superior to ASCs in this regard. Scans can be visualized on ASC systems for approximately ten minutes before they begin to deteriorate; however, as long as the power stays on, they may be viewed indefinitely on a DSC.

Display Modes

Echo signals from a transducer can be displayed in a number of formats, depending upon whether amplitude, time, or spatial distribution are of interest. In the A-mode, or amplitude mode, the target depth and amplitude are displayed either on the horizontal and vertical scales or on a cathode ray tube (CRT), respectively. The entire vertical scale of the CRT may be used to display about 40 dB of amplitude information. The anatomical origin of the signal being displayed is difficult to determine, since only the depth information is present on the horizontal axis. The A-mode display is commonly used in ophthalmology (fig. 1.20), echoencephalography, echocardiology, and as an adjunct to B-mode displays for more accurate measurement.

In the M-mode, or motion-mode display, the position and pattern of movement of reflecting surfaces are displayed. Depth information is displayed vertically, with a slow horizontal sweep tracing out the motional pattern of the target (for example, the swinging pendulum in figure 1.21). Amplitude information is encoded into the shades of gray on the display. As figure 1.21 shows, the displayed traces are highly dependent on the orientation of the target in the beam and on the type of target motion. The M-mode display is used primarily in echocardiology and as an adjunct to B-mode displays to determine the pulsatile nature of a mass or the fetal heart motion.

The B-mode, or brightness mode display, gives a two-dimensional cross-sectional spatial representation of the examined tissue on the horizontal and vertical axes while encoding echo amplitude information in gray levels. It is the primary display mode of noncardiac ultrasound.

Character Generator

Many systems now have typewriter keyboards available to the operator for placing patient or scan information directly on the television image. Such a system helps insure that all scans are properly identified.

Permanent Image Recording Techniques

Several recording methods are used for B-scan images. Film, especially Polaroid film, is most popular. The initial expense of a Polaroid camera system is relatively low, but the film is expensive. Spatial and gray scale resolution are satisfactory, but the exposure latitude of Polaroid films necessitates a precise adjustment of the television monitor controls and camera settings. Since the brightness and contrast of many television monitors are unstable, poor Polaroid pictures may result, unless a photometer is used to monitor the light output.

"Multi-image cameras" are a popular alternative to Polaroid recording. They make four, nine, or more images on a standard 8- × 10-in film. Despite the inconvenience of wet processing and film handling, they offer superior image quality, better gamma and latitude reproducibility than the Polaroid, and they produce a transparency which may be viewed on a light box. Roll film systems have similar advantages over Polaroid. The processing is, however, less convenient, more expensive, and subject to errors not present in the other systems.

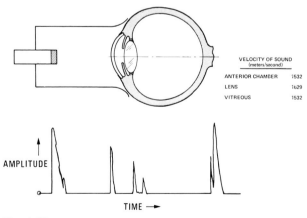

VELOCITY OF SOUND	
(meters/second)	
ANTERIOR CHAMBER	1532
LENS	1629
VITREOUS	1532

Fig. 1.20

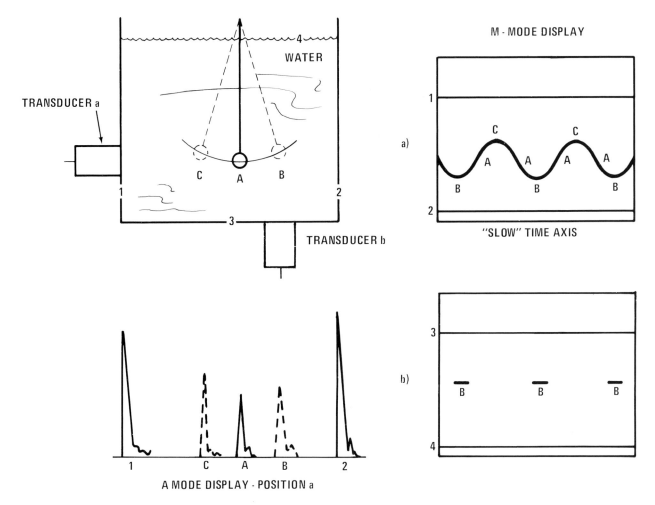

Fig. 1.21

Since the output signal from the scan converter systems is in video form, video tape or video disk recording is also possible. This is particularly important for teaching purposes, but relatively expensive.

With all present film recording systems, the major limiting factor is the quality and stability of the television display monitor. As a result, a high quality television monitor is one of the most important components of the overall system and is frequently neglected.

Practical Considerations

A clear understanding of the fundamental principles of sound waves and ultrasound instrumentation represents more than an intellectual exercise for the expert ultrasonographer. In no other medical imaging modality is this basic knowledge of physics used so extensively

on a day-to-day basis. The ultrasonographer must continuously and rapidly integrate anatomic information and sound–tissue interaction phenomena in order optimally to adjust the instrumentation variables so that high quality images can be obtained and artifacts recognized.

In order to illustrate the practical aspects of acoustic physics and instrumentation, a conceptual phantom was developed which contains most of the various sound–tissue interactions encountered in biological tissues (fig. 1.22). The simplified simulated gray scale B-scan below the phantom shows how these effects would be recorded in an actual B-scan. These interactions provide the information from which diagnoses are made. The phantom is divided into specific areas, A–I, to illustrate particular interactions with important underlying physical principles. The direction of sound beam propagation is indicated by arrows and appropriately num-

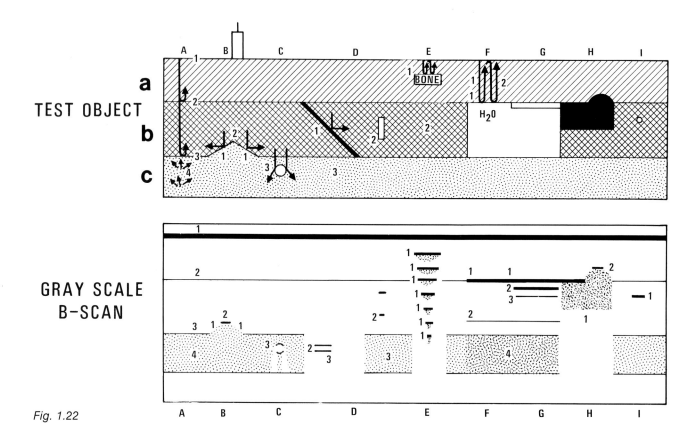

TEST OBJECT

GRAY SCALE
B-SCAN

Fig. 1.22

bered so that the effect can be appreciated on the simulated scan. Each area will be discussed, and clinical examples illustrating the significance of the interaction will be demonstrated.

Regions a and b of the phantom represent uniform regions of material in which no small scatterers are present to produce a gray level signal. Region c does produce a consistent gray level. Regions such as a and b are not likely to be encountered during actual scanning of the body. They were included in this conceptual phantom for clarity.

Areas A and B in the test object illustrate how a sound beam interacts with interfaces of different size and orientation. A_1 represents the excitation pulse or "main bang" of ultrasound. It is a large overloading signal and usually produces a thick line artifact at the skin. Specular reflecting interfaces, A_2 and A_3, perpendicular to the sound beam are recorded on the scan. The diffuse scatterers in the deeper portion of the phantom (A_4) are recorded on the scan regardless of the orientation. Specular reflectors with an inclined orientation (B_1) to the beam are not recorded on the scan. B_2 presents a wedge discontinuity which scatters sound from the tip

despite its inclined sides. The edge of the wedge is displayed as a line due to the transducer beamwidth. Note that despite the absence of a specular interface at B_1, an interface can be inferred from the change of texture.

The practical drawback of using specular reflectors is the necessity for the ultrasonographer to anticipate the shape of specular interfaces and thereby keep the scanning beam perpendicular to the interfaces throughout the scanning motion in order to record them and to prevent refractive and critical-angle phenomena. Sometimes this requires changing the position of the patient, the degree of inspiration, the degree of bladder filling, and so forth. This accounts for some of the difficulties encountered in the bistable systems used before the introduction of the gray scale.

The importance of these two basic types of tissue interfaces lies in the fact that ultrasound images portray not only the elasticity and density composition of tissues but also the structural organization of the components. For example, the orientation of interfaces within the kidney allows for distinction between the renal cortex and pyramids, but the sound beam must be scanned perpendicular to the renal capsule to accentuate these internal differences.

The critical-angle phenomena associated with curved structures (C_3) are encountered frequently in clinical scans. Many such interfaces within the body lead to shadowing effects which conceal the underlying acoustic texture, for example, the upper pole of the kidney, the edges of fluid areas, or some gallstones. One distinguishing feature of these shadows is the absence of any signals since the totally reflected beams never return to the transducer.

Another interesting reflection phenomenon, often seen near the diaphragm, is shown in region D. In this case, the tilted reflector (D_1) directs the energy to target D_2, but the system is "fooled" and incorrectly places the target directly below the reflector. As the scan continues to the right, the correct location is also displayed. A key to interpreting this phenomenon is the unexplained change in texture in region D_3, or in the case of targets near the diaphragm, the display of targets where they are anatomically implausible.

Region E in the phantom represents the interposition of a complete reflector, such as air or bone, or especially a rib, in the path of the sound beam. The acoustic impedance mismatch is so great that virtually all the sound is reflected back and forth from the target to the transducer when the beam is perpendicular to the reflector. No information is recorded distal to the interface in region E_2 except for reverberation (E_1) and ring-down artifacts.

The reverberations created by highly reflecting interfaces represent the bouncing of the sound back and forth between the transducer and the interface. Each successive reflection is weaker and later in time and is, therefore, misinterpreted by the instrument as arising from a deeper region within the body. Reverberations are usually easily recognized and characterized by their periodic quality and by the fact that the apparent interfaces are progressively narrower and thinner (E_1). Ring down is related to the damping mechanisms in the transducer and appears as a mist following each reverberation.

The situation commonly arises in the abdomen, where only a single reverberation is recorded; this gives the apparent impression of through transmission. When performing scans, the ultrasonographer must notice all highly reflective interfaces, anticipate where reverberation artifacts might occur, and analyze the

regions for noise and subtle shadowing effects. This type of analysis usually will distinguish artifacts related to total reflectors from pathological processes causing shadowing through absorption, critical angle, or refraction.

The interface between the upper area and the water-filled area in region F_1 produces stronger interface reflection than the same interface in regions A–E. This is due to the larger change of acoustic impedance across the interface. This change is generally masked by gray level compression of specular interfaces.

Regions F and G of the phantom also illustrate additional effects of strong specular boundaries, with a variety of reverberation artifacts being created (F_2, G_2, G_3). The reverberation artifacts sometimes can give the appearance of masses some distance from the region of low attenuation. The artifactual nature of these reflections usually can be determined by noting how the recorded echoes change as the receiver gains are adjusted and the scanning path is changed. Reverberation artifacts G_2 and G_3 often are seen from the bladder wall or the proximal wall of the aorta.

In practice, the edges of large fluid-filled areas will be poorly resolved by the lateral resolving capability of the equipment, especially if compound scanning motions are used. The resulting beamwidth artifacts can mimic solid projections from the wall and can thereby change the differential diagnosis. If the depth-resolving capabilities of the system are used by scanning limited portions of the wall with simple motions at normal incidence, the true edge characteristics will be recorded.

Regions F and G illustrate another important phenomenon caused by the lack of attenuation in the water-filled area. The TGC is adjusted for continuous attenuation with depth. The transmitted signal level arriving at region C is, therefore, higher than expected by the instrument because the attenuation in the fluid is much lower than in tissue, producing stronger echoes. This distal enhancement is the primary method of determining a cystic or fluid-filled region.

Region H contains an area of increased absorption compared with average biological tissue. This leads to distal reflections that do not produce high enough levels to be displayed correctly with the TGC function (H_1). This pattern is sometimes the only indicator of a mass, unless the mass alters an adjacent normal boundary structure (H_2), and it is clinically important in detecting dermoids, myomata, calculi, and diffuse liver abnormalities. Some normal anatomical structures such as superficial scars or the ligamentum teres in the liver, for example, show unusual absorption which can shadow areas the sonographer wishes to see. Positional changes which alter the scan path usually will circumvent the problem. The shadowing effect of a highly absorbant material usually can be distinguished from that of a total reflector by means of the lack of reverberation noise.

In region I, a small specular reflector has been interposed along the path of the sound beam in order to demonstrate relative lateral and depth resolution. In general, even with focused sound beams, the lateral resolution is worse than the depth resolution, as indicated by the relative thickness and width of the recorded reflection on the scan (I_1).

The above discussion emphasizes the importance, for the ultrasonographer, of constantly thinking about physics and instrumentation while performing and interpreting sonograms. It is hoped that the reader will analyze the subsequent effects of the various sound-tissue interactions.

References

American Institute of Ultrasound in Medicine. Standard 100 mm test object and recommended procedures for its use. *Reflections* 1:74, 1975.

Bernardi, R. B. et al. A dynamically focused annular array. Ultrasonics Symposium Proceedings, *IEEE Trans. Biomed. Eng.* 76:157–159, 1976.

Busey, H. W., and Rosenblum, L. T. Physical aspects of gray scale ultrasound. Pp. 559–566 in *Ultrasound in medicine*, vol. 1. White, D. N. ed. New York: Plenum Press, 1976.

Carlsen, E. N. Ultrasound physics for the physician: a brief review. *J. Clin. Ultrasound* 3:69–75, March 1975.

Carson, P. L. Rapid evaluation of many pulse echo system characteristics by use of a triggered pulse burst generator with exponential decay. *J. Clin. Ultrasound* 4:259–263, August 1976.

Carson, P. L. Gray scale ultrasound: understanding an innovation in imaging to speed realization of its potential. *Appl. Radiol.* 6:185–189, May–June 1977.

Goldstein, A. Gray scale shifts in ultrasound displays. *Radiology* 121:157–162, October 1976.

Graham, R. L. Principles of ultrasonography in diagnostic ultrasound. Gottlieb, S., Viamonte, M., Jr., Eds. American College of Radiology, 1976.

Hileman, R. E., and McLain, J. A. Image improvement with second generation gray scale. Pp. 527–536 in *Ultrasound in medicine.* White, D. N. ed. New York: Plenum Press, 1976.

Hileman, R. E. Shades of gray. Sonix 1:30–36, April 1975.

Kossoff, G.; Robinson, D. E.; and Garrett, W. J. Ultrasonic two-dimensional visualization for medical diagnosis. *J. Acoust. Soc. Amer.* 44:1310–1318, 1968.

Kossoff, G. The ultrasonic transducer. *Int. Ophthalmol. Clin.* 9:523–541, Fall 1969.

Kossoff, G. Improved techniques in ultrasonic cross sectional echography. *Ultrasonics* 10:221–227, 1972.

Kossoff, G. Display techniques in ultrasound pulse echo investigation: a review. *J. Clin. Ultrasound.* 2:61–72, March 1974.

McDicken, W. N. *Diagnostic ultrasonics*. New York: John Wiley & Sons, 1975.

Nigam, A. K. Standard phantom object for measurements of gray scale and dynamics range of ultrasonic equipment. *Acoustical Holography* 6:689–710, 1976.

Robinson, D. E. Ultrasonic systems for medical diagnostic visualization. *MIT Quart. Prog. Report*, 104: 289–305, January 1972.

Robinson, D. E., and Kossoff, G. Performance tests of ultrasonic echo scopes for medical diagnosis. *Radiology* 104:123–132, July 1972.

Smith, S. W. Diagnostic ultrasound: a review of clinical applications and the state of the art of commercial and experimental systems. HEW Publication *FDA 76–8055*, 1976.

Steidley, K. D. An introduction to the physics of diagnostic ultrasound. *Appl. Radiol.*, 6:155–164, 170, March–April 1977.

Wells, P. N. T. *Physical principles of ultrasonic diagnosis*. New York: Academic Press, 1969.

White, D. N. *Ultrasound in medical diagnosis*. Kingston, Ontario: Ultramedison, 1976.

CASES
Dennis A. Sarti, M.D.
W. Frederick Sample, M.D.

Sound-Tissue Interactions

Figure 1.23 represents a phantom developed by Dr. Nabil F. Maklad and Dr. Jonathan Ophir at the University of Kansas Medical Center, Kansas City, Kansas. The background material within the phantom has acoustic properties similar to those of liver tissue. Inserted within the phantom are various circular materials of varying size with different acoustic properties. In the upper row are a series of 1.6-cm diameter substances; in the lower row 0.6-cm diameter structures are interposed. In Sections A and B of the phantom the material has a decreased attenuation. In addition, in section A the material is surrounded by a membrane across which a velocity change occurs. The velocity of sound in the background material is 1540 meters per second whereas the velocity of sound within the membrane is 2000 meters per second. In section C of the phantom the material has an increase of 30% in attenuation and in section B of the phantom the material has an increase of 200% in attenuation without any change in velocity of the sound.

In section A of the phantom, where velocity changes occur at the membrane, its shadowing effects are observed. In general, when critical angular refractive phenomenon take place, the sound beam is bent towards the side of the interface with the lower velocity.

In area B of the phantom, where no velocity changes take place, only the enhancement of the sound beyond the region is appreciated; this is related to the lower attenuation through the area. In section C of the phantom, the material causing the increased attenuation can be visualized, as well as the deeper shadowing effects related to the attenuation. In contrast, in region D of the phantom, the actual material causing the attenuation cannot be visualized; however, the shadowing effects of the attenuation are appreciated.

A clinical example of velocity changes is provided in figure 1.24. This longitu-

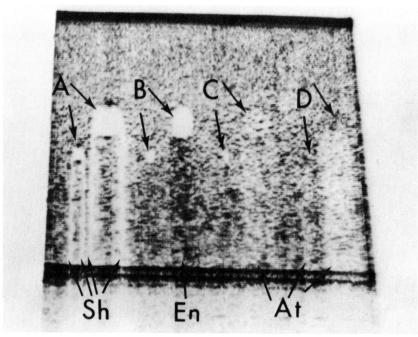

Fig. 1.23

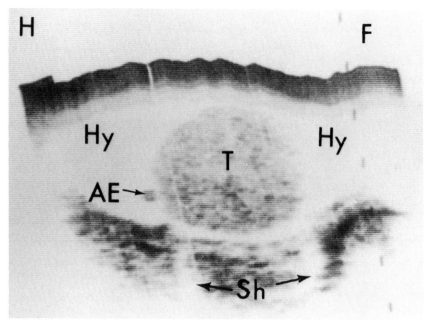

Fig. 1.24

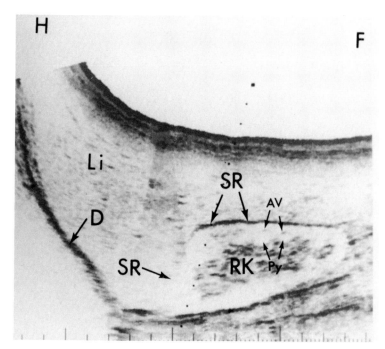

Fig. 1.25

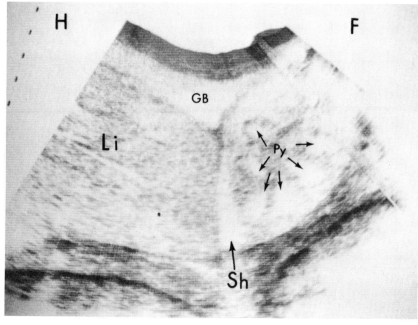

Fig. 1.26

dinal scan of a scrotum shows a testicle surrounded by a hydrocele. The difference in velocities in the two materials leads to the shadowing effects. Figures 1.25 and 1.26 represent clinical examples of the inclination dependence of specular reflectors demonstrated in the conceptual phantom (fig. 1.23). The interface between the kidney and the liver represents a specular reflector. It is, however, variable in contour so that only when the scanning beam is pointed relatively perpendicular to the interface is the tissue plane recorded. The tissue plane frequently is lost in the upper pole of the kidney, since the reflections that occur never return to the transducer. Instead, they are reflected back to an area on the skin surface, where the transducer is not present, and are not recorded.

In figure 1.26 the beneficial effects of the inability to see specular reflectors when they are parallel or inclined to the sound beam is demonstrated by the ability to differentiate the pyramids of the kidney from the surrounding cortex. Generally, when the scanning beam is kept perpendicular to the renal capsule, the interfaces within the pyramids are parallel or sufficiently inclined in relation to the sound beam so that they are not recorded. In contrast, the rather haphazardly organized interfaces within the renal cortex, many of which are diffuse reflectors, are recorded regardless of the inclination of the beam. A shadowing effect is also demonstrated secondary to the velocity changes that occur at the liver and gallbladder renal interfaces.

AE	=	Appendix epididymis
At	=	Attenuation
AV	=	Arcuate vessels
D	=	Diaphragm
En	=	Enhancement
F	=	Feet
GB	=	Gallbladder
H	=	Head
Hy	=	Hydrocele
Li	=	Liver
Py	=	Renal pyramids
RK	=	Right kidney
Sh	=	Shadowing
SR	=	Specular reflector
T	=	Testis

Sound-Tissue Interactions Related to Velocity Changes

In this set of clinical examples, the potentially detrimental effects of shadowing related to velocity changes are illustrated. In figure 1.27 the amniotic fluid surrounding the fetal head and extremities represents interfaces with major velocity changes. Shadows occur at the edges of these curvilinear surfaces and are related to critical-angle phenomena. The shadowed area deep to the edges may make localization of the placenta difficult. In many instances, moving the position of the mother in order to change the position of the fetal head is necessary in order to determine the exact location of the placenta in relationship to the endocervical canal.

In figure 1.28 the shadowing effect of the bladder-uterine interface in this longitudinal scan of a postpartum mother prevents visualization of the acoustic texture of the uterus in this region. Since this area is the region where cesarean sections are performed and is susceptible to various complications, such as hematoma or abscess, the sound beam must be manipulated to avoid this interface and shadowing effect.

Figure 1.29 represents a common shadowing effect related to velocity changes. At the edges of the gallbladder and, most importantly, near the neck where multiple surfaces created by the spiral valves are present, shadowing on the basis of critical-angle or refractive phenomena can occur. These shadows can mimic stones unless this normal variant is appreciated. In these situations movement of the patient to try to alter the orientation of the sound beam, and therefore the shadowing, is necessary before stones can be excluded.

A similar situation is created when the gallbladder is folded upon itself or has an incomplete septation such as is demonstrated in figure 1.30. The velocity change occurring at the bile-infolding interface can lead to a shadow which simulates a calculus. Generally, the movement of the patient into various positions will cause an unfolding of the gallbladder, and this normal variant will be recognized.

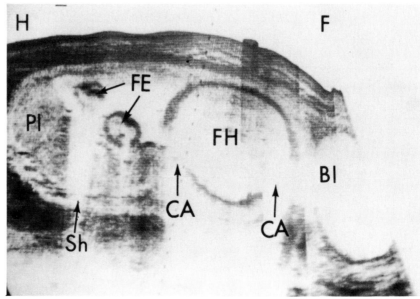

Fig. 1.27

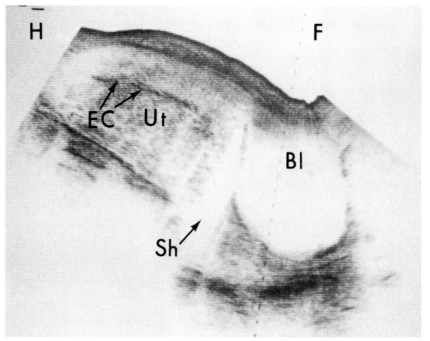

Fig. 1.28

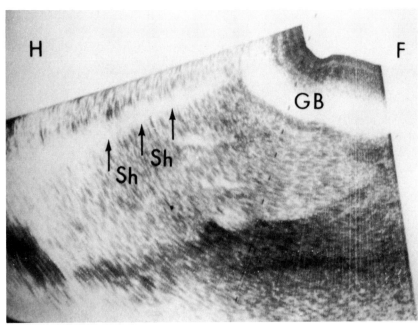

Fig. 1.29

Bl = Bladder
CA = Critical angle
EC = Endometrial canal
F = Foot
FE = Fetal extremities
FHe = Fetal head
GB = Gallbladder
H = Head
In = Infolding
Li = Liver
Pl = Placenta
Sh = Shadowing
Ut = Uterus

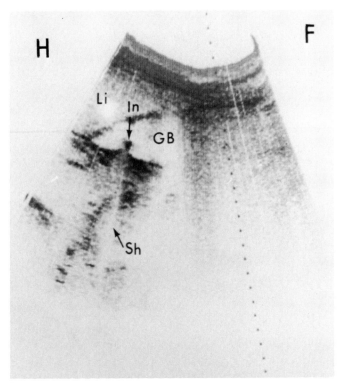

Fig. 1.30

Sound-Tissue Interactions Related to Velocity Changes

The shadowing effects related to velocity changes at curvilinear specular interfaces may provide differentially diagnostic information. In figure 1.31 an amebic abscess is present within the liver. The lower attenuation of the abscess, in spite of the internal solid elements, is indicated by the enhancement in the deeper region of the liver. The presence of its shadowing also indicates that velocity changes are occurring. The importance of the shadowing effects of various types of masses may be related to wall characteristics that could have differential diagnostic significance. Considerably more work in this area is necessary to determine the exact nature of this differential diagnostic information.

In figure 1.32 a limited high-resolution scan using a high-frequency real-time system (Biodynamics Incorporated) demonstrates two shadowing effects relating to velocity changes in the region of the common carotid artery. The shadowing effects allow the sonographer actually to visualize the thickness of the carotid wall, which cannot be visualized by means of acoustic impedance differences alone. The outer shadowing effect is probably related to critical-angle phenomena, whereas the inner shadowing effect is related to refraction.

An important differentially diagnostic aspect of shadowing related to velocity changes frequently is observed in the gallbladder area. A gallbladder filled with stone may be difficult to outline. The shadowing effects related to what are probably velocity changes at the stone interfaces, however, lead to a type of shadowing that is distinctly different from the gas-containing nearby duodenum (fig. 1.33). In the case of the former, where the reflections or refractions of the sound related to the velocity never return to the transducer, the shadowing has little reverberation or noise within it. In contrast, at the air interface of the duodenum, which is a total reflector returning the sound to the transduc-er, a series of reverberation and ring-

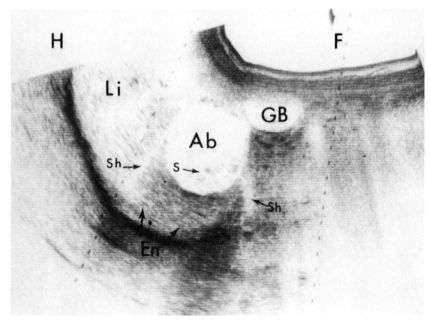

Fig. 1.31

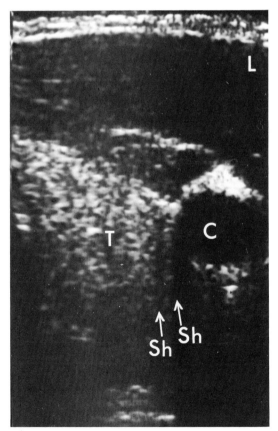

Fig. 1.32

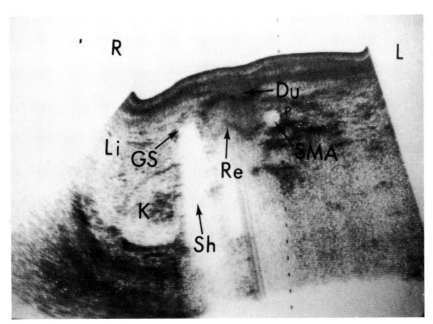

Fig. 1.33

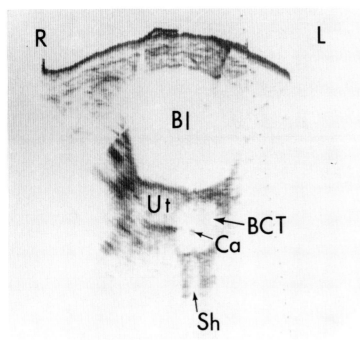

Fig. 1.34

down artifacts leading to a noisy or "dirty" type of shadowing is observed. Therefore, the different types of shadowing resulting from the different interreactions of the sound beam allow proper identification of an abnormal gallbladder even though the gallbladder itself is not visualized.

Figure 1.34 illustrates a relatively nonspecific appearing adnexal mass, which could have an extensive differential diagnosis. The presence of an interface within the mass, however, is related to a significant velocity change resulting in shadowing and suggests the presence of calcification. This places the mass in a more limited differentially diagnostic grouping that includes benign cystic teratoma which was proven at surgery.

Ab	=	Abscess
BCT	=	Benign cystic teratoma
Bl	=	Bladder
C	=	Common cartoid artery
Ca	=	Calcium
CCA	=	Common carotid artery
Du	=	Duodenum
En	=	Enhancement
F	=	Foot
GB	=	Gallbladder
GS	=	Gallstone
H	=	Head
K	=	Kidney
L	=	Left
Li	=	Liver
P	=	Pancreas
R	=	Right
Re	=	Reverberation
S	=	Solid elements
SCM	=	Sternocleidomastoid muscle
Sh	=	Shadowing
SMA	=	Superior mesenteric artery
T	=	Thyroid
Ut	=	Uterus

Total Ultrasonic Reflectors

The major complete reflector within the body represents air. In addition to the shadowing effect, the very strong reflections lead to a series of reverberation and ring-down artifacts. In figure 1.35, the typical appearance of artifacts associated with a total reflector is seen. In this case, a linear cap of gas in the stomach overlying the pancreas is illustrated. Each reverberation has regular periodic qualities and is associated with a tail ring-down artifact. Each subsequent reverberation is narrower, thinner, and associated with a smaller ring-down tail.

Figure 1.36 illustrates an additional feature of a reverberation artifact. Since it represents the bouncing back and forth between two surfaces, the configuration of the reverberation is the summation effect of the configuration of the two interfaces. In this case, the configurations of the skin and the linear cap of gas are different; as a result, the configuration of the reverberation is significantly different from that of the total reflector. The source of the reverberation is still easily identified by the associated shadowing and the tail of ring down.

When a gas pocket is spherical in shape, the total reflection is inclined and never returns to the transducer, leading to a clean type of shadowing (fig. 1.37). This most frequently occurs in the small bubble of gas in the duodenal bulb and can mimic the clean shadowing resulting from velocity changes in an abnormal gallbladder. Therefore, when the diagnosis of an abnormal gallbladder, based on shadowing related to velocity changes, is entertained, the duodenum must be specifically identified.

In general, artifacts related to total reflectors are easily identified, but they still may cause problems in scan interpretation. In figure 1.38, the artifacts associated with the total reflectors make determination of the extent of the aneurysm difficult. If the gas pockets were more generalized, the aneurysm could be entirely obscured.

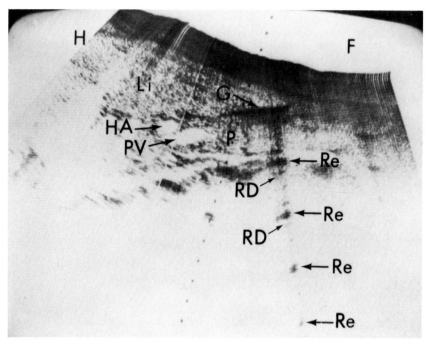

Fig. 1.35

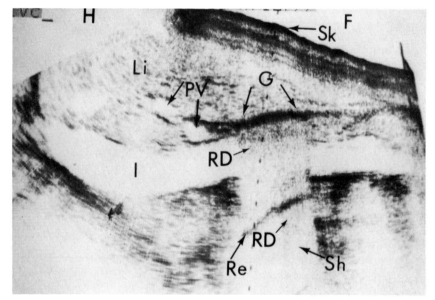

Fig. 1.36

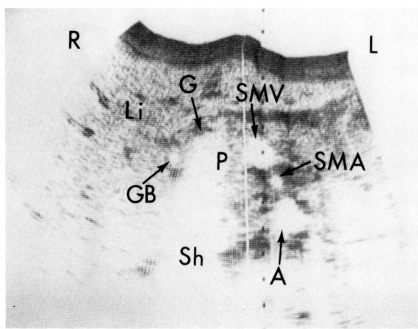
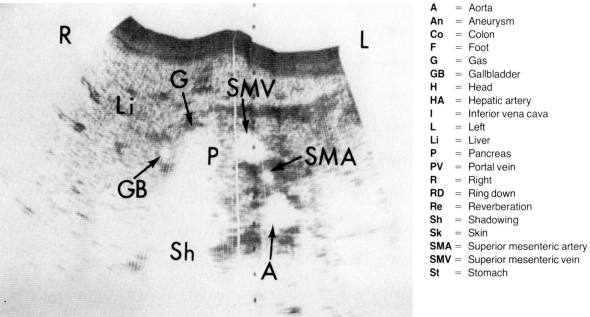

A	=	Aorta
An	=	Aneurysm
Co	=	Colon
F	=	Foot
G	=	Gas
GB	=	Gallbladder
H	=	Head
HA	=	Hepatic artery
I	=	Inferior vena cava
L	=	Left
Li	=	Liver
P	=	Pancreas
PV	=	Portal vein
R	=	Right
RD	=	Ring down
Re	=	Reverberation
Sh	=	Shadowing
Sk	=	Skin
SMA	=	Superior mesenteric artery
SMV	=	Superior mesenteric vein
St	=	Stomach

Fig. 1.37

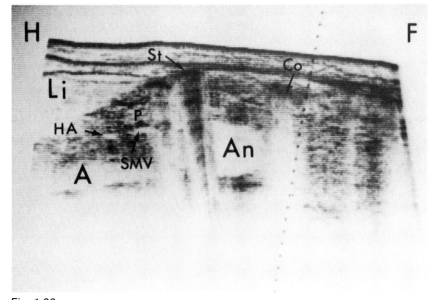

Fig. 1.38

Total Sound Reflectors

In some cases, the reverberation phenomena created by total reflectors are more difficult to recognize. In figures 1.39 and 1.40 the transverse and longitudinal scans of a patient being evaluated for pancreatic disease are provided. A flat cap of gas within the duodenal bulb has resulted in a single reverberation artifact which mimics a true, more deeply situated interface. The resulting through transmission sign is seemingly satisfied, and a mass is misinterpreted in the pancreatic region. The different inclination of the reverberation in figure 1.40 that results from the differing configurations of the skin and gas pocket further confuses the issue. These types of reverberative phenomena usually can be recognized if multiple scanning approaches are directed at the same interface. Different types of reverberative phenomena usually can be elicited and will allow proper recognition.

Another place where phenomena reverberating off total reflectors frequently occur is in the pelvis. The fluid-filled bladder allows a path of decreased attenuation for such a reverberation even if the total reflecting surface is deep within the pelvis. The apparent mass effect created by reverberation off the gas in the rectal sigmoid portion of the colon passing beneath the adnexa is shown in figure 1.41. Since the reverberation was associated with very little ring-down noise, a cystic-appearing mass with apparent through transmission was simulated. The apparent through transmission, however, represents the reverberation plus its accompanying ring-down noise.

If the reverberation artifact from gas beneath the bladder is associated with a large amount of noise, a solid-appearing mass within the pelvis can be simulated, as demonstrated in figure 1.42. The mass in this case mimics an enlarged uterus adjacent to an adnexal fluid collection. Careful questioning of the patient, however, revealed that the uterus had been removed some years ago and led to alternative scanning approaches that demonstrated the artifactual nature of the mass.

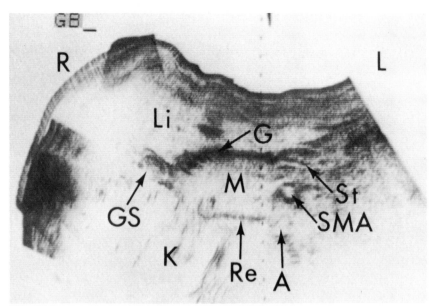

Fig. 1.39

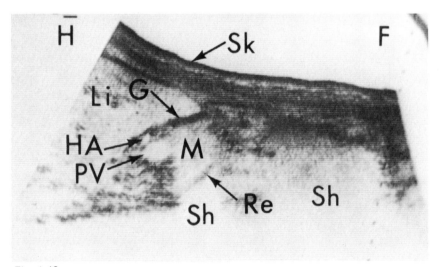

Fig. 1.40

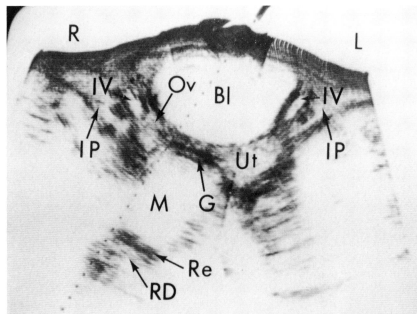

Fig. 1.41

A   = Aorta
Bl   = Bladder
F   = Foot
Fl   = Fluid
G   = Gas
GS   = Gallstone
H   = Head
HA   = Hepatic artery
IP   = Iliopsoas muscle
IV   = Iliac vessels
K   = Kidney
L   = Left
Li   = Liver
M   = Mass
Ov   = Ovary
PV   = Portal vein
R   = Right
RD   = Ring down
Re   = Reverberation
Sh   = Shadowing
Sk   = Skin
SMA = Superior mesenteric artery
St   = Stomach
Ut   = Uterus

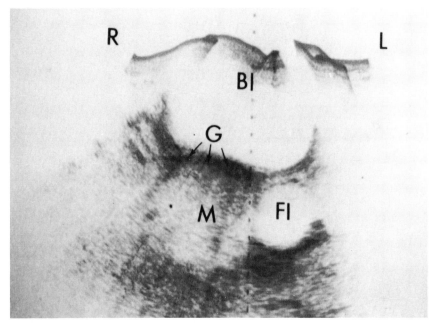

Fig. 1.42

Effects of Areas of Diminished Attenuation

The time gain compensation curve of the contact B scanner compensates for the average attenuation of tissues. The effects on the ultrasound image of an intervening area of diminished attenuation have certain characteristics which are basic to cyst-solid determinations. In figure 1.43, the classical differences between a cystic and solid lesion are demonstrated. In this instance there was no velocity change across the interfaces, and therefore, shadowing effects related to refractive or critical-angle phenomena are not observed. Nevertheless, fluid areas of lower attenuation are associated with sharp posterior walls and apparent enhancement of the underlying echo amplitude.

To demonstrate enhancement, however, reflecting surfaces must be beneath the area of decreased attenuation that allows this phenomenon to be observed. In figure 1.44, two amebic abscesses are present within the liver. The more superficial abscess in the left lobe is associated with shadowing related to velocity changes at the edges as well as enhancement effects related to the lower attenuation demonstrated in the deeper retroperitoneal tissues. The even larger abscess in the deep right lobe abuts directly on the diaphram-air interface which does not allow the enhancement to be observed, since the interface represents a total reflector.

In some regions of the body, such as the pelvis, even though a normal fluid collection is present for comparison (bladder), total reflectors, such as bowel gas or bone, prevent the enhancement phenomenon from being observed (fig. 1.45). For cyst-solid differentiation, other features must be sought, such as the relative anterior ring-down phenomenon and the presence of reflections from internal solid components. In this case the different reflectivity of the solid components is readily visible in this complex benign cystic teratoma.

The enhancement phenomenon associated with lower attenuating regions (usually fluid) is still, however, the most reliable sign of a lower attenuator. Therefore, when a mass meets all of the

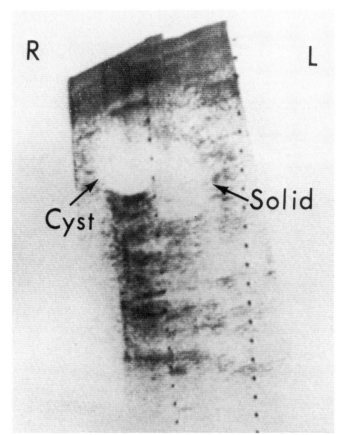

Fig. 1.43

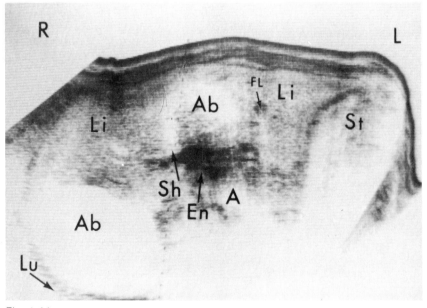

Fig. 1.44

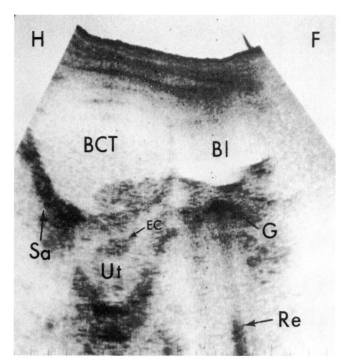

Fig. 1.45

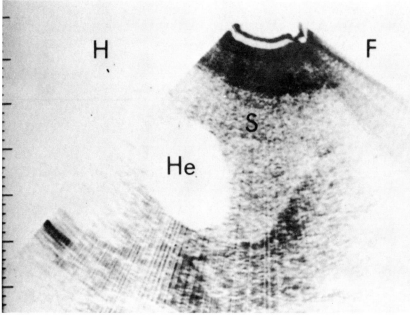

Fig. 1.46

other criteria of a lower attenuator, such as smooth margins or absence of internal echoes, the absence of enhancement where sufficient tissue is present deep to the area is still the most reliable sign that the mass is not a fluid. This is demonstrated by the clotted hematoma within the spleen in figure 1.46, which demonstrates all of the characteristics of a fluid mass, with the exception of the enhancement phenomenon. Sufficient splenic tissue and retroperitoneal structures are present deep to the mass, so that enhancement should have occurred if it were, in fact, fluid in nature.

A	=	Aorta
Ab	=	Abscess
BCT	=	Benign cystic teratoma
Bl	=	Bladder
EC	=	Endometrial canal
En	=	Enhancement
F	=	Foot
FL	=	Falciform ligament
G	=	Gas
H	=	Head
He	=	Hematoma
L	=	Left
Li	=	Liver
Lu	=	Lung
R	=	Right
Re	=	Reverberation
S	=	Spleen
Sa	=	Sacrum
Sh	=	Shadowing
St	=	Stomach
Ut	=	Uterus

Artifacts Associated with Regions of Low Attenuation

Interposed regions of low attenuation are associated with a number of artifacts. The acoustic impedance differences at the junction of an average and a low-attenuating tissue usually are substantial and generate relatively strong reflections. When the region of low attenuation is, therefore, close to the transducer, a series of reverberation and ring-down artifacts can be generated within the low-attenuating area. These regions have been recognized in ultrasound as the echoes in the near side of the fluid region (figure 1.47) and usually are easily identified. However, when the region of low attenuation occurs very superficially, the noise and ring-down phenomena, particularly if the gain settings are somewhat high, can totally obscure the region unless careful attention is paid to underlying enhancement. A typical clinical example is illustrated in figure 1.48, in which a very superficial renal cyst easily could be missed.

More deeply situated regions of diminished attenuation also can lead to artifacts if there is a nearby strong reflecting surface. A common place for such an artifact to occur is in a cystic or fluid mass within the liver adjacent to the diaphragm. Reverberation artifacts result and give the apparent appearance of a similar mass on the other side of the diaphragm, as indicated in figure 1.49.

An experimental situation simulating this phenomenon is demonstrated in figure 1.50. A water bath containing a balloon filled with water is placed midway along the ultrasound beam but adjacent to the highly reflective water-bath wall. While the sound beam is insonating the water-bath wall at an inclination, reflections are set up which reverberate off the balloon and simulate a similarly configured mass in the air outside of the container. This experiment was conducted by Fred Gardner, one of our technicians at the University of California School of Medicine, Los Angeles, California.

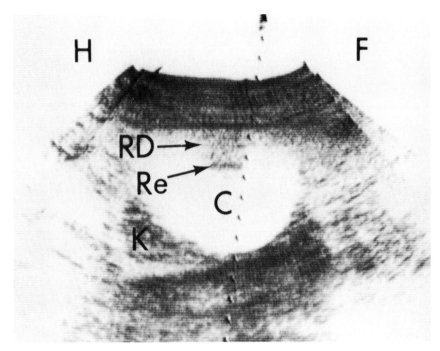

Fig. 1.47

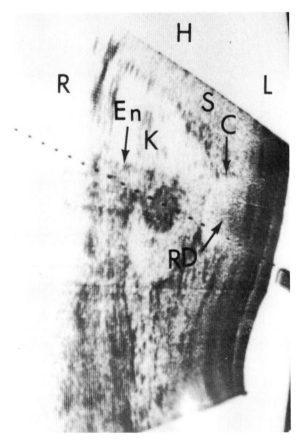

Fig. 1.48

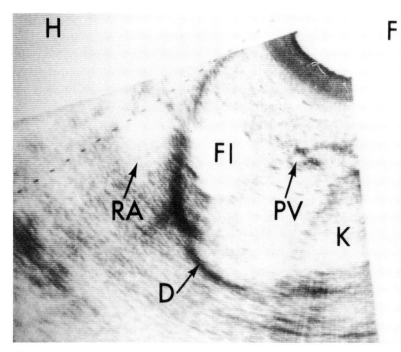

Fig. 1.49

B	=	Balloon
C	=	Cyst
D	=	Diaphragm
En	=	Enhancement
F	=	Foot
FI	=	Fluid
H	=	Head
K	=	Kidney
L	=	Left
PV	=	Portal vein
R	=	Right
RA	=	Reverberation artifact
RD	=	Ring down
Re	=	Reverberation
S	=	Spleen

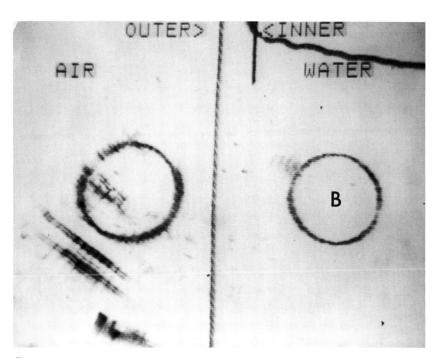

Fig. 1.50

Effects of Regions of Diminished Attenuation

The comparison of the acoustic textures of various organs has become an important part of ultrasonography. In general, the relative reflectivity of various organs compared at the same depth within the body can be a reliable indicator of certain diseases. If an area of diminished attenuation is present between the transducer and one of the tissues, however, fallacious overamplification of the acoustic texture will occur. If this is not recognized, the appearance of an abnormal organ texture can be simulated. A typical example is illustrated in figures 1.51 and 1.52. Normally the amplitude of echoes arising from the renal cortex is slightly less than that of the liver. In figure 1.51, however, the texture comparison is made with the lower-attenuating gallbladder intervening between the sound beam and the kidney. The apparently abnormal, greater-amplitude echoes of the renal parenchyma, as compared to the liver, suggest some form of generalized renal disease. In figure 1.52, however, the patient has been moved into the decubitus position, throwing the lower-attenuating gallbladder out of the field of comparison. As a result, a more appropriate relative amplitude texture comparison between the kidney and liver can be made.

Similarly, difficulty in recognizing certain components of a gestation may result from the intervening amniotic fluid, as demonstrated in figures 1.53 and 1.54. In figure 1.53, because of the overamplification resulting from the intervening amniotic fluid as well as from an inappropriately high gain setting, it is impossible to tell whether the thickened posterior wall of the gestation represents a placental tongue or a uterine contraction. In figure 1.54 the gain settings and time gain compensation have been readjusted, so that the proper acoustic texture of the posterior gestational wall can be analyzed. The texture is seen to be different from that of the anterior placenta and, therefore, identified as a uterine contraction.

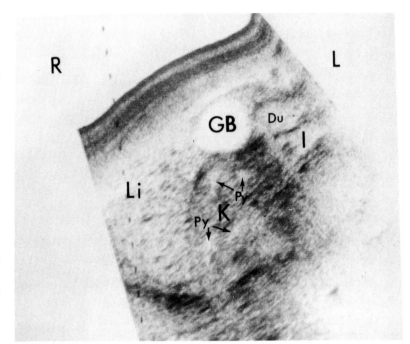

Fig. 1.51

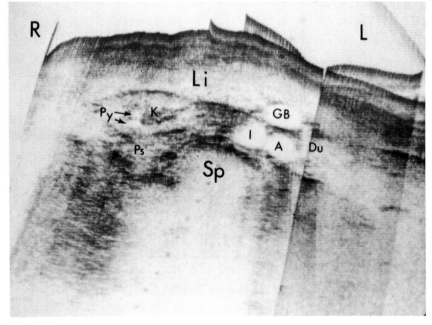

Fig. 1.52

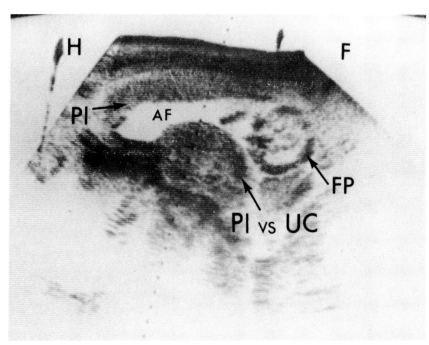

Fig. 1.53

A	=	Aorta
AF	=	Amniotic fluid
Du	=	Duodenum
F	=	Foot
Fh	=	Fetal head
FP	=	Fetal parts
GB	=	Gallbladder
H	=	Head
I	=	Inferior vena cava
K	=	Kidney
L	=	Left
Li	=	Liver
Pl	=	Placenta
Pl vs Uc	=	Placenta vs uterine contractions
Ps	=	Psoas muscle
Py	=	Renal pyramids
R	=	Right
Sp	=	Spine
UC	=	Uterine contraction

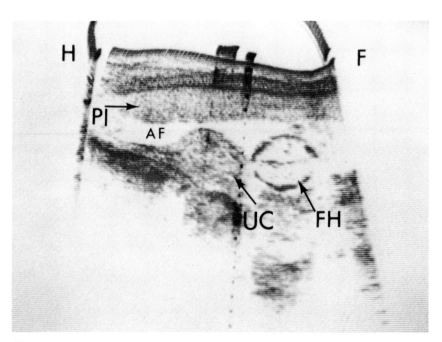

Fig. 1.54

Effects of Regions of Increased Attenuation

A number of areas of increased attenuation occur normally and pathologically within the body. In normal cases, if the resulting phenomena of the increased attenuation are not appreciated, an incorrect diagnosis can be made. A common high attenuator within the upper abdomen is the falciform ligament, accompanied by its extension within the liver, the ligamentum teres. This represents a dense fibrous band which is highly attenuative of the ultrasound beam. As a result, the underlying ultrasonic textures are of a lower amplitude than usual. The effects of this phenomenon are illustrated in figure 1.55. The head of the pancreas is identified precisely by anatomic landmarks that include the gallbladder, duodenum, common bile duct, superior mesenteric vein, and superior mesenteric artery. In addition, the scanning around the falciform ligament has provided through transmission, so that the prevertebral vessels, the crus of the diaphragm, and the anterior surface of the spine are visualized. Due to the attenuation process in the falciform ligament, the acoustic texture and relative amplitude of the pancreas are not, however, properly registered. As a result, a pancreatic abnormality might be suspected if the effects of the falciform ligament are not realized.

A similar situation is created by scars in the skin and subcutaneous tissues. These often are difficult to see, yet their effects on the attenuation of the sound and the underlying acoustic texture are dramatic. In figure 1.56, a small scar in the subcutaneous tissues has caused a dramatic attenuation and shadowing effect which has resulted in a wide area of abnormal texture throughout the underlying liver. In figure 1.57, the patient has been rescanned, and the scar area was avoided during the scanning process. The more normal hepatic acoustic texture, as well as the clear visualization of interhepatic vascular anatomy, is appreciated. For this reason, when scanning portions of the body where scars are likely to occur, it is best to hold the transducer between the

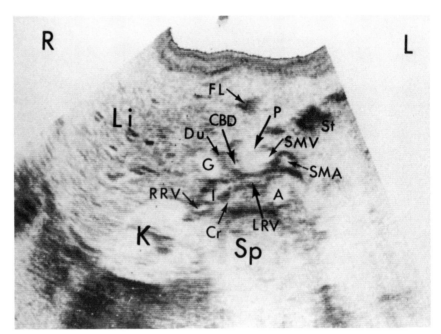

Fig. 1.55

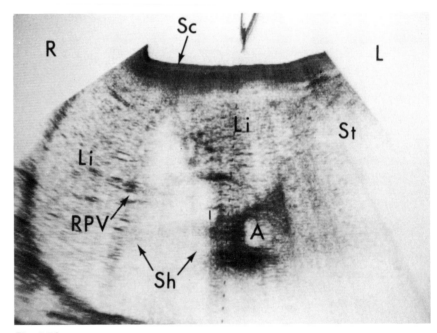

Fig. 1.56

thumb and index finger and slide the third, fourth, and fifth digits in contact across the skin in order to palpate the scar.

Figure 1.58 represents an excellent example of the combined effects of the presence of areas of increased and decreased attenuation. In this transverse scan of a gestational uterus, a remarkable difference in the acoustic texture of the placenta is appreciated. The normal acoustic texture of the placenta is ap-

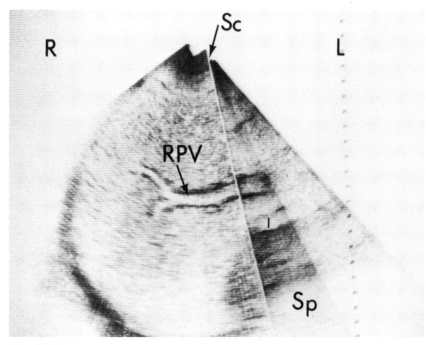

Fig. 1.57

section scar. Finally, the placental texture of the left side of the uterus is noted to be slightly higher in amplitude than that of the right, with no intervening fluid. This demonstrates the effect of the scanning speed on the acoustic texture in analog systems. Since most analog systems use a peak detection system, the actual amplitudes of the reflections received from an area are subject to a sampling error. The faster the sonographer scans, the less likely the optimal reflection from that area will be achieved. Therefore, when comparing various textures with analog systems, a constant scanning speed is required.

A	=	Aorta
AF	=	Amniotic fluid
CBD	=	Common bile duct
Cr	=	Crus of the diaphragm
Du	=	Duodenum
En	=	Enhancement
FL	=	Falciform ligament
G	=	Gallbladder
I	=	Inferior vena cava
K	=	Kidney
L	=	Left
Li	=	Liver
LRV	=	Left renal vein
My	=	Myometrium
P	=	Pancreas
Pl	=	Placenta
R	=	Right
RPV	=	Right portal vein
RRV	=	Right renal vein
Sc	=	Scar
Sh	=	Shadowing
SMA	=	Superior mesenteric artery
SMV	=	Superior mesenteric vein
Sp	=	Spine
St	=	Stomach

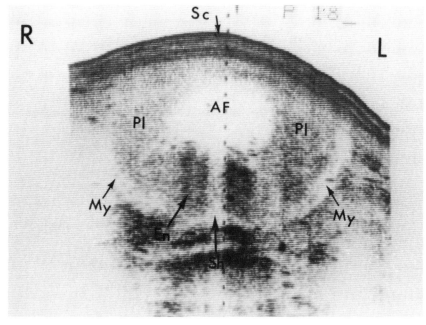

Fig. 1.58

preciated on the right side of the uterus. A higher amplitude acoustic texture is noted in the region deep to the amniotic fluid. This has resulted from an inappropriate amplification related to the standard time gain compensation. In addition, a shadowed area of decreased placental texture is noted within this region. It is secondary to the attenuation resulting from a superficial cesarean-

Effects of Areas of Increased Attenuation

The increased attenuation process is an important sign of pathology. Depending upon the region of the body, however, the appreciation of the increased attenuation may be difficult. Furthermore, the entire path of the sound beam must be appreciated if this sign is to be used as an indicator of disease.

A common entity which may only be recognized by an area of increased attenuation is the presence of a benign cystic teratoma within the pelvis. Figure 1.59 demonstrates, in the left adnexal region, an area of increased attenuation which is associated with a deformity of the bladder wall. This could be related to a large gassy area within the colon; however, the rectosigmoid region is identified on the opposite side of the pelvis. Figure 1.60 demonstrates in another case how the posterior wall of a highly attenuative mass may still be demonstrated by appropriate changes in the gain settings.

Another area where increased attenuation is associated with disease is in cirrhosis of the liver. In figure 1.61, a small liver surrounded by ascitic fluid should normally have a consistent strong acoustic texture. This liver, however, has been markedly scarred from the cirrhotic process, and the decreased texture in the deeper parts of the liver, a result of the attenuation process, can be appreciated. In the deeper regions of the liver, underlying the gallbladder which counteracts this attenuation by the lower attenuation of the bile, the two processes offset one another and give rise to an apparently normal liver texture.

Therefore, when assessing attenuation, it is important to try to compare organs with similar textures of the same size. Figure 1.62 is also a patient with cirrhosis and ascites. The sections of the liver and spleen are similar in size and surrounded by similar amounts of ascites. Therefore, the decreased attenuation seen in the deeper areas of the liver is real and aids in the differential diagnosis of the ascites.

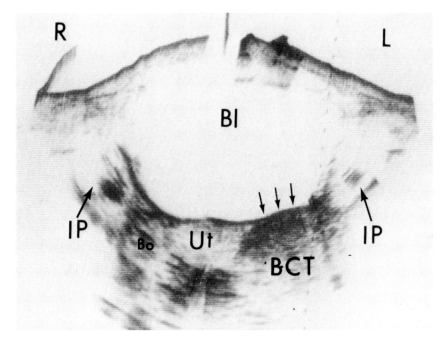

Fig. 1.59

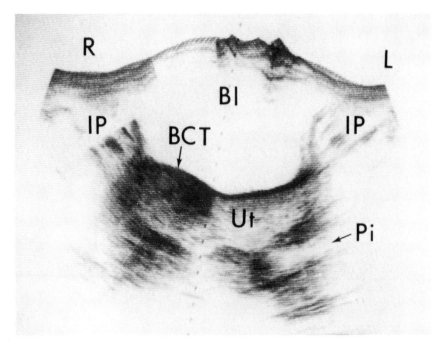

Fig. 1.60

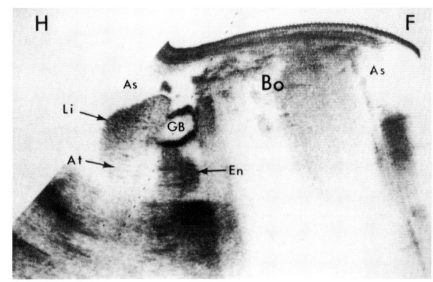

Fig. 1.61

A	=	Aorta
Arrows	=	Bladder wall indentation
As	=	Ascites
At	=	Attenuation
BCT	=	Benign cystic teratoma
Bl	=	Bladder
Bo	=	Bowel
En	=	Enhancement
F	=	Foot
GB	=	Gallbladder
H	=	Head
I	=	Inferior vena cava
IP	=	Iliopsoas muscle
K	=	Kidney
L	=	Left
Li	=	Liver
Pi	=	Piriformis muscle
Ps	=	Psoas muscle
R	=	Right
S	=	Spleen
Sp	=	Spine
Ut	=	Uterus

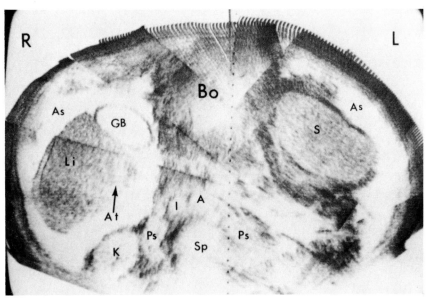

Fig. 1.62

Effects of Beam Profile Characteristics

Consideration of the beam profile must concern both its spatial resolution and its intensity characteristics. Using the phantom illustrated in figure 1.63 and developed by Nabil F. Maklad, M.D., and Jonathan Ophir, Eng. D., both aspects of the beam characteristics can be appreciated. The phantom background material simulates the acoustic properties of liver. In region A, a series of five wires, 3.5 cm from the scanning surface and separated by a decreasing distance, are present. A similar set of wires separated by the same distance are situated more deeply in the phantom, 9.5 cm from the scanning surface. Additional wires are seen by their high reflectivity and the acoustic shadowing at the periphery. A 3.5-MHz transducer, 19 mm in diameter, was used to scan the phantom. The maximal focal point was 9.0 cm. The relative resolving capabilities of the beam can be appreciated by the relative size of the echoes in both regions A and B of the wires, as well as by the background texture pattern which appears as three distinct bands. In the near- and far-field regions the echoes are larger than those seen in the focal zone region. The pattern of the beam-intensity profile can be appreciated due to the somewhat higher-intensity echoes in the focal zone, in spite of the fact that average time gain compensation was used on the receiver board. The phantom shows that the exact textures seen within different organs of the body are very much dependent upon the spatial and intensity profiles of a given transducer.

A clinical example of the transducer's characteristics is appreciated in figure 1.64. This transverse scan of the testis shows the higher intensity echoes in the focal zone of this 5-MHz, short internal focus transducer, 7 mm in diameter. If the beam-intensity profile is known for a transducer, and there is substantial flexibility in the time gain compensation control, some of the texture in homogeneities can be corrected by manipulations of the time gain compensation.

Although the spatial resolution of the transducer is limited by the frequency

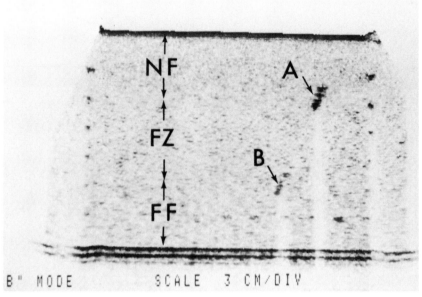

Fig. 1.63

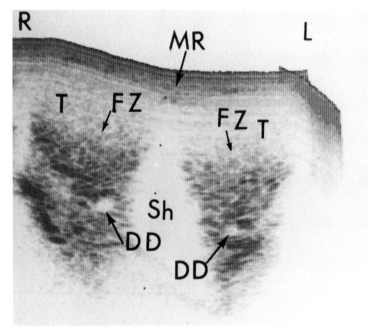

Fig. 1.64

and other characteristics, the spatial resolution can be further deteriorated by manipulation of the gain control. This can be appreciated in figures 1.65 and 1.66, where a phantom made up of a single interface is scanned. The time gain compensation was constant, and the same transducer was used. In figure 1.65, the receiver gain was placed at a low setting, and the resulting recorded interface can be seen to be quite thin. In figure 1.66, the receiver gains were increased, resulting in a thicker recorded echo and a decreased axial resolution. In general, it is best to work at the lowest gains in order to obtain a consistent texture in that portion of the gray scale where subtle differences and gray shades can be appreciated by the eye.

A	=	Echoes arising from wires at different depths in the phantom
B	=	Echoes arising from wires at different depths in the phantom
DD	=	Ductus deferens
FF	=	Far field
FZ	=	Focal zone
HG	=	High gain
L	=	Left
LG	=	Low gain
MR	=	Median raphae
NF	=	Near field
R	=	Right
Sh	=	Shadowing
T	=	Testis

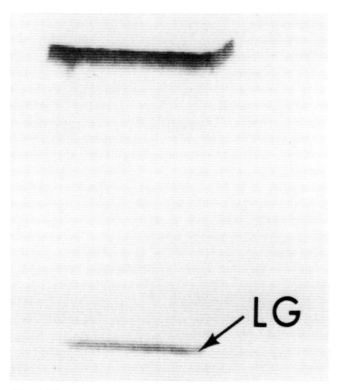

Fig. 1.65

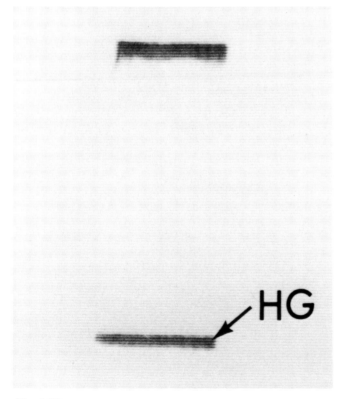

Fig. 1.66

Effects of Beamwidth

Since the beamwidth characteristics of a transducer lead to the writing of the echo as a line rather than a dot, the wall characteristics of a mass should be analyzed with the better resolving axial resolution of the system. In figure 1.67, a large cystic mass anterior to the uterus is identified. Portions of its wall, however, are imaged with the lateral resolving capabilities of the beam leading to linear projections into the cyst. These can be mistaken for solid components and thus lead to misinterpretation. The proper scanning technique for such a large cystic mass is demonstrated in figures 1.68–1.70. Each segment of the wall is scanned with the axial resolution of the system by keeping the scanning path perpendicular to the wall contour. The beamwidth artifacts are no longer visualized, and the proper conclusion of a simple fluid area is made.

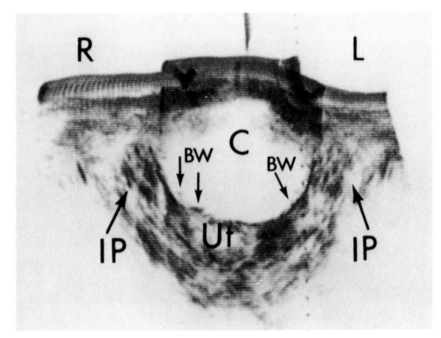

Fig. 1.67

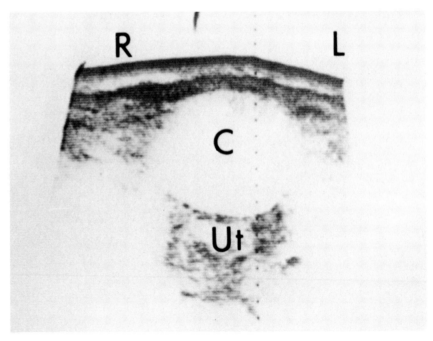

Fig. 1.68

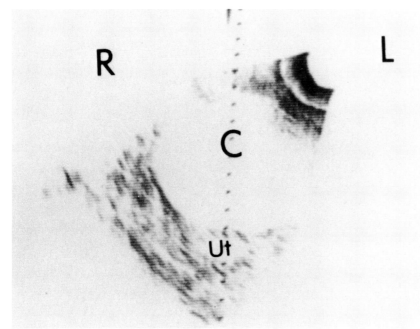

Fig. 1.69

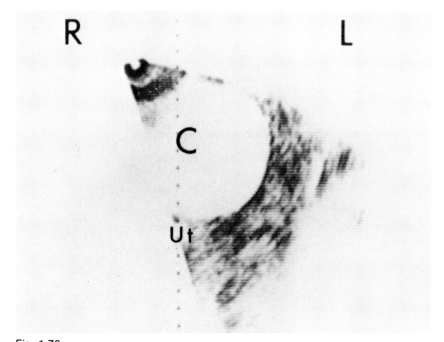

Fig. 1.70

BW = Beamwidth artifacts
C = Cyst
Ip = Iliopsoas muscle
L = Left
R = Right
Ut = Uterus

Effects of Beamwidth

In contrast to the previous case, figures 1.71 and 1.72 show two different cases of fluid masses within the liver. Proper scanning technique in each case demonstrates solid projections within the fluid areas. Such a finding alters the differential diagnosis, indicating a complex rather than a simple fluid collection which in both of these cases was secondary to metastatic cystic ovarian carcinoma. Another commonly encountered effect of the different resolving capabilities in the lateral and depth dimensions is illustrated in figures 1.73 and 1.74. The long curvilinear interface between the kidney and the liver will, depending upon the course of the scanning beam, be resolved either with the axial resolution or with the azimuthal resolution. The sharpness of the depth resolution is appreciated in the midportions of the kidney, and the inferior lateral resolution, in the upper pole region. If the interface represents a weak specular reflector, as in the upper pole region of the kidney in figure 1.74, it may not be resolved at all.

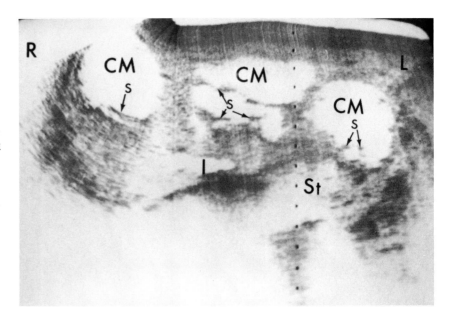

Fig. 1.71

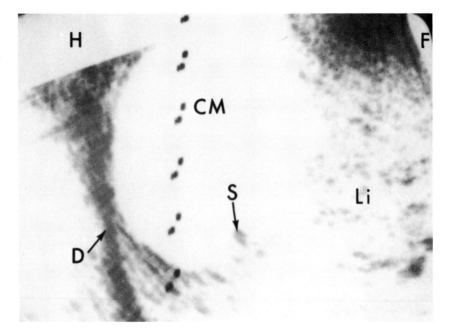

Fig. 1.72

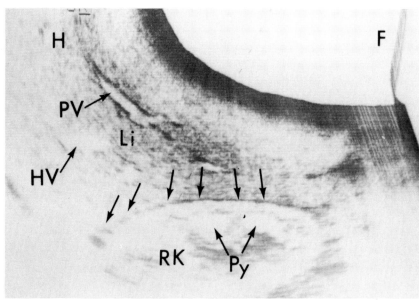

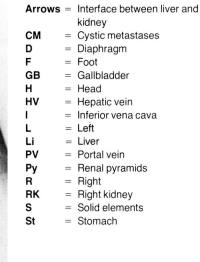

Arrows = Interface between liver and kidney
CM = Cystic metastases
D = Diaphragm
F = Foot
GB = Gallbladder
H = Head
HV = Hepatic vein
I = Inferior vena cava
L = Left
Li = Liver
PV = Portal vein
Py = Renal pyramids
R = Right
RK = Right kidney
S = Solid elements
St = Stomach

Fig. 1.73

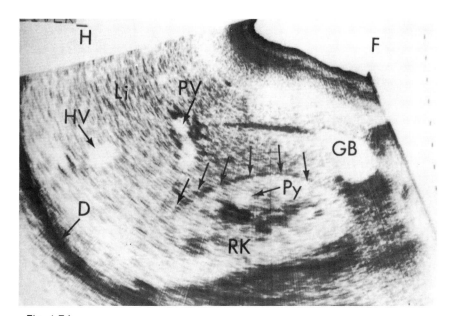

Fig. 1.74

Effects of the Compression Amplifier

One of the most important aspects of the signal processing is the method of compression amplification. The exact type of compression can be widely varied, but in analog systems it is set by the manufacturer. Four different compression amplification systems are indicated by the gray scale bar curves in figure 1.75. According to the compression system, an echo of given amplitude X can be represented by a variable shade of gray.

The effects of the compression amplification curve can best be appreciated by observing the changes in the image while scanning the phantom described in figure 1.23. As we study figures 1.76–1.78, the effects of the different compression curves on various sound interactions within the phantom can be appreciated. In figure 1.76, which represents a more even compression of the entire dynamic range, the shadowing effects related to velocity changes as well as the enhancement resulting from regions of lower attenuation are easily appreciated. In figure 1.77, where the lower portions of a dynamic range are represented by darker shades of gray, the appreciation of enhancement is diminished, and the appreciation of attenuation is accentuated. In figure 1.78, where the maximal accentuation of the low portion of the dynamic range has occurred, further deterioration of the enhancement phenomenon occurs, the shadowing effects resulting from velocity changes are beginning to become obscured, and the high-attenuating area accounting for the shadow in region D is more easily appreciated. It can, therefore, be seen that in analog systems the exact form of compression amplification is critical to the differentiation of a number of normal as well as the abnormal tissue acoustic textures. Since the exact compression curves used by different manufacturers varies, and since these represent an unstable portion of the system, it is not suprising that image quality varies from institution to institution and from day to day.

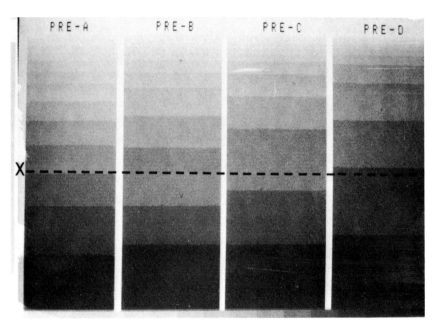

Fig. 1.75

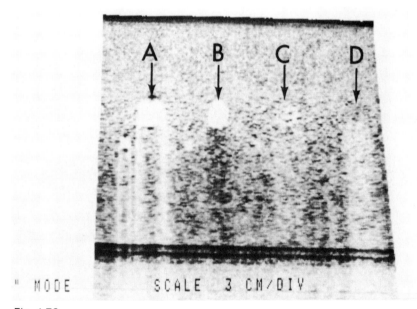

Fig. 1.76

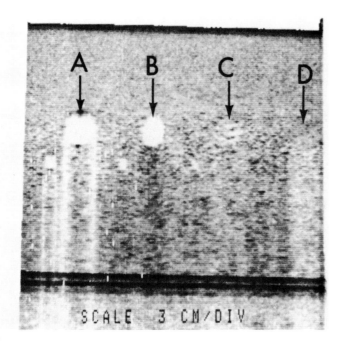

Fig. 1.77

A = Region where velocity changes occur at the membrane; shadowing effects are observed.

B = Area where no velocity changes take place; only the enhancement of the sound beyond the region is appreciated. This is related to the lower attenuation through the area.

C = In this section of the phantom, the material causing the increased attenuation can be visualized, as well as the deeper shadowing effects related to the attenuation.

D = In this region the actual material causing the attenuation cannot be visualized; however, the shadowing effects of the attenuation are appreciated.

X = A given echo amplitude.

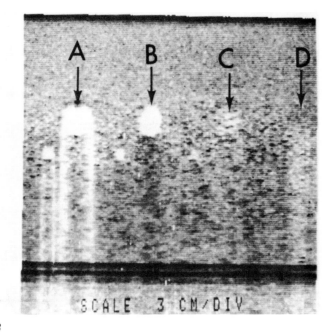

Fig. 1.78

Effects of Compression Curve Assignment

With analog scan converter systems, the compression curve assignment is critical to high-quality scans. The appropriate gray scale mapping, gain settings, and scanning technique lead to the type of spatial and contrast resolution indicated by figure 1.79. In this longitudinal scan of the liver, intricate detail of the vascular anatomy is seen. A relatively homogeneous acoustic texture pattern is also possible, in spite of the beam intensity profile effects. In addition, the echo amplitude differences between the kidney and the liver can be appreciated. Only with this type of technique can subtle, solid abnormalities and acoustic texture, such as those seen with a slightly more reflective metastasis, be appreciated (fig. 1.80).

Similarly, the variety of acoustic textures and gray tones within the gestational uterus (fig. 1.81) requires proper compression curve assignment, machine setup, and scanning technique. Only then can subtle differences in acoustic texture indicating such abnormalities as a myoma in conjunction with a gestation (fig. 1.82) be recognized.

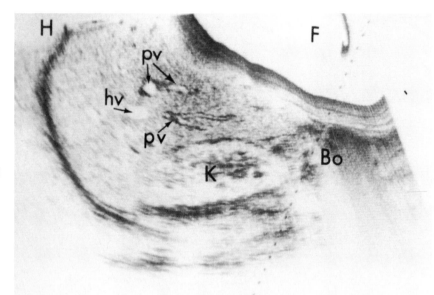

Fig. 1.79

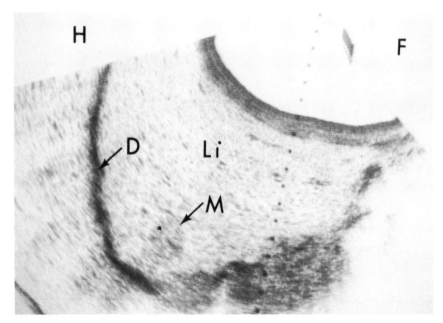

Fig. 1.80

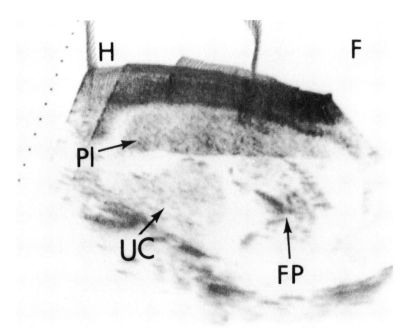

Fig. 1.81

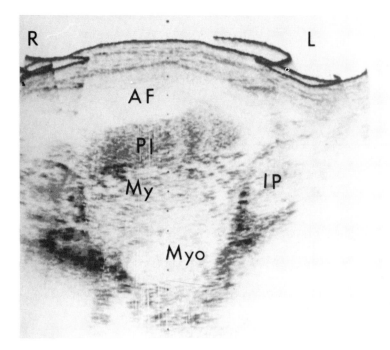

Fig. 1.82

Digital Signal Processing

With the advent of digital signal processing, the ultrasonographer has, for the first time, gained flexible control over the compression amplification portion of the signal processing. Figures 1.83–1.86 represent scans of the same area, using the same transducer and the same gain settings but with different compression signal processing. Close analysis of the image reveals that variations in this portion of the signal processing lead to visual changes in the image, some of which are detrimental and some of which are beneficial. For example, in the format used in figure 1.83, the subdiaphragmatic abscess is clearly visualized with a minimal amount of ringdown artifact and a good appreciation of the enhancement. The relative texture differences between the kidney and the overlying liver are not, however, as well appreciated.

As we progress from figure 1.84 through figure 1.86, a compression format that increasingly augments the lower-level echoes into higher shades of gray is instituted. Although both the abscess and the acoustic enhancement become less evident, the acoustic texture of the kidney in relation to the liver is better appreciated. Therefore, with digital capabilities, scans of the same area using different compression formats may, in fact, lead to an increased information content for the overall study.

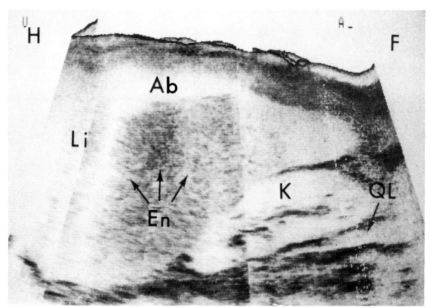

Fig. 1.83

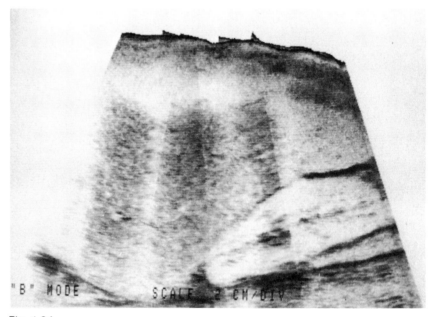

Fig. 1.84

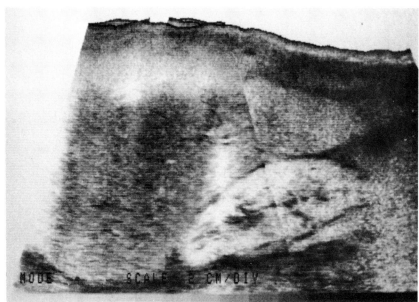

Fig. 1.85

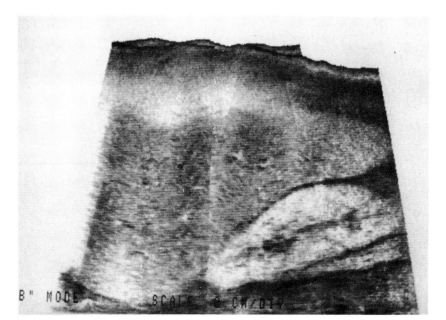

Fig. 1.86

Ab = Abscess
En = Enhancement
F = Foot
H = Head
K = Kidney
Li = Liver
QL = Quadratus lymborum muscle

Digital Signal Processing

One of the initial questions regarding digital scanning systems was whether or not the image quality would be comparable to a well-tuned analog system. Such a comparison required an instrument that could display both analog and digital formats while keeping the other scanning parameters constant. These included the scanning rate and path. Such a protocol system was designed by Rohe Scientific, Incorporated, for our clinical evaluation. In figures 1.87 and 1.88, analog and digital images, respectively, of the same transducer path are illustrated. The overall differences in the image are almost impossible to detect, but the slight effect of the pixel format can be appreciated in figure 1.88. Nevertheless, the subtle acoustic texture differences within the ovary, representing small cysts and scars, is equally appreciated with both formats. The compression curve portion of the signal processing and the postprocessing gray scale mapping are identical in both images.

In figures 1.89 and 1.90, the equality in spatial resolution between the two systems is also demonstrated. Subtle anatomic detail in the retroperitoneal structures is similarly displayed. Furthermore, the texture artifact in the superficial portions of the liver related to an inappropriate time gain compensation is evident in both formats, indicating that even with digital systems, proper machine setup is critical.

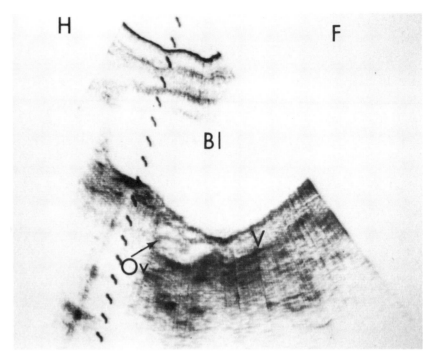

Fig. 1.87

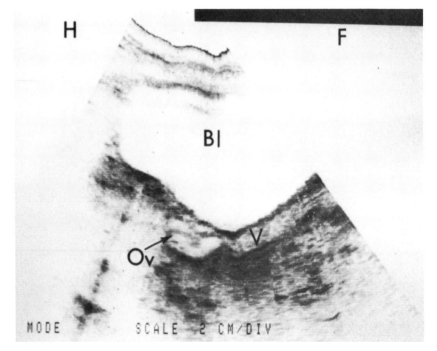

Fig. 1.88

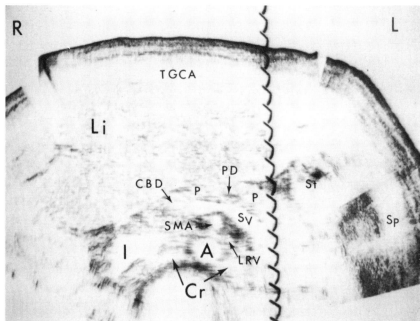

Fig. 1.89

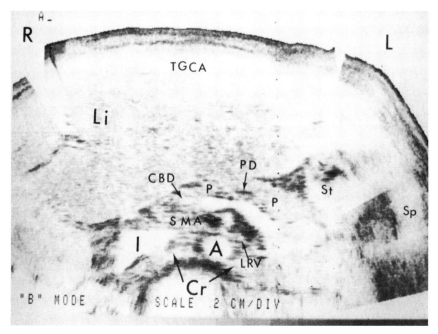

Fig. 1.90

A   = Aorta
Bl = Bladder
CBD = Common bile duct
Cr = Crus of the diaphragm
F   = Foot
H   = Head
I   = Inferior vena cava
L   = Left
Li = Liver
LRV = Left renal vein
Ov = Ovary
P   = Pancreas
PD = Pancreatic duct
R   = Right
SMA = Superior mesenteric artery
Sp = Spleen
St = Stomach
SV = Splenic vein
TGCA = Time gain compensation artifact
V   = Vagina

Digital Signal Processing

The imaging quality of digital and analog systems is further illustrated in figures 1.91 and 1.92. This longitudinal scan of a second-trimester pregnancy with an incompetent cervix demonstrates similar spatial and contrast resolution. On the digital display represented in figure 1.92, ring-down and beamwidth artifacts are unchanged, and the shadowing effects related to velocity alterations can still be appreciated.

One feature of the digital systems which has become evident is the decreased dependence of image quality on scanning speed. Figures 1.93 and 1.94 represent analog and digital scans, respectively, in which the same transducer path was used for the pelvis in a woman with a large ovarian cyst. Although the overall topography is similar, the skip lines resulting from the incomplete sampling, secondary to the rapid scanning speed, are evident on the analog image. Furthermore, the decreased texture within the uterus is secondary to a similar phenomenon. The more rapid data acquisition capabilities of the digital systems allow not only for less dependence on scanning speed but also for the capability of a rapid survey mode type of scanning.

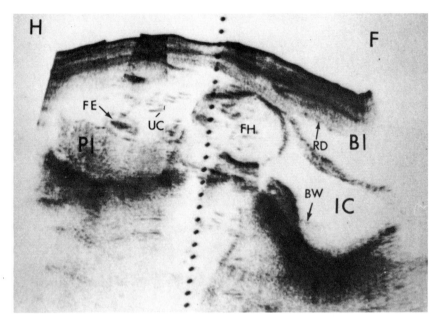

Fig. 1.91

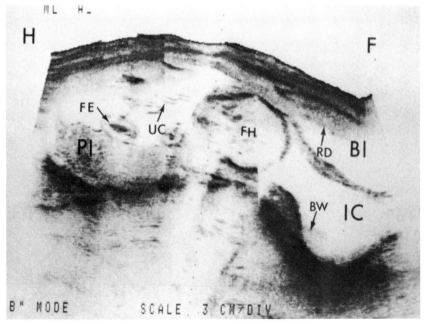

Fig. 1.92

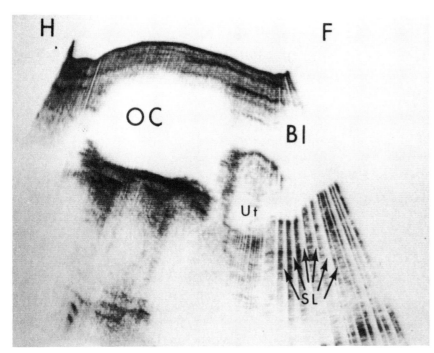

Fig. 1.93

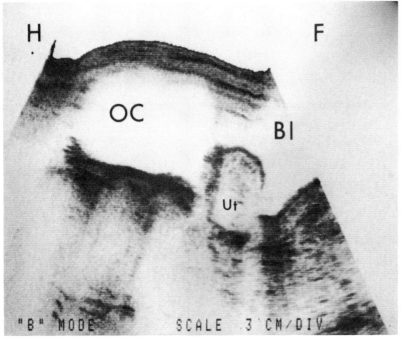

Fig. 1.94

BI	=	Bladder
BW	=	Beamwidth artifact
F	=	Foot
FE	=	Fetal extremity
FH	=	Fetal head
H	=	Head
IC	=	Incompetent cervix
OC	=	Ovarian cyst
PI	=	Placenta
RD	=	Ring down
SL	=	Skip lines
UC	=	Umbilical cord
Ut	=	Uterus

Digital Postprocessing

Retaining an image in a digital memory allows for considerably more flexibility in postprocessing, although it is important to know this has certain limitations when compared with the preprocessing associated with the compression curve. In digital signal processing, the dynamic range of returning echoes is divided into packets, the number of which is determined by the depth of the digital memory (bits). We can take a small region of the dynamic range and divide it into very small packets, or we can take a large portion of the dynamic range and divide it into larger packets. Once the image is stored in memory in this fashion, however, postprocessing will never be able to separate information that has been placed into a single packet. Postprocessing may involve a variable gray scale assignment to the already predetermined packets.

An example of the effects of postprocessing involving the gray scale assignment is illustrated in figures 1.95 and 1.96. This transverse scan of an abdominal aneurysm illustrates textural differences between the thrombus and the lumen of the aneurysm. In figure 1.95, the lower level information is given relatively higher gray shades; the upper part of the dynamic range has been assigned only a few shades of gray. The resulting image highlights the difference between lumen and thrombus as well as the areas of calcification. The outer margin of the aneurysm, however, is not well seen. A different postprocessing gray scale assignment demonstrated in figure 1.96 for the same image demonstrates more clearly the external contours of the aneurysm, whereas some of the textural features of the internal aspect of the aneurysm are not as well appreciated.

In figure 1.97, a longitudinal scan of the left-upper quadrant demonstrates a hydronephrotic left kidney. The postprocessing mapping, however, is set up to delineate the textural differences between the kidney and the spleen. A different postprocessing gray scale assignment of the same image is demonstrated in figure 1.98. The lower amplitude information has been assigned

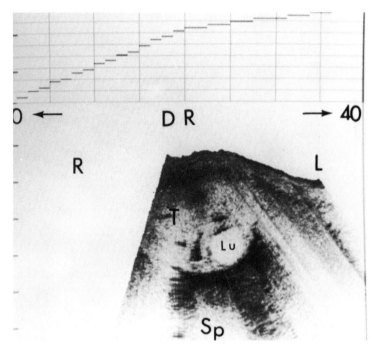

Fig. 1.95

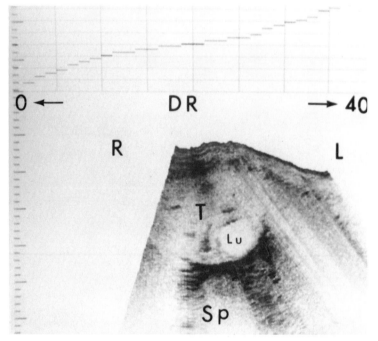

Fig. 1.96

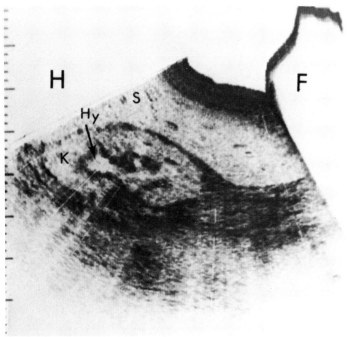

Fig. 1.97

relatively fewer lighter shades of gray; the upper portion of the dynamic range has been assigned the majority of the gray shades. The resulting image better demonstrates the calcifications in the calices and their accompanying shadowing. How beneficial this type of postprocessing will be for all pathologies is still unclear. Nevertheless, in our initial experience, the ability to manipulate the image in this fashion may bring out additional information on the scans.

DR	=	Dynamic range in decibels
F	=	Foot
H	=	Head
Hy	=	Hydronephrosis
K	=	Kidney
L	=	Left
Lu	=	Lumen
R	=	Right
Sh	=	Shadowing
Sp	=	Spine
S	=	Spleen
St	=	Stones
T	=	Thrombus

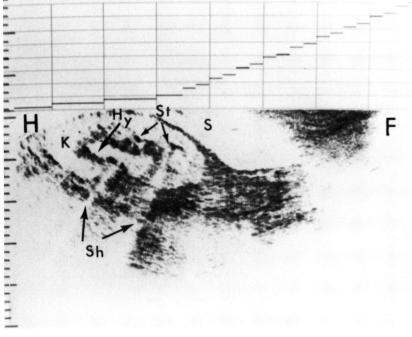

Fig. 1.98

Digital Postprocessing

The digital storage system allows for a number of other postprocessing techniques. By means of various software programs, the relative percentage of amplitude distribution for echoes within the entire scan, or within selected areas of the scan, can be displayed with a histogram format. Such a technique allows the operator to look at the actual echo distributions within a given area. This may be important in comparing the acoustic textures of different organs, if such comparisons can lead to the detection of focal or generalized diseases. This type of processing also overcomes the optical illusion of a higher shade of gray and implies higher echo amplitude in a specific area. This higher amplitude is due simply to the number of written echoes within the area rather than to their actual increased amplitude.

Figures 1.99–1.100 demonstrate a transverse scan of the upper abdomen that attempts a comparison between pancreatic and liver tissue. No definite difference in the echo amplitudes between the two organs is present. In figure 1.99, an amplitude distribution histogram for a small area of the pancreas (0.2 sq cm, indicated by the arrow at the bottom right-hand corner of the digital readout) is indicated at the top of the screen. The first derivative of this histogram is seen in figure 1.100, indicating that the mean amplitude echo within this area is approximately 15 dB. A similar area of analysis was performed in the liver at the same depth of the scan in order to overcome time gain compensation corrections. The relative percent amplitude histogram is indicated in figure 1.101. The first derivative of this histogram distribution is indicated in figure 1.102, which shows a mean echo amplitude of 10 dB. Therefore, although visually the echo amplitudes—as indicated by the visual gray shades—appeared similar, the mean echogenicity of the pancreas is, in fact, greater than the liver.

The ultimate value of this type of postprocessing has yet to be determined, for the effects on these types of histograms and first derivatives by differences in

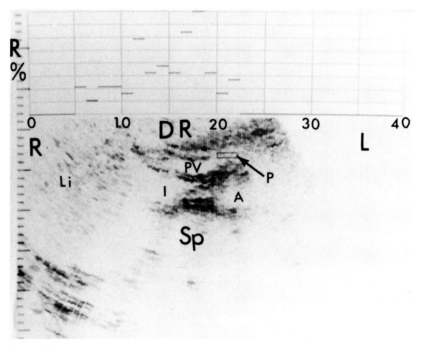

Fig. 1.99

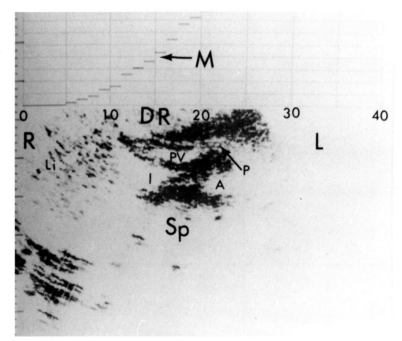

Fig. 1.100

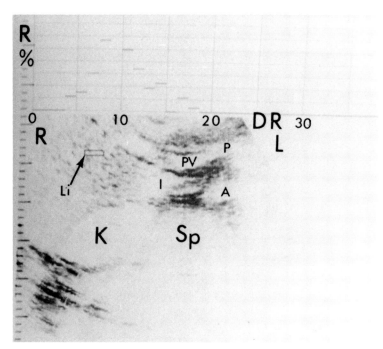

Fig. 1.101

scanning parameters and scanning
speeds still must be evaluated.

A	=	Aorta
Arrow	=	Digital readout of area
DR	=	Dynamic range in decibels
I	=	Inferior vena cava
K	=	Kidney
L	=	Left
Li	=	Liver
M	=	Mean amplitude echo
P	=	Pancreas
PV	=	Portal vein
R	=	Right
R%	=	Relative percentage
Sp	=	Spleen

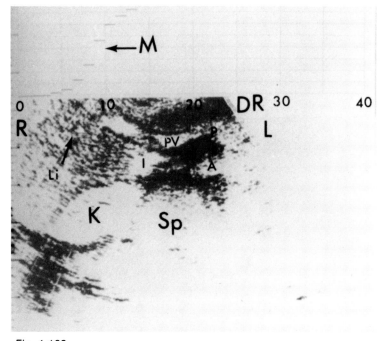

Fig. 1.102

2.
Hepatic Ultrasonography

Barry Green, M.D.
Harvey M. Goldstein, M.D.

Prior to the advent of gray scale technology, ultrasound evaluation of the internal structure of the liver was inaccurate. Only the gross hepatic contours could be assessed; intrahepatic abnormalities were diagnosed only with the greatest of difficulty. During the past several years, it has been successfully demonstrated that the internal structure of the liver and parenchymal abnormalities could be easily identified and assessed with gray scale techniques (Bryan et al. 1977; Carlsen 1975; Green et al. 1977; McArdle 1976; Scheible, Gosink, and Leopold 1977; Taylor, Carpenter, and McCready 1973; Taylor et al. 1976). This section describes the technique, normal ultrasonic hepatic anatomy, and ultrasonic appearance of various intrahepatic disorders.

Hepatic Ultrasound Technique

No specific patient preparation is necessary unless elective examination of the gallbladder is also to be attempted. If so, an eight-hour fast prior to the examination is required. The patient is examined in the supine position, in both the longitudinal and transverse planes, with sections obtained at 1-cm intervals across the liver. The longitudinal scans are best performed with a subcostal single pass technique with respirations suspended in deep inspiration in order to displace the liver inferiorly (Carlsen 1975; Taylor and Hill 1975). This maneuver further serves to displace the bowel gas below the organ of interest and helps to eliminate rib artifacts. The transducer is placed under the costal margin and is angled cephaladly. To visualize the anterior liver, the transducer face is pushed gently onto the patient's abdomen beneath the costal margin. The transducer tip is used as a fulcrum, as its face is rotated caudally while maintaining constant contact with the skin surface. The transducer face is smoothly arced in sequence, perpendicular first to the diaphragm, then to the right kidney, and finally to the inferior edge of the liver. Occasionally, reversing the sequence of the arc will result in a more satisfactory scan (Albertson and Leopold 1977). The transverse scans are performed with a combined compound scanning and sectoring technique. Oblique views will sometimes add further information, particularly when evaluating the portal vasculature and bile ducts. The right lateral dome of the liver can be an extremely difficult area to evaluate and can be examined with 45° oblique sections obtained somewhat parallel to the porta hepatis.

The highest-frequency transducer that can entirely "fill in" the liver with echoes is used. This is currently a 3.5-MHz, medium- or long-focus transducer. Occasionally, a 5-MHz transducer can be used over thin areas—the lateral segment of the left lobe, for example, or in smaller patients. Obese or muscular patients may require a 2.25-MHz transducer. The critical objective of longitudinal scans is to demonstrate a uniform parenchymagram that is interrupted only by the portal vessels and hepatic veins. Echoes must be recorded from every portion of the liver. The normal parenchymal echo pattern is dependent upon the particular patient, type of equipment, and transducer used. Most of the pertinent parenchymal information is obtained from the longitudinal scans, since the rib and respiratory artifacts encountered on transverse views are avoided, and more meaningful interpretation of the parenchymal pattern can be made. On occasion, central vascular anatomy and visualization of the lateral segment of the left lobe is better appreciated on the transverse views. (See also p. 68 for additional comments on the technique for liver examination.)

Normal Ultrasonographic Anatomy of the Liver

All imaging techniques indicate that the size and shape of the liver is quite variable. The right lobe comprises the greatest bulk. It generally has a rounded contour with rather smooth margins, although frequently a tongue of liver tissue will extend caudally; this is the so-called Riedel's lobe. Nearer the midline, the normal liver size is gradually reduced until it merges into the lateral segment of the left lobe which normally extends 3–4 cm to the left of the midline as a thin wedgelike structure. Often, this segment extends further into the left anterior abdomen, but in the normal state it will continue to taper as it extends toward the left. The medial segment of the left lobe is situated between the right lobe and the lateral segment of the left lobe and usually cannot be discerned as a separate anatomic entity. The falciform ligament, situated between the medial and lateral segments of the left lobe, will frequently be appreciated as a distinct echogenic structure just to the right of midline. In a small percentage of normal livers it will have a sharply circumscribed, rounded configuration and should not be confused with a hepatic mass (Bryan et al. 1977; Prando et al. 1979).

The caudate lobe, a posterior portion of the medial segment of the left lobe, can be seen as a distinct structure in both longitudinal and transverse views. It usually straddles the midline, cephalic to the head of the pancreas and anterior to the inferior vena cava (IVC). This should not be confused with a true mass since it is always in this characteristic location, and its texture is usually that of the remainder of the liver. The diaphragm is a sharply circumscribed, curvilinear, echogenic line that demarcates the cephalic and posterior margins of the liver and separates the liver from the right lung.

The parenchymagram should be quite uniform with a homogeneous echo pattern that is interrupted only by the echoes emanating from the various vascular structures. All areas of the liver should have essentially the same echo texture. The normal intrahepatic biliary tree and hepatic arteries are not visualized, although the portal and hepatic veins are always seen.

The gross ultrasonic anatomy of the intrahepatic vascular structures has been described in detail (Carlsen and Filly 1976; Leopold 1975; Sanders, Conrad, and White 1977; Taylor and Carpenter 1975). On parasagittal sections, just to the left of midline, the aorta can be seen as it courses posterior to the lateral segment of the left lobe. Just to the right of the midline, the wider IVC can be identified, especially with Valsalva's maneuver. The more cephalic portion of this vessel curves ventrally as it nears its insertion through the diaphragm to enter the right atrium.

The larger portal venous structures course through the liver transversely and are better assessed on transverse views, where greater lengths of the portal veins are depicted on a single scan. The main portal vein crosses just anterior to the inferior vena cava. Frequently, branching of the portal vein into the main right and left channels is observed. The left portal vein is seen as a narrower caliber trunk coursing transversely through the left lobe. The portal veins also are seen on longitudinal scans, but their distribution is difficult to appreciate. The intrahepatic portal branches will appear as small, dense, echogenic streaks or dots or as branching, parallel dense lines, depending upon the plane of section.

All of the major hepatic vein trunks and some of their tributaries can be recognized on longitudinal scans. They will present as tubular, oval, or round, thin-walled sonolucencies in the liver parenchyma. Their lack of an echogenic border enables them to be distinguished from thicker-walled highly echogenic portal branches.

The appearance of the portal vein walls is felt to be secondary to the presence of surrounding fibrous tissue within the portal triads. The hepatic veins can vary remarkably in size and can be quite large with strenuous Valsalva maneuver or right heart failure. Serial scanning in oblique planes enables us to trace these back to their junction with the IVC.

Hepatic Pathology

Ultrasonography of the liver is most useful in the evaluation of intrahepatic mass lesions. These include primary and secondary neoplasms, cysts, abscesses, hematomas, and other less commonly encountered entities (Carlsen 1975; Doust, Quiroz, and Stewart 1977; Green et al. 1977; Lawson 1977; Maklad, Doust, and Baum 1974; Scheible, Gosink, and Leopold 1977; Taylor et al. 1976).

Ultrasonography is also a very sensitive, excellent means of assessing dilation of the biliary tree. This topic will be discussed in another chapter. To date, the value of ultrasonography in the evaluation of hepatocellular disorders, such as cirrhosis and hepatitis, has been limited.

Malignant Neoplasms

Metastatic liver disease represents the most common intrahepatic neoplasm and presents a varied gray scale echographic appearance (Green et al. 1977; McArdle 1976; Scheible, Gosink, and Leopold 1977). Three patterns are most commonly encountered: (1) relatively well-defined hypoechoic masses containing fewer echoes than the adjacent, surrounding parenchyma; (2) relatively well-defined echogenic masses containing higher-amplitude echoes than the surrounding parenchyma; and (3) diffuse distortion of the normal homogeneous parenchymal pattern without focal masses. Multiple echogenic and hypoechoic areas without dominant focal lesions may be present in this latter pattern. The pattern is the most difficult to identify and requires good technique and familiarity with the normal parenchymal appearances as produced with the clinician's own equipment. Various combinations of these patterns can be seen simultaneously. For example, it is not unusual to see a diffuse alteration of internal echo architecture along with focal hyperechoic and/or hypoechoic masses.

Although not as helpful diagnostically as parenchymal evaluation, assessment for liver enlargement and/or contour alterations may be useful. This is particularly evident in the region of the lateral segment of the left lobe which can appear enlarged and bulbous when compared to its normal triangular tapering configuration. Lesions may be solitary or multiple and can vary greatly in size. With modern gray scale technology, detection of lesions as small as 1.5–2 cm is possible. The margins of the masses can be sharp or ill-defined, but most are round. This may reflect the hematogenous origin of most liver metastases.

Aside from these frequently encountered basic patterns, other variations are also seen with some regularity. Less than 5% of liver metastases present as totally sonolucent masses (Wooten, Green, and Goldstein 1978). This appearance is not specific for one type of tumor, although in our experience approximately half have been seen with metastatic leiomyosarcomas of gastrointestinal origin. Presumably, most of these represent lesions with central liquefaction necrosis to account for the sonolucency. On an ultrasonic basis alone they can be difficult to differentiate from cysts, although they tend to have irregular inner margins. Other more typical metastatic lesions frequently are seen in adjacent portions of the liver. Occasionally, a small central lucency will be seen within echogenic metastases. "Bulls-eye" lesions are those in which an echogenic central focus is surrounded by a more lucent margin. This appearance can also be seen with a wide variety of primary tumors (Scheible, Gosink, and Leopold 1977). Calcified liver metastases are highly echogenic, with posterior acoustic shadowing (Katragadda, Goldstein, and Green 1977). This distinctive appearance usually is seen with mucinous tumors of the colon.

In our experience, tumor histology or degree of vascularity does not correlate with ultrasonographic appearances (Green et al. 1977). Others feel, however, that the majority of echogenic lesions represent adenocarcinoma, usually arising from the colon (Scheible, Gosink, and Leopold 1977). We have seen metastases from virtually all organs present in this fashion. The same primary lesion may even result in sonolucent and echogenic hepatic metastases simultaneously (Green et al. 1977).

Lymphoma deserves particular attention in this discussion, since it affects the liver in various ways. Many lymphoma patients demonstrate hepatomegaly, though with a normal internal sonographic parenchymagram. Others show hepatomegaly with a diffuse alteration of echo architecture but without focal masses. Occasionally, focal sonolucent or echogenic masses will be seen. It is virtually impossible to tell these lesions from metastatic disease of a nonlymphomatous nature. The concomitant presence of splenomegaly and/or retroperitoneal adenopathy may be an aid in this differentiation. Leukemia will demonstrate hepatomegaly but not other hepatic abnormalities. We have not encountered focal hepatic masses in this latter entity.

Primary liver malignancies are most often hepatomas in adults and hepatoblastomas in young children. As with metastases, these can present as focal echogenic or hypoechoic masses or as diffuse disturbances of hepatic sonographic parenchyma. This latter presentation may be subtle and is usually seen with the multifocal variety of hepatoma. In our experience, the majority of hepatocellular cancerous lesions present as echogenic masses. Angiography and usually biopsy are needed to differentiate these lesions from metastatic disease.

In addition to the initial evaluation, ultrasonography is an excellent modality for following the progress of liver metastases while the patient undergoes therapy. Changes in size, contour, distribution, number, and internal characteristics may be accurately assessed.

Benign Neoplasms

Benign liver neoplasms are less commonly observed than malignant tumors. Among the more common are cavernous hemangiomas, hepatic adenomas, and focal nodular hyperplasia. Reports of the ultrasonic appearances of these lesions are scanty. Not enough have been studied to allow definitive comment on their sonographic appearance. We would, however, expect these lesions to have similar nonspecific appearances as described above for other liver neoplasms. It is of interest that all four of the cavernous hemangiomas we studied had a highly echogenic pattern secondary to their highly vascular structure.

Cystic Disease

Ultrasound technique has the well-known ability to distinguish between cystic and solid lesions and is thus an excellent modality for identifying intrahepatic cysts (Albertson and Leopold 1977; McCarthy et al. 1969; Weaver et al. 1978). It is more accurate in detecting small cysts than solid lesions of comparable size, because the change in acoustic impedance between the cyst and normal parenchyma is greater than between solid lesions and parenchyma.

Cysts of the liver may be congenital or acquired and may occur singly or multiply. They often are encountered as an incidental finding during abdominal sonography or are discovered during the evaluation of a positive radionuclide liver scan in a patient without any clinical evidence of significant liver disease. Classically, they are described as round, sonolucent masses with sharply defined regular borders and with definite posterior wall acoustical enhancement. It has been our experience, however, that these findings are not always present. Cystic contours may be lobular or ovoid, the walls minimally irregular, and the degree of sound transmission quite variable (Weaver, et al. 1978). As in other cystic lesions, septations may be present. The appearance, including the size of the cysts, remains relatively stable on follow-up examinations. In the case of polycystic liver disease, the kidneys and pancreas also should be examined for associated cysts.

Abscess

Intrahepatic, subphrenic, and subhepatic abscesses can be identified by ultrasound (Albertson and Leopold 1977; Carlsen 1975; Doust 1977; Doust, Quiroz, and Stewart 1977; Gosink and Leopold 1975; Kressel and Filly 1978; Landay and Harless 1977; Lawson 1977; Maklad, Doust, and Baum 1974; Taylor et al. 1976). Collaborative clinical information, including fever, elevated white blood cell count, and right upper-quadrant pain, usually is present and will facilitate this diagnosis. Intrahepatic abscesses usually are solitary but can occur multiply. They have been described as sonolucent with somewhat thick, irregular margins and accentuated posterior wall transmission. They may contain some internal echoes, due to the presence of necrotic debris.

This may be a particularly prominent feature of amebic abscesses. This sonographic appearance is not, however, diagnostic of abscess and may be seen with hematoma, necrotic metastasis, or hemorrhagic cyst. Gas-containing liver abscesses may appear as densely echogenic masses with or without acoustic shadowing and may be confused with solid intrahepatic lesions (Kressel and Filly 1978). This appearance may be due to a "microbubble" contrast effect.

There is probably a spectrum of presentation related to the evolution of the inflammatory process. In the early stages, before frank necrosis, the abnormal area will appear as a focal zone of altered parenchyma. With progressive necrosis, the abscess will gradually assume its classic, well-defined sonolucent appearance. Bacterial as well as amebic abscesses will have this variable appearance.

Subphrenic abscesses lie between the diaphragm and liver and present as sonolucent collections which depress the liver surface away from the diaphragm. The major differential consideration is pleural fluid at the right-lung base (Landay and Harless 1977). With attention to anatomic detail and visualization of the diaphragm, pleural effusion will be identified cephalad to the diaphragm. Subhepatic abscesses present as sonolucent masses inferior to the liver and anterior to the upper pole of the right kidney. Ascitic fluid accumulated in this space must be differentiated from a purulent collection in this same region. Ascitic fluid will be echo-free, whereas a subhepatic abscess usually will have irregular, thick margins and some internal echoes arising from debris.

Hematoma

Hematomas may be intrahepatic or subcapsular in location. They usually are the result of trauma, although occasionally spontaneous rupture of an intrahepatic neoplasm can result in a hematoma. This phenomenon is characteristically seen with hepatic adenoma, metastatic choriocarcinoma, and cavernous hemangioma. Within the liver, a hematoma will appear as a relatively sonolucent mass. It usually is not sharply circumscribed and may contain scattered internal echoes representing clots and areas of organization. Over several weeks or months, the hematoma should become smaller; this should allow it to be distinguished from tumors or cysts.

Without clinical information, they cannot be differentiated from abscesses.

Subcapsular collections of blood will present as an echo-free area, either focal in nature or more diffusely surrounding a larger portion of the liver. The focal variety is found more commonly after liver biopsy procedures. It is often difficult to detect a sharp line of demarcation between the edge of the compressed parenchyma and the blood because of the numerous rib reverberation artifacts. The diffuse variety of subcapsular hematomas must be distinguished from ascitic fluid collections around the liver. While a subcapsular hematoma will be confined strictly to the margins of the liver ascitic fluid should be seen elsewhere in the abdomen, aside from the perihepatic regions. If rupture of the capsule has occurred with free spillage of blood into the peritoneal cavity, it can be impossible to differentiate between these entities.

Hepatocellular Disorders

Very little has been written concerning the gray scale appearances of primary hepatocellular disease (Albertson and Leopold 1977). Ultrasonographically, an abnormality is appreciated only in the presence of severe changes of either fatty metamorphosis or fibrosis. This produces a diffuse increase in echogenicity at standard gain settings. Poor penetration of sound may also exist secondary to increased absorption and scattering by the fibrotic liver. As a result, the posterior aspect of the liver can be difficult to demonstrate. In the case of cirrhosis, helpful ancillary findings include prominence of the portal vasculature, splenomegaly, and ascites. We have encountered one case of diffusely infiltrating Hodgkin's disease which presented with this identical pattern. Regenerating nodules may be detected and can become a confusing diagnostic problem, for they can present as focal masses (Albertson and Leopold 1977). In this situation, isotope scan, angiography and/or biopsy can be used to distinguish these nodules from true tumor masses.

References

Albertson, K. W., and Leopold, G. R. Liver. Pp. 103–136 in *Abdominal Gray Scale Ultrasonography.* Goldberg, B. ed. New York: Wiley Medical Publications, 1977.

Bryan, P. J. et al. Correlation of computed tomography, gray scale ultrasonography and radionuclide imaging of the liver in detecting space-occupying processes. *Radiology*. 124:387–393, 1977.

Carlsen, E. N. Liver, gallbladder and spleen. *Radiol. Clin. North. Am.* 13:543–556, 1975.

Carlsen, E. N., and Filly, R. A. Newer ultrasonographic anatomy in the upper abdomen: the portal and heaptic venous anatomy. *J. Clin. Ultrasound* 4:85–90, 1976.

Doust, B. D. Abscesses, hematomas and other fluid collections. In *Abdominal gray scale ultrasonography*, ed. B. Goldberg. New York: Wiley Medical Publications, 1977, pp. 231–259.

Doust, B. D.; Quiroz, F.; and Stewart, J. M. Ultrasonic distinction of abscesses from other intra-abdominal fluid collections. *Radiology* 125:213–218, 1977.

Gosink, B. B., and Leopold, G. R. Abdominal echography. *Semin. Roentgenol.* 10:229–304, 1975.

Green, G. et al. Gray scale ultrasound evaluation of hepatic neoplasms: patterns and correlations. *Radiology* 124:203–208, 1977.

Katragadda, C. S.; Goldstein, H. M.; and Green, B. Gray scale ultrasonography of calcified liver metastases. *Am. J. Roentgenol.* 129:591–593, 1977.

Kressel, H. Y., and Filly, R. A. Ultrasonographic appearance of gas-containing abscesses in the abdomen. *Am. J. Roentgenol.* 130:71–73, 1978.

Landay, M., and Harless, W. Ultrasonic differentiation of right pleural effusion from subphrenic fluid on longitudinal scans of the right upper quadrant: importance of recognizing the diaphragm. *Radiology* 123:155–158, 1977.

Lawson, T. L. Hepatic abscess: ultrasound as an aid to diagnosis. *Am. J. Dig. Dis.* 22:33–37, 1977.

Leopold, G. R. Gray scale ultrasonic angiography of the upper abdomen. *Radiology* 117:665–671, 1975.

Maklad, N. F.; Doust, B. D.; and Baum, J. K. Ultrasonic diagnosis of postoperative intra-abdominal abscess. *Radiology* 113:417–422, 1974.

McArdle, C. R. Ultrasonic diagnosis of liver metastases. *J. Clin. Ultrasound* 4:265–268, 1976.

McCarthy, C. F. et al. The use of ultrasound in the diagnosis of cystic lesions of the liver and upper abdomen and in the detection of ascites. *Gut* 10:904–912, 1969.

Prando, A. et al. Ultrasonographic pseudolesions of the liver. *Radiology* 130:403–407, 1979.

Sanders, R. C.; Conrad, M. R.; and White, Jr., R. I. Normal and abnormal upper abdominal venous structures as seen by ultrasound. *Am. J. Roentgenol.* 128:657–662, 1977.

Scheible, W.; Gosink, B. B.; Leopold, G. R. Gray scale echographic patterns of hepatic metastatic disease. *Am. J. Roentgenol.* 129:983–987, 1977.

Taylor, K. J. W., and Carpenter, D. A. The anatomy and pathology of the porta hepatis demonstrated by gray scale ultrasonography. *J. Clin. Ultrasound* 3:117–119, 1975.

Taylor, K. J. W. et al. Gray scale ultrasound imaging. The anatomy and pathology of the liver. *Radiology* 119:415–423, 1976.

Taylor, K. J. W.; Carpenter, D. A.; and McCready, V. R. Gray scale echography in the diagnosis of intrahepatic disease. *J. Clin. Ultrasound* 1:284–287, 1973.

Taylor, K. J. W. and Hill, C. R. Scanning techniques in gray scale ultrasonography. *Br. J. Radiol.* 48:918–920, 1975.

Weaver, R. et al. Gray scale ultrasonic evaluation of hepatic cystic disease. *Am. J. Roentgenol.* 130:849–852, 1978.

Wooten, W. B.; Green, B.; and Goldstein, H. M. Ultrasonography of necrotic hepatic metastases. *Radiology* 128:447–450, 1978.

CASES

Dennis A. Sarti, M.D.
W. Frederick Sample, M.D.

Technique for Liver Examination

Liver examinations usually start with the patient in the supine position. Transverse scans are obtained in the epigastric region with a single-sweep scan between the costal margins. We obtain the best visualization of the left lobe of the liver and a portion of the right lobe in this fashion. The lateral aspect of the right lobe of the liver, however, will be difficult to visualize because of the costal margins. Artifacts from the overlying ribs will cause some difficulty in evaluating the lateral aspect of the right lobe. Figure 2.1 is an example of the transducer path obtained during transverse scanning. The lateral aspect of the right lobe of the liver can be visualized by making small sector scans in the intercostal spaces. Scanning is begun with a single-sweep scan over the epigastric region. The lateral aspect of the right lobe is filled in by these small intercostal sector scans. It is important to have the patient in deep inspiration to place the liver as caudal as possible and to avoid the costal margins and ribs. Scans are usually obtained at 1-cm intervals. Often a cephalic angulation will increase the ability to visualize the cephalad portion of the liver.

Longitudinal scans as demonstrated in figure 2.2 are obtained at 1-cm intervals until the entire liver parenchyma is covered. The left lobe of the liver is quite easily identified, because the epigastric region has no ribs obscuring the view. The right lobe of the liver, however, is much more difficult to visualize because of the overlying ribs. We can begin the longitudinal scans on the right side with the transducer underneath the right costal margin. The transducer initially is arched so that it is parallel to the right hemidiaphragm. It continues straight down the right lateral abdomen parallel to the skin's surface.

The right lateral and superior portions of the liver are often missed with the normal transverse and longitudinal scanning technique. This is because it is

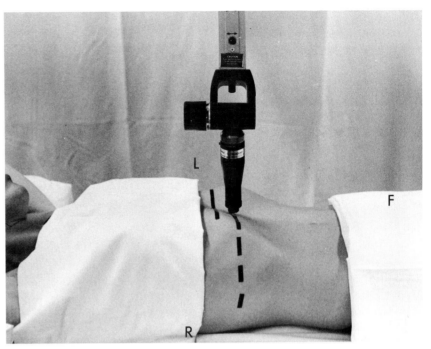

Fig. 2.1

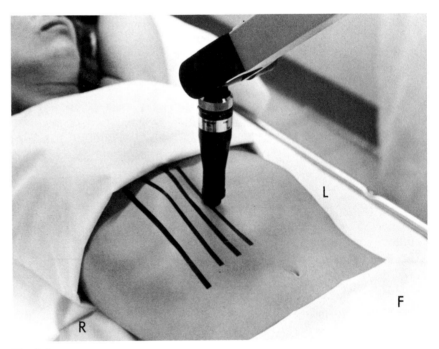

Fig. 2.2

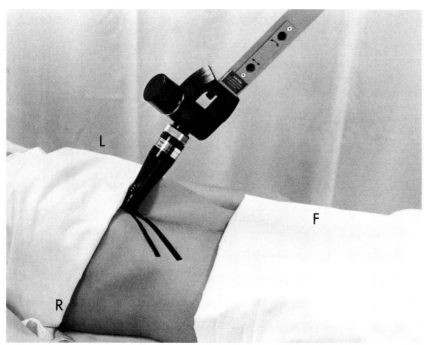

Fig. 2.3

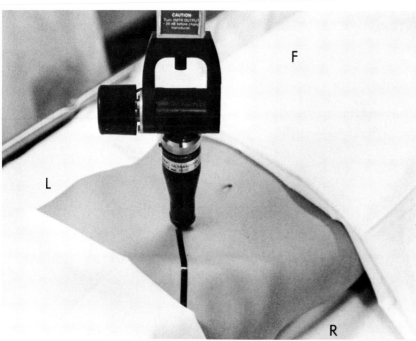

Fig. 2.4

difficult to get under the right costal margin. Figure 2.3 is an oblique eephalad-angled scan underneath the right costal margin; it yields better visualization of the right lateral dome of the liver. Placing the transducer face underneath the right costal margin, with a marked cephalad angulation, we can pick up numerous lesions that are routinely missed in the normal transverse and longitudinal scanning planes. Another method for evaluating the right superior lateral portion of the liver is a scan parallel to the porta hepatis. Figure 2.4 is an example of the scanning plane aimed 45° toward the superior right lateral dome of the liver. This is in close proximity to the portal vein and can yield important information about the peripheral anatomy. This scanning technique is also extremely valuable in evaluating the portal venous system, the common bile duct, and the biliary tree.

F = Foot
L = Left
R = Right

Normal Hepatic Transverse Scans

Transverse sections of the liver are best obtained with the patient in deep inspiration. This drives the liver caudal so that it can be visualized beneath the right costal margin. In some individuals with very high diaphragms, adequate liver studies are not possible unless we scan laterally through the intercostal spaces.

Figure 2.5 is a transverse scan with cephalad angulation of the transducer. The inferior vena cava is seen anterior to the spine. Hepatic veins are noted draining into the inferior vena cava. The echo pattern of the liver is fairly homogeneous. This even echo pattern is interrupted by tubular structures throughout the liver. Some of the tubular structures have high-amplitude echoes surrounding them. These arise from the fibrous tissue surrounding the portal triad. The tubular structures with the strong surrounding echoes represent branches of the portal venous system. The hepatic veins are also tubular structures coursing through the liver, but they do not have this high-amplitude surrounding echo. Therefore, they can be distinguished from the portal venous system.

Figure 2.6 demonstrates some portal veins with the strong surrounding echoes and a hepatic vein without the strong surrounding echoes. The crus of the diaphragm is seen anterior to the aorta as a thick lucent band.

Figures 2.7 and 2.8 are transverse sections of the liver using some sector scanning through the intercostal spaces over the right lateral aspect of the abdomen. The major portion of the scan is done in a single-sector sweep anteriorly over the epigastrium. The lateral aspects of the liver, however, are filled in with small sector scans through the intercostal spaces. The left portal vein is seen in both figures 2.7 and 2.8 in the mid portion of the left lobe of the liver. This can usually be identified in most studies. Figure 2.8 demonstrates the right portal vein in the mid portion of the right lobe of the liver, separating the anterior and posterior portions of this lobe.

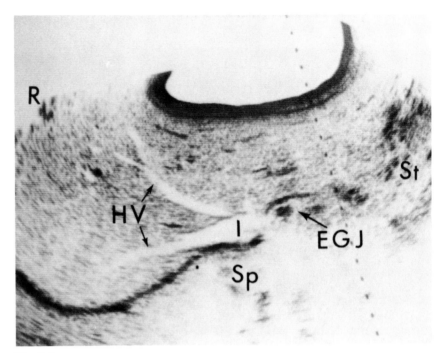

Fig. 2.5

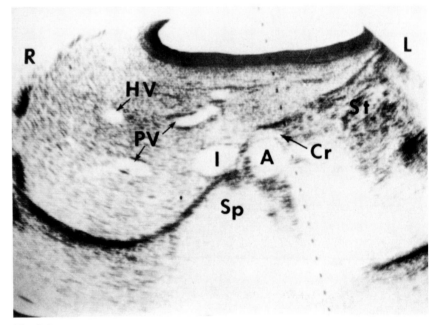

Fig. 2.6

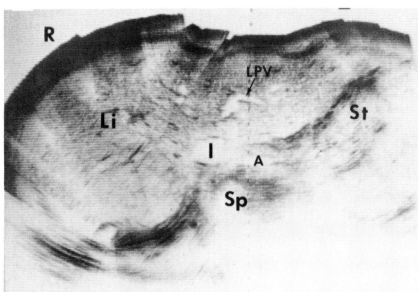

Fig. 2.7

A = Aorta
Cr = Crus of the diaphragm
EGS = Esophagogastric junction
HV = Hepatic vein
I = Inferior vena cava
K = Kidney
L = Left
Li = Liver
LPV = Left portal vein
PV = Portal vein
R = Right
RPV = Right portal vein
Sp = Spine
St = Stomach

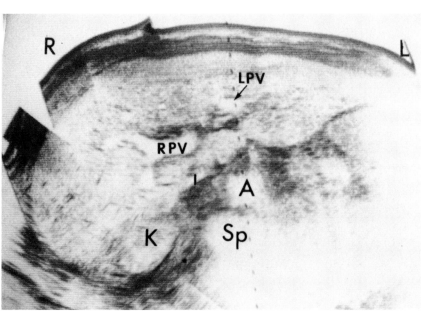

Fig. 2.8

Normal Hepatic Transverse Sections

Occasionally, the portal vein can be seen in its entirety, as in figure 2.9. This occurs when it has a horizontal orientation. It can be seen situated anterior to the inferior vena cava. High-level echoes surround the portal vein, secondary to fibrous tissue. This is well seen in figure 2.10 as dark echoes surround the portal vein and separate the caudate lobe from the anterior portion of the left lobe of the liver. It is important to recognize the caudate lobe as arising from the liver. It can occasionally be confused as a mass in the head of the pancreas. The echogenicity arising from the caudate lobe, however, is similar to that of the liver.

Figures 2.11 and 2.12 demonstrate an increased echo amplitude arising from the liver when compared to the kidney. The echoes arising from the renal parenchyma are usually several shades of gray lighter than the liver parenchyma. The pancreas seen in figure 2.12 has a darker echo appearance when compared to the liver. This is the normal echo amplitude relationship of the three organs: pancreas > liver > kidney. The gallbladder can be seen within the liver parenchyma; it is usually lateral to the inferior vena cava, as seen in figures 2.11 and 2.12. The left lateral border of the liver is often demarcated by a strong C-shaped echo arising from the medial wall of the stomach.

A strong circular echo, seen in the left lobe of the liver, arises from the falciform ligament as is present in figure 2.12. Shadowing behind the falciform ligament is also seen in many instances.

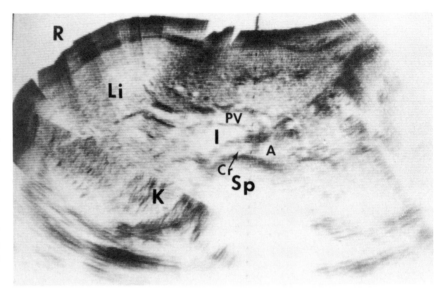

Fig. 2.9

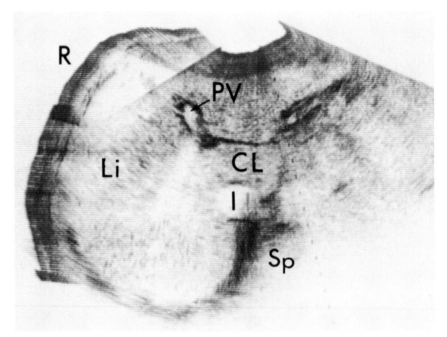

Fig. 2.10

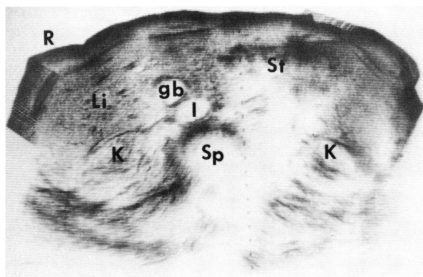

Fig. 2.11

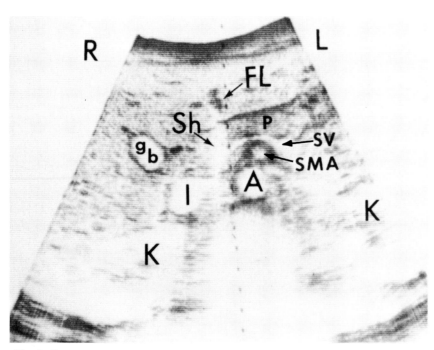

Fig. 2.12

Normal Hepatic Longitudinal Scans

Evaluation of liver echogenicity and texture is best performed by longitudinal scans. A single sweep of the liver can be obtained approximately parallel to the diaphragm and continuing down over the abdominal surface. This yields an even texture to the liver parenchyma except for the tubular structures coursing through it. Figure 2.13 is an example of a longitudinal scan obtained quite laterally, over the right abdomen. The diaphragm is a strong curvilinear echo which provides the superior border to the liver echo pattern. Because of the single-sweep technique, an even parenchymagram of the liver can be obtained. This is not possible on transverse scans because of the overlying ribs on the lateral aspect of the liver. As we continue to scan more medially, the right kidney comes into view (fig. 2.14). Numerous tubular structures secondary to the hepatic and portal veins are present within the liver.

Figures 2.14 and 2.15 demonstrate the normal echo relationship of the renal to the liver parenchyma. The echoes arising from the renal cortex and medulla are of a lower amplitude than those arising from the liver. Furthermore, the hepatic veins do not contain the strong high-level surrounding echoes that are present around the portal venous system. As we continue more medially, the gallbladder will come into view, as seen in figures 2.15 and 2.16.

The inferior vena cava is a large tubular structure present on the posterior aspect of the liver. Figure 2.16 demonstrates the hepatic vein draining into the inferior vena cava. Around the porta hepatis are seen several circular lucencies which represent the right portal vein, the hepatic artery, and the common bile duct. As we scan longitudinally on the right side, the gallbladder also is visible as a lucent structure just posterior to the right lobe of the liver.

Occasionally, some echoes can be seen above the diaphragm, as are present in figure 2.13. These are reverberations off the diaphragm and also represent liver parenchyma duplication artifacts which are placed in the lowe

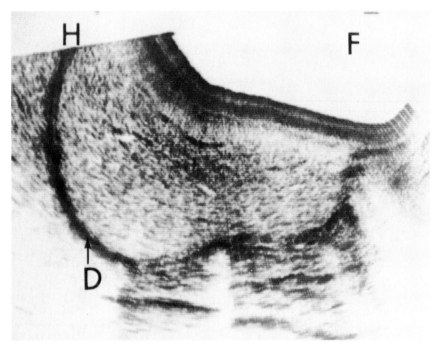

Fig. 2.13

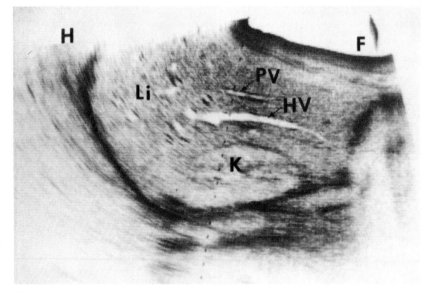

Fig. 2.14

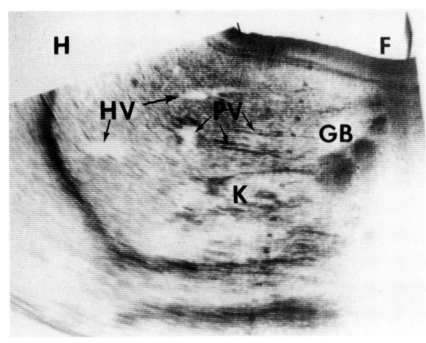

Fig. 2.15

lung field (see chapter 1). It is important to note that the posterior thoracic wall is not seen above the diaphragm in any of these cases. In chapter 8, the posterior thoracic wall will be shown secondary to the presence of right pleural effusions.

The longitudinal scans provide excellent visualization not only of the liver parenchyma but also of the subdiaphragmatic, subhepatic, and hepatorenal spaces.

CBD	=	Common bile duct
D	=	Diaphragm
F	=	Foot
GB	=	Gallbladder
H	=	Head
HA	=	Hepatic artery
HV	=	Hepatic vein
I	=	Inferior vena cava
K	=	Kidney
Li	=	Liver
PV	=	Portal vein
RPV	=	Right portal vein

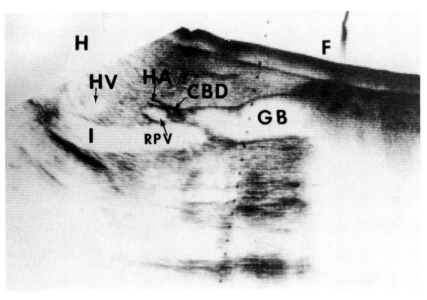

Fig. 2.16

Normal Hepatic Longitudinal Scans

As we scan to the right, the inferior vena cava is seen as a posterior tubular structure with the liver situated anteriorly. We can visualize a small circular structure indenting the posterior aspect of the inferior vena cava. This is the right renal artery (figs. 2.17–2.19). The liver maintains its fairly even echo pattern except in the region of the porta hepatis where numerous tubular structures are identified. The largest of these are secondary to various branches of the portal venous system. Figure 2.17 demonstrates the caudate lobe as seen on longitudinal scans. It is situated anterior to the inferior vena cava. There is also a strong echogenic region just posterior to the liver which arises from the mucosa of the duodenum. We can notice a small lucent area surrounding the mucosa of the duodenum which represents its muscular wall. Some posterior shadowing is noted. The pancreas is evident slightly caudal to the portal vein.

Figure 2.18 demonstrates a small tubular structure coming out of the porta hepatis and situated posterior to the head of the pancreas. This represents the common bile duct. The pancreas often is seen just posterior to the left lobe of the liver. Caudal to this is the strong echo of the air-filled stomach. Figure 2.20 is a longitudinal scan further to the left, in which we see a fairly homogeneous left lobe of the liver. There, a few highly echogenic circular structures represent the portal venous system. Just posterior to the liver we can see the echoes of the pancreas which are situated anterior to the splenic vein and splenic artery.

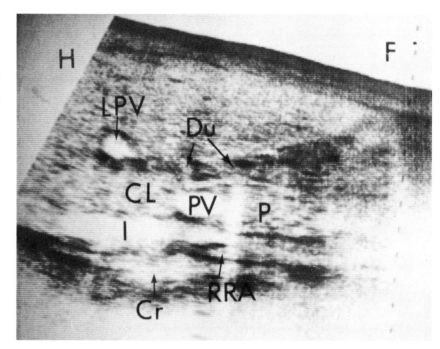

Fig. 2.17

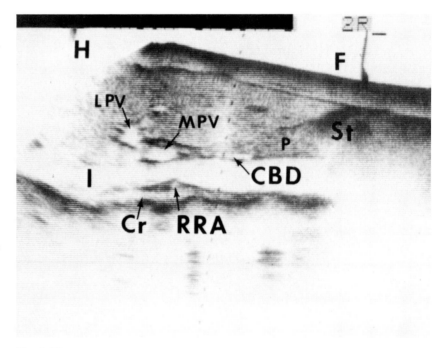

Fig. 2.18

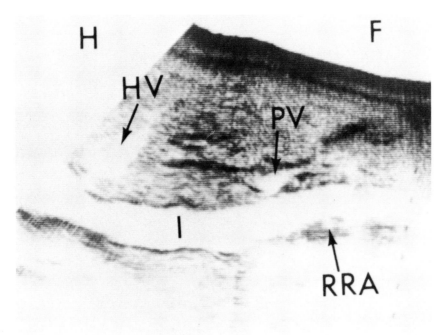

Fig. 2.19

CBD = Common bile duct
CL = Caudate lobe
Cr = Crus of the diaphragm
Du = Duodenum
F   = Foot
H   = Head
HV = Hepatic vein
I   = Inferior vena cava
Li = Liver
LPV = Left portal vein
MPV = Main portal vein
P   = Pancreas
PV = Portal vein
RRA = Right renal artery
SA = Splenic artery
St = Stomach
SV = Splenic vein

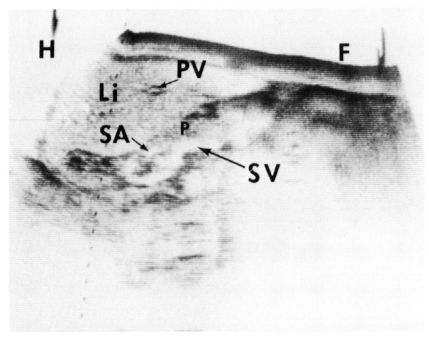

Fig. 2.20

Dilated Portal Vein, Hepatomegaly, and Cirrhosis

Figures 2.21 and 2.22 are examples of a patient with a dilated portal vein. The portal vein can be extremely variable in size. Its size is affected by Valsalva maneuvers and respiratory changes. The most dramatic dilatations, however, are found in cases of portal venous hypertension. The portal vein in figure 2.21 is markedly dilated when compared to the inferior vena cava. Very often a filling defect on the liver spleen scan will be noted in the porta hepatis. Ultrasound examination of this region can be extremely helpful if a large portal vein is diagnosed. This will explain the defect in the porta hepatis. Furthermore, dilated hepatic veins can give defects on the nuclear medicine study near the medial portion of the dome of the right hemidiaphragm. Figure 2.21 demonstrates a rather prominent left lobe of the liver, indicating some hepatomegaly.

Hepatomegaly is best evaluated on a liver-spleen scan. Unless we do volume determinations, hepatomegaly can be difficult to evaluate on ultrasound, but massively enlarged livers such as is present in figure 2.23 are easily demonstrated. Figure 2.23 is a longitudinal scan of the right lobe of the liver which extends caudal to the lower pole of the right kidney. There is even evidence of abdominal distention, as is demonstrated by the protuberance of the anterior abdominal wall (arrows).

The ultrasonic findings in cirrhotic changes of the liver are mainly those of severe attenuation to the sound. Figure 2.24 is an example of cirrhosis in which strong echoes are noted in the near field, with marked attenuation present more distally. The echoes arising from the liver are fairly even and small, but of high amplitude in the near field. We are barely able to penetrate the liver to visualize the lateral aspects of the spine and aorta. The marked attenuation of sound is felt to be secondary to fibrotic changes within the liver, but other causes of attenuation, such as fatty infiltration, may give an ultrasonic picture somewhat similar to cirrhosis.

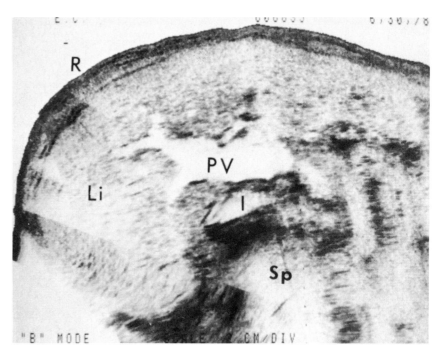

Fig. 2.21

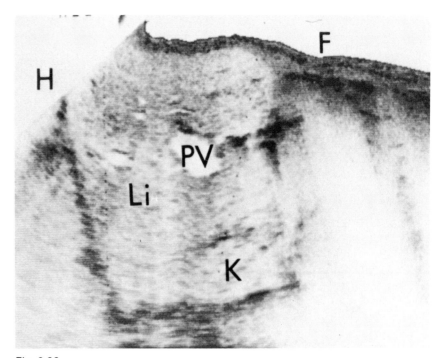

Fig. 2.22

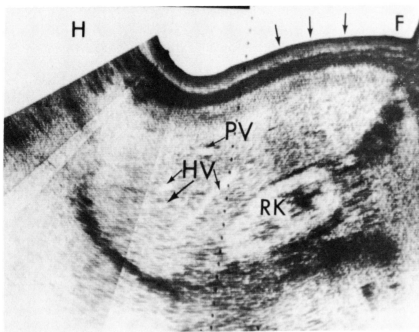

A	=	Aorta
Arrows	=	Protuberance of the anterior abdominal wall
F	=	Foot
H	=	Head
HV	=	Hepatic veins
I	=	Inferior vena cava
K	=	Kidney
L	=	Left
Li	=	Liver
PV	=	Portal vein
R	=	Right
RK	=	Right kidney
Sp	=	Spine

Fig. 2.23

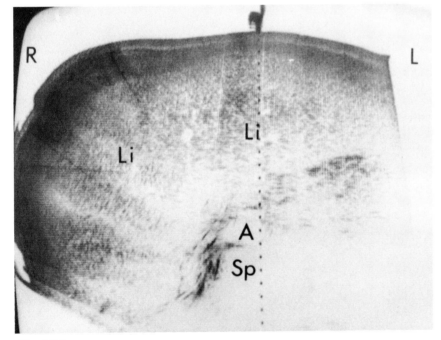

Fig. 2.24

Cirrhosis and Fatty Infiltration

Figure 2.25 is a longitudinal scan of a patient with ascites and marked cirrhotic changes of the liver. The capsule of the liver is seen adjacent to the ascites. The near echoes of the liver are quite dark. Penetration of sound through the liver, however, is extremely poor, as is indicated by the dramatic drop-off of echoes. This finding is compatible with marked fibrotic changes in a liver involved with cirrhosis. The severe attenuation of sound is evident in this case.

Fatty infiltration of the liver can demonstrate an ultrasonic appearance quite similar to cirrhotic changes. Figures 2.26–2.28 are of a patient who had fatty involvement of the liver. Figure 2.28 is a CT scan of the liver in which we see that the density of the liver is much less than the spleen secondary to fatty infiltration. The portal vein is seen within the liver as a much denser structure. Figures 2.26 and 2.27 are transverse and longitudinal ultrasound scans of the same patient. There is marked attenuation of sound by the liver due to the fatty infiltration. The transverse sections in figure 2.26 demonstrate poor visualization of the spine. The echoes arising from the spine are much weaker than we would usually expect. The longitudinal scan of the liver in figure 2.27 again demonstrates marked attenuation of sound by the fatty infiltration of the liver. The diaphragm (arrows) is barely seen because of this marked attenuation.

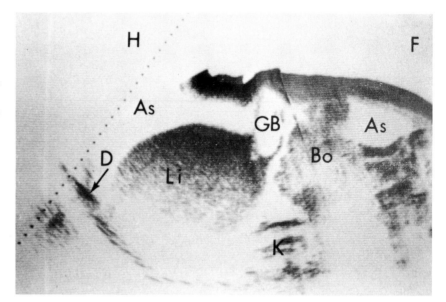

Fig. 2.25

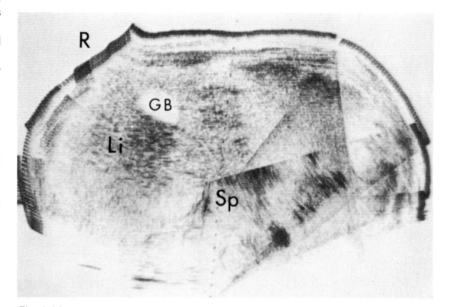

Fig. 2.26

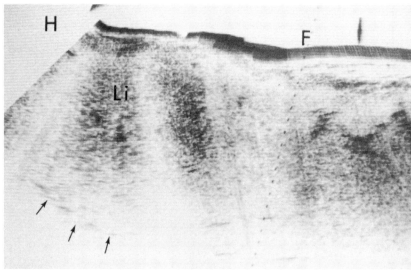

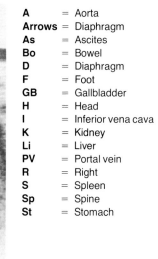

A	= Aorta
Arrows	= Diaphragm
As	= Ascites
Bo	= Bowel
D	= Diaphragm
F	= Foot
GB	= Gallbladder
H	= Head
I	= Inferior vena cava
K	= Kidney
Li	= Liver
PV	= Portal vein
R	= Right
S	= Spleen
Sp	= Spine
St	= Stomach

Fig. 2.27

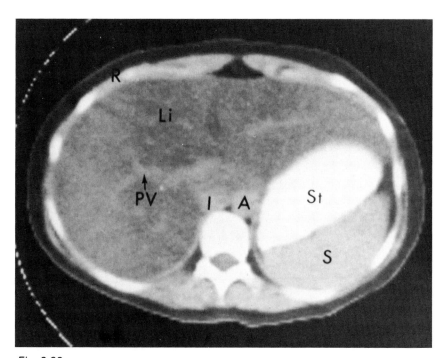

Fig. 2.28

Hypoechotic Liver Metastases

Metastatic lesions of the liver can present with a variety of ultrasonic patterns. The following examples demonstrate liver metastases that are decreased in echo amplitude compared to the rest of the liver. Figure 2.29 is a longitudinal scan of the lateral right lobe of the liver from a middle-aged woman with a known gastric carcinoma. A relatively sonolucent mass is seen within the liver. The borders are slightly irregular with no evidence of enhanced through transmission. Soft echoes are noted within the mass, indicating a solid rather than a fluid nature. The patient was placed on several months of chemotherapy; the liver metastasis, however, continued to enlarge. Figure 2.30 is the same patient approximately three months later. The liver metastasis has markedly enlarged. The borders have become more irregular, and numerous echoes are noted within. This is an example of a solitary hypoechotic liver metastasis that did not respond to chemotherapy.

Figure 2.31 is a longitudinal scan of the right lobe of the liver in a patient who had a transitional cell carcinoma of the urinary bladder. A filling defect on liver-spleen scan was noted near the dome of the liver on the right side. Ultrasound demonstrated a relatively sonolucent mass (arrows) with a slightly echogenic center. The patient underwent laparoscopy and liver biopsy. Frozen section revealed metastatic transitional cell carcinoma. This scan serves as an example of hypoechotic liver metastasis with some increased echogenicity centrally.

Figure 2.32 is a scan from a 39-year-old woman undergoing treatment for breast carcinoma. Isotopic liver scan showed numerous cold areas in both lobes. Percutaneous liver biopsy confirmed metastatic adenocarcinoma. The scan demonstrates multiple hypoechotic areas (arrows) throughout the liver. The normal liver echogenicity is of greater amplitude than the metastatic lesions.

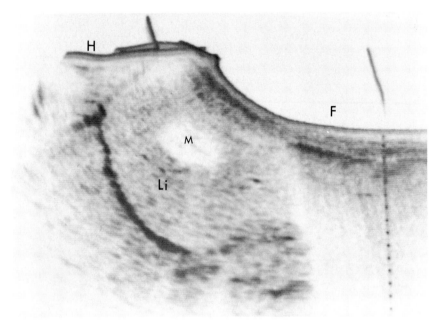

Fig. 2.29

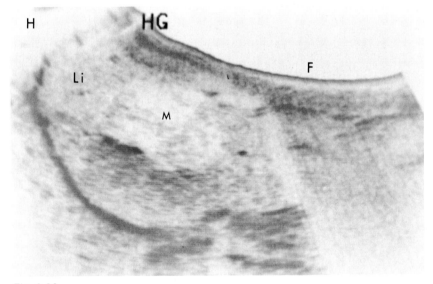

Fig. 2.30

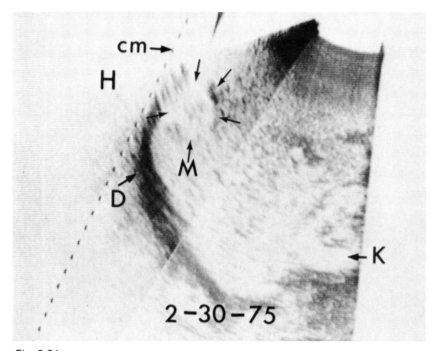

Fig. 2.31

SOURCE: Figures 2.29, 2.30, and 2.32 are provided through the courtesy of Dr. B. Green and Dr. H. Goldstein, M.D. Anderson Hospital, Texas Medical Center, Houston, Texas.

Arrows = Metastatic lesions
cm = Centimeter markers
D = Diaphragm
F = Foot
H = Head
K = Kidney
Li = Liver
Me = Metastases

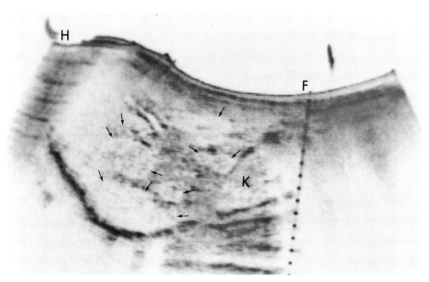

Fig. 2.32

Echogenic Liver Metastasis

Figure 2.33 is a longitudinal scan of the right lobe of the liver in a 58-year-old woman with colonic carcinoma. The scan demonstrates a highly echogenic area in the posterior aspect of the right lobe (arrows) which indicates a single metastatic lesion from the colon. Colonic metastases are often highly echogenic lesions. This may be secondary to their increased vascularity or mucinous nature. Tumors usually do not yield a characteristic echo pattern within the liver. However, colonic tumors often are highly echogenic. The patient was placed on combined chemotherapy; the metastatic disease, however, progressed. Figure 2.34 is a longitudinal scan of the right lobe of the liver four months later. Multiple echogenic masses are present throughout the liver (arrows). They are quite varied in size and echogenicity.

Figure 2.35 is a transverse scan of another patient's liver which demonstrates a large, well circumscribed echogenic mass lateral to the portal vein. This patient also had a carcinoma of the transverse colon. As noted, the echo amplitude of the metastatic lesion is much greater than that of the surrounding normal liver parenchyma. Figure 2.36 is a longitudinal scan of the right lobe of the liver of a 72-year-old woman with known carcinoma of the cecum. She had abnormal liver function studies and a markedly abnormal liver-spleen scan. Liver biopsy confirmed metastatic adenocarcinoma. The scan demonstrates multiple highly echogenic lesions (arrows) within the normal, less echogenic, liver parenchyma. We can see the varying sizes of the liver tumors. They are of a much higher amplitude than the surrounding liver parenchyma. All of these cases are examples of echogenic liver metastasis arising from the colon.

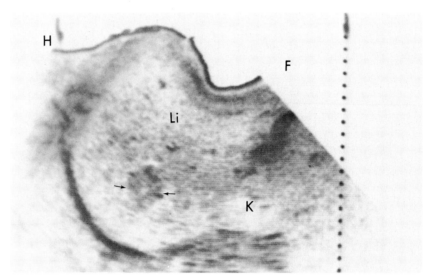

Fig. 2.33

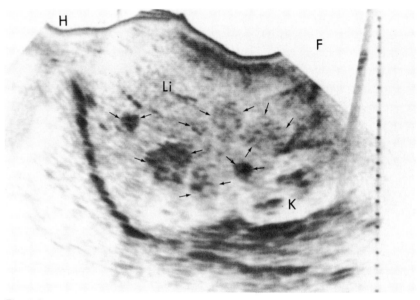

Fig. 2.34

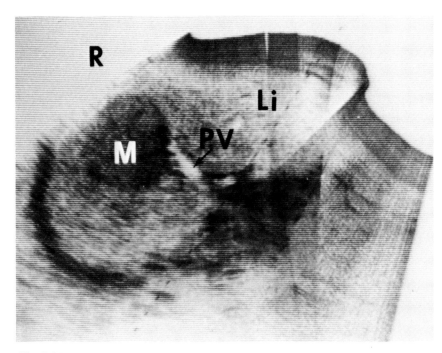

Fig. 2.35

SOURCE: The cases in figures 2.33, 2.34, and 2.36 are provided through the courtesy of Dr. B. Green and Dr. H. Goldstein, M. D. Anderson Hospital, Texas Medical Center, Houston, Texas.

Arrows = Echogenic liver metastasis
F   = Foot
H   = Head
K   = Kidney
Li   = Liver
M   = Echogenic mass
PV   = Portal vein
R   = Right

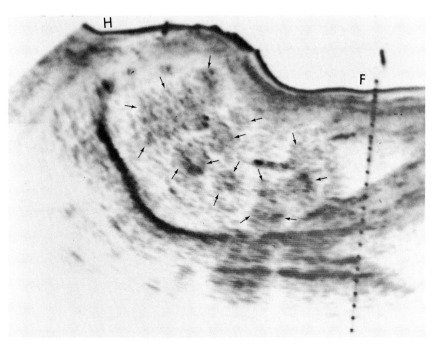

Fig. 2.36

Various Liver Metastases

Figure 2.37 is a longitudinal scan obtained from a 43-year-old woman with metastatic melanoma. A previous liver ultrasound was found to be normal. The present examination demonstrates multiple small echogenic masses within the liver parenchyma (arrows). These range from 0.5 to 1.0 cm in size. The remainder of the liver has a fairly even echogenicity, except for the strong echogenic metastasis.

Figure 2.38 is a transverse scan obtained from a 59-year-old woman with adenocarcinoma of the transverse colon. A prominent focal lesion with a bull's-eye configuration (arrows) is present on this section. There is a hypoechotic periphery with an echogenic area more central and finally, a hypoechotic area in the center of the lesion. The central decreased echogenicity may be secondary to necrosis or decreased vascularity. The increased echogenic areas are most likely secondary to hypervascular regions of the tumor.

Figure 2.39 is a longitudinal scan obtained from a 70-year-old woman with carcinoma of the breast. This scan demonstrates a large metastatic lesion (arrows) of the inferior aspect of the right lobe of the liver. The echo amplitude of the metastatic lesion is not that markedly different from the remainder of the liver. A slight hypoechotic rim, however, demonstrates a separation between the metastatic lesion and the liver. If it were not for this hypoechotic rim, the mass would be quite difficult to distinguish from the surrounding liver parenchyma. To identify liver metastasis, it is necessary to detect either a difference in echogenicity from the surrounding liver parenchyma or a capsular echo which will separate it from the remainder of the liver.

Figure 2.40 is a longitudinal scan obtained from a 53-year-old man with poorly differentiated carcinoma of the left superior pulmonary sulcus. A large liver metastasis is present involving only the caudate lobe (arrows). Again the echo amplitude from the metastatic lesion is approximately the same as the normal liver situated anteriorly. The

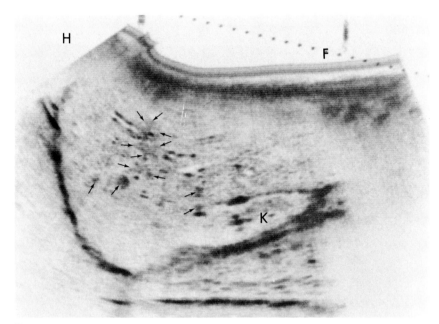

Fig. 2.37

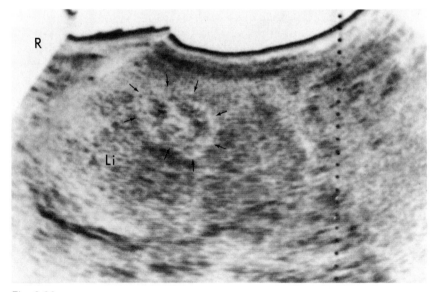

Fig. 2.38

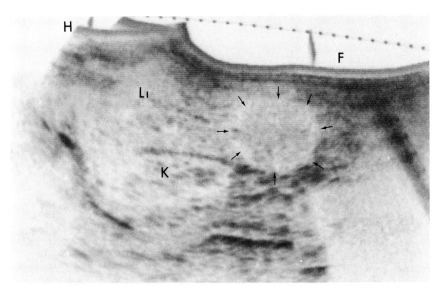

Fig. 2.39

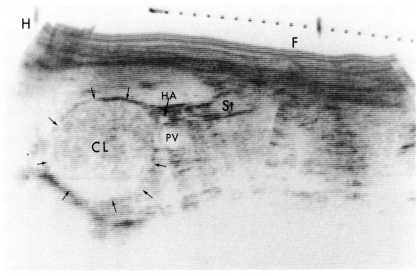

Fig. 2.40

echoes arising from the metastatic lesion are somewhat coarser than those from the normal liver and are markedly enlarging the caudate lobe, which led to the diagnosis.

Source: The cases for Figures 2.37–2.40 are provided through the courtesy of Dr. B. Green and Dr. H. Goldstein, M. D. Anderson Hospital, Texas Medical Center, Houston, Texas.

Arrows	=	Metastatic lesions
CL	=	Caudate lobe
F	=	Foot
H	=	Head
HA	=	Hepatic artery
K	=	Kidney
Li	=	Liver
PV	=	Portal vein
R	=	Right
St	=	Stomach

Necrotic Liver Metastases

The case shown in figures 2.41–2.44 is of a 66-year-old man with proven rectal carcinoid tumor metastatic to the lungs and liver. The initial ultrasound was performed after several courses of combination chemotherapy. The metastatic lesions of the liver are noted to be in various stages of necrosis. Figure 2.41 is a transverse scan over the upper liver demonstrating a highly echogenic metastasis (arrows) in the posterior aspect of the left lobe. Fluid-filled necrotic metastases are noted in the right lobe.

Figure 2.42 is a longitudinal scan through the lateral aspect of the right lobe demonstrating numerous fluid-filled masses which are secondary to necrosis within the tumors. Notice the two larger sonolucent masses have markedly irregular and ratty-appearing borders. Figure 2.43 is a longitudinal scan near the midline through the main portion of the large echogenic metastasis (arrows). Figure 2.44 is a longitudinal scan, through the left lobe of the liver, which demonstrates echogenic metastases. Necrotic areas are also noted within the echogenic metastases on the inferior aspect of the left lobe of the liver. An unusual finding of a fluid-fluid level is present in one of the metastatic lesions noted on the inferior aspect of the left lobe of the liver.

This case is an unusual manifestation of liver metastases in which marked necrotic changes are present. Necrosis has brought about liquefaction of the tumor in which fluid is noted in the central portion of many of these metastatic lesions. The irregular borders rule out a simple cyst. The fluid structures could possibly indicate abscess or hematomas. In light of the echogenic metastatic lesions, however, they are consistent with necrosis of the central portion of the tumor.

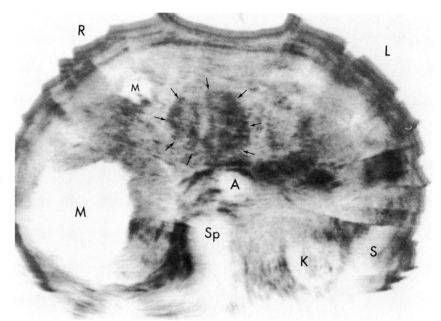

Fig. 2.41

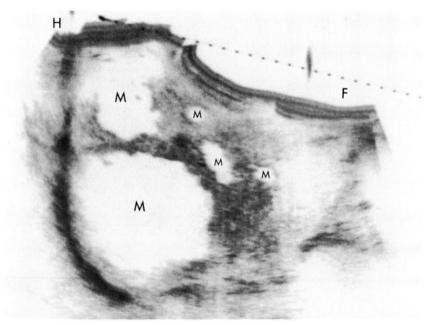

Fig. 2.42

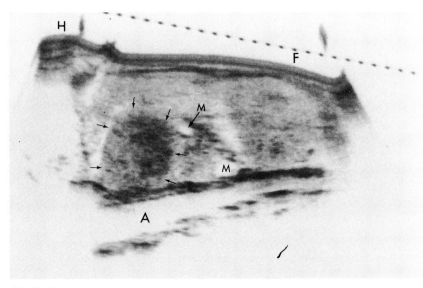

SOURCE: Figures 2.41–2.44 are provided
through the courtesy of Dr. B. Green and
Dr. H. Goldstein, M. D. Anderson Hospital,
Texas Medical Center, Houston, Texas.

A	=	Aorta
Arrows	=	Echogenic metastases
F	=	Foot
FF	=	Fluid-fluid layer
H	=	Head
K	=	Kidney
L	=	Left
M	=	Necrotic metastasis
R	=	Right
S	=	Spleen
Sp	=	Spine

Fig. 2.43

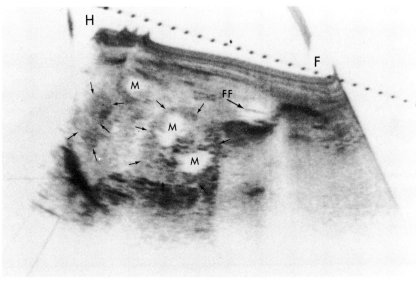

Fig. 2.44

Unusual Liver Metastases

Figures 2.45 and 2.46 are scans obtained from a 24-year-old man with embryonal cell carcinoma of the testes. The initial scan in figure 2.45 demonstrated a large necrotic metastasis involving most of the right lobe of the liver. The borders are irregular and ratty in appearance. The size of the mass involves most of the right lobe. The patient was placed on combined chemotherapy over several months' duration.

Figure 2.46 is a longitudinal scan of the right lobe of the liver several months after the scan in figure 2.45. The entire right lobe of the liver is now filled in with normal liver parenchyma. There is no evidence of the large fluid-filled necrotic mass which was noted earlier. Repeat biopsy of the liver showed no evidence of residual tumor. This was a remarkable disappearance of a large necrotic tumor following chemotherapy.

Figure 2.47 is a transverse section of the liver from a 53-year-old woman with leiomyosarcoma resected from the small intestine eight years previously. An isotopic scan of the liver was positive, and biopsy confirmed metastatic disease. This scan demonstrates a fluid-filled mass in the left lobe of the liver. A horizontal line represents a fluid-filled layer within the mass. A longitudinal scan in figure 2.48 demonstrates two mass lesions which are fluid filled.

The fluid-fluid layer is again noted in the larger mass. This layer most likely represents debris within the tumor which is layering out in the fluid.

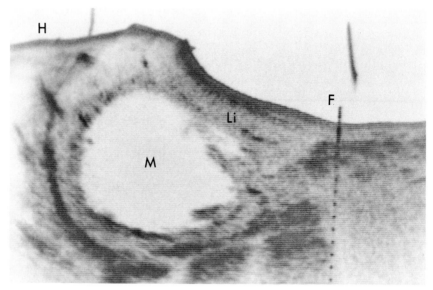

Fig. 2.45

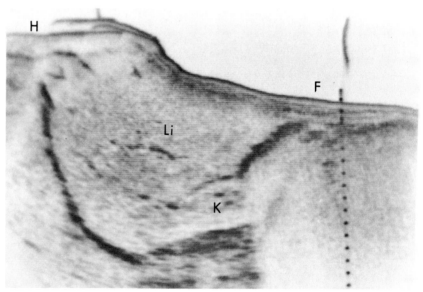

Fig. 2.46

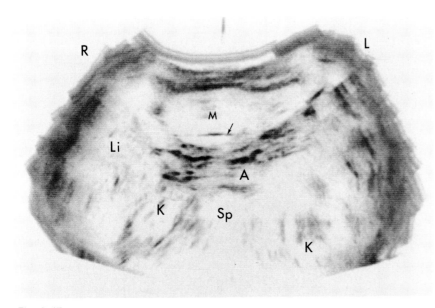

Fig. 2.47

SOURCE: The cases for figures 2.45–2.48 are provided through the courtesy of Dr. B. Green and Dr. H. Goldstein, M. D. Anderson Hospital, Texas Medical Center, Houston, Texas.

A	=	Aorta
Arrows	=	Fluid-fluid layer
F	=	Foot
H	=	Head
K	=	Kidney
L	=	Left
Li	=	Liver
Me	=	Necrotic metastases
R	=	Right
SA	=	Splenic artery
SMV	=	Superior mesenteric vein
Sp	=	Spine

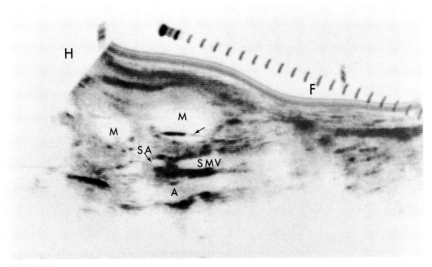

Fig. 2.48

Metastatic Disease of the Liver with Diffuse Abnormality

Often liver involvement is difficult to detect ultrasonically because of the diffuse nature of metastatic disease. The liver parenchymagram does not have its even texture. Instead disruption and disorganization of the liver parenchyma are apparent with ultrasound, and although no discreet lesion can be detected, this disorganization is evident in the liver echoes.

Figure 2.49 is a longitudinal scan of the right lobe of the liver obtained from a 65-year-old woman with metastatic melanoma. The right lobe of the liver is markedly enlarged. The echo pattern arising from the liver demonstrates diffuse distortion of the usual normal architecture. Although no discreet lesions are easily visualized, destruction of the normal parenchymal echo pattern is evident.

Figure 2.50 is a longitudinal scan of the right lobe of the liver obtained from a 56-year-old woman with metastatic colonic carcinoma. Ultrasound demonstrates a lack of normal homogeneous hepatic pattern, indicating diffuse metastatic disease. Increased echoes are noted posteriorly within the liver and are disorganized in nature. However, the anterior, less echogenic half of the liver also appears disrupted.

Figure 2.51 is a longitudinal scan of the liver obtained from a 65-year-old woman with metastatic sigmoid colon carcinoma. Again, diffuse extensive disruption of the ultrasonic parenchymal pattern is present with no discreet lesions noted.

Figure 2.52 is a longitudinal scan of the right lobe of the liver obtained from a 66-year-old man with metastatic melanoma. The scan demonstrates a subtle inhomogeneous echo architecture of the posterior half of the liver. The anterior half of the liver appears to have a fairly even echo pattern that is characteristic of normal liver. The area in the posterior half of the liver (arrows), however, is less echogenic and much coarser in appearance, an indication of diffuse involvement with the liver in this section.

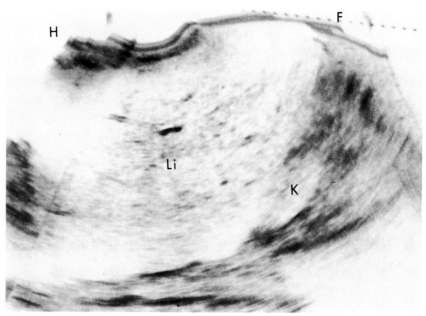

Fig. 2.49

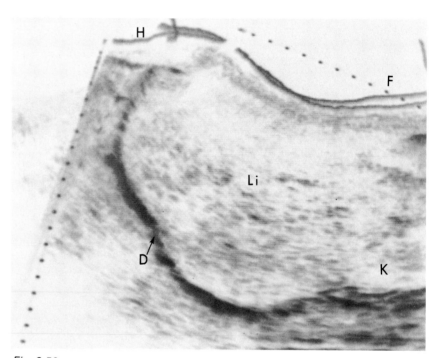

Fig. 2.50

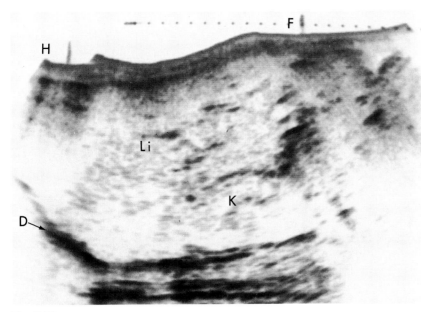

Fig. 2.51

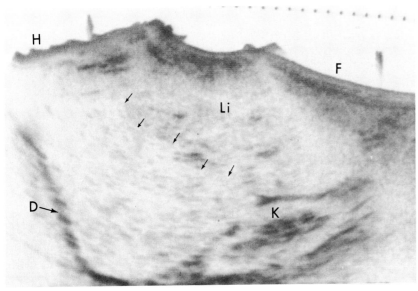

Fig. 2.52

This is a good example of a comparison of the normal, soft, even echo pattern of the liver with the diffuse, irregular echogenicity of metastatic disease.

SOURCE: The cases for figures 2.49–2.52 are provided through the courtesy of Dr. B. Green and Dr. H. Goldstein, M. D. Anderson Hospital, Texas Medical Center, Houston, Texas.

Arrows = Demarcation between normal and abnormal liver
D = Diaphragm
F = Foot
H = Head
K = Kidney
Li = Liver

Calcification of Liver Metastasis

Liver metastasis can occasionally calcify and lead to characteristic ultrasonic findings. Figure 2.53 is a longitudinal scan obtained from a 56-year-old woman with metastatic colonic carcinoma. Two highly echogenic areas are noted within the inferior posterior portion of the liver. Shadows are noted behind the strong echoes. Figure 2.54 is an X-ray of the right-upper quadrant demonstrating the calcifications within the liver arising from the metastatic colonic lesions.

Figure 2.55 is a transverse scan obtained from a 60-year-old woman with colon carcinoma known to be metastatic to the liver. The scan in figure 2.55 demonstrates a highly echogenic region (arrows) in the lateral posterior aspect of the right lobe of the liver. The left lobe of the liver has a fairly even echo pattern to it. Figure 2.56 is a longitudinal scan of the same patient. Again, a high-amplitude echogenic region (arrows) is noted in the anterior aspect of the right lobe of the liver. Quite evident behind these strong echoes is an acoustic shadow arising from the calcified metastatic lesions.

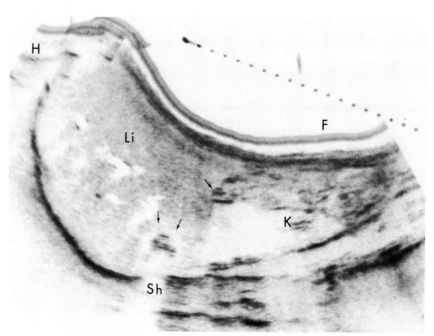

Fig. 2.53

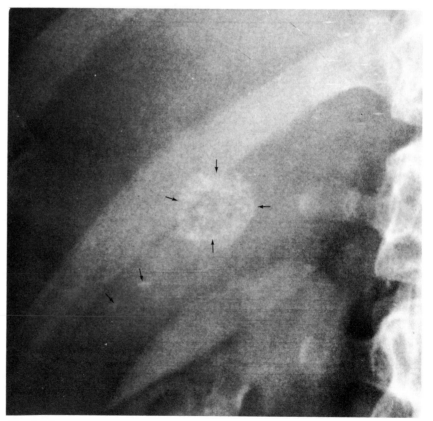

Fig. 2.54

SOURCE: The cases for Figures 2.53–2.56 are presented through the courtesy of Dr. B. Green and Dr. H. Goldstein, M. D. Anderson Hospital, Texas Medical Center, Houston, Texas.

A	=	Aorta
Arrows	=	Highly echogenic metastatic regions and calcified regions
F	=	Foot
GB	=	Gallbladder
H	=	Head
K	=	Kidney
L	=	Left
Li	=	Liver
R	=	Right
Sh	=	Shadowing
Sp	=	Spine

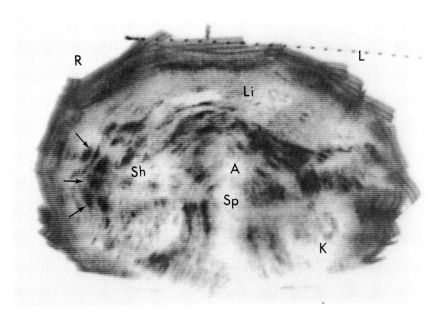

Fig. 2.55

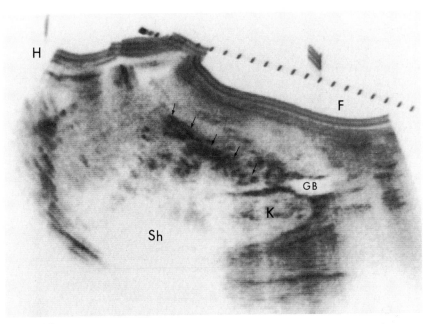

Fig. 2.56

Involvement of the Liver with Lymphoma

This 40-year-old man had a long history of lymphocytic lymphoma with spread to the neck, oropharynx, lungs, and liver. Figure 2.57 is a transverse scan of the liver in which a relatively sonolucent mass is noted within the left lobe. There are internal echoes within it, indicating a solid structure. A CT scan demonstrates a decreased density (arrows) in figure 2.58; this corresponds to the site of lymphomatous involvement.

Figure 2.59 is a longitudinal scan of the right lobe of the liver obtained from a 22-year-old man with progressive Hodgkin's disease. A 15-cm hypoechotic mass (arrows) is seen to occupy much of the right lobe of the liver. Soft echoes are present within the mass. They are somewhat disorganized when compared with a normal liver parenchymagram.

Figure 2.60 is a longitudinal scan of the right lobe of the liver obtained from a 54-year-old woman with non-Hodgkin's lymphoma. In this case, a large echogenic nodule (arrows) is present in the right lobe of the liver. The other two cases demonstrated hypoechotic masses when lymphoma involved the liver. This case is somewhat unusual in that the mass is extremely echogenic. Lymph node involvement around the periaortic region is usually sonolucent. Lymphoma of the liver tends generally to be hypoechotic. The case in figure 2.60 is an unusual example of an echogenic lesion.

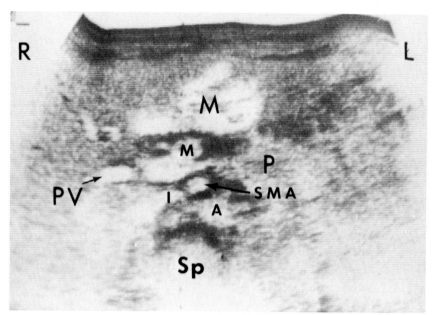

Fig. 2.57

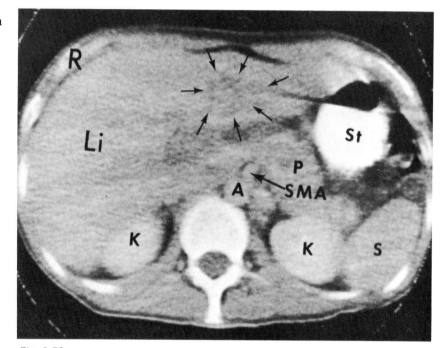

Fig. 2.58

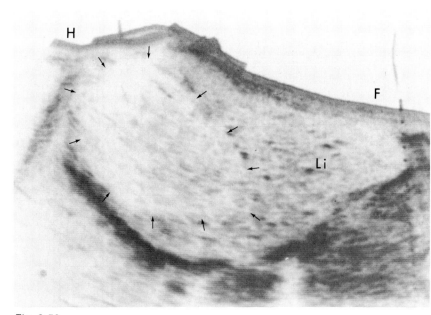

Fig. 2.59

SOURCE: The cases for figures 2.59 and 2.60 are provided through the courtesy of Dr. B. Green and Dr. H. Goldstein, M. D. Anderson Hospital, Texas Medical Center, Houston, Texas.

A	=	Aorta
Arrows	=	Lymphoma involvement of the liver
F	=	Foot
H	=	Head
I	=	Inferior vena cava
K	=	Kidney
L	=	Left
Li	=	Liver
M	=	Mass
P	=	Pancreas
PV	=	Portal vein
R	=	Right
S	=	Spleen
SMA	=	Superior mesenteric artery
Sp	=	Spine
St	=	Stomach

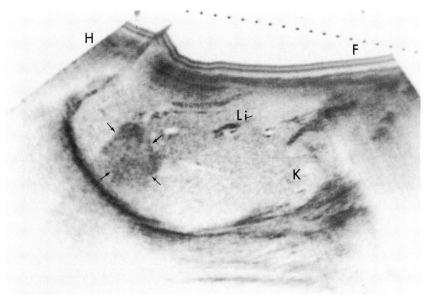

Fig. 2.60

Hepatoma

The case in figures 2.61 and 2.62 is a 36-year-old man with a long history of heavy ethanol abuse. Approximately three months prior to admission, he noted the onset of nausea, vomiting, and sharp abdominal pain. While in the hospital, a liver isotope study demonstrated a large filling defect in the right lobe of the liver. Figure 2.61 is a transverse scan of the upper abdomen in which we see a large echogenic mass (arrows) in the posterior aspect of the right lobe of the liver. The portal vein is displaced anteriorly. Figure 2.62 is a longitudinal scan of the entire abdomen. The echogenic mass is seen in the superior aspect of the right lobe of the liver. Also noted on this scan is fluid in the pelvis secondary to ascites. The high echogenicity of this mass suggests a vascular lesion. Angiography determined that this was true. The patient had a diagnosis of hepatoma.

The case in figures 2.63 and 2.64 is a 60-year-old man with multifocal hepatoma involving both lobes of the liver. The isotope study (fig. 2.63) shows diffuse irregular uptake throughout the liver. Ultrasound examination indicated marked irregular echogenicity to the liver, which is evident in figure 2.64. Normal liver echoes are noted anteriorly only in a small portion. The posterior aspect of the liver demonstrates somewhat increased echogenicity along with an irregular, coarser pattern than is seen in a normal liver. This patient's liver had diffuse involvement with multifocal hepatoma.

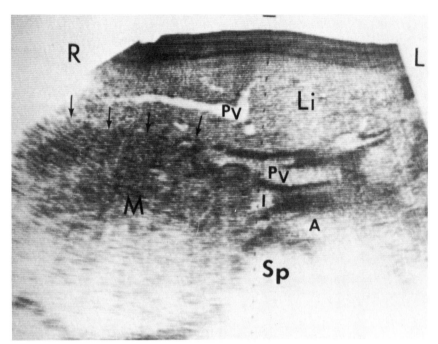

Fig. 2.61

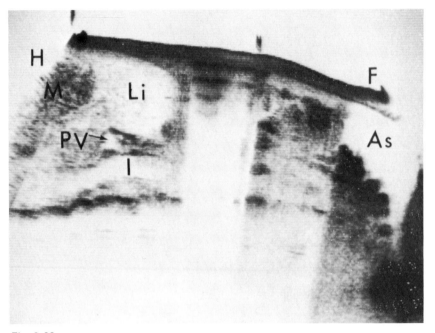

Fig. 2.62

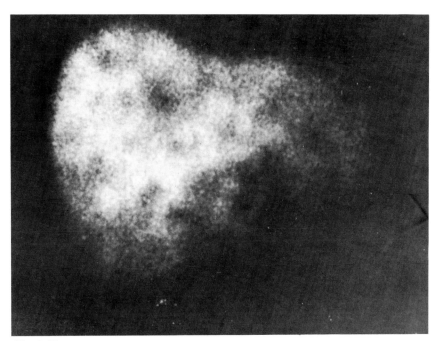

SOURCE: The case for figures 2.63 and 2.64 is provided through the courtesy of Dr. B. Green and Dr. H. Goldstein, M. D. Anderson Hospital, Texas Medical Center, Houston, Texas.

A	=	Aorta
Arrows	=	Hepatoma
As	=	Ascites
F	=	Foot
H	=	Head
I	=	Inferior vena cava
K	=	Kidney
L	=	Left
Li	=	Liver
M	=	Hepatoma
PV	=	Portal vein
R	=	Right
Sp	=	Spine

Fig. 2.63

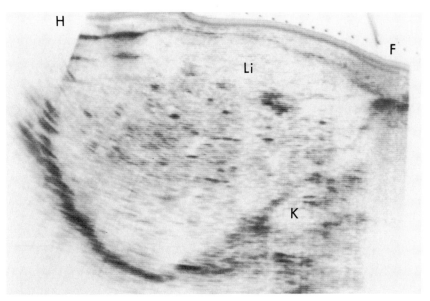

Fig. 2.64

Hepatoblastoma and Cavernous Hemangioma

The case for figures 2.65 and 2.66 is of a two-year-old boy with proven hepatoblastoma of the liver. Figure 2.65 is a transverse section of the liver in which we can see a highly echogenic mass (arrows) in the central portion of the liver. The mass is much more echogenic than the surrounding normal liver. Increased echogenicity within the liver, or within any other mass, is often highly suggestive of a vascular lesion. Figure 2.66 is an angiogram of the liver lesion in which marked increased vascularity throughout most of the right and left lobe can be seen. The angiogram corresponds accurately with the increased echogenic area noted on ultrasound.

Figures 2.67 and 2.68 are obtained from a 58-year-old man. Physical examination demonstrated a large right lobe of the liver. Isotope liver scan indicated a large filling defect within the liver. Figure 2.67 is a transverse scan of the liver with an echogenic area (arrows) within the right lobe. Again, the echoes arising from this mass are of a higher amplitude than the normal surrounding liver, which suggests a vascular lesion. Figure 2.68 is a hepatic artery angiogram that demonstrates pooling of contrast material at many sites within the tumor. At surgery this was found to be a cavernous hemangioma. The increased vascularity is manifested by increased echogenicity on ultrasound.

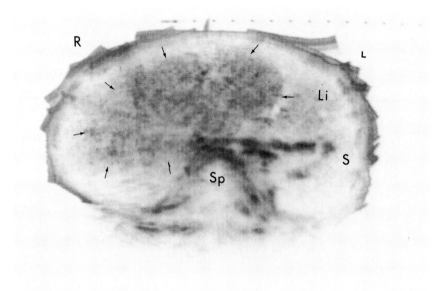

Fig. 2.65

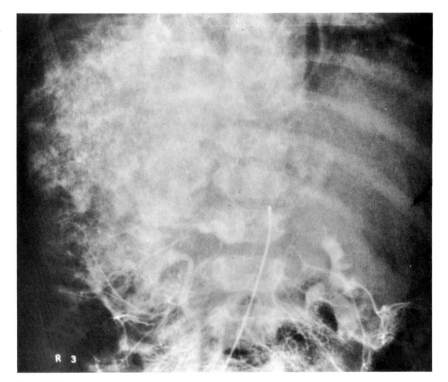

Fig. 2.66

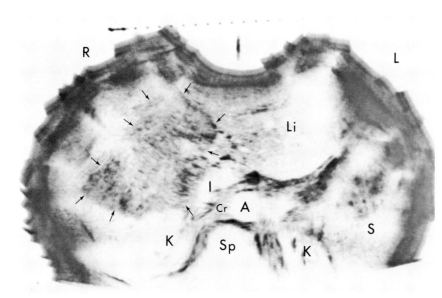

Fig. 2.67

SOURCE: The cases in figures 2.65–2.68 are provided through the courtesy of Dr. B. Green and Dr. H. Goldstein, M. D. Anderson Hospital, Texas Medical Center, Houston, Texas.

A	=	Aorta
Arrows	=	Echogenic mass
Cr	=	Crus of the diaphragm
I	=	Inferior vena cava
K	=	Kidney
L	=	Left
Li	=	Liver
R	=	Right
S	=	Spleen
Sp	=	Spine

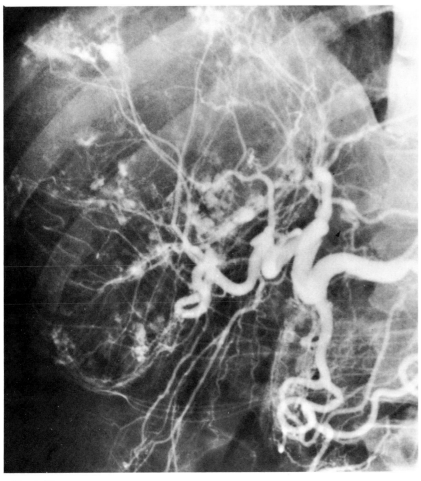

Fig. 2.68

False Liver Masses ; Polycystic Liver Disease

Occasionally, ultrasound examination of the liver will yield an area of decreased echogenicity secondary to technical factors. Figure 2.69 is an example of a false liver mass in the anterior lateral aspect of the right lobe of the liver. This occurs quite commonly over the right costal margin. Since ultrasound cannot penetrate bone well, the area deep to the right costal margin will not echo normally. The anterior portion of the liver over the epigastric region can be filled in quite well since no ribs are present. The technologist can sector scan through the costal spaces laterally. This will often leave an area of decreased echogenicity just beneath the right costal margin that can simulate a hypoechotic liver mass. The sharpness of the borders, however, will be an important clue that this is a technical artifact. We can also scan underneath the costal margin with the patient in deep inspiration to rule out such a mass.

Figure 2.70 is an example of an area of decreased echogenicity within the liver secondary to attenuation from a midline scar from previous surgery. Since scar tissue has a large amount of fibrous tissue present, this will lead to marked attenuation of the sound beam. Therefore, the echoes arising deep to the scar tissue will appear less echogenic than those of the surrounding liver parenchyma. Figure 2.70 is an excellent example of a false liver mass in the left lobe of the liver that actually is a technical problem arising from attenuation posterior to scar tissue.

Frequently, an isotope liver scan will yield multiple filling defects within the liver that will be highly suspicious for diffuse metastatic disease. Ultrasound will, however, elicit a characteristic appearance of numerous sonolucent masses present diffusely throughout the liver. Figures 2.71 and 2.72 are of a patient with polycystic liver disease. The liver is markedly enlarged; this is best seen on the longitudinal scan in figure 2.72. Dispersed throughout the liver are numerous fluid-filled cysts filling nearly the entire liver parenchyma. This char-

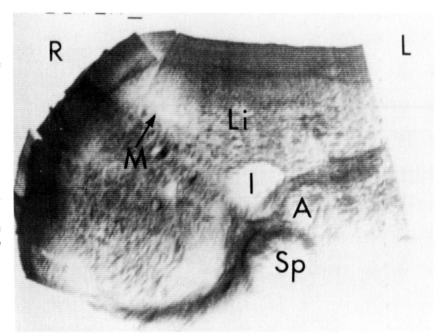

Fig. 2.69

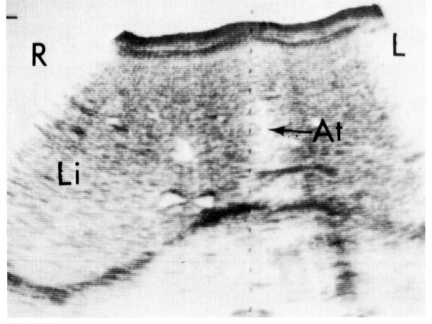

Fig. 2.70

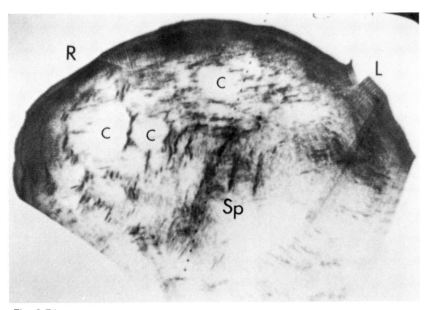

Fig. 2.71

acteristic echo pattern is fairly easy to diagnose by ultrasound because of the prominent sonolucencies caused by the liver cysts. When examining a patient with such a finding, it is also important to examine the kidneys and pancreas to see if these organs are involved with cystic disease.

A	=	Aorta
At	=	False mass due to scar attenuation
C	=	Cysts
H	=	Head
I	=	Inferior vena cava
L	=	Left
Li	=	Liver
M	=	False mass behind the right costal margin
R	=	Right
Sp	=	Spine
U	=	Umbilical level

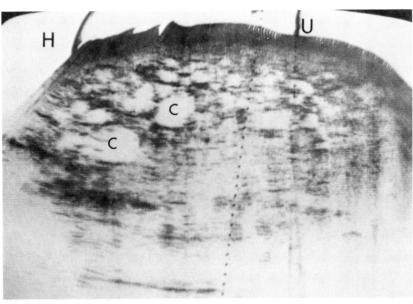

Fig. 2.72

Liver Cysts

The case in figures 2.73–2.75 is a 30-year-old woman referred for ultrasound examination because of an area of decreased uptake in the right lobe of the liver on isotopic scan. Ultrasound demonstrated a fluid-filled mass within the posterior aspect of the right lobe of the liver. Figure 2.73 is a transverse section showing the liver cyst to be echo-free except for one linear echo (arrow) on its medial aspect. Longitudinal scan of the same area demonstrated a fluid-filled mass with through transmission (fig. 2.74). The walls are fairly smooth except for the suggestion of a small septum on the superior aspect (arrow). A percutaneous needle puncture was performed, and contrast was instilled. Figure 2.75 demonstrates a liver cyst with some small septations (arrows) which correspond to the ultrasonic findings. The through transmission noted on the longitudinal scan in figure 2.74 is excellent confirmation of the fluid-filled nature of the mass.

Figure 2.76 is another ultrasound examination of a patient who had a filling defect on the isotope study. This longitudinal scan over the left lobe of the liver demonstrates a fluid-filled mass representing a liver cyst. Posterior to the liver cyst is increased through transmission, indicating the fluid-filled nature of the mass. This was somewhat difficult to obtain because of the high position beneath the costal margin. With angulation of the transducer head high underneath the costal margin, however, a scan through the cephalad portion of the liver and through the mass was possible. Liver cysts usually are smooth-walled, with fairly sharp borders and excellent through transmission. The cases of necrotic metastases presented earlier demonstrated much more ratty and irregular borders compared with these present examples of liver cysts.

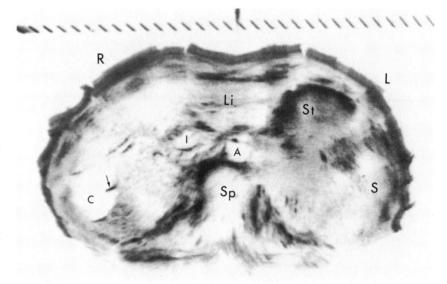

Fig. 2.73

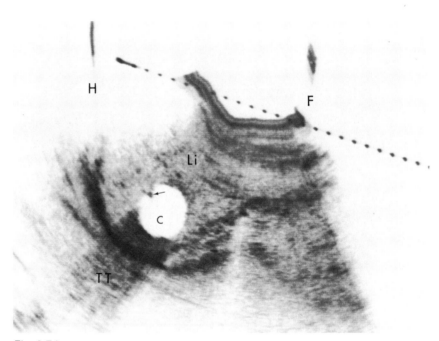

Fig. 2.74

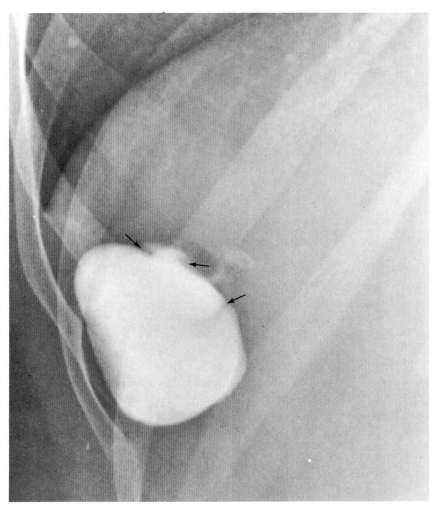

Fig. 2.75

SOURCE: The case in figures 2.73–2.75 is provided through the courtesy of Dr. B. Green and Dr. H. Goldstein, M. D. Anderson Hospital, Texas Medical Center, Houston, Texas.

A	=	Aorta
Arrows	=	Septations in the liver cysts
C	=	Cyst
CA	=	Celiac axis
F	=	Foot
H	=	Head
I	=	Inferior vena cava
L	=	Left
Li	=	Liver
p	=	Pancreas
R	=	Right
S	=	Spleen
S	=	Splenic artery
SMA	=	Superior mesenteric artery
SMV	=	Superior mesenteric vein
Sp	=	Spine
St	=	Stomach
TT	=	Through transmission

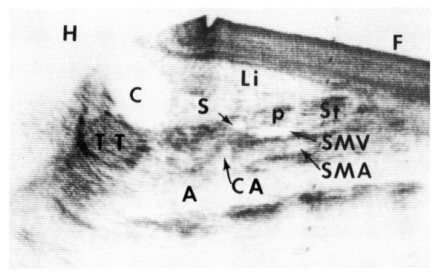

Fig. 2.76

Amebic and Sterile Abscesses

The ultrasonic findings in amebic abscesses can present as a spectrum. Very often the abscesses are relatively sonolucent with good through transmission. When debris is present, however, they can yield large masses with numerous soft internal echoes. Figures 2.77 and 2.78 are scans obtained on a 52-year-old Mexican-American man who had a three-week history of sore throat and steadily increasing right upper-quadrant pain. About one day prior to admission, the patient developed the onset of diarrhea with some blood-tinged stools. A liver-spleen scan demonstrated two large filling defects in the right lobe of the liver. Ultrasound examination demonstrated two large abscesses within the right lobe of the liver (figs. 2.77 and 2.78). Echoes are noted within the abscesses, especially the more anterior and medial one. The more posterior abscess was noted to be somewhat more lucent.

The patient was treated with metronidazole (Flagyl) and developed rapid improvement in his symptoms. Amebic serologies revealed an amebic fluorescent antibody which was markedly positive. This case demonstrates two amebic abscesses in the liver with slightly different echo appearances. The anterior abscess had more echoes within it, indicating debris.

The patient in figures 2.79 and 2.80 is a 36-year-old man working in Saudi Arabia, with a three-month history of weight loss, right upper-quadrant and pleuritic pain. He had developed fever and leukocytosis, along with pleural effusion, while in Saudi Arabia and had been treated with a course of antibiotics in that country. Further workup in the United States demonstrated a mass in the right lobe of the liver which was seen in ultrasound (figs. 2.79 and 2.80). The mass was relatively sonolucent with an echogenic center highly suggestive of an abscess. The patient was treated for a period of time with antibiotics. He eventually underwent surgery for drainage of the abscess. The abscess was found to be sterile, with all cultures re-

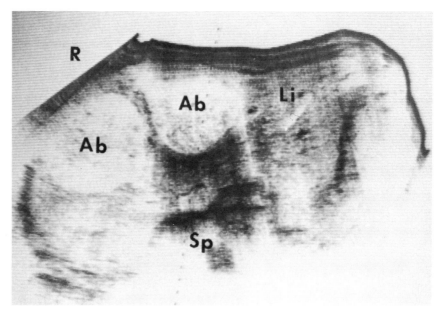

Fig. 2.77

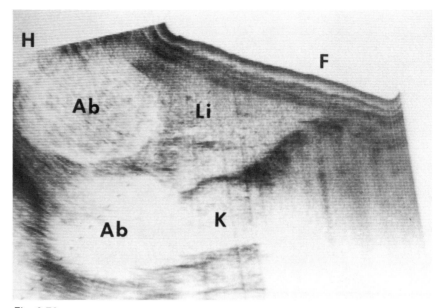

Fig. 2.78

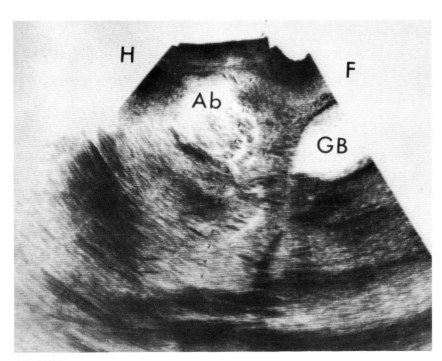

Fig. 2.79

maining negative. Biopsy of the abscess wall also was negative.

This is an example of a sterile abscess in which a large amount of debris was found. Figure 2.80 demonstrates shadowing on the lateral borders of the abscess wall similar to that seen in other circular sonolucent structures (see chapter 1).

Ab	=	Abscess
F	=	Foot
GB	=	Gallbladder
H	=	Head
K	=	Kidney
Li	=	Liver
PV	=	Portal vein
R	=	Right
Sh	=	Shadowing
Sp	=	Spine

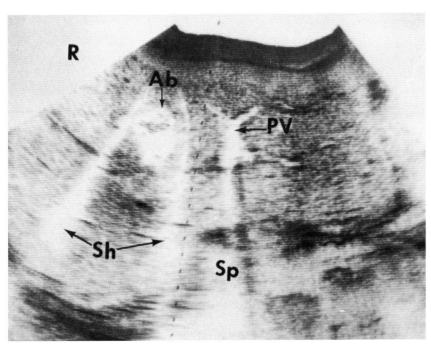

Fig. 2.80

Liver Abscess

The patient in figures 2.81 and 2.82 is a 72-year-old woman who had developed a fever of undetermined etiology. At hospitalization, a liver scan demonstrated a defect in the superior dome of the right lobe of the liver. Figure 2.81 is a longitudinal scan of the area corresponding to the defect on the liver scan. The ultrasound examination demonstrates a relatively sonolucent mass near the dome of the liver on the right side. Soft echoes are present within the mass, but it is mainly sonolucent. A pleural effusion is noted in the right pleural space. The patient had a history of chronic congestive heart failure. A portion of the base of the right lung (arrows) is also seen on the scan. The patient was treated with IV antibiotics over a three-week period, with marked clinical improvement and no further fever. An ultrasound examination performed at that time is seen in figure 2.82. The abscess has markedly decreased in size; soft echoes, however, are still present within the central portion. Fluid is still noted in the right pleural space.

Figures 2.83 and 2.84 are scans obtained from a 65-year-old woman with multiple medical problems including previous pulmonary emboli and cerebral vascular accident. She had developed an acute onset of mid epigastric pain which was knifelike and radiated toward the right flank. She developed a fever and signs of peritonitis and was taken to the operating room where a perforated jejunum in the proximal portion was found. On the seventh postoperative day, the patient had a persistent right pleural effusion along with fever spikes. The possibility of an abscess was considered. Because of this, an ultrasound examination was performed, and figures 2.83 and 2.84 represent longitudinal scans of the right lobe of the liver. There is evidence of a relatively sonolucent mass representing an abscess in the liver and subdiaphragmatic region. The borders are slightly irregular, and soft echoes are noted within. A pleural effusion is also seen above the right hemidiaphragm. The patient underwent a repeat operation, and a subdiaphragmatic

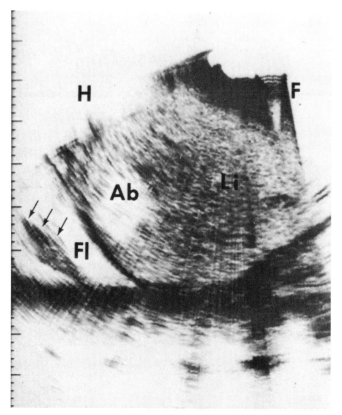

Fig. 2.81

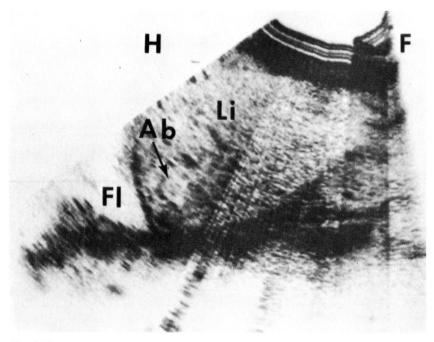

Fig. 2.82

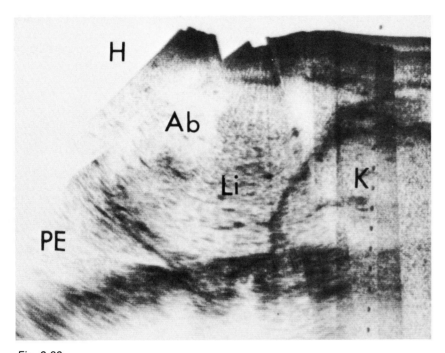

Fig. 2.83

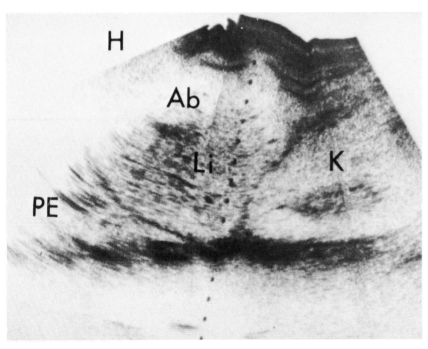

Fig. 2.84

and intrahepatic abscess was confirmed.

Ab   = Abscess
Arrows = Inferior portion of the collapsed
             right lung
F   = Foot
Fl   = Pleural fluid
H   = Head
K   = Kidney
Li   = Liver
PE   = Pleural effusion

Hepatic Hematoma

Figures 2.85 and 2.86 are transverse scans of a patient with sickle cell anemia and multiple complications. He was admitted for a progressive rise in serum bilirubin. An ultrasound study was initially performed to rule out an obstructive cause for his jaundice. Figure 2.85 is a transverse scan obtained at that time which did not show any evidence of a dilated biliary tree within the liver, although we did see prominent portal venous structures at the time. The patient underwent a transhepatic cholangiogram, which was followed by a drop in hematocrit. He was felt to have sustained a liver laceration, and a repeat ultrasound examination was performed.

Figure 2.86 demonstrates a transverse scan from the follow-up study. We now see a relatively sonolucent mass on the lateral aspect of the right lobe of the liver which represents a liver hematoma. Soft echoes are noted within the hematoma. There is also peritoneal fluid, indicative of an extrahepatic bleed. The liver echoes posterior to the hematoma are increased, indicating some through transmission. These findings are an example of an intrahepatic and extrahepatic bleed diagnosed by ultrasound.

Figures 2.87 and 2.88 are of a 22-year-old woman with uterine choriocarcinoma which was found to be metastatic to the liver. The liver tumor underwent spontaneous hemorrhage with the development of a subcapsular hematoma. Figure 2.87 is a transverse scan of the liver in which we see the hematoma involving the lateral posterior aspect of the right lobe. The normal liver parenchymagram is present in the left lobe. The echoes of the medial aspect of the right lobe are increased noticeably. This may be due to two factors. First of all, there is most likely through transmission through the hematoma, increasing the echogenicity of the liver. Secondly, tissue compression of the liver parenchyma may be present, yielding compressed echogenicity.

Figure 2.88 is from a selective hepatic arteriogram which demonstrates gross hepatomegaly along with numerous hypervascular tumor nodules scattered

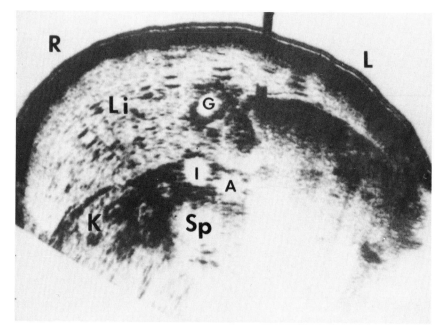

Fig. 2.85

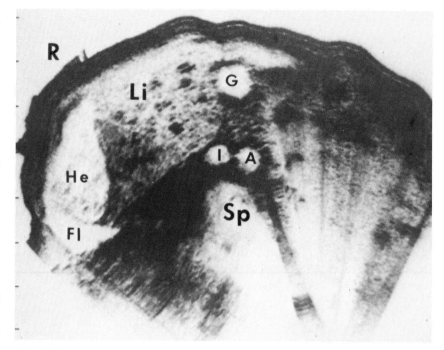

Fig. 2.86

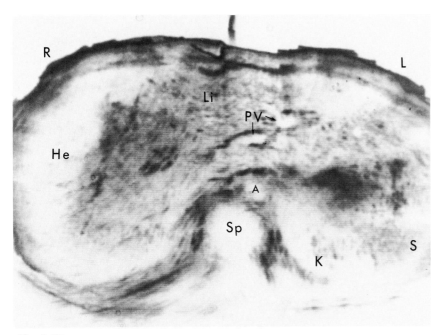

Fig. 2.87

throughout the liver. The parenchymal blush is deviated to the left side by a totally avascular area in the right lateral abdomen representing the site of the hematoma.

SOURCE: The case in figures 2.87 and 2.88 is provided through the courtesy of Dr. B. Green and Dr. H. Goldstein, M. D. Anderson Hospital, Texas Medical Center, Houston, Texas.

A	=	Aorta
Arrows	=	Medial border of the hematoma
Fl	=	Fluid
G	=	Gallbladder
He	=	Hematoma
I	=	Inferior vena cava
K	=	Kidney
L	=	Left
Li	=	Liver
PV	=	Portal vein
R	=	Right
S	=	Spleen
Sp	=	Spine

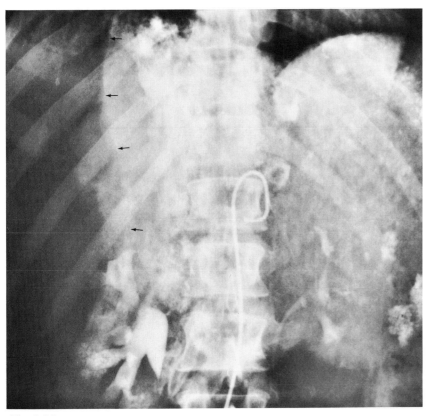

Fig. 2.88

Echinococcal Cysts

The following case is an excellent example of the different manifestations of an echinococcai cyst. Figures 2.89–2.92 are from the same patient, a three-year-old male child. An echinococcal cyst was diagnosed one year previously, with removal of a cyst from the right lung. Three weeks prior to admission, he developed high temperature associated with abdominal pain. There was no vomiting or diarrhea. Ultrasound examination demonstrated a fluid-filled mass in the anterior portion of the left lobe of the liver (figs. 2.89 and 2.91). Through transmission is present posterior to the fluid on the images. Also noted during the course of examination was a highly echogenic region in the posterior aspect of the right lobe of the liver (figs. 2.90 and 2.92). This was secondary to a calcified inactive echinococcal cyst from the previous episode.

Chest X-rays demonstrated a lesion in the right lobe of the lung which was well circumscribed, circular, and consistent with an echinococcal cyst of the lung. The patient was taken to the operating room where a right lobectomy of the lung was performed, along with a removal of the left lobe of the liver. The findings were consistent with echinococcal cysts of both lung and liver.

This case demonstrates the ultrasonic findings of an echinococcal cyst in different stages of activity. The left lobe cyst represents a fluid-filled mass with through transmission and fairly sharp borders. This would be difficult to distinguish from a simple liver cyst. The lesion in the posterior aspect of the right lobe represented calcification within an inactive echinococcal cyst from a previous infection. Abdominal films at the time of admission demonstrated calcification in the right upper quadrant that corresponded to the lesion in the liver.

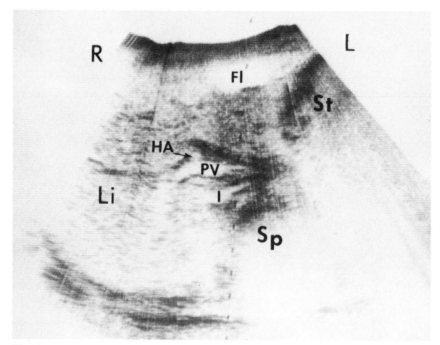

Fig. 2.89

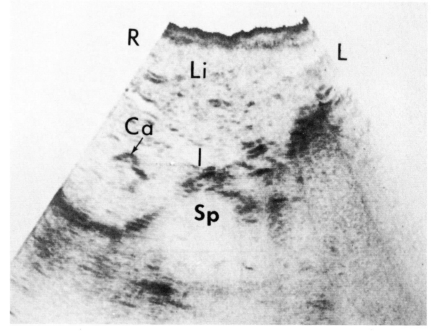

Fig. 2.90

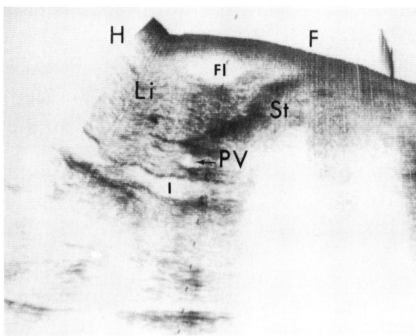

Fig. 2.91

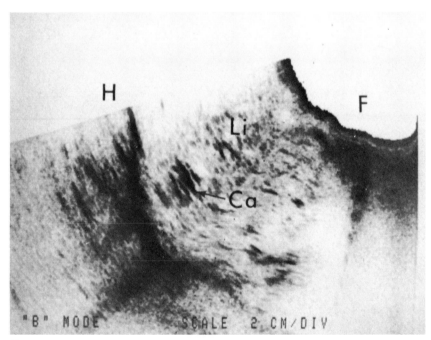

Fig. 2.92

Ca = Calcified echinococcal cyst
F = Foot
Fl = Echinococcal cyst with fluid
H = Head
HA = Hepatic artery
I = Inferior vena cava
L = Left
Li = Liver
PV = Portal vein
R = Right
Sp = Spine
St = Stomach

Echinococcal Cyst

The patient in figures 2.93–2.95 had a left lower lung echinococcal cyst removed 17 years prior to the present admission. She had done well until approximately one month prior to admission when she began experiencing right shoulder and back pain which radiated to the right flank. Ultrasound examination and CAT scan studies were performed. Figure 2.93 is an ultrasound scan of the liver in a longitudinal plane. There is a large calcified echinococcal cyst noted in the superior aspect of the liver just beneath the diaphragm. The mass is strongly echogenic, which indicates its solid nature. It also has decreased transmission secondary to the calcified walls. Figure 2.94 is a transverse scan with cephalad angulation to visualize the echinococcal cyst.

A CAT scan was performed, and figure 2.95 demonstrates the calcified wall of the echinococcal cyst. The mass is present in the superior portion of the right lobe of the liver. The patient was taken to the operating room where an echinococcal cyst of the right lobe of the liver was removed.

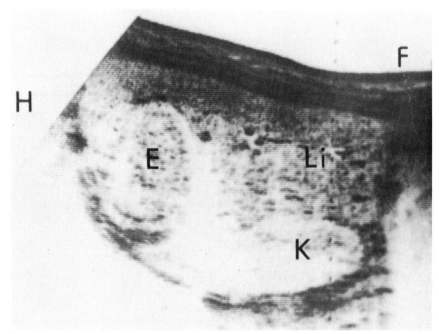

Fig. 2.93

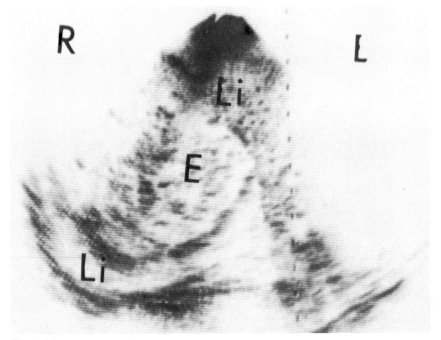

Fig. 2.94

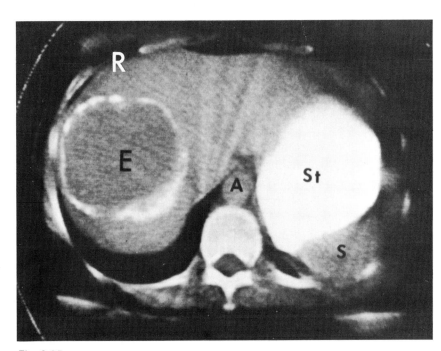

Fig. 2.95

A = Aorta
E = Echinococcal cyst
F = Foot
H = Head
K = Kidney
L = Left
Li = Liver
R = Right
S = Spleen
St = Stomach

3.
Ultrasonography of the Gallbladder and Biliary System

Michael M. Raskin, M.D.

Ultrasound Technique

The gallbladder is frequently visualized during the routine study of the upper abdomen, but it is more consistently detected if the patient has been fasting for at least 12 hours prior to the examination. In addition, the patient should take a fat-free meal on the evening prior to the examination. If maximal distention of the gallbladder is to be achieved, it is important that the patient receive nothing by mouth after the evening meal and that the ultrasound examination of the gallbladder be performed as early in the morning as possible. An early examination will minimize the effects of bowel gas due to air swallowed by an anxious patient. In some emergency situations, however, an examination may be performed at any time, since fasting will not alter the size of the gallbladder if obstruction is not present. It can be especially helpful in cases of suspected acute cholecystitis.

The examination is performed routinely with the patient in the supine position. An oblique ultrasound scan usually provides the best delineation of the long axis of the gallbladder. In order to obtain the proper obliquity, however, scans often must be obtained initially in the transverse and longitudinal planes.

Transverse scans are usually begun at the level of the xiphoid, scanning laterally to the right subcostal area. Serial scans are obtained at 1-cm intervals in a caudal direction until the rounded sonolucent area that represents the gallbladder is obtained. Serial scans are continued in a caudal direction until the gallbladder no longer is visible. In order to obtain a more precise scan of the long axis of the gallbladder, it often is helpful to indicate the lateral borders of the gallbladder on the patient's scan with a marking pen.

If good visualization of the gallbladder is achieved on transverse scanning, true longitudinal scans (parallel to the sagittal plane) usually are not necessary. Longitudinal oblique scans, parallel to the long axis of the gallbladder, are obtained at 5-mm intervals, starting at the medial border of the gallbladder and continuing through its lateral border. When the transducer makes contact with the right costal margin, it is often advantageous to angle it deeply under the ribs so that the beam is directed in a cephalad direction, rather than to move the transducer in a linear direction over the ribs. The ribs will cause acoustic shadowing and obviate the possibility of obtaining an optimal examination. This technique avoids artifacts produced by absorption and reverberation. In many instances, real-time B-scan ultrasonography can be used to great advantage. It can rapidly localize the gallbladder and determine its longitudinal axis prior to actually obtaining B-scan ultrasonograms.

It should be emphasized that compound sector scanning of the gallbladder should be avoided to reduce the possibility of filling an area of true acoustic shadowing. In addition, each scan should be performed with the patient in suspended respiration in order to reduce respiratory artifacts. In order to prevent changes in the position of the gallbladder during scanning, the approximate same level of suspended respiration should be achieved each time. The most reproducible phase of respiration is at the end of a normal expiration, as this is achieved by the normal elastic recoil of the lung.

At times it may be difficult to obtain adequate visualization of the entire gallbladder when it is high in the right upper quadrant or when the right costal margin is low. In these cases, it is often helpful to have the patient suspend respiration after a maximal inspiratory effort. This maneuver will lower the right hemidiaphragm and liver and displace the gallbladder caudally. On occasion, the examination can be performed with the patient in the erect position or in the left lateral decubitus position when the routine supine position fails to produce optimal visualization of the gallbladder (Albarelli 1975; Foster and McLaughlin 1977). All gallbladder studies should require a few scans with the patient in the left decubitus position. This maneuver will often displace those stones lodged near the cystic duct during a supine study.

Although ultrasonography can determine the anatomical configuration and morphology of the gallbladder in normal and diseased states, it does not indicate much about the function of the gallbladder. A normal physiological mechanism resulting in gallbladder contraction is initiated by the ingestion of food. This produces neural and hormonal stimuli, resulting in the release of cholecystokinin from the duodenal mucosa which produces contraction of the gallbladder and simultaneous relaxation of the sphincter of Oddi. In a clinical setting, contraction of the gallbladder is usually achieved by having the patient ingest a fatty meal, although the response of the gallbladder to a fatty meal is unpredictable and varies according to the rate of release of endogenous cholecystokinin. In addition, the patient often ingests large quantities of air along with the meal; this results in suboptimal visualization of the gallbladder. Further-

more, ingestion of food may prevent obtaining other examinations for which the patient is fasting.

The gallbladder can be provoked to contract with either oral ingestion of a fatty meal or intravenous administration of sincalide. Either of these two procedures will cause the gallbladder to contract within 5–30 minutes. Sincalide has been shown to give more uniform contraction and quicker results than does a fatty meal.

Sincalide (Kinevac®) is a synthetic, sterile, lyophilized powder of the C-terminal octapeptide of cholecystokinin which reproduces all the known biological activities of the intact molecule of cholecystokinin. The powder is reconstituted with sterile water for injection. The dose is based on the patient's weight and injected intravenously. It results in an early, predictable contraction of the normal gallbladder, with a 40% or greater reduction in size, within 5 to 15 minutes after intravenous injection (Sargent, Meyers, and Hubsher 1976). It should be noted that sincalide is contraindicated in patients sensitive to the drug, and its safety for use in pregnant women or in children has not yet been established.

The normal common bile duct rarely can be visualized in its entirety. It is not uncommon, however, to visualize a small portion of the common bile duct by performing longitudinal scans at 5-mm intervals, starting just medial to the gallbladder.

The normal intrahepatic biliary radicles rarely are visualized, but they become easier to demonstrate as they dilate. The intrahepatic portion of the biliary radicles becomes more tortuous and can be demonstrated in both the transverse and longitudinal planes. (See also p. 122 for additional comments on technique for examination of the gallbladder and biliary system.)

Normal Anatomy

The biliary radicles of each lobe unite to form a right and left hepatic duct which emerge near the hilum of the liver and form the common hepatic duct. The common hepatic duct joins the cystic duct from the gallbladder to form the common bile duct which then passes posterior to the first portion of the duodenum, through the head of the pancreas, to enter the ampulla of vater in the second portion of the duodenum.

The gallbladder is an ovoid-shaped sac lying in the gallbladder fossa of the inferior aspect of the right lobe of the liver. The position of the gallbladder is variable but is usually quite close to the anterior abdominal wall. If the gallbladder is elongated, it may extend below the inferior edge of the liver. Occasionally, the gallbladder is in the right lower quadrant or even in the pelvis. Rarely, a totally intrahepatic gallbladder will be encountered. Although the position of the gallbladder may be quite variable, it is almost never situated to the left of midline, except in patients with abdominal situs inversus.

In transverse sections, the gallbladder is seen as a circular sonolucency in the right upper quadrant. Longitudinal oblique sections parallel to the long axis of the gallbladder give the characteristic pear-shaped sonolucent appearance. The caudal portion of the gallbladder has an oval contour, while the cephalic portion narrows down to a tubular appearance as the gallbladder joins the cystic duct.

Ultrasound allows adequate visualization of the gallbladder in 75–92% of normal patients (Doust and Maklad 1974; Goldberg, Harris, and Broocker 1974). This is best performed with gray scale ultrasonography, prior fasting of the patient, additional positions, and gallbladder contraction. The gallbladder can then be visualized routinely in over 90% of all normal patients (Hublitz, Kahn, and Sell 1972; Leopold et al. 1976). Nevertheless, and despite all known attempts to visualize the gallbladder, a small percentage of gallbladders cannot be visualized adequately with ultrasound. These include the following conditions:

1. A normal but small gallbladder may be present but contracted. When the gallbladder is less than 2 cm in diameter, the normal sonolucent appearance may be lost.
2. The gallbladder may be shrunken, secondary to chronic inflammation.
3. A stone may be filling the entire gallbladder.
4. Bowel gas in the duodenum or hepatic flexure may be anterior to the gallbladder and, therefore, prevent visualization of the gallbladder.
5. The gallbladder may not be in its normally expected position.
6. The patient may have had a cholecystectomy.

Gallbladder size varies considerably among patients and within the same patient, depending upon the fasting or nonfasting state of the patient. A normal anatomical variant may be an extremely elongated gallbladder. A diameter greater than 5 cm is generally accepted as abnormally large. It should be noted, however, that scans not performed perpendicular to the long axis of the gall-

bladder may elongate the true diameter of the gallbladder and produce a falsely larger transverse diameter.

The function of the gallbladder is to receive, store, and concentrate bile produced from the liver and to release it, upon demand, into the common bile duct. Bile from the liver reaches the gallbladder through the funnel-shaped cystic duct that widens toward the gallbladder. The course of the cystic duct appears serpentine because its lumen is ridged by a series of folds called the valves of Heister. This explains why only a small portion of the cystic duct is visible with ultrasound.

When the bile ducts dilate, the intrahepatic biliary radicles become tortuous. The dilated biliary radicles are not difficult to differentiate from dilated hepatic veins since the hepatic veins usually can be seen near the diaphragm extending in a vertical direction and entering the inferior vena cava. Furthermore, hepatic veins do not have the high-amplitude circumferential echo of the portal and biliary systems. It is somewhat more difficult to differentiate dilated intrahepatic biliary ducts from dilated portal veins. Since the common bile duct has a more vertical course, and the portal vein has a more horizontal course, demonstration of communication between the dilated intrahepatic structures and their extrahepatic component usually will result in the correct interpretation.

Real-time equipment can expedite determination of dilated biliary radicles. The dilated structure easily can be traced centrally to the region of the porta hepatis so that differentiation of dilated common hepatic duct from portal vein can be made (Perlmutter and Goldberg 1976). If real-time equipment is not available, however, or if the dilated structure cannot be traced centrally, other indirect signs aid in distinguishing dilated biliary radicles from dilated portal venous structures.

Anatomically, bile ducts are situated anterior to portal venous structures. Dilated biliary radicles may, however, be extremely difficult to differentiate from normal intrahepatic portal veins on anatomical appearance alone. Furthermore, since the two structures are intimately related within the liver, they cannot be distinguished on the basis of location or orientation. A relatively high volume of blood flows through the portal venous system, which parallels the intrahepatic biliary radicles. The portal venous systems are often demonstrated in the normal individual while the biliary radicles are not. Dilatation of the intrahepatic biliary radicles, however, will often result in the "parallel channel" sign of biliary dilatation. This is produced by the dilated intrahepatic biliary radicle's lying anterior to the posterior portal venous structure. Another feature, although less characteristic, is the greater transmission of sound through bile-filled dilated biliary radicles than through blood-filled portal venous structures.

Pathological States

Cholelithiasis

Gallstones most often form in the gallbladder, but occasionally they may occur in the biliary ducts. The normal constituents of bile (cholesterol, calcium bilirubinate, and calcium carbonate) are the three principal stone-forming substances. Gallstones may be composed almost entirely of any one of these substances or of a mixture of them in varying proportions. Pure gallstones, composed almost entirely of a single substance, represent less than 10% of all gallstones and usually produce no changes in the gallbladder wall. Mixed gallstones are by far the most common and are composed of varying proportions of all three of the stone-forming constituents of bile. Radiographically, the plain-film demonstration of gallstones depends upon their calcium content. Most often, multiple stones, which can vary greatly in size, are encountered. Multiple stones, if larger than 5 mm, are often multifaceted.

The overall accuracy of gallbladder ultrasound is approximately 90% (Arnon and Rosenquist 1976). If the gallbladder is visualized as a sonolucency, stones as small as 1 mm can be detected. If the gallbladder is shrunken and its walls are thickened, however, large stones can be missed. The classic gallstone, as originally described in the literature, is an echogenic area in the dependent portion of the gallbladder with an acoustic shadow distal to the echogenic area within the gallbladder. The increased echoes within the dependent portion of the gallbladder are produced by virtue of the large difference in acoustic impedance between the two media (Crow, Bartrum, and Foote 1976). Despite the fact that considerable scattering occurs, the acoustic interface is so strong that the gallstone is seen as a highly echogenic structure. The acoustic shadow is produced by the high attenuation and scattering of the sound beam by the stone. The degree of acoustic shadowing depends primarily on the size of the stone and not on the calcium content.

Occasionally, gallstones of uniform density may float in a single layer, suggesting only thickening of the gallbladder wall. If the patient is then scanned in the erect position, the layering gallstones will shift to the dependent portion of the gallbladder and clarify the problem. Stones within the cystic duct may be difficult to demonstrate. Occasionally, a stone within the cystic duct may produce a target-shaped echo pattern (Anderson and Harned 1977). Shadowing is often noted in the cystic duct region but without a stone present. This is generally secondary to the spiral valves of Heister, which scatter the reflected sound in all directions. Patients should be examined in the left lateral decubitis position in order to displace the stone, if any question exists.

The acoustic shadow is produced by the high attenuation and scattering of the sound beam by the stone. In order to produce shadowing, there must be a difference in acoustic impedance of sufficient area to cause visible attenuation of the sound beam. An extremely small stone, not apparent as an echogenic structure in the dependent portion of the gallbladder, may be indirectly visualized because of its acoustic shadow.

The following factors will affect the production of an acoustic shadow:

1. The size of the stone. In general, the larger the stone, the larger the acoustic shadow.
2. Tissues posterior to the gallbladder. It is axiomatic that in order to demonstrate acoustic shadowing from gallstones, the gallbladder must be overlying either the liver or the right kidney. If the gallbladder is overlying the bowel, not only may the acoustic shadow be masked, but a false acoustic shadow may be created.
3. Stones in a contracted gallbladder. If the gallbladder is completely filled with stones, the normal sonolucency of the bile-filled gallbladder cannot be demonstrated. Therefore, the only indication that stones are present may be the acoustic shadow produced by the gallstones.
4. Impacted stones. If the stone is impacted in the cystic duct, its direct visualization may be difficult, due to the lack of sonolucent bile. The acoustic shadow, however, will be produced even though the stone itself may not be visualized directly.

The cystic duct, if visualized at all, will have more irregular contours than the common bile duct, which has a linear appearance. The common bile duct is often not visualized because of overlying bowel gas in the duodenum. In addition, when the common bile duct does contain small stones, the stones often are apparent only by their acoustic shadowing. If the common bile duct is dilated proximal to the stone, the common bile duct and biliary radicles usually are well recorded because of distention from the bile, which produces a highly echo-free area.

Polyp

A polyp frequently presents as an echo-producing structure within the sonolucent lumen of the gallbladder. It usually is not, however, of higher increased echogenicity than the gallbladder wall, and it rarely will produce an acoustic shadow (Goldberg 1977). Although this condition is rare, the position of the polyp will not change between the supine and erect positions of the patient, and will confirm its diagnosis.

Segmental Adenomyomatosis

This condition is one of the hyperplastic cholecystoses in which a segmental narrowing of the gallbladder often presents as a septation within the sonolucent bile-filled lumen. This condition is readily diagnosed by oral cholecystography. It is characterized by segmental constriction, dense opacity, and hypercontractility. This condition should be distinguished from a folded gallbladder which is not completely distended, or a phrygian cap.

Biliary Sludge

Biliary sludge most often presents as fine homogeneous echoes that layer out in the dependent portion of the gallbladder (Goldberg 1977). These fine echoes will change with the position of the patient and do not cause any degree of significant acoustic shadowing. Biliary sludge can exist by itself or may be associated with gallstones or chronic cholecystitis.

Cholecystitis

Acute cholecystitis occasionally is caused by cystic duct obstruction from stones. The gallbladder often is enlarged, and stones usually can be seen within it. The walls of the gallbladder may appear somewhat indistinct and thickened due to edema. Often, a double rim effect will be produced due to reflections from both the inner and outer walls of the inflamed gallbladder. Though seen in acute cholecystitis, this pattern is more commonly associated with chronic cholecystitis (Goldberg 1977).

In chronic cholecystitis, there can be many repeated episodes of acute cholecystitis. The walls of the gallbladder appear thickened, and its overall size is usually, although not always, contracted.

In both acute and chronic cholecystitis, the gallbladder characteristically fails to contract. It should be understood, however, that the diagnosis of acute or chronic cholecystitis with ultrasound may not be revealing and is often misleading. The history and clinical condition of the patient must be studied carefully.

Carcinoma

Carcinoma of the gallbladder may produce thickening of its walls. In addition, the carcinoma may project into the lumen of the gallbladder and appear similar to a polyp or even to stones. The wall is usually thickened and has an irregular, indistinct border. It often presents as a large ill-defined mass in the gallbladder bed.

Jaundice

Using ultrasound, jaundice due to intrahepatic disease can be differentiated from jaundice due to extrahepatic obstruction (Malini and Sabel 1977; Taylor, Carpenter, and McCready 1974). If careful scanning reveals neither dilated intrahepatic ducts nor a dilated common bile duct, jaundice is most likely due to a nonobstructive cause. This would most often be secondary to diffuse intrahepatic disease, such as hepatitis or cirrhosis.

The majority of patients with obstructive jaundice will have dilated intrahepatic biliary radicles. The most sensitive diagnostic indicator, however, is early extrahepatic biliary dilatation. Recent studies suggest that the size criterion of the common bile duct, which would optimize the nosological probabilities important to a screening procedure, is 7 mm for patients without previous biliary surgery (Sample et al. 1978). It is important to search for both the common bile duct and dilated intrahepatic biliary radicles, as some cases of obstructive jaundice will have dilatation of the common bile duct as the only abnormal finding. Jaundiced patients with prior common duct bypass surgery, however, are just as likely to have a nondiagnostic ultrasound examination (Sample et al. 1978).

Dilated biliary radicles usually indicate extrahepatic obstruction. If a dilated common bile duct is seen, the obstruction must be distal to the porta hepatis. This is most likely due to choledocholithiasis or pancreatic carcinoma. If dilated intrahepatic biliary radicles are found, and careful scanning fails to reveal a dilated common bile duct, the site of obstruction may be in the region of the porta hepatis (Taylor and Carpenter 1975). The overall accuracy of ultrasound technique in differentiating obstructive from nonobstructive jaundice is 82–90% (Isikoff and Diaconis 1977; Malini and Sabel 1977; Neiman and Mintzer 1977; Sample et al. 1978).

Dilated Gallbladder

A dilated gallbladder that does not contract usually indicates obstruction distal to it in either the cystic duct or the common bile duct. A stone in either the cystic duct or the common bile duct can cause dilatation of the gallbladder, but only a common bile duct stone will result in dilatation of the biliary radicles. Therefore, demonstrating a dilated gallbladder requires examination of the liver in order to determine whether dilated biliary radicles exist. A small carcinoma of the cystic duct or the common bile duct can cause similar findings and be indistinguishable with ultrasound.

Extrinsic obstruction resulting in a dilated gallbladder can be produced by a mass in the region of the porta hepatis or by a mass in the head of the pancreas (Cunningham 1977). A mass in the region of the porta hepatis, usually due to enlarged nodes, may cause extrinsic compression of the cystic duct. A mass in the head of the pancreas, whether it is from carcinoma or it is secondary to edema from pancreatitis, may cause obstruction of the common bile duct. As with a stone in the common bile duct, there is dilatation of both the biliary radicles and the gallbladder.

The finding of a dilated gallbladder secondary to a pancreatic carcinoma has often been incorrectly called Courvoisier's sign. Courvoisier syndrome, first described in the literature in 1890, is the eponym for ampulla of Vater obstruction associated with painless jaundice and distention of the gallbladder (Goldberg 1977). Courvoisier further indicated that pain, chills, and fever indicate the presence of common bile duct calculi; their absence indicates tumor of the head of the pancreas.

References

Albarelli, J. N. Erect cholecystosonography. *J. Clin. Ultrasound* 3:309, December 1975.

Anderson, J. C., and Harned, R. K. Gray scale ultrasonography of the gallbladder: an evaluation of accuracy and report of additional ultrasound signs. *Am. J. Roentgenol.* 129:975–977, December 1977.

Arnon, S., and Rosenquist, C. J. Gray scale cholecystosonography: an evaluation of accuracy. *Am. J. Roentgenol.* 127:817–818, 1976.

Crow, H. C.; Bartrum, R. J.; and Foote, S. R. Expanded criteria for the ultrasonic diagnosis of gallstones. *J. Clin. Ultrasound* 4:289–292, August 1976.

Cunningham, J. J. Atypical cholesonograms in primary and secondary malignant disease of the biliary tract. *J. Clin. Ultrasound* 5:264–267, August 1977.

Doust, B. D., and Maklad, N. F. Ultrasonic B-mode examination of the gallbladder. *Radiology* 110:643–647, 1974.

Foster, S. C., and McLaughlin, S. M. Improvement in the ultrasonic evaluation of the gallbladder by using the left lateral decubitus position. *J. Clin. Ultrasound* 5:253–256, August 1977.

Goldberg, B. B. Gallbladder and bile ducts. In *Abdominal gray scale ultrasonography,* ed. B. B. Goldberg, pp. 137–165. New York: John Wiley & Sons, 1977.

Goldberg, B. B.; Harris, K.; and Broocker, W. Ultrasonic and radiographic cholecystography—a comparison. *Radiology* 111:405–409, May 1974.

Hublitz, U. F.; Kahn, P. C.; and Sell, L. A. Cholecystosonography: an approach to the non-visualized gallbladder. *Radiology* 103:645–649, June 1972.

Isikoff, M. B., and Diaconis, J. N. Ultrasound—a new diagnostic approach to the jaundiced patient. *JAMA* 238:221–223, July 18, 1977.

Leopold, G. R.; Amberg, J.; Gosink, B. B.; and Mittelstaedt, C. Gray scale ultrasonic cholecystography: a comparison with conventional radiographic techniques. *Radiology* 121:445–448, November 1976.

Malini, S., and Sabel, J. Ultrasonography in obstructive jaundice. *Radiology* 123:429–433, May 1977.

Neiman, H. L., and Mintzer, R. A. Accuracy of biliary

duct ultrasound: comparison with cholangiography. *Am. J. Roentgenol.* 129:979–982, December 1977.

Perlmutter, G. S., and Goldberg, B. B. Ultrasonic evaluation of the common bile duct. *J. Clin. Ultrasound* 4:107–111, April 1976.

Sample, W. F.; Sarti, D. A.; Goldstein, L. I.; Weiner, M.; and Kadell, B. M. Gray scale ultrasonography of the jaundiced patient. *Radiology* 128:719–725, 1978.

Sargent, E. N.; Meyers, H. I.; and Hubsher, J. Cholecystokinetic cholecystography: efficacy and tolerance study of sincalide. *Am. J. Roentgenol.* 127:267–271, 1976.

Tabrisky, J.; Lindstrom, R. R.; Herman, M. W.; Castagna, J.; and Sarti, D. Value of gallbladder B-scan ultrasonography. *Gastroenterology* 68:1246–1252, May 1975.

Taylor, K. J. W., and Carpenter, D. A. The anatomy and pathology of the porta hepatis demonstrated by gray scale ultrasonography. *J. Clin. Ultrasound* 3:117–119, June 1975.

Taylor, K. J. W.; Carpenter, D. A.; and McCready, V. R. Ultrasound and scintigraphy in the differential diagnosis of obstructive jaundice. *J. Clin. Ultrasound* 2:105–116, June 1974.

CASES

Dennis A. Sarti, M.D.
W. Frederick Sample, M.D.

Technique for Gallbladder Examination

Gallbladder examination usually follows overnight fasting. At least a 12-hour fast is necessary to distend the gallbladder enough for ultrasonic visualization. Figure 3.1 shows the transverse scanning planes used in initially evaluating the gallbladder. The patient is studied in the supine position with transverse scans obtained in the right upper quadrant. The normal circular structure of the gallbladder can be seen in the right-upper quadrant. It is most helpful to map the medial and lateral borders of the gallbladder with a grease pencil while doing the transverse scans, as is demonstrated in figure 3.1. Transverse scans should be obtained at 1-cm intervals, paying careful attention to the thickness of the gallbladder wall and the gallbladder lumen. Once the transverse scans are finished, we should have an outline of the gallbladder on the patient's skin.

Oblique longitudinal scans are obtained parallel to the long axis of the gallbladder mapped on the patient's skin (fig. 3.2). The patient should be asked to take in a deep breath using the same respiratory pattern each time, so that the gallbladder is in a similar position for the longitudinal and the transverse scans. Longitudinal scans should be obtained at 5-mm intervals parallel to the long axis of the gallbladder. Scans can be started medial to the gallbladder and continue through the gallbladder until the lateral aspect of the gallbladder is completely covered. By scanning at 5-mm intervals, small stones will not be missed. At larger intervals, this can easily happen.

Occasionally, the gallbladder will be difficult to visualize in the right subcostal margin, because the liver is not caudally extended enough. In these instances, scanning through the intercostal space may yield the normal sonolucency of the gallbladder. Figure 3.3 is an example of an intercostal scan made in an effort to visualize a highly positioned gallbladder.

It is important routinely to place the patient in the decubitus position with the right side up as is shown in figure 3.4. This is done so that cystic duct stones will not be missed. Often, the gallbladder will appear normal in the supine position. By turning the patient to the decubitus position, however, numerous stones in the cystic duct region of the gallbladder will be displaced and can then be visualized by ultrasound. Figure 3.4 is an example of scanning beneath the right costal margin with the patient in the decubitus position. The gallbladder will be in a somewhat different location on these scans. It may be necessary to begin surveying the right upper quadrant to locate its actual position.

A = Anterior
F = Foot
H = Head
L = Left
P = Posterior
R = Right

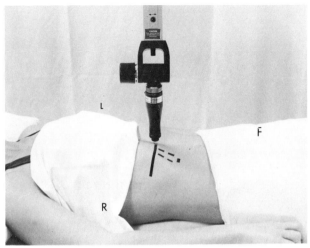

Fig. 3.1

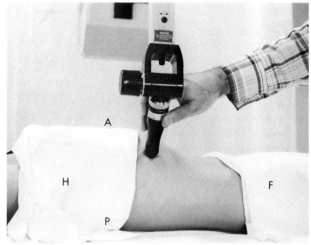

Fig. 3.3

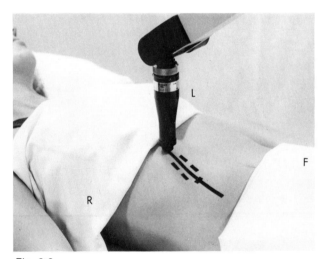

Fig. 3.2

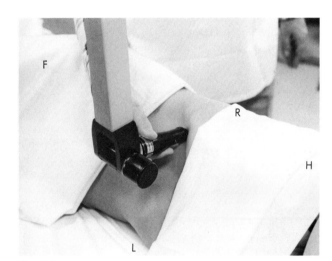

Fig. 3.4

Normal Gallbladder

Ultrasonic examination of the gallbladder usually is performed following overnight fasting. Fasting will allow normal distention of the gallbladder with bile and, therefore, will enhance ultrasonic visualization of this organ. If the patient has eaten recently, the gallbladder will contract and often may not be seen on ultrasound examination. Recent reports have stated that the inability to visualize the gallbladder with ultrasound indicates gallbladder disease if the patient has, in fact, been fasting. Therefore, it is extremely important to perform gallbladder examinations following an overnight fast.

The gallbladder is initially examined in the transverse plane with the medial and lateral borders marked on the skin. Longitudinal exams of the gallbladder at 5-mm intervals will rule out any gallbladder pathology. Figures 3.5–3.8 are examples of longitudinal scans of the normal gallbladder. The gallbladder walls are fairly smooth, sharp, and not markedly thickened. Figure 3.5 demonstrates the gallbladder with liver parenchyma noted both anterior and posterior to the gallbladder. The characteristic pear shape of the gallbladder is seen anterior to the right kidney.

The gallbladder is easily recognizable in the right upper quadrant because of the sonolucent bile. Figure 3.6 demonstrates a longitudinal scan of the gallbladder with liver parenchyma again noted posteriorly. Very often, the right kidney can be seen through the gallbladder (fig. 3.7). This often can facilitate examination of the right kidney. Figure 3.8 demonstrates a tubular structure anterior to the portal vein and representing the common hepatic duct. This structure often is visualized coursing over the portal vein before it joins with the cystic duct to form the common bile duct. Figure 3.8 also demonstrates echoes on the anterior wall of the fundal region of the gallbladder; they are secondary to the reverberation artifacts commonly seen in sonolucent masses on the anterior wall (see chapter 1).

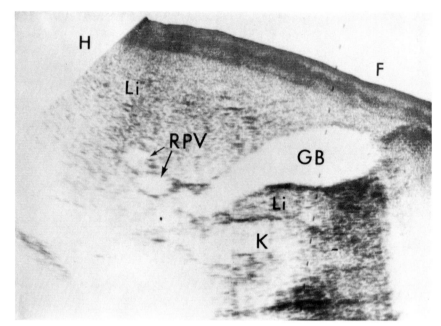

Fig. 3.5

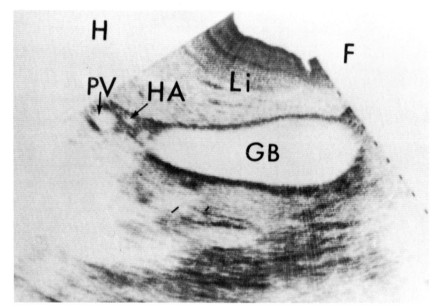

Fig. 3.6

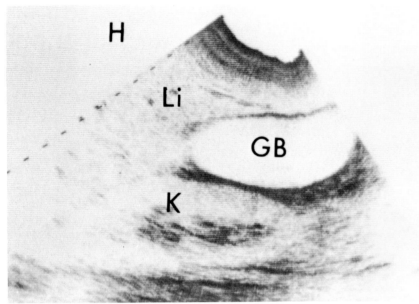

Fig. 3.7

Ad	=	Adrenal gland
CHD	=	Common hepatic duct
CL	=	Caudate lobe
F	=	Foot
GB	=	Gallbladder
H	=	Head
HA	=	Hepatic artery
HV	=	Hepatic vein
I	=	Inferior vena cava
K	=	Kidney
Li	=	Liver
PV	=	Portal vein
RPV	=	Right portal vein

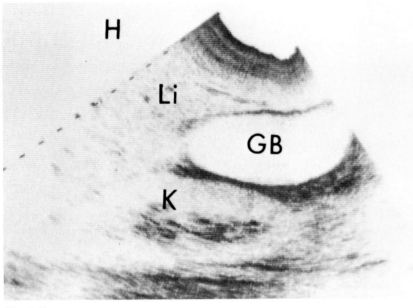

Fig. 3.8

Normal Gallbladder

Since the gallbladder is a fluid-filled structure, through transmission is seen posterior to the gallbladder when liver parenchyma or kidney is visualized. This is present in figure 3.9 where the gallbladder is seen as the characteristic pear structure in the right upper quadrant with increased echogenicity present in the liver posterior to the gallbladder. On transverse sections, the gallbladder appears as a circular or oval structure in the right upper quadrant. It is most often seen anterior to the right kidney as in figures 3.10 and 3.11. Figure 3.10 demonstrates the characteristic circular echo of the gallbladder in the right upper quadrant. The borders are sharp and distinct. The gallbladder can be used as an ultrasonic window for visualization of the right kidney.

Figure 3.11 demonstrates slight decreased visualization of the medial wall of the gallbladder secondary to overlying bowel gas. Since the duodenum is adjacent ot the medial aspect of the gallbladder, this border often may be indistinct or may not be seen, because it has become obscured by bowel air. Occasionally, the gallbladder may be in a slightly unusual position (fig. 3.12). Here the gallbladder is situated more laterally than is usual. This scan may be misinterpreted as ascitic fluid in the hepatorenal angle.

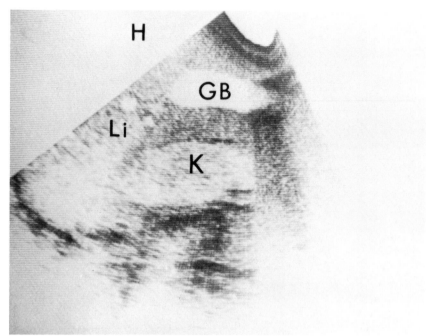

Fig. 3.9

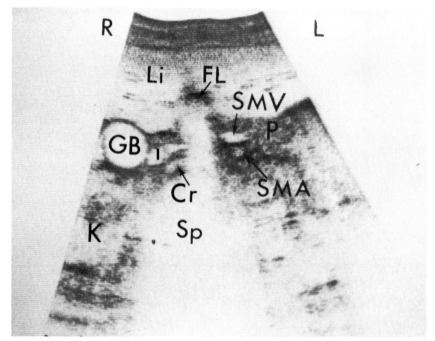

Fig. 3.10

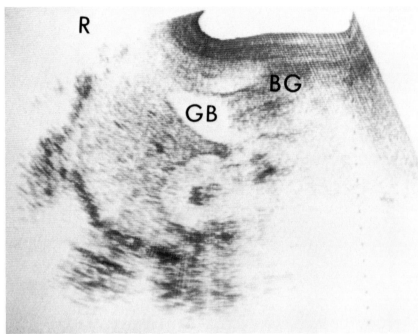

Fig. 3.11

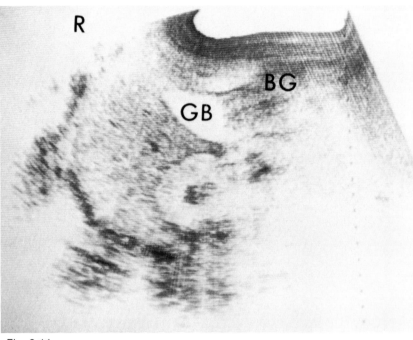

A   = Aorta
BG   = Bowel gas
Cr   = Crus of the diaphragm
FL   = Falciform ligament
GB   = Gallbladder
H   = Head
I   = Inferior vena cava
K   = Kidney
L   = Left
Li   = Liver
P   = Pancreas
PV   = Portal vein
R   = Right
SMA = Superior mesenteric artery
SMV = Superior mesenteric vein
Sp   = Spine

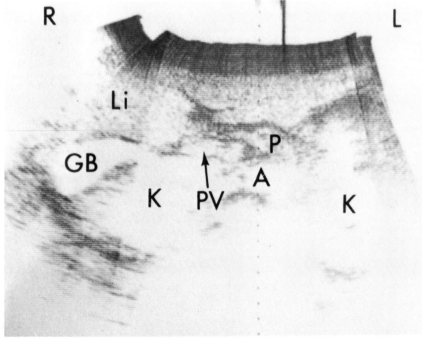

Fig. 3.12

Normal Gallbladder and Anatomic Variants

Occasionally the gallbladder can assume a rather unusual configuration, which may be confusing. Figures 3.13 and 3.14 are examples of rather long gallbladders that are kinked or bent. These often can be confusing in the transverse plane, but marking the medial and lateral borders on the patient's skin, while doing transverse scans, will markedly facilitate the longitudinal scans. By taking longitudinal scans parallel to the long axis of any sonolucent mass in the right upper quadrant, we can usually determine whether or not it is a gallbladder or another mass such as an abscess, pseudocyst, or loculated ascites.

Figure 3.15 shows a gallbladder with a phrygian cap (arrows). The fundus of the gallbladder is noted distal to the phrygian cap. Occasionally, a mass will be noted adjacent to the gallbladder. Fluid around the gallbladder may represent abscess or loculated ascites, but we must also consider fluid within a loop of bowel such as is present in figure 3.16. Here the duodenum is present as a fluid-filled mass posterior to the normal gallbladder. The duodenum is recognized by the highly echogenic mucosa forming the irregular border of the duodenal loop.

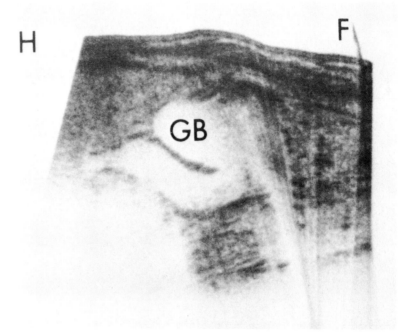

Fig. 3.13

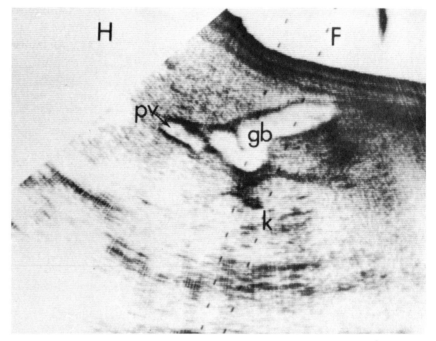

Fig. 3.14

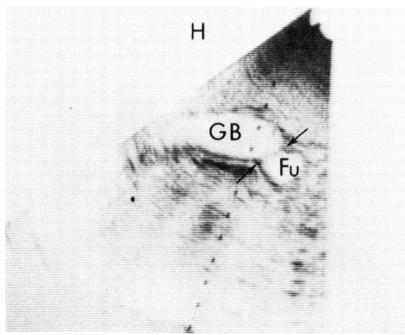

Fig. 3.15

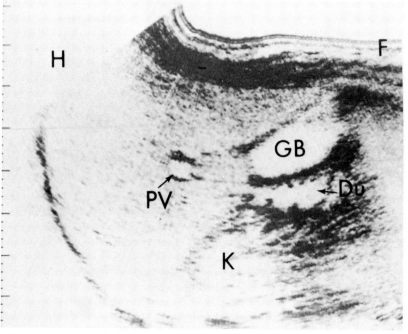

Fig. 3.16

Arrows = Phrygian cap
Du = Duodenum
F = Foot
Fu = Fundus of the gallbladder
GB = Gallbladder
gb = Gallbladder
H = Head
K = Kidney
k = Kidney
PV = Portal vein
pv = Portal vein

Cholelithiasis

The most common pathology of the gall-bladder to be diagnosed by ultrasound is cholelithiasis. It characteristically presents as a strong echo within the sonolucent lumen of the gallbladder (figs. 3.17 and 3.18). The strong echogenicity of a gallstone is due to the marked acoustic mismatch between the stone and the bile. Posterior to the majority of the stones will be acoustic shadowing. This often aids in distinguishing between a gallstone and a polyp. Figures 3.17 and 3.18 are scans of a patient with multiple stones. Figure 3.18 demonstrates the numerous strong echoes consistent with cholelithiasis in the posterior aspect of the gallbladder.

When the gallbladder is well distended, visualization of the gallstones is quite easy. Often, the gallbladder is not markedly distended in the presence of cholelithiasis, and so the diagnosis becomes more difficult. Figure 3.19 is an example of cholelithiasis with a somewhat smaller gallbladder. Because fluid is still present in the gallbladder, however, the gallstones stand out quite easily. Two gallstones are seen in figure 3.19.

One of the more difficult areas for detection of a gallstone is near the cystic duct region of the gallbladder. Figure 3.20 shows a gallstone that casts a shadow in the cystic duct area. In all of the examples in this section (figs. 3.17–3.20), the gallbladder wall remains fairly sharp. Therefore, we cannot make a diagnosis of coincident cholecystitis based on these examinations.

Since the gallbladder is adjacent to the duodenum and hepatic flexure, we may have difficulty in visualizing a gallstone in the fundal region adjacent to the bowel gas. Fairly characteristic findings from bowel gas, however, may be present. Figure 3.17 is an example of bowel gas adjacent to the fundal region of the gallbladder. The highly reflective surface of the bowel gas gives a "dirty" shadow, as compared with the rather "clean" shadow of the gallstone. Behind the bowel gas echo are reverberation artifacts, along with ring down of the transducer (see chapter 1).

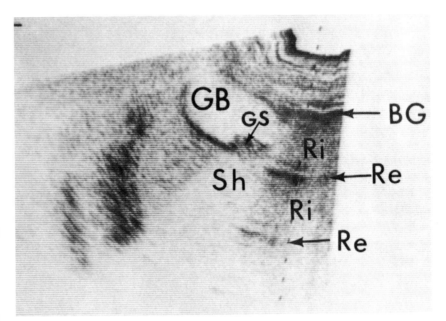

Fig. 3.17

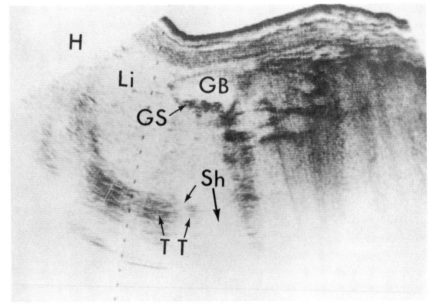

Fig. 3.18

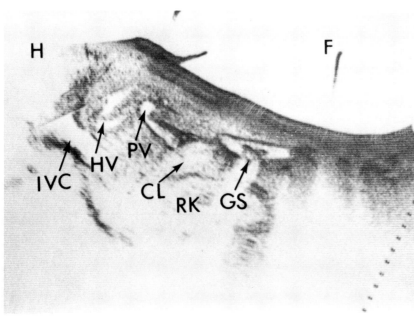

BG = Bowel gas
CL = Caudate lobe
F   = Foot
GB = Gallbladder
H   = Head
HV = Hepatic vein
IVC = Inferior vena cava
Li = Liver
PV = Portal vein
Re = Reverberation
Ri = Ring down
RK = Right kidney
Sh = Shadowing
TT = Through transmission

Fig. 3.19

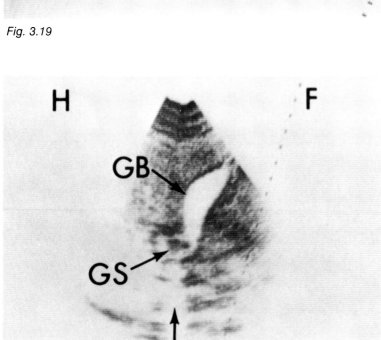

Fig. 3.20

Cholelithiasis with Shadowing and Layered Stones

Do all gallstones shadow? There has been disagreement and growing investigation into this problem without uniformity in opinion to date. Dr. Roy Filly of the University of San Francisco Medical Center in San Francisco, California, has performed an excellent experiment in a liver phantom model with varying sizes of gallstones in a gallbladder phantom. He has demonstrated that even very small stones (down to 1 mm in thickness) will shadow if the frequency of the transducer is high enough and if the center of the transducer beam is accurately positioned over the stone. The case shown in figures 3.21–3.23 appears to support his contention.

Figure 3.21 is a longitudinal scan of the gallbladder with a small echogenic mass (arrow) on the posterior wall, suggesting a gallstone. However, there is no evidence of shadowing on this scan. Most likely, we had the transducer beam slightly off center in relation to the gallstone. By minutely altering the transducer path on longitudinal scans, we were able to demonstrate the shadowing in figure 3.22. Figure 3.23 is a transverse scan of the same patient, again demonstrating shadowing when the transducer beam path is directly situated over this small stone. This appears to support Dr. Filly's contention that all stones do shadow if the technologist uses a high enough frequency transducer and meticulously attempts to place the center of the transducer beam directly over the stone itself.

Figure 3.24 is an example of multiple gallstones layering out within the gallbladder. This is a longitudinal scan in which a line of gallstones is seen in the mid portion of the gallbladder, almost as a linear echo. This finding is similar to the oral cholecystogram in which layered gallstones are seen when the patient is in the upright position.

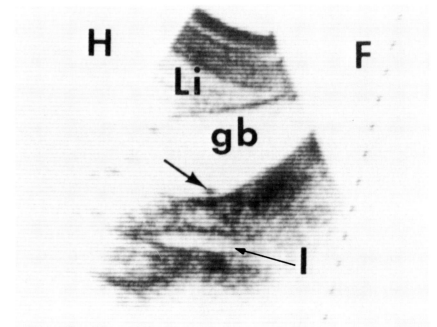

Fig. 3.21

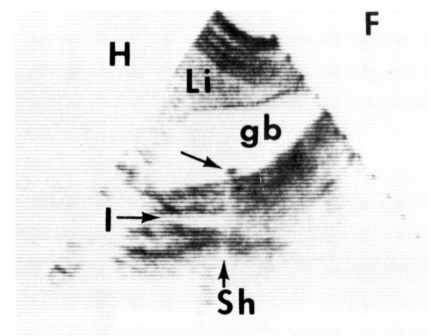

Fig. 3.22

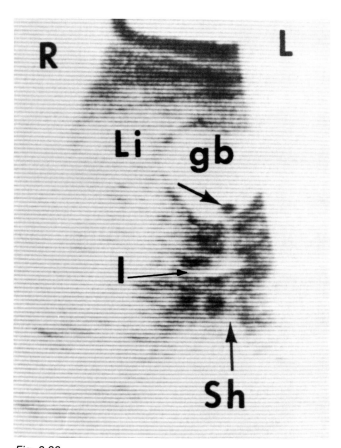

Arrow	=	Gallstones
CHD	=	Common hepatic duct
cm	=	Centimeter markers
F	=	Foot
GB	=	Gallbladder
GS	=	Gallstones
H	=	Head
I	=	Inferior vena cava
L	=	Left
Li	=	Liver
PV	=	Portal vein
R	=	Right
Sh	=	Shadowing

Fig. 3.23

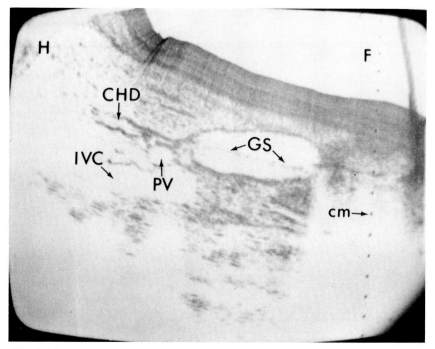

Fig. 3.24

Cholelithiasis near the Cystic Duct

Often, gallstones are embedded in the cystic duct region of the gallbladder and are consequently difficult to visualize with ultrasound. It is important to establish the habit of scanning the patient in a decubitus view to displace any stones that may be lodged in the cystic duct. By turning the patient to the left lateral decubitus position, with the right side up, the gallbladder will usually be situated more medially and will often allow a better visualization of the cystic duct region. Very often, a questionable stone in this region will be displaced into the gallbladder lumen and will become more readily visible.

The case in figures 3.25 and 3.26 is a 27-year-old woman with a one-month history of right upper quadrant pain. This pain lasted up to two hours and usually followed meals. She did not have any evidence of obstruction of her biliary tract, and there was no chemical evidence of jaundice. Figure 3.25 is a longitudinal scan with the patient in the supine position. The gallbladder is well distended but is within normal limits for its size. Any diameter of the gallbladder less than 5 cm is considered within normal limits. There is tremendous variation within the normal range, so the diagnosis of an obstructed gallbladder by ultrasound is an extremely difficult one. Figure 3.25 does demonstrate strong echoes in the region of the cystic duct that correspond to gallstones. Posterior to the gallstones is evidence of shadowing. This is a difficult area to assess, since the cystic duct itself may cause shadowing secondary to the spiral valves of Heister. Because of this problem, the patient is placed in a decubitus position (fig. 3.26). The numerous stones floating within the proximal portion of the gallbladder lumen can be seen; they are more easily evident in this position. Therefore, examination of this patient in the decubitus view was extremely helpful in demonstrating a definite diagnosis of cholelithiasis in the cystic duct area.

Figures 3.27 and 3.28 are of a 77-year-old woman who presented with an acute onset of right upper quadrant pain

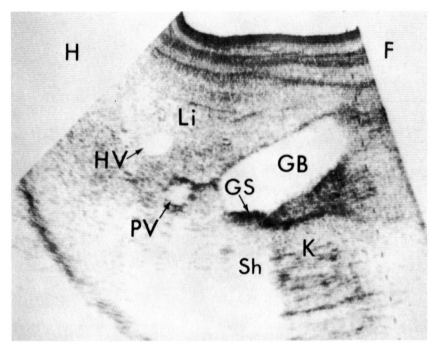

Fig. 3.25

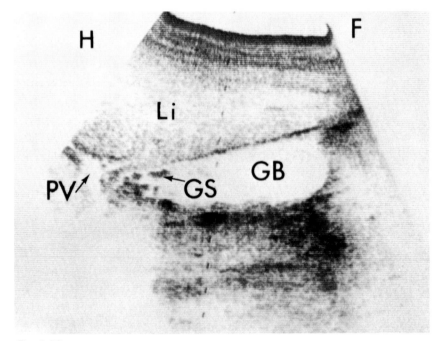

Fig. 3.26

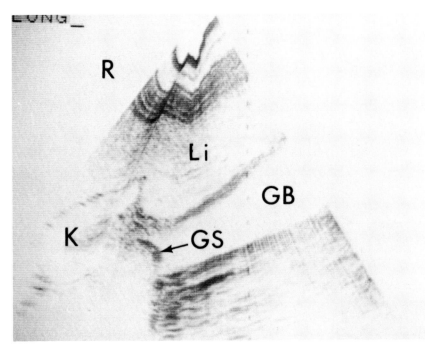

Fig. 3.27

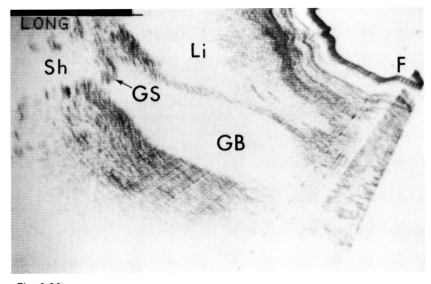

Fig. 3.28

occurring within two hours after dinner on the evening of admission. She had no previous history of abdominal pathology. A longitudinal scan (fig. 3.27) demonstrated a strong curvilinear echo in the cystic duct region and represented a cystic duct stone. In the decubitus view (fig. 3.28) the gallstone remained in the cystic duct region, suggesting the possibility of an impacted stone. Shadowing is seen posterior to the gallstone. The patient was taken to the operating room, and a cystic duct stone was found at surgery. The gallbladder was felt to be enlarged due to the obstruction from the cystic duct stone.

Since ultrasonic criteria for gallbladder obstruction necessitates a gallbladder diameter of greater than 5 cm, we did not definitely diagnose gallbladder distention. With the evidence of an impacted cystic duct stone, however, the diagnosis suggested this, even though the absolute size of the gallbladder was within normal limits. This is a major shortcoming of ultrasound technique. The high degree of variability in gallbladder size makes a diagnosis of obstruction very difficult.

F	=	Foot
GB	=	Gallbladder
GS	=	Gallstones
H	=	Head
HV	=	Hepatic vein
K	=	Kidney
L	=	Left
Li	=	Liver
PV	=	Portal vein
R	=	Right
Sh	=	Shadowing

Cholelithiasis without a Fluid-filled Gallbladder

Frequently, cholelithiasis will be present when there is no evidence of bile within the gallbladder. This is secondary to chronic inflammation of a gallbladder completely filled with stones. The case shown in figures 3.29 and 3.30 is a 64-year-old woman with chronic right upper quadrant pain. Ultrasound examination demonstrated a strong shadow in both the longitudinal and transverse sections. Figure 3.29 is a longitudinal scan in which the superficial border of the gallstones is seen as very highly reflective echoes. Behind the stones is a clear shadow. Figure 3.30 is a transverse scan of the gallbladder adjacent to the duodenum. Here we see a "dirty" appearance to the shadowing noted by the duodenum, whereas there is a "clean" shadow behind the gallstone. Furthermore, it is quite evident in this case that the superficial border of the gallstone is easily visible.

The case shown in figures 3.31 and 3.32 is a similar finding of a gallbladder completely filled with gallstones. No fluid is evident within the gallbladder. Here the superficial borders of the gallstones are more easily evident as a strong curvilinear echo. Again posterior to the gallstones is a clean shadowing area. It is important to recognize that a gallbladder filled with stones is not easily visualized and that the diagnosis of cholelithiasis can be easily misinterpreted for bowel gas in the area.

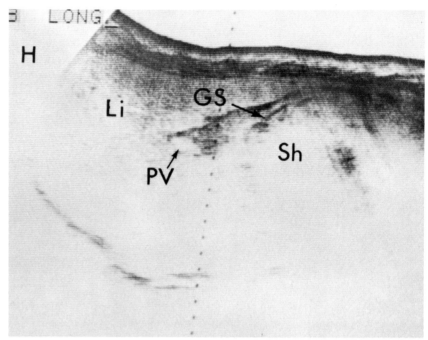

Fig. 3.29

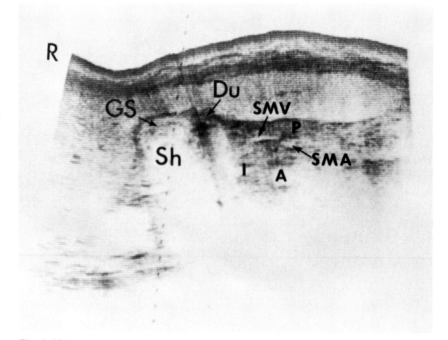

Fig. 3.30

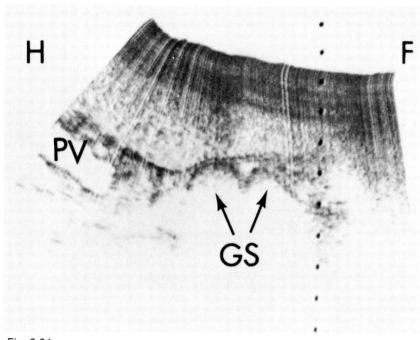

Fig. 3.31

A	=	Aorta
Du	=	Duodenum
F	=	Foot
GS	=	Gallstones
H	=	Head
I	=	Inferior vena cava
K	=	Kidney
L	=	Left
Li	=	Liver
P	=	Pancreas
PV	=	Portal vein
R	=	Right
Sh	=	Shadowing
SMA	=	Superior mesenteric artery
SMV	=	Superior mesenteric vein

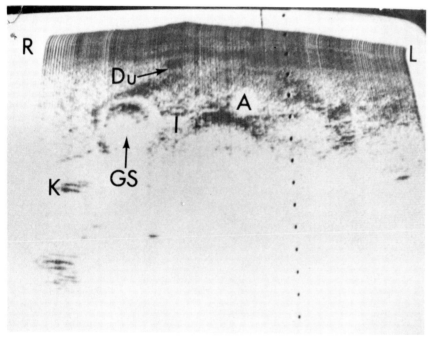

Fig. 3.32

Cholelithiasis with a Clean Shadow

The diagnosis of cholelithiasis often is extremely difficult to make, because it frequently is impossible to visualize the gallbladder, or even a large stone. Often, a gallstone will be present with a border that cannot be seen, and only the shadow from the stone itself will be visible. This usually will appear as a "clean" shadow, as opposed to the "dirty" shadow noted by the reflection from bowel air. Figures 3.33 and 3.34 are of a patient with a large shadow present in the right upper quadrant on ultrasound examination. The longitudinal scan in figure 3.33 demonstrates the clear shadowing behind the gallstone as opposed to the bowel air which has a dirty shadow posteriorly. The border of the gallstone is very difficult to see secondary to its irregular surface. The transverse scan in figure 3.34 again demonstrates the clean shadowing, obscuring visualization of the medial portion of the right kidney, as compared with the dirty shadowing present behind the duodenum.

Figure 3.35 shows another case in which clean shadowing appears again behind a gallstone. This time there is a suggestion of visualization of the anterior border of the gallstone, but the important information here is the contrast to be made between the echoes behind the duodenum, which are secondary to ring down and reverberation, and the extremely clean shadow behind the gallstone.

Figure 3.36 is another example of clean shadowing seen behind a right upper quadrant gallstone. There is only slight suggestion of a curvilinear echo at the superficial border of the gallstone. Without this clean shadowing, the diagnosis easily would be missed. This right upper quadrant finding cannot be overemphasized since many gallbladders completely filled with gallstones will present in this manner.

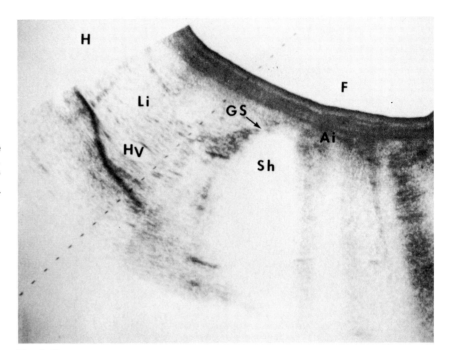

Fig. 3.33

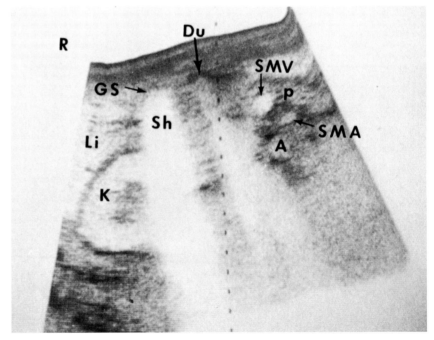

Fig. 3.34

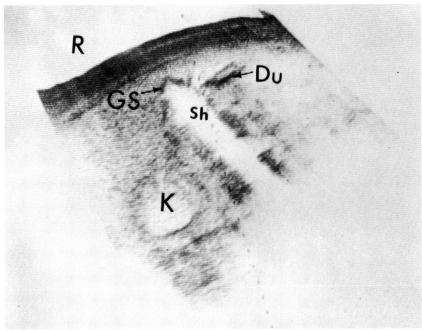

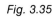
Fig. 3.35

A	=	Aorta
Ai	=	Air
Du	=	Duodenum
F	=	Foot
GS	=	Gallstone
H	=	Head
HV	=	Hepatic vein
K	=	Kidney
Li	=	Liver
P	=	Pancreas
R	=	Right
Sh	=	Shadowing
SMA	=	Superior mesenteric artery
SMV	=	Superior mesenteric vein

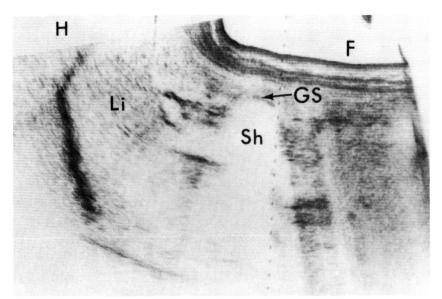

Fig. 3.36

Biliary Sludge

Biliary sludge is similar to a new children's toy called "Slime." Both are a result of modern technology, and until recently, both were unheard of. They can cause abdominal pain in the young to middle-aged woman, but biliary sludge may predispose to stone and, therefore, cause right upper quadrant pain. Slime, in the hands of children, can lead to discolored carpets and also cause abdominal pain in the young mother. Both are thick, viscous, and slow-moving. Therefore, the parallel is significant.

Figures 3.37 and 3.38 are transverse scans of a patient with findings consistent with biliary sludge. On the back wall of the gallbladder is material evident in figure 3.37 as soft echoes. These are consistent with the diagnosis of biliary sludge. There also is fluid in the duodenum. One of the diagnostic features of thick viscous biliary sludge is that it layers out quite slowly. The patient was turned to the left posterior oblique position, and a scan was obtained within a few seconds. Figure 3.38 demonstrates the slow movement of the biliary sludge, which has not layered out immediately.

Figures 3.39 and 3.40 are two more examples of biliary sludge. There the entire posterior half of the gallbladder is filled with echoes compatible with sludge. There is no evidence of shadowing which is consistent with the presence of biliary sludge. The patient was again placed in the decubitus position (fig. 3.40), and there is no evidence of immediate layering of the fluid. This confirms a thickened, viscous material.

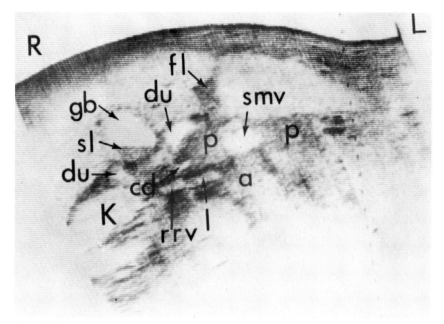

Fig. 3.37

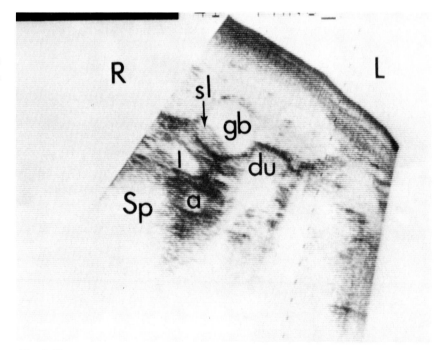

Fig. 3.38

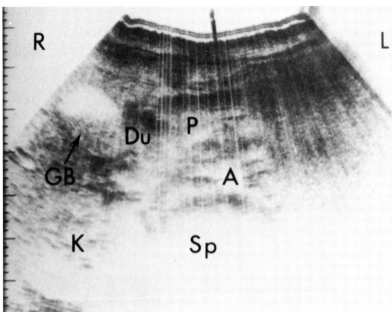

Fig. 3.39

A	=	Aorta
a	=	Aorta
cd	=	Common bile duct
Du	=	Duodenum
du	=	Duodenum
fl	=	Falciform ligament
GB	=	Gallbladder
gb	=	Gallbladder
I	=	Inferior vena cava
K	=	Kidney
L	=	Left
P	=	Pancreas
p	=	Pancreas
R	=	Right
RRV	=	Right renal vein
sl	=	Sludge
SMV	=	Superior mesenteric vein
Sp	=	Spine

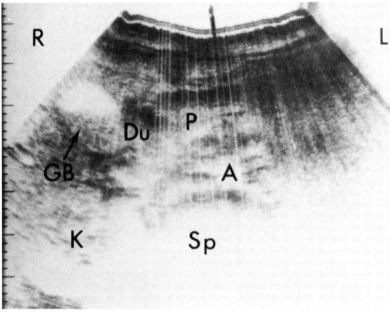

Fig. 3.40

Cholelithiasis Accompanied by Biliary Sludge

It is not unusual to find cholelithiasis in the presence of biliary sludge. The case shown in figures 3.41–3.43 is an example. Figure 3.41 is an excellent example of a gallbladder filled with "alphabet soup." Also noted are gallstones and biliary sludge. The patient was turned to the decubitus position, and the gallstone changed position much more quickly than the biliary sludge (fig. 3.42). The gallstone is notably closer to the fundus of the gallbladder than it is to the biliary sludge when compared with figure 3.41. Note that shadowing is present only behind the gallstone, but is not posterior to the biliary sludge. The transverse section in figure 3.43 was obtained over the area of the sludge, but not the gallstone. The soft echoes in the posterior aspect of the gallbladder do not cast a shadow when they are not over a gallstone.

Figure 3.44 is another example of cholelithiasis accompanied by biliary sludge. The soft echoes on the posterior aspect of the gallbladder wall are secondary to the biliary sludge, and the stronger echo is secondary to a gallstone. Posterior to the gallstone is an acoustic shadow. Shadowing is not present behind biliary sludge. This is important in distinguishing sludge from cholelithiasis.

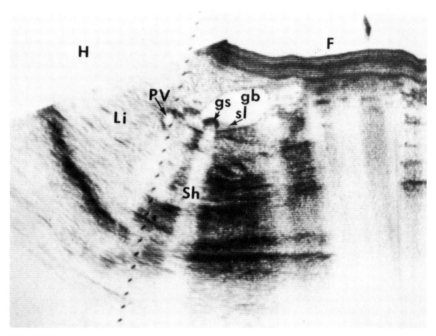

Fig. 3.41

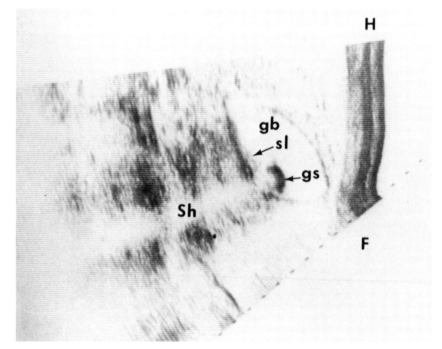

Fig. 3.42

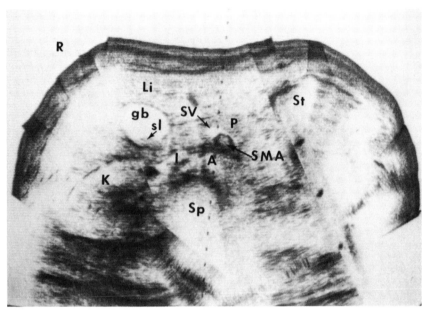

Fig. 3.43

A	=	Aorta
F	=	Foot
GB	=	Gallbladder
gb	=	Gallbladder
GS	=	Gallstone
gs	=	Gallstone
H	=	Head
I	=	Inferior vena cava
K	=	Kidney
Li	=	Liver
P	=	Pancreas
PV	=	Portal vein
R	=	Right
Sh	=	Shadowing
Sl	=	Biliary sludge
sl	=	Biliary sludge
SMA	=	Superior mesenteric artery
Sp	=	Spine
St	=	Stomach
SV	=	Splenic vein

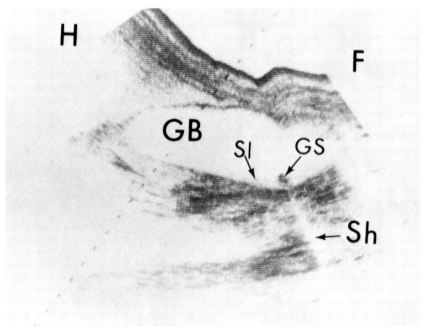

Fig. 3.44

Gallbladder Polyps ; Cholecystitis

Often, internal echoes not secondary to gallstones are noted within the gallbladder. Figure 3.45 is a scan of a patient who had a gallbladder polyp on OCG. There is an internal echo within the gallbladder. Several important features are present which helped to distinguish this from a stone. First, the size of the polyp is approximately 8 mm. Most gallstones of this size will shadow. There is no shadow distal to the gallbladder polyp. This indicates that the polyp is composed of soft tissue. Furthermore, the polyp is notably adherent to the lateral gallbladder wall. If this were a stone, it would most likely be in the dependent portion of the gallbladder adjacent to the posterior wall. Most polyps will present as soft internal echoes within the gallbladder and without evidence of shadowing. By changing the patient's position, in an effort to cause the stone to drop into a dependent position in the gallbladder, the diagnosis of a gallstone can be made. If the internal echo does not fall into a posterior position, the diagnosis of a polyp is quite likely. If there also is a lack of shadowing, we are fairly safe in diagnosing a gallbladder polyp.

Also of interest is the manner in which the scan in figure 3.45 was performed. We can see a small sector scan through an intercostal space, yielding a great deal of information. When we attempted to scan this patient anteriorly we were unable to visualize the gallbladder, due to the fact of overlying bowel air in the hepatic flexure.

Diagnostic ultrasound can assist in the diagnosis of cholecystitis. Very often, a fuzzy irregular wall is present surrounding the gallbladder. In more severe cases, we can actually see a lucent rim outlining the gallbladder wall. This is most likely secondary to severe inflammation and edema. Figure 3.46 is of a 66-year-old man who had a sudden onset of epigastric and right upper quadrant pain just prior to admission. An ultrasound examination demonstrated biliary sludge without evidence of a stone. Of importance was the appearance of the gallbladder wall (arrows). It is markedly thickened with a sonolucent

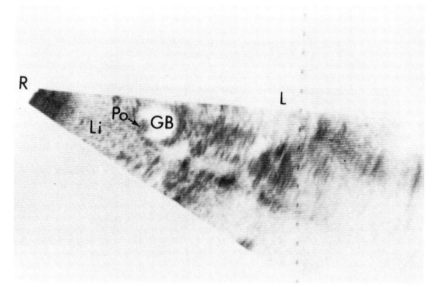

Fig. 3.45

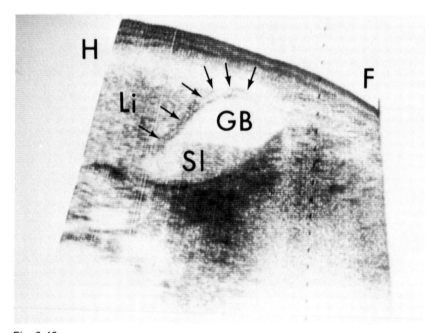

Fig. 3.46

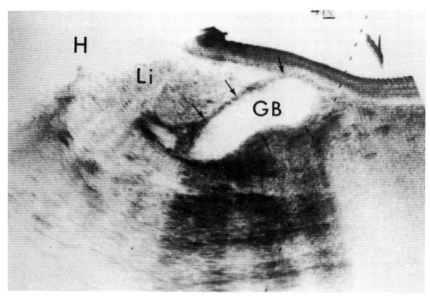

Fig. 3.47

rim outlining the echogenic interior of the gallbladder wall. The findings were compatible with cholecystitis. We did not find any evidence of a stone at the time of examination. The patient was taken to the operating room and a markedly inflamed gallbladder was found, although without evidence of cholelithiasis.

Figures 3.47 and 3.48 are of another patient who underwent surgery for cholecystitis. In this instance, the ultrasound examinations demonstrate a fuzzy thickened ill-defined wall (arrows) of the gallbladder. The lucent rim noted in the previous case is not seen. The gallbladder wall itself, however, is not sharp; it is thickened and slightly irregular. This is seen in both the longitudinal and transverse scans.

Arrows	=	Thickened irregular gallbladder wall consistent with cholecystitis
F	=	Foot
GB	=	Gallbladder
H	=	Head
L	=	Left
Li	=	Liver
Po	=	Gallbladder polyp
R	=	Right
Sl	=	Biliary sludge
Sp	=	Spine
SMV	=	Superior mesenteric vein

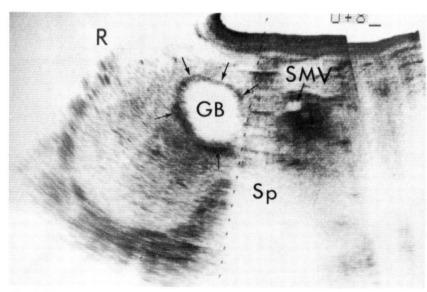

Fig. 3.48

Acute Cholecystitis

Figure 3.49 shows another thickened gallbladder wall. We see a strong linear echo of this wall, which is in contact with the sonolucent bile. The thickness of the gallbladder wall, however, is approximately 3–4 mm, and its rim is much more lucent than we would usually expect. The normal surrounding gallbladder wall is a fairly sharp linear echo. This was consistent with the inflamed gallbladder wall due to cholecystitis, which was found at surgery.

Figures 3.50–3.52 are ultrasound scans from another patient taken a few weeks apart. The patient, a 20-year-old woman, had had a cesarian section three days earlier. One day after the section, she had an episode of epigastric pain which shifted to the right upper quadrant. Subsequently, an ultrasound study was performed on the third postoperative day. Figure 3.50 is a transverse scan of the right upper quadrant. A gallstone near the cystic duct region is present in the gallbladder. Posterior to the gallstone is a shadow. Although the gallbladder wall is not extremely sharp, there is no evidence of marked thickening or lucency around the gallbladder wall. The thickness of the gallbladder wall could be within normal limits. The patient's upper-quadrant pain subsided, and she was discharged home.

Approximately three weeks after the initial scan, she returned to the emergency room with an acute episode of right upper quadrant pain. An ultrasound exam was performed at that time (figs. 3.51 and 3.52), showing evidence of marked gallbladder wall thickening (arrows). This is best seen on the anterior surface of the gallbladder in contact with the liver. The sonolucent rim surrounding the central echogenic gallbladder wall is also noted. This is markedly abnormal, since there should be no sonolucency surrounding the gallbladder wall. The ultrasound findings indicated a gallbladder wall approximately 4–5 mm in thickness. Also noted in figure 3.52 is a strong echo just lateral to the gallbladder. This was secondary to a cystic duct stone. Shadowing is noted posterior to the stone.

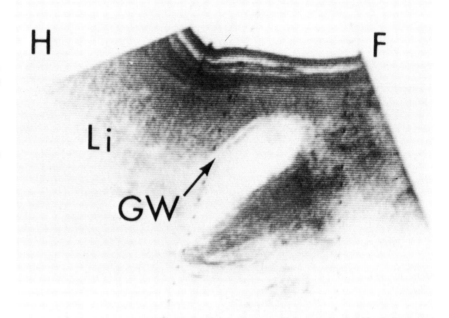

Fig. 3.49

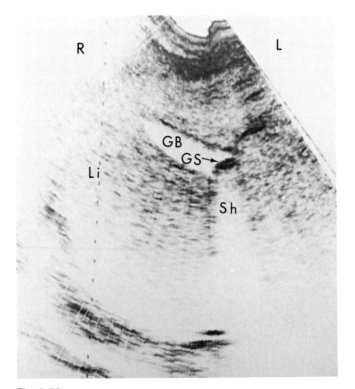

Fig. 3.50

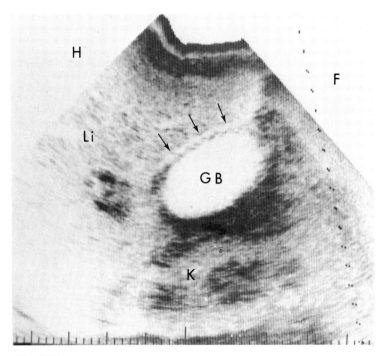

Fig. 3.51

The patient was taken to surgery following the ultrasound examination. Severe acute cholecystitis was present, with a gallbladder wall, which ranged from 3 to 4 mm in thickness. A gallstone was found impacted in the cystic duct; it measured 1.5 cm. This case is an excellent example of the progression of gallbladder wall thickening over a 3-week period, as documented by ultrasound.

Arrows = Markedly thickened gallbladder
wall and acute cholecystitis
F   = Foot
GB   = Gallbladder
GS   = Gallstone
GW   = Thickened gallbladder wall
H   = Head
K   = Kidney
L   = Left
Li   = Liver
R   = Right
Sh   = Shadowing

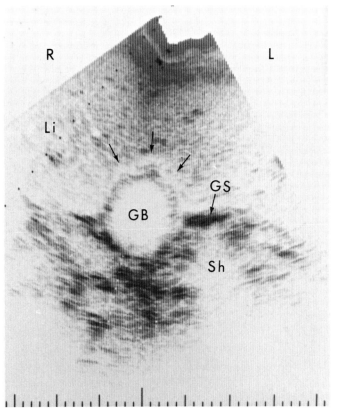

Fig. 3.52

Gangrenous Cholecystitis with Gallbladder Hematoma

The case shown in figures 3.53–3.56 is a 44-year-old man with carcinoma of the cecum. An ultrasonic examination performed near the time of his diagnosis (figs. 3.53 and 3.54) demonstrates a gallbladder in the right upper quadrant. The walls are fairly sharp, and there is no evidence of any internal echoes indicating stones. This was felt to be a normal study. The longitudinal scan in figure 3.53 also demonstrates an interesting finding of pleural fluid in the right lower pleural space. The posterior thoracic wall can be seen due to the fluid in the pleural space. This should not be seen under normal circumstances. The patient underwent a hemicolectomy for his carcinoma of the cecum a few days after the initial ultrasound study.

Approximately six weeks later, the patient experienced sudden onset of abdominal pain, and his white count became elevated. Because of the possibility of a postoperative abscess, an ultrasound study was performed. The findings (figs. 3.55 and 3.56) show a dramatic change in the gallbladder, as compared to the study performed six weeks earlier. The gallbladder is completely filled with echoes, and there is hardly any evidence of sonolucent bile. The walls are minimally thickened, as compared to the previous study. Because of the elevated white blood count and the findings with ultrasound, the patient was taken to the operating room. At operation, a gangrenous gallbladder was found, and on opening the gallbladder, the lumen was entirely filled with a hematoma. This case is an excellent example of the rapid development of cholecystitis followed by hemorrhage into the gallbladder lumen. Figures 3.55 and 3.56 show the soft internal echoes nearly completely filling the gallbladder lumen, secondary to a hematoma.

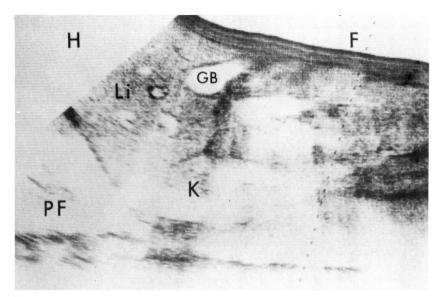

Fig. 3.53

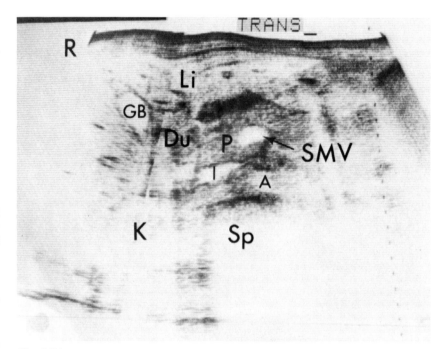

Fig. 3.54

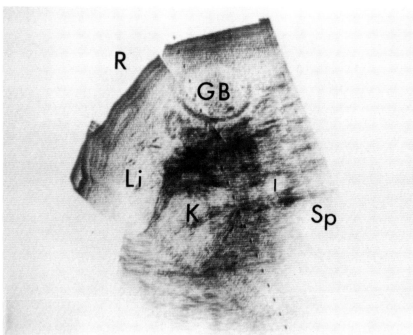

Fig. 3.55

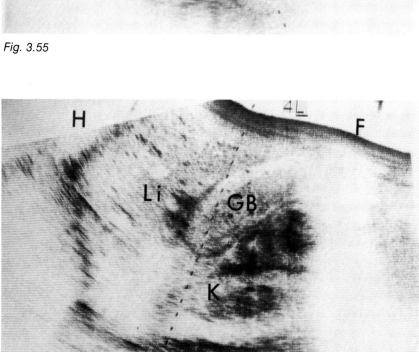

Fig. 3.56

A	=	Aorta
Du	=	Duodenum
F	=	Foot
GB	=	Gallbladder
H	=	Head
I	=	Inferior vena cava
K	=	Kidney
Li	=	Liver
P	=	Pancreas
PF	=	Pleural fluid
R	=	Right
SMV	=	Superior mesenteric vein
Sp	=	Spine

Gallbladder Perforation with Inflammation; Gallbladder Carcinoma

Figure 3.57 is a longitudinal scan of a 32-year-old man with a long history of lupus and steroid treatment. The patient had experienced increasing discomfort in the right upper quadrant for several months. Ultrasound examination demonstrated a gallbladder displaced somewhat posteriorly by a large mass that eventually turned out to be inflammatory tissue from bile perforation. The patient was taken to the operating room, and a gangrenous gallbladder with perforation was noted with marked inflammatory tissue surrounding the gallbladder. This coincided with the ultrasound findings. This case is an example of gangrenous cholecystitis in which perforation produced a mass adjacent to the gallbladder.

Figure 3.58 is a longitudinal scan obtained from a 79-year-old woman who had a three- to four-week history of right-sided abdominal pain, nausea, and vomiting. She also had noticed some recent weight loss. Ultrasound examination demonstrated a large mass in the region of the gallbladder. This mass was solid, since numerous echoes were present. Shadowing noted in the gallbladder bed indicated calcification. The patient was taken to the operating room, and she was found to have gallbladder carcinoma which was actually metastatic squamous cell carcinoma. The primary tumor was unknown. Necrosis within the gallbladder tumor was evident.

Figures 3.59 and 3.60 are ultrasound scans of a 77-year-old woman who had right upper quadrant pain that had become progressively worse over a two- to three-week period. Ultrasound examinations demonstrated a solid mass in the gallbladder bed (arrows). The mass was solid in nature; echoes were noted throughout. The longitudinal scan in figure 3.60 demonstrates the gallbladder mass situated anterior to the kidney. The patient was taken to the operating room where an adenocarcinoma of the gallbladder was found. Figures 3.58–3.60 are examples of solid masses with-

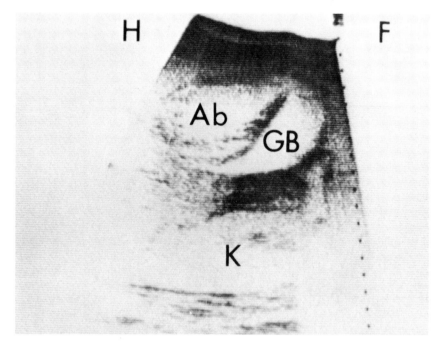

Fig. 3.57

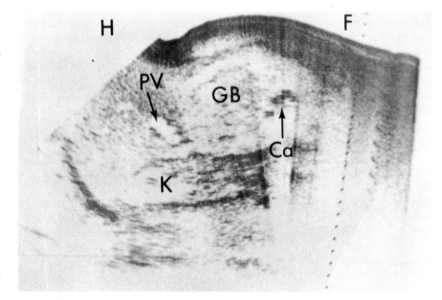

Fig. 3.58

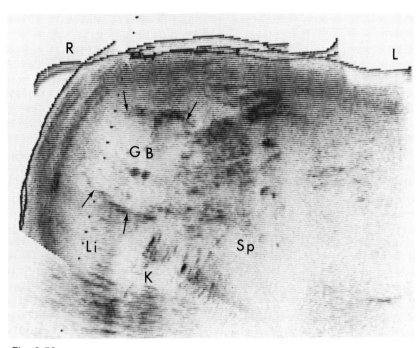

Fig. 3.59

in the gallbladder bed. The possibility of severe cholecystitis could not be ruled out.

Ab	=	Adjacent abscess
Ca	=	Calcification
F	=	Foot
GB	=	Gallbladder
GB and arrows	=	Gallbladder carcinoma
H	=	Head
K	=	Kidney
L	=	Left
Li	=	Liver
PV	=	Portal vein
R	=	Right
Sp	=	Spine

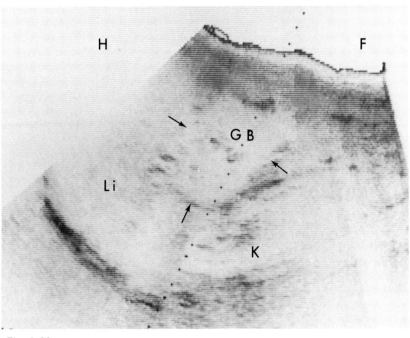

Fig. 3.60

Normal Biliary System

In examination of the biliary system, it is important to understand the anatomy of the portal venous system. Normally, the portal venous system yields the largest tubular structures within the parenchyma of the liver. These vessels are surrounded by strong echoes arising from the fibrous tissue. The hepatic veins are the second tubular structures seen within the liver. They have less of an echogenic surrounding because there is less fibrous tissue. We do not usually see the biliary system within the parenchyma of the liver. When, on occasion, it is visualized within the parenchyma of the liver, it presents as a second tubular structure, adjacent to the portal venous system yielding the "parallel channel" sign.

Figures 3.61 and 3.62 are transverse sections of the same patient and demonstrate the normal anatomy of the portal venous system. The vertical lines, numbered 1–4, correspond to the longitudinal scans in figures 3.63–3.66.

The main portal vein is formed by the left portal vein and the right portal vein. Figure 3.61 shows bifurcation of the right portal vein in the lateral aspect of the right lobe of the liver. Figure 3.63 is a longitudinal scan corresponding to the vertical line, number 1, in figure 3.61. In figure 3.63 we see bifurcation of the right portal vein. This is important to recognize so as not to misdiagnose biliary dilatation. The longitudinal scans should demonstrate a second tubular structure, parallel to the portal vein, which will aid in the diagnosis of biliary obstruction. We do, however, see bifurcation of the portal venous system at certain anatomical sites. Peripheral bifurcation at one of these sites is seen at the right portal vein. If we follow the right portal vein medially, we will see only one circular structure in the porta hepatis. Figure 3.64 is a longitudinal scan corresponding to the vertical line, number 2, in figure 3.61. Here we see the juncture of the right portal vein as it approaches a single circular structure.

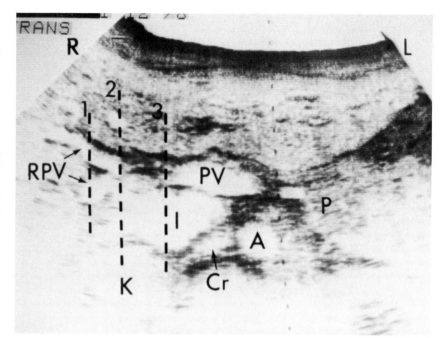

Fig. 3.61

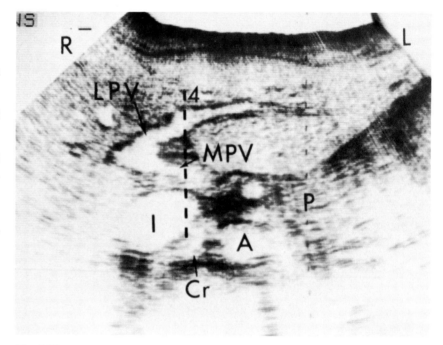

Fig. 3.62

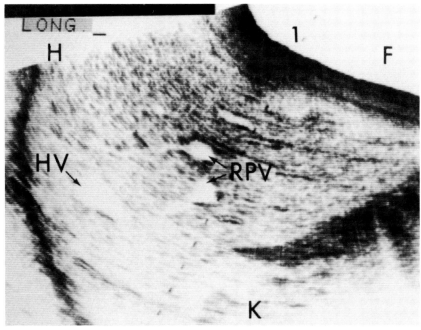

Fig. 3.63

A	=	Aorta
Cr	=	Crus of the diaphragm
F	=	Foot
4	=	longitudinal scan corresponding to figure 3.66
H	=	Head
HV	=	Hepatic vein
I	=	Inferior vena cava
K	=	Kidney
L	=	Left
LPV	=	Left portal vein
MPV	=	Main portal vein
1	=	longitudinal scan corresponding to figure 3.63
P	=	Pancreas
PV	=	Portal vein
R	=	Right
RPV	=	Right portal vein
2	=	longitudinal scan corresponding to figure 3.64
3	=	longitudinal scan corresponding to figure 3.65

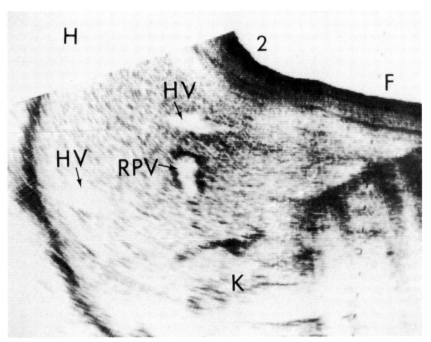

Fig. 3.64

Normal Biliary System

Figure 3.65 is a longitudinal scan through the liver corresponding to the vertical line, number 3, in figure 3.61. Here we are scanning through the main portion of the right portal vein, which appears as a single circular sonolucency. This is the important part of an examination to rule out biliary obstruction. At this point, we should see only one circular sonolucency on longitudinal scans within the porta hepatis. This corresponds to that segment of the right portal vein before bifurcation and before the left portal vein can be seen. If we do not see a single circular sonolucency, but instead see two or three, we have evidence consistent with biliary obstruction. As we move medially, we will see two circular sonolucencies once we encounter the left portal vein (fig. 3.66). Figure 3.66 is a longitudinal scan corresponding to the vertical line, number 4, in figure 3.62. The left portal vein is situated anterior to the main portal vein. Again, there are two circular sonolucencies. This is a normal finding and not to be mistaken for biliary obstruction.

This conception of the portal venous system is extremely important in order not to misdiagnose biliary obstruction. There are certain anatomical positions where two large circular sonolucencies on longitudinal scans, corresponding to bifurcations in the portal venous system, can be seen. The segment of the right portal vein where we should see only a single sonolucency on longitudinal scan corresponds to figure 3.65. It is important to look for this site in order to rule out biliary obstruction. If two circular sonolucencies of approximately the same size are seen consistently, biliary obstruction is most likely present.

Transverse scans in the region of the porta hepatis often demonstrate several circular sonolucencies situated anterior to the portal vein. Figures 3.67 and 3.68 examplify this. Usually the hepatic artery is the medial sonolucency, with the common bile duct or common hepatic duct representing the lateral sonolucency. Ordinarily, these are only 3–4 mm in diameter. If they are greater in size, then obstruction should be sus-

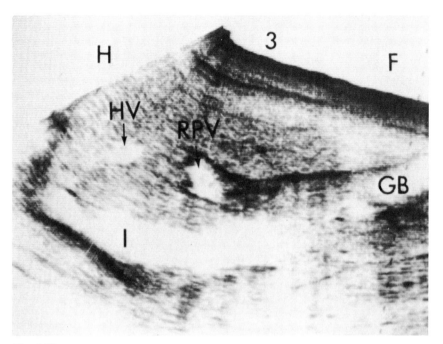

Fig. 3.65

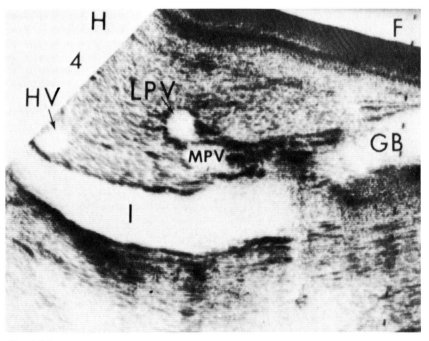

Fig. 3.66

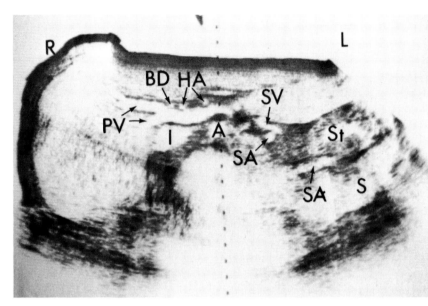

Fig. 3.67

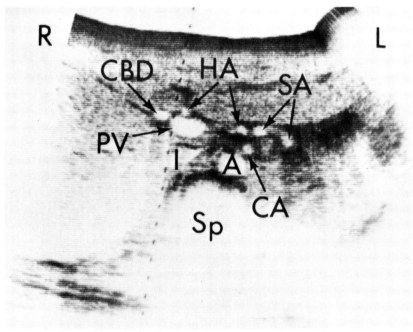

Fig. 3.68

pected. The portal vein is the larger sonolucency noted posteriorly. This is best evident in figure 3.68 which demonstrates the portal triad of the common bile duct, hepatic artery, and portal vein.

A	=	Aorta
BD	=	Bile duct
CA	=	Celiac axis
CBD	=	Common bile duct
F	=	Foot
4	=	longitudinal scan corresponding to the vertical line in figure 3.62
GB	=	Gallbladder
H	=	Head
HA	=	Hepatic artery
HV	=	Hepatic vein
I	=	Inferior vena cava
L	=	Left
LPV	=	Left portal vein
MPV	=	Main portal vein
PV	=	Portal vein
RPV	=	Right portal vein
S	=	Spleen
SA	=	Splenic artery
Sp	=	Spine
St	=	Stomach
SV	=	Splenic vein
3	=	longitudinal scan corresponding to the vertical line in figure 3.61

Normal Biliary System

Transverse scans of the porta hepatis are continued in a caudal direction until the head of the pancreas is visualized. Occasionally, a circular sonolucency corresponding to the common bile duct can be seen just lateral to the head of the pancreas. Often, however, this is obscured by air in the duodenum. The upper normal limits for the common bile duct in a patient who has not had a previous cholecystectomy is in the range of 6–7 mm. Figure 3.69 is a transverse scan with the common bile duct and gastroduodenal artery situated between the duodenum and head of the pancreas. The lumen of this common bile duct measures approximately 3–4 mm, measuring only the sonolucent portion. This is within normal limits. In a patient who has had a cholecystectomy the common bile duct can be larger without obstruction present. We are presently using 1 cm as the upper limit of normal in those instances, but more data is necessary. Obstruction of the common bile duct often can be seen in this area and will present as a large circular sonolucency just lateral to the head of the pancreas.

It is important to attempt to visualize the common bile duct on longitudinal scans. Figure 3.70 is a longitudinal scan in the region of the porta hepatis in which we see the common hepatic duct anterior to the portal vein. The common hepatic duct is draped over the portal vein and begins its course posteriorly, so that it may end up posterior and lateral to the head of the pancreas. Figure 3.71 is a longitudinal scan which demonstrates the common bile duct coursing more posteriorly and situated behind the head of the pancreas. A tubular sonolucency, coursing anterior to the head of the pancreas, is secondary to the gastroduodenal artery. These two tubular structures surround the head of the pancreas on longitudinal scans and provide excellent anatomical landmarks. The common bile duct in this case (fig. 3.71) is approximately 2–3 mm in diameter. Figure 3.72 is another example of the common bile duct and gastroduodenal artery surrounding the head of the pancreas. The common bile

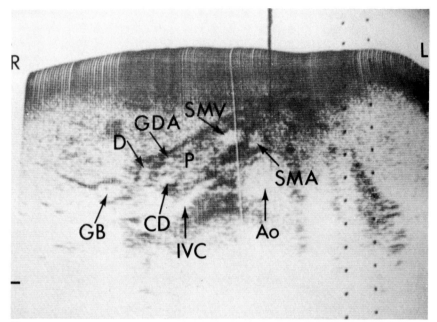

Fig. 3.69

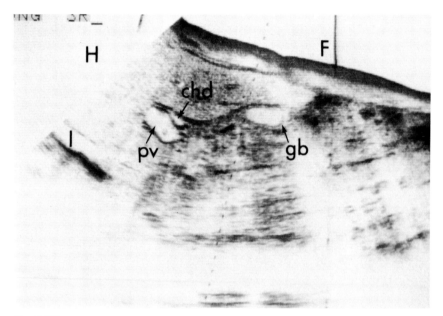

Fig. 3.70

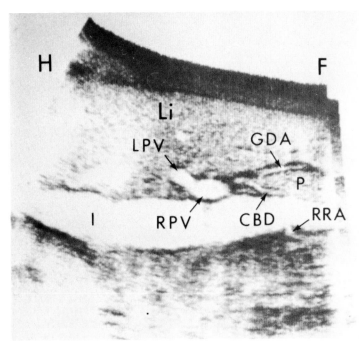

Fig. 3.71

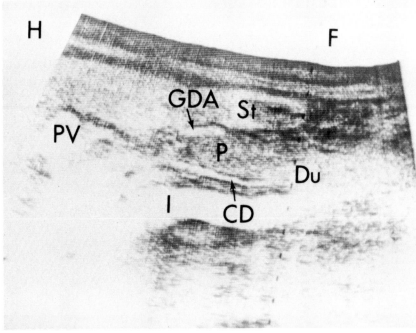

Fig. 3.72

duct here is approximately 2–3 mm in diameter, within the normal range. The common bile duct courses anterior to the portal vein and dips posteriorly behind the head of the pancreas, frequently just anterior to the inferior vena cava. In order to confirm the diagnosis of biliary obstruction, it is necessary to visualize the common bile duct in longitudinal scans draping over the portal vein and posterior to the pancreas. The technologist must be certain he or she is not visualizing the superior mesenteric vein.

A	=	Aorta
CBD	=	Common bile duct
CD	=	Common bile duct
chd	=	Common hepatic duct
D	=	Duodenum
Du	=	Duodenum
F	=	Foot
GB	=	Gallbladder
gb	=	Gallbladder
GDA	=	Gastroduodenal artery
H	=	Head
I	=	Inferior vena cava
L	=	Left
Li	=	Liver
LPV	=	Left portal vein
P	=	Pancreas
PV	=	Portal vein
pv	=	Portal vein
R	=	Right
RPV	=	Right portal vein
RRA	=	Right renal artery
SMA	=	Superior mesenteric artery
SMV	=	Superior mesenteric vein
St	=	Stomach

Biliary Obstruction

When biliary obstruction is present, a second tubular structure adjacent to the portal vein will be identified. This has been described as the "parallel channel" sign. Figure 3.73 is an example of this sign in a patient with extrahepatic jaundice secondary to choledocholithiasis. The portal vein is seen posterior to a second tubular structure that represents a dilated intrahepatic biliary duct. Normally, only the portal vein would be seen, without evidence of the second tubular structure anterior to it.

Very often, the dilated biliary ducts present as knobby irregular branching tubular patterns within the liver. Usually, the portal venous system has a fairly even, smooth, branching pattern. Figure 3.74 is an example of a dilated biliary tree secondary to carcinoma of the pancreas in a 53-year-old man. The tubular structures within the liver have a "knotty" appearance, rather than the even branching noted in the normal portal venous system.

Figure 3.75 shows a 64-year-old woman who also had carcinoma of the head of the pancreas. Again, an irregular "knotty" appearance to the dilated bile ducts is noted in the anterior half of the liver on this longitudinal scan. The common bile duct is also markedly dilated. This was approximately 2 cm in diameter.

Figure 3.76 is a transverse section near the region of the head of the pancreas. The portal triad is seen with the portal vein noted posteriorly. Anterior and medial to the portal vein is the hepatic artery. Lateral and anterior to the portal vein is the dilated common bile duct. The portal triad is easily recognized within the porta hepatis of the liver. The common bile duct should be approximately the size of the hepatic artery or slightly smaller. Here it is approximately 2–3 times the size of the hepatic artery. The pancreas is less echogenic than the liver. This is consistent with pancreatitis which was the cause of the biliary obstruction (see chapter 4).

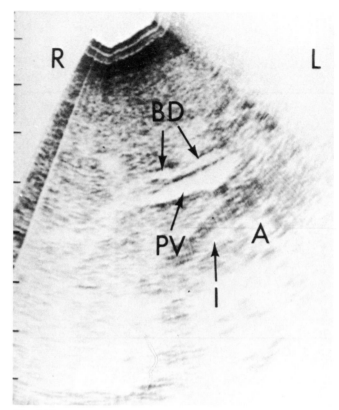

Fig. 3.73

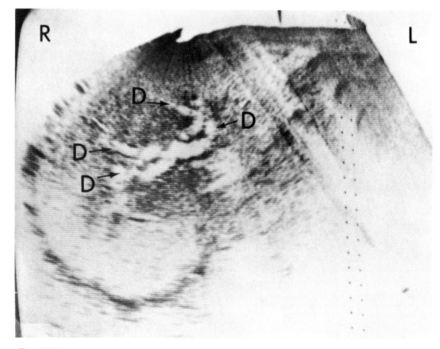

Fig. 3.74

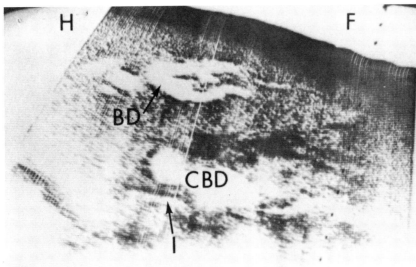

A   = Aorta
BD = Dilated bile ducts
CBD = Common bile duct
D   = Dilated bile ducts
F   = Foot
H   = Head
HA = Hepatic artery
I   = Inferior vena cava
K   = Kidney
L   = Left
P   = Pancreas
PV = Portal vein
R   = Right
SMA = Superior mesenteric artery

Fig. 3.75

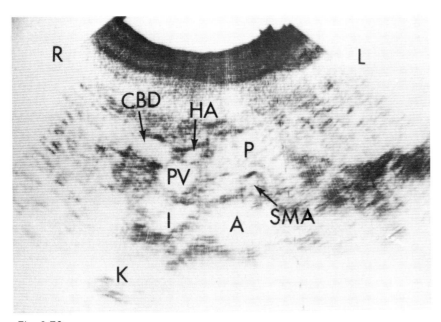

Fig. 3.76

Biliary Obstruction Secondary to Choledocholithiasis

Figures 3.77–3.80 are of a 26-year-old woman with an 8-day history of right upper quadrant pain. Two days prior to admission, she developed nausea and vomiting. Transverse scans demonstrated dilated biliary ducts within the liver (fig. 3.77). The portal vein is well seen. Anterior to the portal vein is a second tubular structure representing a dilated bile duct. Also noted more peripherally in the liver are numerous dilated tubular structures (arrows) which represent further dilatation of the bile duct within the liver. Transverse scans were continued more caudally to determine the level of the obstruction. Figure 3.78 is a transverse section near the head of the pancreas. A circular sonolucency is noted anterior to the inferior vena cava and secondary to a markedly dilated common bile duct. The relative size of the common bile duct when compared to the aorta and the superior mesenteric vein is of interest. It measured 1.2 × 1.4 cm at this level.

A longitudinal scan through the dilated common bile duct was obtained and is present in figure 3.79. A large tubular structure representing the dilated common bile duct is noted posterior to the head of the pancreas. Again, the dilated biliary structures within the liver (arrows) are readily seen on this longitudinal section. The obstruction was secondary to choledocholithiasis. A longitudinal scan of the gallbladder in figure 3.80 demonstrates multiple gallstones.

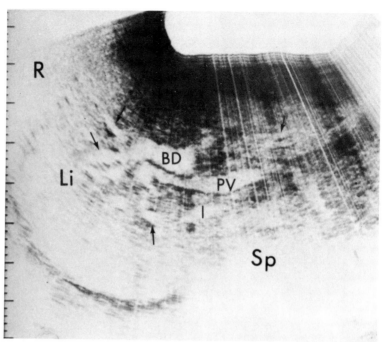

Fig. 3.77

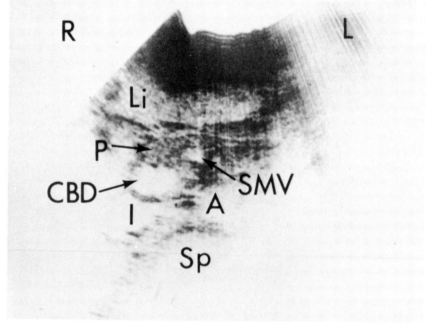

Fig. 3.78

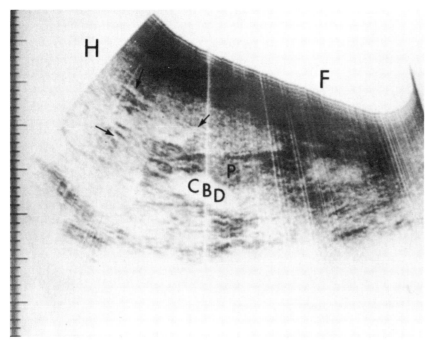

A	=	Aorta
Arrows	=	Dilated bile duct
BD	=	Dilated bile duct
CBD	=	Dilated common bile duct
F	=	Foot
GB	=	Gallbladder
GS	=	Gallstones
H	=	Head
I	=	Inferior vena cava
K	=	Kidney
L	=	Left
Li	=	Liver
P	=	Pancreas
PV	=	Portal vein
R	=	Right
Sh	=	Shadowing
SMV	=	Superior mesenteric vein
Sp	=	Spine
Tt	=	Through transmission between the gallstones

Fig. 3.79

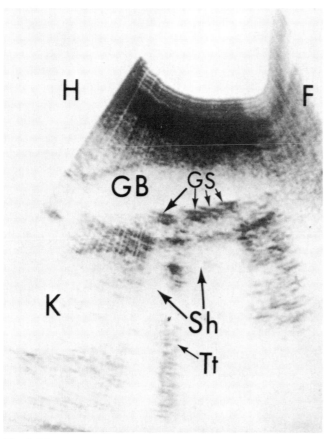

Fig. 3.80

Biliary Obstruction with Choledocholithiasis

This 20-year-old woman was 10 weeks pregnant. She had experienced colicky right upper quadrant pain for 4 weeks. This was episodic in nature and usually came after eating. Ultrasound exam demonstrated a dilated biliary tree which is seen in a transverse section of the liver (fig. 3.81). The portal vein is seen on transverse section with a dilated biliary duct situated anterior to it. A transverse scan more caudal and near the region of the head of the pancreas (fig. 3.82) indicated a circular sonolucency lateral to the head of the pancreas, measuring approximately 15 mm, and representing a dilated common bile duct. A longitudinal scan following this circular structure is seen in figure 3.83. The common bile duct is seen nearly in its entirety with a circular echo noted in its distal portion. This circular echo was found at surgery to be a common bile duct stone.

It is interesting to realize that during the early part of ultrasound examination the patient experienced a large amount of pain and that the transverse scan in figure 3.82 was obtained while the patient was in a great deal of pain. During the latter half of the ultrasound examination, the patient volunteered the fact that the pain had disappeared. Because of this, a repeat transverse scan was obtained.

Figure 3.84 is a transverse section near the head of the pancreas obtained a few minutes after figure 3.82. The only difference was the cessation of the patient's pain. The common bile duct is still visible adjacent to the head of the pancreas. It has, however, decreased dramatically in size, as compared to figure 3.82. Figure 3.84 demonstrates a common bile duct approximately 9 mm in diameter. The patient had most likely decompressed herself during the course of the examination and thereby relieved her pain temporarily. This surely is a therapeutic triumph for ultrasound.

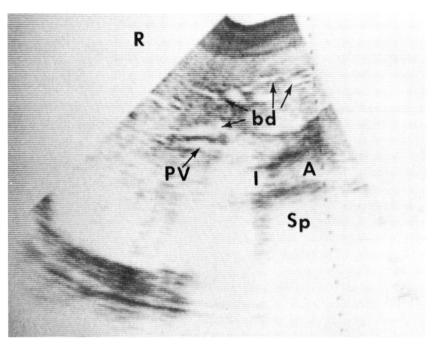

Fig. 3.81

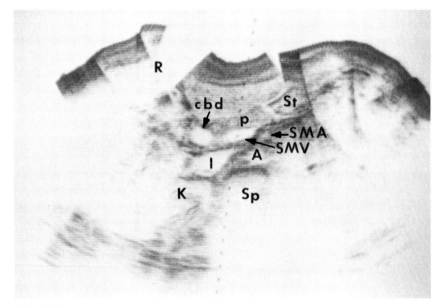

Fig. 3.82

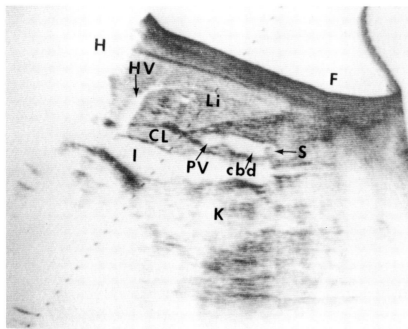

Fig. 3.83

A   = Aorta
BD   = Dilated bile duct
cbd = Common bile duct
CL   = Caudate lobe
Cr   = Crus of the diaphragm
F   = Foot
H   = Head
HV   = Hepatic vein
I   = Inferior vena cava
K   = Kidney
Li   = Liver
LRV = Left renal vein
P   = Pancreas
PV   = Portal vein
R   = Right
S   = Stone
SC   = Spinal canal
SMA = Superior mesenteric artery
SMV = Superior mesenteric vein
Sp   = Spine
St   = Stomach

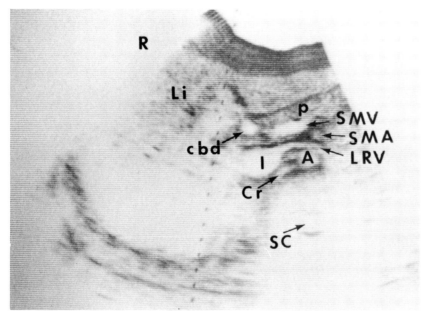

Fig. 3.84

Biliary Duct Stones ;
Biliary Duct Air

Figures 3.85–3.87 are from an unusual 14-year-old patient who had multiple abdominal aneurysms present on angiography. After an upper-GI bleed, surgery was performed, and a large hepatic artery aneurysm with fistula formation to the common bile duct was found. The aneurysm was resected. A choledochojejeunostomy was performed. Approximately 6 months after the surgery, the patient returned, and an ultrasound examination was performed. Figures 3.85–3.87 are scans from that examination. We see evidence of a dilated biliary tree in figure 3.85. Also noted within the dilated biliary segments are circular and oval internal echoes consistent with intrahepatic bile stones. A transverse scan, a little more cephalad than figure 3.85, was performed. Figure 3.86 demonstrates a strong echo arising from a bile stone; posterior to this stone is shadowing. Figure 3.87 is a longitudinal scan which again demonstrates a dilated bile duct with stones present. The patient had an intravenous cholangiogram in which numerous biliary stones were noted, corresponding to the ultrasound findings.

Figure 3.88 is a transverse scan obtained from an 83-year-old man with a history of cholelithiasis. As a result, a cholecystectomy had been performed along with a choledochojejeunostomy, 3 years previously. Since that time there had been repeated episodes of ascending cholangitis. The patient was found to have had reflux of intestinal contents into the biliary tree which had resulted in cholangitis. In numerous instances, air also was noted in the biliary tree. Figure 3.88 is a transverse section of the liver with numerous strong circular echoes (arrows). These findings were consistent with the X-ray findings of air in the biliary tree. Air in the biliary system will yield high-amplitude echoes similar to stones.

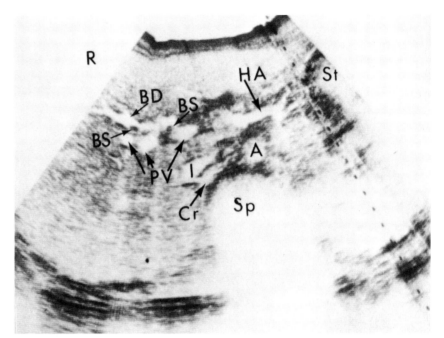

Fig. 3.85

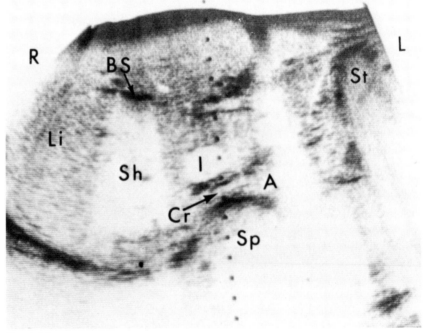

Fig. 3.86

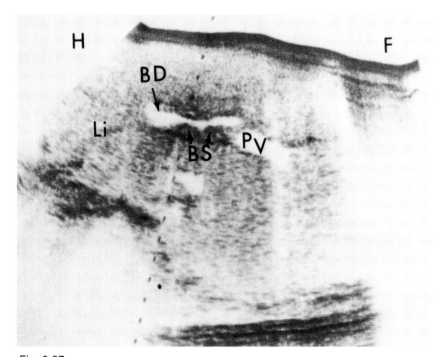

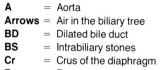

A   = Aorta
Arrows = Air in the biliary tree
BD   = Dilated bile duct
BS   = Intrabiliary stones
Cr   = Crus of the diaphragm
F   = Foot
H   = Head
HA   = Hepatic artery
I   = Inferior vena cava
L   = Left
Li   = Liver
PV   = Portal vein
R   = Right
Sh   = Shadowing behind the biliary
             stones
Sp   = Spine
St   = Stomach

Fig. 3.87

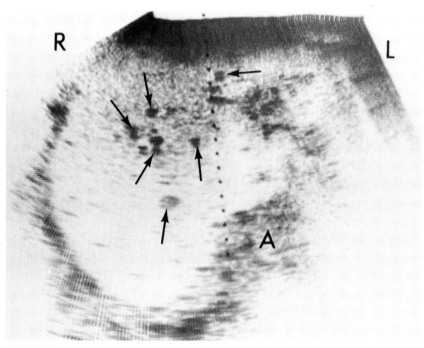

Fig. 3.88

Choledochal Cyst ; Congenital Stenosis of the Common Hepatic Duct

Figures 3.89 and 3.90 are ultrasound scans of a 2-month-old female infant who had experienced jaundice since birth. A rose-bengal study suggested obstruction of the bile ducts. Ultrasound examinations (figs. 3.89 and 3.90) showed a sonolucency near the region of the common bile duct. This sonolucent area was situated just lateral to the pancreas, as is best seen in the transverse scan (fig. 3.89). There was no evidence of marked biliary dilatation. The patient was taken to surgery, and a 1-cm choledochal cyst contiguous with the cystic duct was found. The gallbladder at the time of surgery was notably atretic and contracted.

Figures 3.91 and 3.92 are ultrasound scans obtained from a 22-year-old woman with a recent onset of pruritus and jaundice. She was initially felt to have jaundice secondary to hepatitis. An ultrasound examination, however, demonstrated two large fluid-filled masses in the porta hepatis. Figure 3.91 is a transverse scan in which we see two large dilated ducts situated anterior to the portal vein. Figure 3.92 is a longitudinal scan again showing the dilated ducts anterior to the left portal vein. The patient went to surgery and was found to have congenital stenosis of the common hepatic duct. This stenotic lesion led to massive dilatation of the right and left intrahepatic ducts which yielded the sonolucencies on ultrasound. We can see through transmission behind these ducts on both the transverse and longitudinal scans.

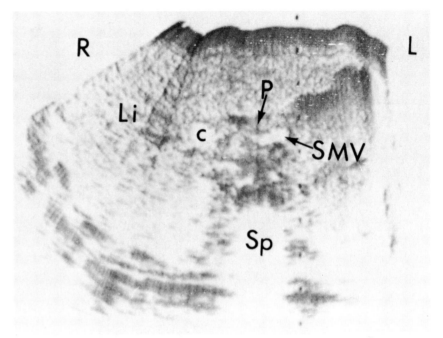

Fig. 3.89

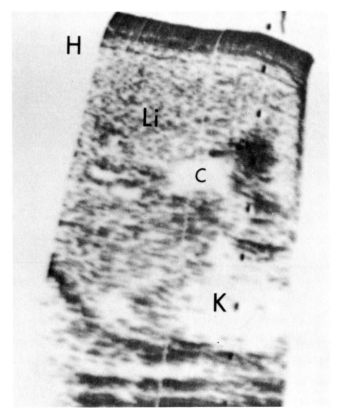

Fig. 3.90

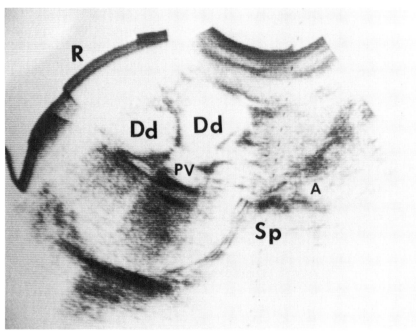

Fig. 3.91

A = Aorta
c = Choledochal cyst
Dd = Dilated intrahepatic ducts
F = Foot
H = Head
I = Inferior vena cava
K = Kidney
L = Left
Li = Liver
LPV = Left portal vein
MPV = Main portal vein
P = Pancreas
PV = Portal vein
R = Right
SMV = Superior mesenteric vein
Sp = Spine
St = Stomach

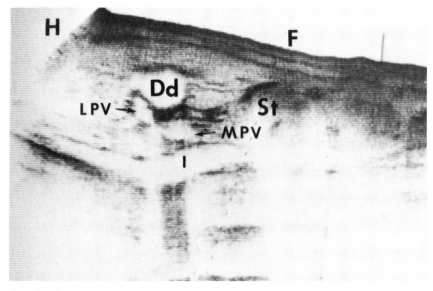

Fig. 3.92

4.
Ultrasonography of the Pancreas

Dennis A. Sarti, M.D.

Introduction

The pancreas is a retroperitoneal organ that has remained hidden to most imaging techniques. An upper-gastrointestinal series is the study most often requested to evaluate pancreatic masses. When pancreatic masses impinge upon the gastrointestinal tract, however, only the "tip of the iceberg" can be seen, and the normal pancreas cannot be visualized by this method. Pancreatic isotope studies also can delineate pancreatic masses, but resolution with this technique is less than optimal, and patchy uptake of the isotope leads to false-positive diagnoses. Selective angiography is another modality used in examination of the pancreas. It gives excellent visualization of this organ. Pancreatic masses and abnormal vascularity are easily detected with the high quality of angiography performed at most centers today. Two drawbacks to this technique, however, still remain. The first is the inherent risk, and the second is the inability routinely to perform serial examinations on patients with suspected pancreatic pathology.

Computed axial tomography (CAT scanning) is a recent technological advance which has increased our ability to visualize the pancreas. It permits direct visualization of the pancreas in both its normal and abnormal states. It is technically easy to perform, and bone and air do not obscure adequate visualization. The disadvantages of CAT scanning are related to cost, ionizing radiation, and the thinness of patients.

Diagnostic ultrasound also permits direct visualization of the pancreas. As with the procedures already mentioned, it has both advantages and disadvantages. Major advantages are that the pancreas can be seen in its normal state and that ultrasound gives information different from X-rays, since it is dealing with acoustic properties. Tissue echogenicity is an important aid in differentiating various masses. As opposed to CAT scanning, thinner patients yield the highest-quality scans. The major disadvantage of ultrasound is related to its high reflectivity at bone and air interfaces. Adequate visualization of the pancreas is often obscured by ribs, stomach, and colon. Even with its inherent drawbacks, diagnostic ultrasound has found an important role in the workup of a patient with suspected pancreatic pathology. Its noninvasive aspect makes serial examination possible, and this allows us to follow the progress of pathological states. Tissue character information can also narrow the diagnostic possibilities.

Normal Anatomy

In a discussion of pancreatic ultrasound examination technique, an anatomical review of those structures adjacent to the pancreas is important. Increased resolution through the development of gray scale and improved transducer technology allows visualization of small, 2–3 mm structures and gives a characteristic echo pattern of the normal pancreas.

Numerous vascular structures are situated in close proximity to the pancreas, and their identification is necessary for adequate localization. Important branches of the aorta to be identified are the celiac axis, hepatic artery, splenic artery, gastroduodenal artery, superior mesenteric artery, and bilateral renal arteries. The celiac axis arises just cephalad to the superior portion of the body of the pancreas and then divides into three major branches: (1) left gastric, (2) common hepatic, and (3) splenic. The first branch of the common hepatic artery is the gastroduodenal artery which courses anterior to the common bile duct and gives off the pancreaticoduodenal artery on the medial aspect of the second portion of the duodenum, adjacent to the head of the pancreas. The splenic artery courses from the celiac axis to the spleen, usually on the dorsal cephalic surface of the pancreas to which it gives off numerous branches. The pancreas is often 1–2 cm caudal to the splenic artery and need not be situated directly anterior to this vessel. The superior mesenteric artery originates at the aorta, approximately 1–2 cm below the celiac axis. It courses inferiorly on the posterior aspect of the junction of the head and body of the pancreas and passes anterior to the uncinate process and third portion of the duodenum. Except for the uncinate process, the pancreas lies anterior to the proximal portion and origin of the superior mesenteric artery. The renal arteries arise from the lateral aspect of the aorta, below the origin of the superior mesenteric artery, and posterior to the head and body of the pancreas.

The portal venous system provides several easily identifiable vessels adjacent to the pancreas that run parallel to smaller arterial structures. The splenic vein arises from the hilum of the spleen and courses from left to right, indenting the superior posterior aspect of the pancreas. It is situated posteriorly from the mid portion to the superior aspect of the pancreas, but seldom on its inferior portion. In these situations the pancreas is directly anterior to the splenic vein. The splenic vein, however, is often found cephalad to the pancreas, and transverse scans must be obtained slightly inferior to the splenic vein in order to detect pancreatic tissue.

The superior mesenteric vein drains the intestines and courses superiorly just to the right of the superior mesenteric artery. Parallel to the artery, it travels anterior to the third portion of the duodenum and uncinate process and posterior to the junction of the head and body of the pancreas. Near the origin of the superior mesenteric artery, the superior mesenteric vein joins the splenic vein, and this confluence of vessels forms the portal vein. The portal vein is approximately 8 cm in length and courses superiorly and to the right, after its formation by the splenic and superior mesenteric veins. It travels upward behind the superior part of the duodenum and enters the porta hepatis posterior to the common bile duct and hepatic artery. As it enters the liver, it divides into right and left with the corresponding branches of the hepatic artery and biliary tree.

The inferior vena cava is situated anterior to the right side of the vertebral bodies and to the right of the aorta. It courses posterior to the duodenum, head of the pancreas, portal vein, and common bile duct. The left renal vein drains the left kidney and courses directly anterior to the aorta just beneath the origin of the superior mesenteric artery. This vessel has a curvilinear shape similar to the splenic vein, with which it may be confused. The left renal vein, however, is in close proximity to the anterior surface of the aorta beneath the superior mesenteric artery, whereas the splenic vein is situated anterior to the superior mesenteric artery. These vessels also can be distinguished by the vessels into which they drain; the left renal vein empties into the inferior vena cava, and the splenic vein empties into the portal vein.

These vessels are important because of their close proximity to the pancreas. Easy recognition of these vessels greatly enhances a pancreatic examination by accurately demarcating the pancreatic bed. Other structures demonstrated by ultrasound can delineate the region of the pancreas. The antrum of the stomach appears as a "bullseye" on a B-scan when it is airless, and the pancreas is often seen directly posterior to this or slightly cephalad and posterior. The C-loop of the duodenum nestles the head of the pancreas and often obscures visualization when it is air-filled. The pancreatic tail is difficult to visualize with the patient in the supine position. This is secondary to the position of the fundus of the stomach and splenic flexure, which are often air-filled. The tail of the pancreas is situated directly anterior to the left kidney and continues on into the hilum of the spleen. This anatomic relation allows visualization of the tail of the pancreas through the left kidney with the patient in the prone position.

Ultrasound Technique for Pancreatic Examination

What is appropriate patient preparation for a pancreatic exam? How do you get rid of bowel air? These questions are repeatedly asked by individuals performing pancreatic studies. There is no really good patient preparation for a pancreatic exam, although various procedures are attempted. Adequate patient hydration is helpful in yielding high-quality studies (Leopold 1975a), but the difficulty in visualizing the pancreas because of bowel air is mainly due to patient anatomy. Those patients with a transverse stomach are difficult to scan, because this air-filled viscus is directly anterior to the pancreas. A small or truncated left lobe of the liver is another important anatomic variant which yields nondiagnostic studies, since we are using the left lobe as an ultrasonic window. Since air is the major culprit in deteriorating a pancreatic scan, the patient is scheduled for examination in the early morning and kept without oral intake to prevent air swallowing. We have had limited success using nasogastric suction overnight on inpatients who have had previously unsuccessful examinations. Others have reported success with the patient drinking large quantities of water prior to the study. We have attempted immobilizing the bowel with glucagon, followed by the ingestion of large quantities of water. This has been unsuccessful since the dilated bowel tends to have large air pockets situated anteriorly. Limited success has been reported using simethicone and other drugs (Sommer and Filly 1977). To date, these numerous efforts have been disappointing. A successful study is most dependent on individual patient anatomy. Ultrasound usually is performed prior to barium examinations because of the high reflectivity of barium (Leopold and Asher 1971). Some penetration is possible if the barium-filled bowel is long-standing (Sarti and Lazere 1978).

The patient is initially scanned in the supine position with adequate mineral oil applied to the upper abdomen for acoustic coupling. Before searching for the pancreas it is important that the output and sensitivity settings are adjusted to yield maximum information from the reflected pancreatic echoes (Filly and Carlsen 1976). This is best accomplished by observing liver echogenicity.

The pancreas is usually slightly more echogenic than the liver; this is due to the greater amount of fibrous tissue. With the liver echo registering in the higher shades of gray, the pancreatic echoes will be in the darkest or highest shade. They will blend in with the high-amplitude echoes of the surrounding fatty retroperitoneum, and the pancreas will be lost. Therefore, when doing a pancreatic exam, it is important to adjust the settings so that the liver echoes are registering in the middle to lighter shades. Thus, the pancreas will register one to two shades darker than the liver but will not be viewed in the darkest shade.

Should compound or single-sector scanning be used? It is important to have facilities for both. Compound scanning is helpful at the beginning of a study, or in a difficult case, for attempting to define organ outlines. Compound scans will not, however, yield the resolution or parenchymal echogenic information that single-sector scanning will. Therefore, compound scans are used for orientation, but single-sector scans are used for the recorded image (Sample et al. 1975). Compound scanning alone invites numerous problems. For example, it is possible to compound scan the splenic vein with the sensitivity set too high and to mistake its irregular border and sonolucency for the pancreas. Decreased resolution from compound scanning will make detection of small lesions less likely. Furthermore, identification of the small vessels surrounding the pancreas, which is necessary for an adequate study, is suboptimal in compound scanning. Therefore, single-sector scanning is the primary scanning technique for pancreatic ultrasonography.

With the correct sensitivity and output setting and proper scanning techniques, the novice is now ready to begin a pancreatic exam. But where should he or she start? In both longitudinal and transverse scans, identification of the portal vein is the first and easiest road sign to look for (Burger and Blauenstein 1974; Sarti, Lindstrom, and Tabrisky 1975).

Let us begin with transverse scans. Since the left lobe is used as an ultrasonic window, the patient should take in a deep breath to drive down the diaphragm and cause the left lobe of the liver to displace the lesser curvature of the stomach as inferiorly as possible. This will not always yield the best anatomic relationship for pancreatic visualization, and various respiratory positions may be better, but it is a good place to start. With the patient in deep inspiration, the technicians start scanning the liver well above the pancreas to identify the portal vein.

The transverse sections continue more caudally while following its course (Carlsen and Filly 1976; Sanders, Conrad, and White 1977). Anterior to the portal vein, two smaller sonolucencies which represent the hepatic artery and common bile duct may be noticed. More inferiorly, the celiac axis arising from the aorta will come into view with its major branches, the splenic and hepatic arteries. The portal vein will join the curvilinear sonolucency of the splenic vein, which is situated anterior to the aorta and the inferior vena cava. It is at this point that the pancreatic echo pattern may come into view. The "cobblestone" echo pattern is often but not always situated directly anterior to the splenic vein (Leopold 1975a).

Occasionally, the technologist may have to continue more caudally before the pancreas is seen. The portal and splenic veins are joined by the superior mesenteric vein which is just to the right of the superior messenteric artery. The pancreas should be seen at this level, and the head of the pancreas will be present on the right if the duodenum is not markedly air-filled. The uncinate process of the pancreas is situated posterior to the superior mesenteric artery and vein and anterior to the inferior vena cava. Just after the origin of the superior mesenteric artery, a second curvilinear lucency, similar in shape to the splenic vein, is seen coursing directly over the aorta behind the superior mesenteric artery and joining the inferior vena cava. This is the left renal vein (Leopold 1975b; Sample 1977; Sarti 1977). It is closer to the aorta than the splenic vein and will not be seen until the superior mesenteric artery comes into view. The origin of the left renal vein is recognizable, because the inferior vena cava loses its oval shape and becomes pointed on the left side.

As all of these vessels come into view, the echo pattern of the pancreas will be seen anterior to them. Occasionally, a linear echo will be present coursing through the center of the pancreatic echoes. This echo arises from the normal pancreatic duct. It is quite difficult to obtain, but meticulous transverse scans at 1–2 mm intervals over the midportion of the pancreas often will yield the pancreatic duct (Sample and Sarti in press). On the right side of the head of the pancreas, at its juncture with the duodenum, a small circular sonolucency which represents the common bile duct can occasionally be seen. More rarely, and anterior to this, is a second circular sonolucency representing the gastroduodenal artery or one of its branches, the superior pancreaticoduodenal artery (Sample 1977).

As already mentioned, air in the stomach obscures visualization of the pancreas. With a large left lobe of the liver this is not usually a problem. However, with a smaller left lobe, sometimes only a portion of the portal vein before it joins the splenic vein or just a little of the celiac axis can be seen before air is encountered. If we could see a few more centimeters caudally, the pancreas would come into view. In these instances, it is helpful to angle the transducer arm 15–20° caudally to increase the use of the left lobe as a window (Sample et al. 1975). This often will enable visualization of the pancreas in a study that would have ordinarily been aborted. Another potential ultrasonic window is the gallbladder, which can be used for visualizing the pancreatic head. Air in the duodenal bulb is a continual irritant when attempting to scan the pancreatic head, and a false mass can be created (Freimanis and Asher 1970). By scanning further to the right side and angling through the gallbladder we can occasionally scan behind the duodenal bulb and encounter the pancreatic head.

Longitudinal scans are also dependent upon understanding the surrounding vascular anatomy. As with transverse scans, the portal vein is an excellent starting point for pancreatic evaluation. On longitudinal scans to the right of midline, the portal vein is a circular sonolucency situated anterior to the inferior vena cava. As the scanning planes progress toward the midline at 1-cm intervals, the pancreatic head will come into view inferior to the portal vein and anterior to the inferior vena cava. The normal common bile duct occasionally can be seen as a tubular sonolucency coursing posterior to the pancreatic head. A second tubular sonolucency will more rarely be seen coursing over the anterior portion of the pancreas. This is the gastroduodenal artery and its caudally continuing branch, the superior pancreaticoduodenal artery (Sample 1977).

As scans progress toward the midline, the portal vein is joined by the superior mesenteric vein which is a longitudinal sonolucency posterior to the neck of the pancreas. A "bull's-eye"-appearing, collapsed stomach is often seen at this point, anterior and slightly caudal to the pancreas. Further scans to the left will slip out of the superior mesenteric vein into the splenic vein which is a circular sonolucency posterior to the cephalad portion of the pancreas. The portal and splenic veins can only be differentiated on longitudinal scans by knowing the location of the superior mesenteric vein. As we progress past midline to the left, a long posterior tubular structure representing the aorta will be easily recognized. The origins of the celiac axis and superior mesenteric artery can be seen off the anterior aorta with the pancreas situated directly anterior to the superior mesenteric artery (Leopold 1975a; Sample 1977; Skolnick and Royal 1976). A slitlike sonolucency occasionally can be seen between the aorta and the superior mesenteric artery, just caudal to the origin of the SMA; this represents the left renal vein. Further to the left, two circular sonolucencies, representing the splenic artery and vein, are situated posterior to the superior aspect of the pancreas.

By marking the superior and inferior borders of the pancreas on the patient's skin during the longitudinal scans, the pancreatic outline can be mapped. The pancreatic head and body are fairly consistent in location, but there is variability in the location of the tail. It is most often situated cephalad in the splenic hilum but also can course straight laterally, anterior to the left kidney, or less commonly, it can turn inferiorly. After mapping the pancreas outline on the patient's skin, the transducer arm is then returned to the transverse side of the bed and aligned parallel to the long axis of the pancreas (Ghorashi and Rector 1977). Oblique transverse scans can be obtained and will yield images containing the pancreatic head, body, and as far into the tail as possible before being obscured by air.

Examination of the pancreatic tail is best performed with the patient prone. In this position, the tail is often situated anterior to the middle portion and upper pole of the left kidney. If the tail is too far cephalad or caudal, it will not be seen anterior to the left kidney. In these instances a diffuse, ill-defined echogenic area is seen and often confused with a pancreatic neoplasm. Computed axial tomography has shown this secondary to loops of proximal jejunum.

Examination of the Normal Pancreas

Bistable examination did not demonstrate the normal pancreas (Filly and Freimanis 1970). With gray scale, the returning pancreatic echoes are equal to, or slightly greater in amplitude than, those in the liver. The pancreas will, therefore, present with slightly darker echoes than the left lobe of the liver under normal circumstances. When comparing the pancreas to the liver it is important that the standard be normal. This necessitates recognizing normal versus abnormal liver echogenicity. The texture of pancreatic echoes is slightly

more irregular than the liver. This has been termed "cobblestoning" (Garrett, Kossoff, and Carpenter 1975; Leopold 1975a). A recent study (Haber, Freimanis, and Asher 1976) reported normal size of the head, body, and tail of the pancreas in craniocaudal (CC) and anteroposterior (AP) dimensions as follows:

	AP	CC
Head	2.7 ± 0.7 cm	3.6 ± 1.2 cm
Body	2.2 ± 0.7 cm	3.0 ± 0.6 cm
Tail	2.4 ± 0.4 cm	2.0 ± 0.4 cm

Size alone is not, however, adequate for the determination of pancreatic pathology. The contour, echogenicity, and "Gestalt" are still most helpful. Furthermore, the tail of the pancreas is not seen routinely in a high percentage of cases. This is a major drawback to the pancreatic exam. (See p. 178 for additional comments on the technique for pancreatic examination.)

Pathology of the Pancreas

Pancreatitis

Acute and chronic pancreatitis has numerous etiologies. Among the most common are alcoholism, gallstones, trauma, and peptic ulcer disease. Less common are complications of pregnancy, mumps, diffuse vascular diseases such as periarteritis nodosa, essential hyperlipemia, hereditary pancreatitis, and hyperparathyroidism. Elevated amylase and white blood count are the pertinent laboratory findings. X-ray films show a "sentinel" loop or, in chronic pancreatitis, calcification in the pancreatic bed.

Acute pancreatitis can be diffuse or localized. Alcoholism leads most often to the generalized form. Diffuse edematous involvement of the pancreas changes the echogenicity of the pancreas which appears more sonolucent than in the uninvolved state (Doust 1975; Hancke 1976; Stuber, Templeton, and Bishop 1972). The normal liver-pancreas echo relationship is reversed. Because of increased pancreatic sonolucency, the liver is more echogenic than the pancreas. This can be a difficult assessment to make in the alcoholic patient, since a cirrhotic liver manifests increased echogenicity. As mentioned earlier, compound scanning of the splenic vein elicits the appearance of a sonolucent pancreas which may be misinterpreted as pancreatic edema. This pitfall can be avoided by single-sector scanning. Pancreatic size may be increased in acute pancreatitis, but the echogenic changes are more helpful than size. Decreased pancreatic echogenicity is also present in pancreatic carcinoma which presents a diagnostic problem. In these instances, clinical history is most helpful to obtain the correct diagnosis. If pancreatitis is suspected, serial scans should be performed with the patient on medical treatment. Successful therapy should demonstrate a decrease in the size and an increase in the echogenicity of the pancreas.

Chronic pancreatitis may be diffuse or localized. The diffuse variety is usually associated with ethanol abuse, whereas localized pancreatitis is commonly secondary to obstruction. The normal "cobblestone" appearance and echogenicity are lost. The pancreas presents with an irregular, more sonolucent picture, but it is more echogenic if marked fibrosis or early calcification is present (Doust 1975; Weill et al. 1975). The borders are often irregular, and distinction from neoplasm is extremely difficult. When the pancreas is calcified, it is difficult, if not impossible, to localize, since the high-level calcific echoes blend with the retroperitoneal fibrofatty echoes. It is not unusual for the clinician to bring an abdominal X-ray film demonstrating pancreatic calcification that had been hidden to ultrasound technique. Calcification will, however, present a coarser, more irregular echo pattern than the retroperitoneum and demonstrate shadowing if the calcification is large enough.

Pancreatic Pseudocysts

The rate of occurrence of pseudocysts in patients with acute pancreatitis ranges from 11 to 18%. Prior to ultrasound, diagnosis of a pancreatic pseudocyst was made by palpation or an upper-GI series. Although these methods show the position of a mass, they do not necessarily confirm its nature. The possibilites of carcinoma, edema, abscess, or other mass should be ruled out. By determining whether a mass is fluid or solid, ultrasound can demonstrate whether or not it is secondary to a pseudocyst (Holmes, Findley, and Frank 1973; Leopold 1972; Sokoloff et al 1974; Walls et al. 1975). Successful surgical drainage of a pancreatic pseudocyst is dependent upon cyst wall maturation for anastomosis to the GI tract. A 4–6 week period has been determined necessary for adequate cyst wall maturity. In the past, however, this was verified by a palpating hand or the gastrointestinal radiologist's eye. With ultrasound we can now follow serially the development and evolution of pancreatic pseudocysts.

Pancreatic pseudocysts are mainly sonolucent masses with enhanced through transmission. Their borders are highly echogenic and somewhat thicker and more irregular than simple cysts of the kidney or ovary. They may be unilocular or multilocular, a distinction which is important to determine for surgical drainage (Duncan, Imrie, and Blumgart 1976). Debris secondary to necrosis and enzymatic action on surrounding tissue presents as echogenic regions within a pseudocyst. In these instances, a solid lesion of the pancreas is suspected. Such unusual locations as the neck and anterior thigh have been reported as sites for pseudocyst migration along tissue planes (Gooding 1977). The majority, however, will be located in close proximity to the pancreatic bed and in contact with the stomach, duodenum, liver, kidneys, and spleen. When a sonolucent structure is noted in the upper abdomen, it is important to rule out a fluid-filled loop of bowel before prematurely diagnosing a pseudocyst (Holm, Rasmussen, and Kristensen 1972). The patient may be kept without oral intake and placed on nasogastric suction, and the study repeated 24 hours later. If the structure remains similar in shape and echogenicity, then fluid-filled bowel is ruled out.

The noninvasive nature of ultrasound allows serial examinations of patients with pancreatic pseudocysts to be performed. We have encountered several cases with spontaneous regression of pseudocysts without the expected morbidity and mortality. Approximately 50% of ruptured pseudocysts drain into the peritoneal cavity, and 50% into the gastrointestinal tract (Clements, Bradley, and Eaton 1976; Leopold, Berk, and Reinke 1972). A mortality of 50% is associated with spontaneous regression into the gastrointestinal tract and a 70% mortality with decompression into the peritoneal cavity (Hanna 1960; Littmann, Pichaczevsky, and Richter 1970). This data was obtained prior to the routine use of diagnostic ultrasound. Serial ultrasound exams have shown that many more patients than originally estimated spontaneously drain their pseudocysts without adverse effect. Serial exams also have demonstrated the rapid development of pseudocysts in patients with acute pancreatitis. An acute episode of pain in a patient with pancreatitis may signal imminent pseudocyst development, and serial ultrasound examinations are indicated. We followed a patient who developed a pseudocyst within a 6-day period after his last negative ultrasound examination (Sarti 1977). The pseudocyst wall was mature enough to anastomose to a loop of jejunum 21 days after the pseudocyst development. Four-to-six weeks' duration is felt necessary for adequate wall maturation.

Congenital pancreatic cysts range from microscopic size to 3–5 cm and are secondary to the anomalous development of pancreatic cysts. Low cuboidal epithelial cells line these cysts, which are found in conjunction with polycystic disease of the liver, kidney, or ovary. When ultrasound detects multiple cysts noted in the liver or kidneys, the pancreatic bed should be examined. Often, this will be normal. Occasionally, numerous cystic lesions also will be evident in the pancreas.

Retention cysts are smaller than congenital cysts, rarely exceeding several centimeters. They are usually secondary to the obstruction of the pancreatic ducts and are rarely of clinical significance.

Pancreatic Abscess

Pancreatic abscesses may arise as a direct extension of a neighboring infection such as perforated peptic ulcer, acute appendicitis, or acute cholecystitis. Bacteria may reach the pancreas through the lymph system. The ultrasonic appearance depends on the amount of suppurative material and debris. If abundant suppuration is present, the mass will appear sonolucent. The walls of an abscess are usually thick, irregular, and highly echogenic. If air bubbles are present, they will yield a highly echogenic region and occasional shadows, depending upon their size.

Pancreatic Neoplasms

Carcinoma of the pancreas has been increasing in frequency and now is the fourth most common malignancy. Detection of this neoplasm is usually late, and medical intervention has not markedly improved survival. Earliest detection occurs in the head of the pancreas where obstruction of the common bile duct occurs. Carcinomas occur twice as often in the head of the pancreas as they do in the body and tail. Gross specimens demonstrate a gray-white scirrhous homogeneous mass which silently grows to a large size. The normal

"cobblestone" appearance of the pancreas is lost and replaced by a less echogenic, coarser mass (Engelhart and Blauenstein 1970; Weill et al. 1975). There is enlargement of the pancreas and often an irregular, nodular border (Stuber, Templeton, and Bishop 1972). Ultrasonic detection is easiest in the pancreatic head where displacement of numerous surrounding vessels is often noted. A dilated common bile duct signals the immediate need for meticulous scanning of the head to determine the cause of obstruction. A dilated pancreatic duct may also be present with tumors of the head of the pancreas. It will present as a tubular sonolucency within the pancreas anterior to the splenic vein with which it may be confused. By demonstrating that it does not join the portal vein and that it is contained within the pancreatic echoes, we can confirm pancreatic duct dilatation (Gosink and Leopold 1978). Tumors of the tail are most difficult to detect secondary to air in the stomach and splenic flexure and are best seen through the left kidney with the patient in the prone position. Increased size of the pancreatic tail alone is not sufficient. Angiography performed on several patients with increased size but normal echogenicity has been negative. This is most likely due to an anteroposterior orientation to the tail as it drapes over the aorta and courses straight back toward the left kidney. Regrettably, a "Gestalt" approach, the feeling of a knobby, less echogenic mass with irregular borders anterior to the left kidney, has been most productive in obtaining the correct diagnosis. Tumors as small as 2 cm have been detected (Otto, Lucke, and Mitzkat 1974). These are usually in locations with abundant vascular anatomy such as the uncinate process. Percutaneous aspiration biopsy under ultrasonic guidance has been found to be useful in the diagnosis and may prevent a laparotomy (Hancke 1976; Hancke, Holm, and Koch 1975; Smith, Bartrum, and Chang 1974; Smith et al. 1975). Ultrasound also may be of assistance in planning radiotherapy and in following tumor response (Brascho 1974).

Islet cell tumors are even more difficult to detect, since they are usually 1–2 cm in size. Again, most success is found in the head of the pancreas; the numerous surrounding anatomic landmarks are very helpful.

Cystadenomas and cystadenocarcinomas have an ultrasonic appearance similar to that of a multiloculated pseudocyst. The mass is mainly sonolucent with numerous curvilinear echoes arising from septae coursing through it (Wolson and Walls 1976). A higher echogenicity may be present about these septae, secondary to the mucous secretions.

Pitfalls in Pancreatic Examination

Numerous problems can arise during the course of an ultrasonic pancreatic examination that can lead to erroneous diagnoses and interpretations. One of the more common errors is producing a false mass in the region of the pancreatic bed. This often occurs around the pancreatic head and is due to air in the duodenum. For example, by compound scanning from different directions, a false mass can be created in the region of the pancreatic head which gives the appearance of a solid carcinoma. It is important to analyze the orientation of the echoes to determine where the transducer was at the time of scanning. The criteria of through transmission is also extremely important in ruling out a mass lesion (Freimanis and Asher 1970). The best way to avoid such an error is to single-sector scan the region of interest once there is a suggestion of a mass on compound scanning. If a mass is truly present, it will show up on single-sector scanning as well as on compound scanning. If not, it will be obscured by air in the duodenum and through transmission is not present. As mentioned earlier, compound scanning of the splenic vein can lead to an erroneous diagnosis of pancreatitis. Its borders become indistinct, and it appears sonolucent. Because of location and contour similar to that of the pancreas, it often can be confused for an edematous pancreas.

One of the more common errors which deserves mention is the misinterpretation of a fluid-filled loop of bowel as a pseudocyst. This is most likely if the stomach is filled with fluid or food. Since the stomach is in close proximity to the pancreatic bed, any sonolocency caused by this structure easily can be misinterpreted for a pancreatic pseudocyst. Therefore, it is wise routinely to reexamine 24 hours later a patient suspected of having a pseudocyst. We often have the patient return the next morning, having been kept without oral intake overnight. If the mass is similar in appearance and contour to the previous study, a fluid-filled loop of bowel is ruled out. Real time examination can be used to detect peristaltic activity.

Many patients will have had surgery prior to an ultrasonic examination. Since there is a preponderance of fibrous tissue within scars, high attenuation can occur. When scanning a patient over the region of a scar, we must be aware that the scan deep to the scar will be less echogenic because of the marked attenuation of sound through the scar tissue. This can often give the appearance of a more lucent mass. Pancreatic tissue will appear less echogenic than the remaining, normal-appearing pancreas and often is confused for edema, neoplasm, or fibrosis. This mistake can be avoided by scanning on either side of the scar with angulation over the area of interest. Scar tissue also may create false masses similar to that noted around the duodenum.

Another problem may arise from a markedly calcified pancreatic bed that is extremely echogenic and may be lost in the high amplitude echoes of the fibrofatty retroperitoneum. The best way to avoid this is by being aware of the vascular anatomy and recognizing the region of the pancreas. If the major vessels in the pancreatic bed can be identified, high-amplitude and extremely coarse echoes of a calcified pancreas will begin to stand out more readily from the usual high-amplitude, even echoes of the fibrofatty retroperitoneum.

Pancreatic echogenicity is affected by the structures situated directly anterior to it. A normally appearing pancreas will have normal structures situated anteriorly. Whenever the liver is cirrhotic it has increased fibrous tissue which attenuates sound. This will give a higher-amplitude echo to the liver but will also yield lower-amplitude echoes to the pancreas because of the attenuation of sound prior to the sound wave's reaching the pancreatic tissue and returning to the transducer. Therefore, a mistaken diagnosis of pancreatitis may be made in the presence of a cirrhotic left lobe of the liver. Furthermore, a fluid-filled mass anterior to the pancreas, such as a pseudocyst, loculated ascites, or fluid-filled stomach, will cause the pancreas to appear more echogenic than usual. This is secondary to the lack of attenuation by a fluid-filled mass. The decreased attenuation will give a higher-amplitude echo returning from the pancreas than is seen in the normal situation. Therefore, a possible erroneous diagnosis of increased echogenicity suggesting chronic pancreatitis may be made. An awareness of those structures anterior to the pancreatic tissue will help avoid these mistakes.

These numerous pitfalls can be very disturbing especially in the early attempts at pancreatic evaluation. With experience, however, they become less troublesome. By paying attention to technique and some basic concepts of physics, the majority of these pitfalls can be avoided.

References

Brascho, D. J. Computerized radiation treatment planning with ultrasound. *Am. J. Roentgenol.* 120:213–223, 1974.

Burger, J., and Blauenstein, V. W. Current aspects of ultrasonic scanning of the pancreas. *Am. J. Roentgenol.* 122:406–412, 1974.

Carlsen, E., and Filly, R. A. Newer ultrasonographic anatomy in the upper abdomen: I. The portal hepatic venous anatomy. *J. Clin. Ultrasound* 4:85–90, 1976.

Clements, J. L.; Bradley, E. L.; and Eaton, S. B. Spontaneous internal drainage of pancreatic pseudocysts. *Am. J. Roentgenol.* 126:985–991, 1976.

Doust, B. D. Ultrasonic examination of the pancreas. *Radiol. Clin. North Am.* 13:467–478, 1975.

Duncan, J. G.; Imrie, C. W.; and Blumgart, L. H. Ultrasound in the management of acute pancreatitis. *Br. J. Radiol.* 49:858–862, 1976.

Engelhart, G., and Blauenstein, V. W. Ultrasound in the diagnosis of malignant pancreatic tumours. *Gut* 11:443–449, 1970.

Filly, R. A., and Carlsen, E. Newer ultrasonic anatomy in the upper abdomen: II. The major systemic veins and arteries with a special note on localization of the pancreas. *J. Clin. Ultrasound* 4:91–96, 1976.

Filly, R. A., and Freimanis, A. K. Echographic diagnosis of pancreatic lesions. *Radiology* 96:575–582, 1970.

Freimanis, A. K., and Asher, W. M. Development of diagnostic criteria in echographic study of abdominal lesions. *Am. J. Roentgenol.* 108:747–755, 1970.

Garrett, W. J.; Kossoff, G.; and Carpenter, D. A. Gray scale compound scan echography of the normal upper abdomen. *J. Clin. Ultrasound* 3:199–204, 1975.

Ghorashi, B., and Rector, W. R. Gray scale sonographic anatomy of the pancreas. *J. Clin. Ultrasound* 5:25–29, 1977.

Gooding, G. A. W. Pseudocyst of the pancreas with mediastinal extension: an ultrasonographic demonstration. *J. Clin. Ultrasound* 5:121–123, 1977.

Gosink, B. B., and Leopold, G. R. The dilated pancreatic duct: ultrasonic evaluation. *Radiology* 126:475–478, 1978.

Haber, K.; Freimanis, A. K.; and Asher, W. M. Demonstration and dimensional analysis of the normal pancreas with gray scale echography. *Am. J. Roentgenol.* 126:624–628, 1976.

Hancke, S. Ultrasonic scanning of the pancreas. *J. Clin. Ultrasound* 4:223–230, 1976.

Hancke, S.; Holm, H. H.; and Koch, F. Ultrasonically guided percutaneous fine needle biopsy of the pancreas. *Surg. Gyn. Obstet.* 140:361–364, 1975.

Hanna, W. A. Rupture of pancreatic cysts. Report of a case and review of the literature. *Br. J. Surg.* 47:495–498, 1960.

Holm, H. H.; Rasmussen, S. N.; and Kristensen, J. K. Errors and pitfalls in ultrasonic scanning of the abdomen. *Br. J. Radiol.* 45:835–840, 1972.

Holmes, J. H.; Findley, L.; and Frank, B. Diagnosis of pancreatic pathology using ultrasound. *Trans. Am. Clin. Climatol. Assoc.* 85:224–234, 1973.

Leopold, G. Echographic study of the pancreas. *JAMA* 232:287–289, 1975a.

Leopold, G. Gray scale ultrasonic angiography of the upper abdomen. *Radiology* 117:665–671, 1975b.

Leopold, G. Pancreatic echography: a new dimension in the diagnosis of pseudocyst. *Radiology* 104:365–369, 1972.

Leopold, G., and Asher, W. M. Deleterious effects of gastrointestinal contrast material on abdominal echography. *Radiology* 98:637–640, 1971.

Leopold, G. R.; Berk, R. N.; and Reinke, R. T. Echographic-radiological documentation of spontaneous rupture of a pancreatic pseudocyst into the duodenum. *Radiology* 120:699–700, 1972.

Littmann, R.; Pichaczevsky, R.; and Richter, R. Spontaneous rupture of a pancreatic pseudocyst into the duodenum. *Arch. Surg.* 100:76–78, 1970.

Otto, P.; Lucke, C.; and Mitzkat, H. J. Sonographische darstellung eines inselzelladenomas. *Dtsch. Med. Wschr.* 99:2344–2347, 1974.

Sample, W. F. Techniques for improved delineation of normal anatomy of the upper abdomen and high retroperitoneum with gray scale ultrasound. *Radiology* 124:197–202, 1977.

Sample, W. F.; Po, J. B.; Gray, R. K.; and Cahill, P. J. Gray scale ultrasonography: techniques in pancreatic scanning. *Appl. Radiol.* 4:63, 1975.

Sample, W. F., and Sarti, D. A. Computed body tomography and gray scale ultrasonography: anatomic correlations and pitfalls in the upper abdomen. *Gastrointestinal Radiology*, in press.

Sanders, R. C.; Conrad, M. R.; and White, R. I. Normal and abnormal upper abdominal venous structures as seen by ultrasound. *Am. J. Roentgenol.* 128:657–662, 1977.

Sarti, D. A. Rapid development and spontaneous regression of pancreatic pseudocysts documented by ultrasound. *Radiology* 125:789–793, 1977.

Sarti, D. A., and Lazere, A. Re-examination of the deleterious effects of gastrointestinal contrast material on abdominal echography. *Radiology* 126:231–232, 1978.

Sarti, D. A.; Lindstrom, R. R.; and Tabrisky, J. Correlation of the ultrasonic appearance of the portal vein with abdominal arteriography. *J. Clin. Ultrasound* 3:263–266, 1975.

Skolnick, M. L., and Royal, D. R. Normal upper abdominal vasculature: a study correlating contact B-scanning with arteriography and gross anatomy. *J. Clin. Ultrasound* 4:399–402, 1976.

Smith, E. H.; Bartrum, R. J.; and Chang, Y. C. Ultrasonically guided percutaneous aspiration biopsy of the pancreas. *Radiology* 112:737–738, 1974.

Smith, E. H.; Bartrum, R. J.; Chang, Y. C.; D'Orsi, C. J.; Lokich, J.; Abbruzzese, A.; and Dantono, J. Percutaneous aspiration biopsy of the pancreas under ultrasonic guidance. *N. Engl. J. Med*. 292 (16):825–828, 1975.

Sokoloff, J. et al. Pitfalls in the echographic evaluation of pancreatic disease. *J. Clin. Ultrasound* 2(4):321–326, 1974.

Sommer, G., and Filly, R. A. Patient preparation to decrease bowel gas: evaluation by ultrasonic measurement. *J. Clin. Ultrasound* 5:87–88, 1977.

Stuber, J. L.; Templeton, A. W.; and Bishop, K. Sonographic diagnosis of pancreatic lesions. *Am. J. Roentgenol.* 116:406–412, 1972.

Walls, W. J.; Gonzales, G.; Martin, N. L.; and Templeton, A. W. B-scan ultrasound evaluation of the pancreas. *Radiology* 114:127–134, 1975.

Weill, F.; Bourgoin, A.; Aucant, D.; Eisencher, A.; and Gallinet, D. Pancreatite chronique cancer du pancreas: differenciation par ultrasons. *Nouv. Presse Med.* 4:567–570, 1975.

Wolson, A. H., and Walls, W. J. Ultrasonic characteristics of cystadenoma of the pancreas. *Radiology* 119:203–205, 1976.

CASES

Dennis A. Sarti, M.D.
W. Frederick Sample, M.D.

Technique for Pancreatic Examination

The pancreatic examination can be started either in the longitudinal or transverse plane. As already mentioned, if the portal vein can be identified, it can eventually be followed to the pancreatic texture. Figure 4.1 is a longitudinal scan in the midline of the pancreas. Scans are usually obtained at 1-cm intervals, starting with the portal vein on the right side and continuing to the midline and to the left until the pancreas is covered in its entirety. The patient usually is asked to take in a deep breath to drive the diaphragm down. This eventually will place the left lobe of the liver anterior to the pancreas and allow visualization of the pancreatic texture.

   Figure 4.2 is a transverse scan over the region of the pancreas. Here we see the transducer arm aligned perpendicular to the tabletop. Transverse scans can be started cephalad to the pancreas in the liver where the portal vein again is identified. They should then be continued caudally at 1-cm intervals or less, until the pancreatic texture comes into view. Again the patient is asked to take in a deep breath to place the left lobe of the liver anterior to the pancreas. In many instances, however, the pancreas may not be seen; this is secondary to bowel air. Rather than aborting the pancreatic examination at this stage, we generally try angling the transducer caudally (fig. 4.3). Transverse scans are continued, but with marked caudal angulation of the transducer arm. This will show several centimeters more of the pancreatic bed through the ultrasonic window of the left lobe of the liver. It is important to realize the number of studies that can be salvaged by using this simple technique. The only difficulty may be poor skin contact because of the angle of the transducer. If this becomes a problem, a gel rather than mineral oil may be used.

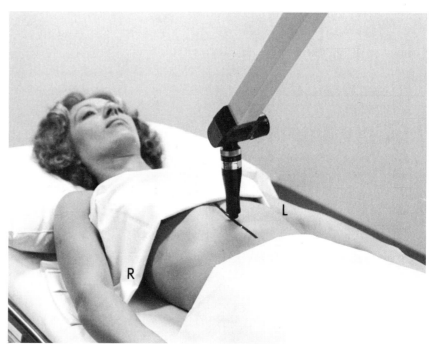

Fig. 4.1

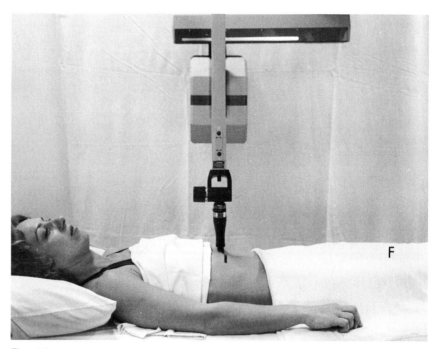

Fig. 4.2

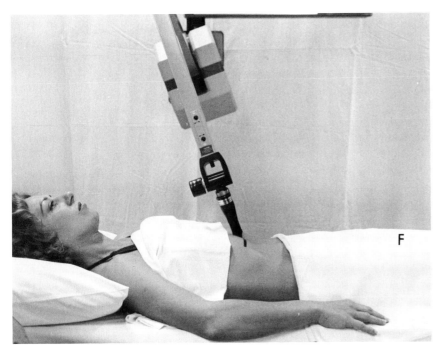

Fig. 4.3

When scanning a patient in the longitudinal plane, it is often helpful to mark the cephalad and caudal borders of the pancreas on the patient's skin. Figure 4.4 shows how we diagrammed the pancreatic anatomy on a patient's skin during the course of a longitudinal examination. Once the topographical anatomy of the pancreas has been placed on the patient's skin, a transverse oblique scan (fig. 4.4) can be obtained. Note that the scanning arm is aligned parallel to the long axis of the pancreas. There is also some caudal angulation of the transducer arm to facilitate using the left lobe of the liver as an ultrasonic window. This transverse oblique scan frequently will yield the best visualization of the pancreas in its entirety.

F   = Foot
L   = Left
R   = Right

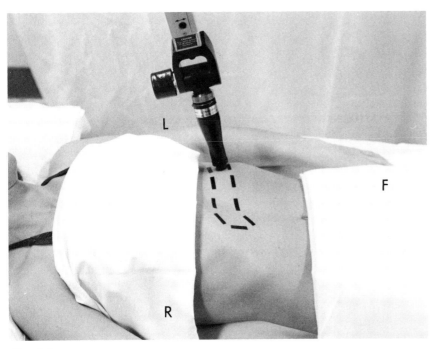

Fig. 4.4

Transverse Scans of the Normal Pancreas

Transverse scans are obtained above the level of the pancreas. We usually start transversely within the liver, progressing caudally until certain vascular structures come into view. Figure 4.5 demonstrates some of the vascular structures seen cephalad to the pancreas. The celiac axis can be seen arising from the anterior surface of the aorta and dividing into the hepatic and splenic arteries. Figure 4.5 also demonstrates the portal vein situated posterior to the hepatic artery. Frequently, air in the stomach will obscure visualization of the pancreas. If the patient takes in a deep breath, the left lobe of the liver can caudally displace the lesser curvature of the stomach. This maneuver often increases visualization of the pancreas.

Near the origin of the hepatic artery, a small vessel will occasionally be noted. This is the left gastric artery (fig. 4.6). Also noted in figure 4.6 is the origin of the superior mesenteric artery. This section was taken with caudal angulation. The hepatic artery situated anterior to the superior mesenteric artery can be seen. This is due to the fact that the transducer is aimed toward the foot of the patient.

Figure 4.7 demonstrates a situation in which too many tubes appear in the region of the head of the pancreas. This occasionally happens when a replaced right hepatic artery is present. The anterior structure represents the portal vein and splenic vein. Posterior to this is the circular superior mesenteric artery. Coming off the superior mesenteric artery and heading toward the right of the patient is the replaced right hepatic artery. A small circular structure posterior to this artery represents the common bile duct, which is only approximately 3 mm in diameter. Just to the right is the gallbladder. The left renal vein can be seen coursing anterior to the aorta and emptying into the inferior vena cava. A relatively lucent structure, posterior to the left renal vein and adjacent to the aorta, represents the crus of the diaphragm. Figure 4.7 represents our first visualization of echoes arising from the pancreas. A portion of the body and tail

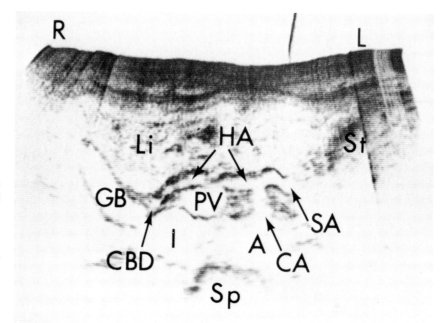

Fig. 4.5

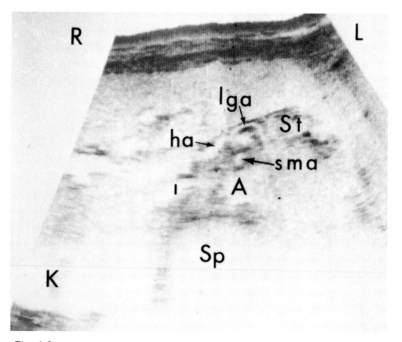

Fig. 4.6

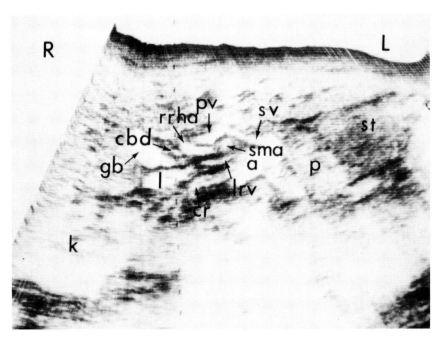

Fig. 4.7

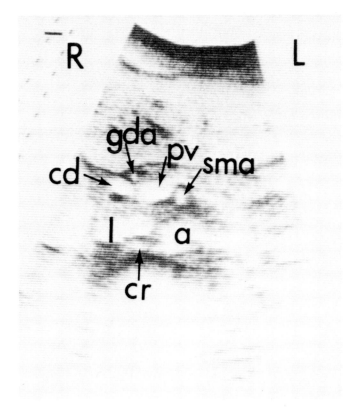

Fig. 4.8

of the pancreas can be seen here. The tail of the pancreas usually comes into view first, since it is often situated more cephalad than is the head of the pancreas. The head of the pancreas will come into view on more caudal sections.

Figure 4.8 demonstrates visualization of the gastroduodenal artery and common bile duct. Just to the left of these vessels a portion of the pancreas situated anterior to the superior mesenteric artery and portal vein can be seen. The pancreatic echoes in figures 4.7 and 4.8 are equal to, or slightly greater in amplitude than, the echoes arising from the liver.

A	=	Aorta
a	=	Aorta
CA	=	Celiac axis
CBD	=	Common bile duct
cbd	=	Common bile duct
cd	=	Common bile duct
Cr	=	Crus of the diaphragm
GB	=	Gallbladder
gb	=	Gallbladder
gda	=	Gastroduodenal artery
HA	=	Hepatic artery
ha	=	Hepatic artery
I	=	Inferior vena cava
K	=	Kidney
k	=	Kidney
L	=	Left
lga	=	Left gastric artery
Li	=	Liver
LRV	=	Left renal vein
p	=	Pancreas
PV	=	Portal vein
pv	=	Portal vein
R	=	Right
rrha	=	Replaced right hepatic artery
SA	=	Splenic artery
sma	=	Superior mesenteric artery
Sp	=	Spine
St	=	Stomach
SV	=	Splenic vein

Transverse Scans of the Normal Pancreas

Figures 4.9–4.12 demonstrate a normal increased echogenicity to the pancreas when compared with the liver. The usual relationship of the pancreas to the liver is that the pancreatic echoes are equal to, or greater in amplitude than, the liver. These figures also demonstrate the various presentations of the duodenum in its relation to the head of the pancreas. The duodenum may be air-filled, fluid-filled, or collapsed. Figure 4.9 demonstrates an air-filled duodenum with posterior shadowing. A portion of the head of the pancreas, just medial to the air-filled duodenum, can still be seen. The level of the pancreas is determined by the visualization of the superior mesenteric vein. A small portion of the head of the pancreas is, however, obscured by the air shadowing of the duodenum (fig. 4.9). There is a normal relationship among the gallbladder, the duodenum, and the pancreas in all of these figures. This relationship is fairly consistent in most ultrasound examinations, where the gallbladder is lateral to the duodenum, and the pancreas is medial.

Figure 4.10 demonstrates a fluid-filled duodenum lateral to the head of the pancreas. The common bile duct can also be seen. The common bile duct along with the gastroduodenal artery (figs. 4.11 and 4.12) are important landmarks in determining the limits of the head of the pancreas. They help to identify the lateral borders of the pancreatic head and allow pancreatic echoes to be distinguished from duodenal echoes. Figures 4.10 and 4.11 show a duodenum with fluid in it. Figure 4.11 demonstrates internal echoes within the duodenum, suggesting some food particles.

Figure 4.12 demonstrates the duodenum in a collapsed presentation. The duodenal bulb and the second portion of the duodenum are seen in their collapsed state. This could suggest a pancreatic mass, but in figure 4.12 the gastroduodenal artery and common bile duct are well visualized, indicating the separation between the head of the pancreas and the collapsed duodenum. Some fluid in the stomach is noted in figure 4.12. The stomach in this view is

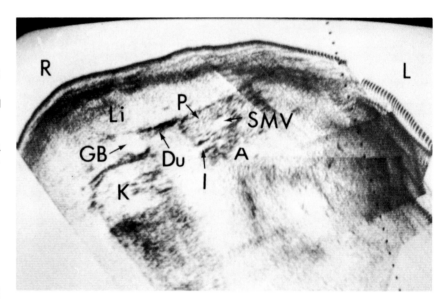

Fig. 4.9

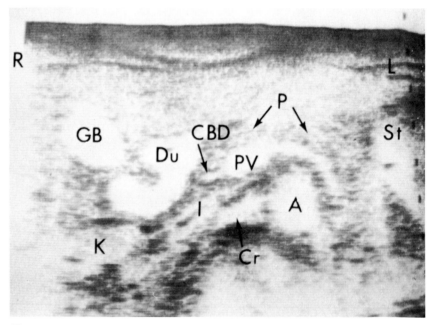

Fig. 4.10

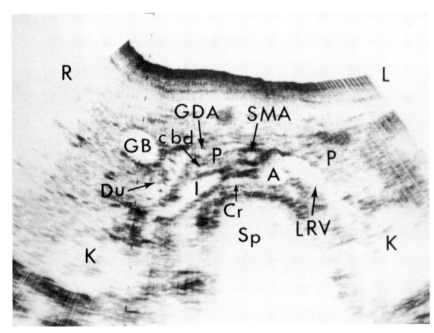

Fig. 4.11

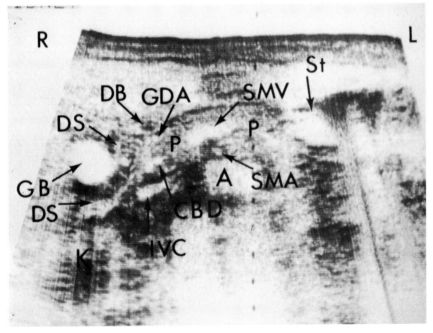

Fig. 4.12

partially air-filled and fluid-filled. The important part of these images is the echogenicity of the pancreas in relation to the liver. A good portion of the head, body, and tail of the pancreas can be seen on all of these studies, with the duodenum in various states of filling. The pancreas is slightly more echogenic than the liver in these four examples.

A = Aorta
CBD = Common bile duct
cbd = Common bile duct
Cr = Crus of the diaphragm
DB = Duodenal bulb
DS = Second portion of the duodenum
Du = Duodenum
GB = Gallbladder
GDA = Gastroduodenal artery
I = Inferior vena cava
IVC = Inferior vena cava
K = Kidney
L = Left
Li = Liver
LRV = Left renal vein
P = Pancreas
PV = Portal vein
R = Right
SMA = Superior mesenteric artery
SMV = Superior mesenteric vein
Sp = Spine
St = Stomach

Transverse Scans of the Normal Pancreas

Often, the most important vascular land-mark for visualizing the pancreas is the splenic vein (fig. 4.13). This curvilinear tubular structure is, however, often confused with the left renal vein. Identification of the splenic vein as distinguished from the left renal vein can be made by recognizing its relation to the aorta and to the superior mesenteric artery. The left renal vein courses directly anterior to the aorta and is situated behind the superior mesenteric artery. The splenic vein is also situated anterior to the aorta, but it courses anterior to the superior mesenteric artery. Therefore, the splenic vein is situated more anteriorly than the left renal vein, with the superior mesenteric artery between them.

In figure 4.13, the left renal vein to the right of the aorta and a tubular structure to the left of the aorta can be seen. This represents the left renal vascular bundle. We are most likely unable to separate the left renal vein and artery on this section. Figure 4.13 demonstrates the body and the tail of the pancreas going posteriorly toward the left kidney. Figure 4.14 is an excellent example of a fairly horizontal pancreas in which we are able to see the head, body, and tail. It is unusual to get a view of the entire pancreas on a single transverse scan. This is because of the unusual configuration of the pancreas where the head is often caudal and the tail cephalad. However, figure 4.14 is an excellent example of the tail of the pancreas anterior to the left kidney, posterior to the stomach, and medial to the spleen.

The superior mesenteric artery and superior mesenteric vein are important landmarks in visualizing the pancreas, because they are in the region of the juncture of the head and body of the pancreas. Occasionally, a strong linear echo can be seen within the confines of the pancreas. This most likely represents the pancreatic duct (fig. 4.15). We must be certain not to conclude that the wall of the stomach is the pancreatic duct. Therefore, it is important to identify pancreatic echoes on each side of this linear echo. It is very difficult to visualize the pancreatic duct during a normal

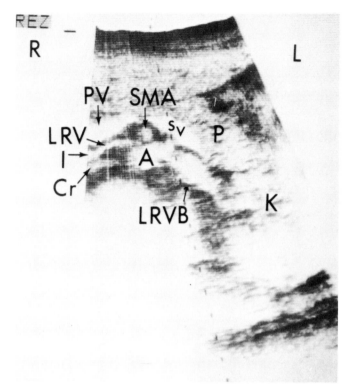

Fig. 4.13

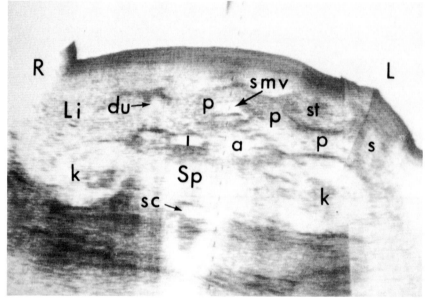

Fig. 4.14

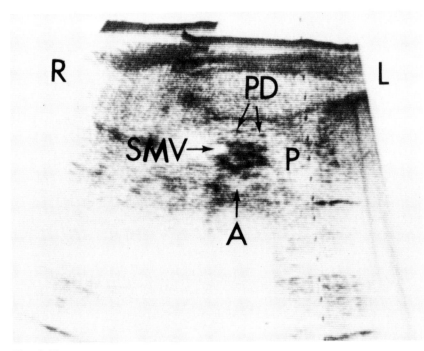

Fig. 4.15

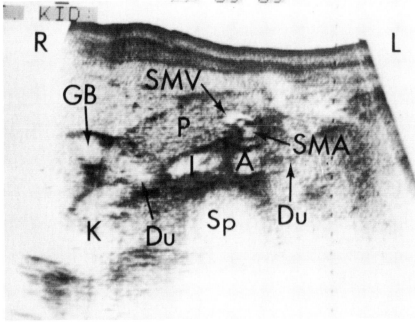

Fig. 4.16

pancreatic exam. In order to see it, a careful study at 1–2-mm intervals over the mid portion of the pancreas must be obtained.

Figure 4.16 demonstrates excellent visualization of the pancreatic head, seen to the right of the superior mesenteric artery and the superior mesenteric vein. Again, we see the normal relationship among the gallbladder, the partially filled duodenum, and the head of the pancreas. We also see some air in the third portion of the duodenum, to the left of the aorta.

A	=	Aorta
a	=	Aorta
Cr	=	Crus of the diaphragm
Du	=	Duodenum
di	=	Duodenum
GB	=	Gallbladder
I	=	Inferior vena cava
K	=	Kidney
k	=	Kidney
L	=	Left
Li	=	Liver
LRV	=	Left renal vein
LRVB	=	Left renal vascular bundle
P	=	Pancreas
p	=	Pancreas
PD	=	Pancreatic duct
PV	=	Portal vein
R	=	Right
s	=	Spleen
sc	=	Spinal canal
SMA	=	Superior mesenteric artery
SMV	=	Superior mesenteric vein
smv	=	Superior mesenteric vein
SP	=	Spine
st	=	Stomach
SV	=	Splenic vein

Longitudinal Scans of the Normal Pancreas

Longitudinal scans are usually started to the right of midline and within the liver. They progress toward the left, until the head of the pancreas comes into view. Again, the best way to find the pancreas is to localize the portal vein and follow it medially. Figure 4.17 is a longitudinal section to the right of the midline in which the head of the pancreas is starting to appear. The left portal vein and the main portal vein can also be seen. Just anterior to the main portal vein is the hepatic artery. The common bile duct is situated anterior to the main portal vein in the porta hepatis. It then courses over the portal vein and continues posteriorly behind the head of the pancreas (figs. 4.17 and 4.18).

The gastroduodenal artery is the first branch of the hepatic artery. It courses anterior to the head of the pancreas. The pancreatic head is located between the posterior common bile duct and the anterior gastroduodenal artery on longitudinal scans. This is well demonstrated in figure 4.18. In order to see the head of the pancreas, either the liver must be anterior to it, or the stomach and duodenum must be airless (fig. 4.19). If air is present in the duodenum and stomach, the pancreas may not be visualized, unless there is a prominent left lobe. Figure 4.20 demonstrates air in the duodenal bulb which obscures a portion of the pancreatic head. The pancreatic head is caudal to the portal vein and the duodenum. The inferior vena cava (fig. 4.20) is seen for almost its entire length, excepting that portion situated posterior to the duodenum. Occasionally, a small circular structure can be seen posterior to the inferior vena cava, displacing it anteriorly. This is due to the position of the right renal artery. Figures 4.18 and 4.19 demonstrate the relation of the pancreas to the stomach and third portion of the duodenum which is caudal to the pancreas. The stomach is often situated anterior to the pancreas. If the stomach were air-filled in these instances, we would be unable to visualize the head of the pancreas.

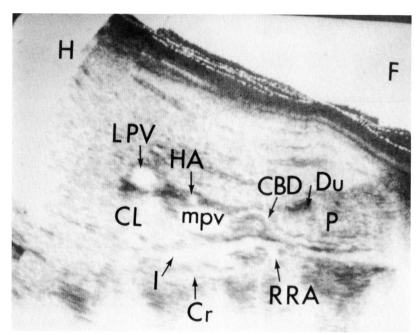

Fig. 4.17

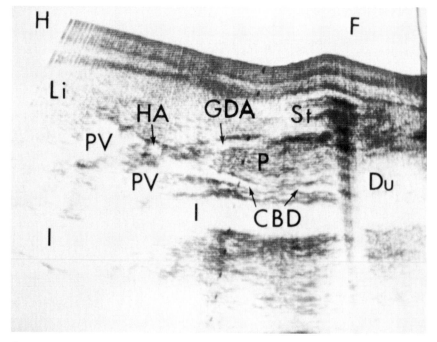

Fig. 4.18

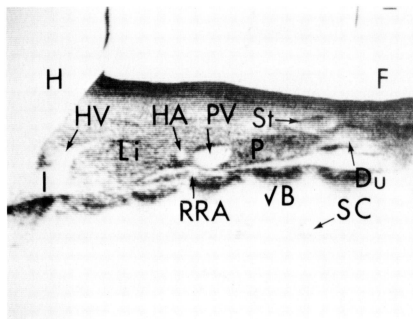

CBD	=	Common bile duct
CL	=	Caudate lobe
Cr	=	Crus of the diaphragm
F	=	Foot
GDA	=	Gastroduodenal artery
H	=	Head
HA	=	Hepatic artery
HV	=	Hepatic vein
I	=	Inferior vena cava
Li	=	Liver
LPV	=	Left portal vein
mpv	=	Main portal vein
P	=	Pancreas
PV	=	Portal vein
RRA	=	Right renal artery
SC	=	Spinal canal
St	=	Stomach
VB	=	Vertebral body

Fig. 4.19

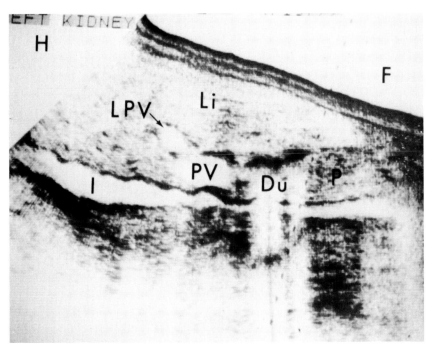

Fig. 4.20

Longitudinal Scans of the Normal Pancreas

As scans progress toward the left, we see the pancreas anterior to the inferior vena cava, the aorta, and the superior mesenteric vein. In figure 4.21 a linear lucency posterior to the inferior vena cava represents the crus of the diaphragm. This should not be confused with a vascular structure. Figure 4.21 also demonstrates the pancreas caudal to the portal vein. Again, the duodenum is seen caudal to the head of the pancreas. The pancreas does not indent the inferior vena cava in figures 4.21 and 4.22. Figure 4.22 shows the hepatic artery and the portal vein cephalad to the head of the pancreas. As we continue to the left, the pancreas is seen anterior to the aorta (fig. 4.23). In an unusual finding, the inferior mesenteric artery (fig. 4.23) is seen caudal to the head of the pancreas and posterior to the stomach. We also visualize the right renal artery toward us, as it is on the right side of the aorta. The head of the pancreas is again situated between the portal vein and the stomach.

The most important longitudinal structure for the identification of the pancreas is the superior mesenteric vein (fig. 4.23). This identifies the juncture of the head and body of the pancreas. The pancreas is usually seen anterior to the superior mesenteric vein as in figure 4.24. There is, also, however, some pancreatic tissue posterior to the superior mesenteric vein (fig. 4.24). This represents the uncinate process of the pancreas. The prominent left lobe of the liver gives excellent visualization of the body of the pancreas. The stomach is somewhat airless and caudal to the body of the pancreas. The duodenum is situated posterior to the stomach with air present. The transverse colon can be seen even more caudally to this.

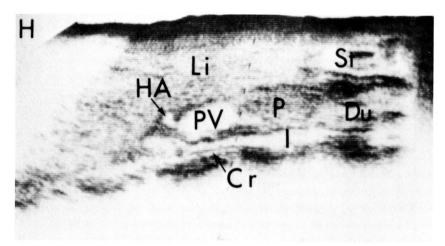

Fig. 4.21

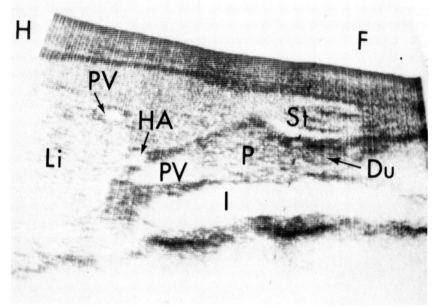

Fig. 4.22

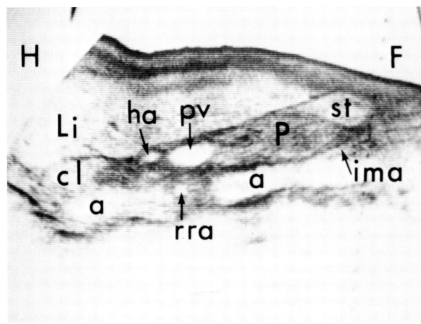
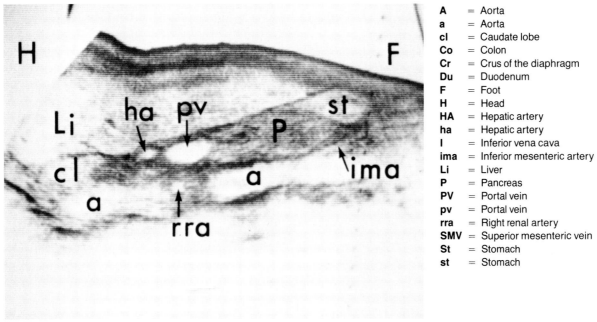

A   = Aorta
a   = Aorta
cl = Caudate lobe
Co = Colon
Cr = Crus of the diaphragm
Du = Duodenum
F   = Foot
H   = Head
HA = Hepatic artery
ha = Hepatic artery
I   = Inferior vena cava
ima = Inferior mesenteric artery
Li = Liver
P   = Pancreas
PV = Portal vein
pv = Portal vein
rra = Right renal artery
SMV = Superior mesenteric vein
St = Stomach
st = Stomach

Fig. 4.23

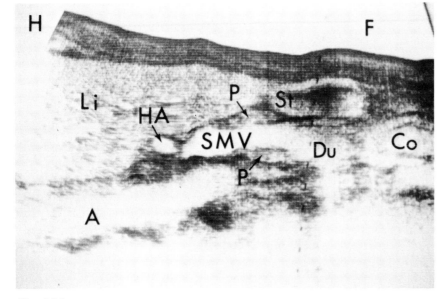

Fig. 4.24

Longitudinal and Prone Scans of the Normal Pancreas

Continuing toward the left, the vessels arising from the aorta can be seen. Figure 4.25 demonstrates the celiac axis and the superior mesenteric artery as they arise off the aorta. A vessel is seen coming off the celiac axis somewhat anteriorly; it most likely represents the left gastric artery. The splenic vein is seen as a circular lucency situated on the posterior aspect of the cephalad portion of the pancreas. The splenic vein is usually situated posterior to the upper third of the pancreas. Occasionally, it is located completely cephalad to the pancreas. When trying to identify the pancreas, the technologist should find the splenic vein and look directly anterior to it for the characteristic pancreatic echoes. If these are not seen anteriorly, he or she should look somewhat caudally, since the pancreas may be situated slightly caudal to the splenic vein.

It is also important to set the ultrasound unit so that the pancreatic echoes are not in the blackest shade. If the unit is set up with too high an output or sensitivity, the pancreatic echoes will blend in with the dark echoes of the fibrofatty retroperitoneum. Therefore, in an effort to bring out the echoes of the pancreas, it is important to adjust the unit so that the shades of the liver are somewhat light.

Occasionally, we see a mass appearing as a "bull's-eye" just beneath the diaphragm on the left side, which represents the esophagogastric junction (figs. 4.25–4.27). The crus of the diaphragm may be visualized anterior to the aorta (fig. 4.26). Progressing toward the left, the pancreas can be seen anterior to the splenic vein as it approaches the hilum of the spleen. Figure 4.27 demonstrates a large left lobe of the liver which enables us to see the tail of the pancreas situated anterior to the splenic vein and the splenic artery. The stomach is seen with its typical bull's-eye appearance, and the fourth portion of the duodenum is situated just caudal to the tail of the pancreas.

When attempting to visualize the tail of the pancreas it is often necessary to

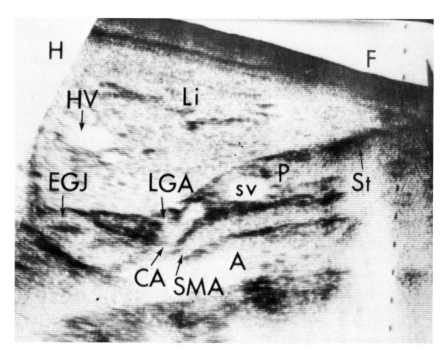

Fig. 4.25

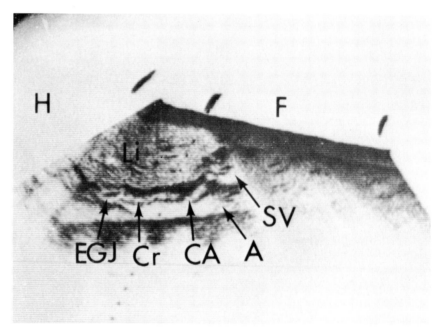

Fig. 4.26

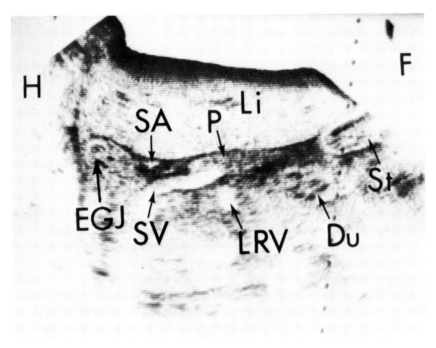

Fig. 4.27

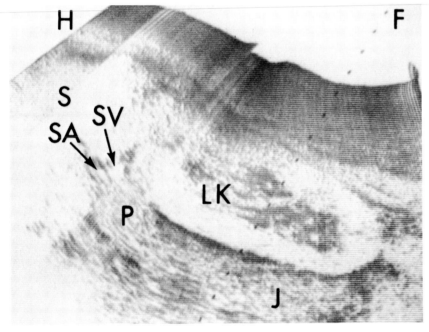

Fig. 4.28

turn the patient to the prone position. Because of air in the stomach and splenic flexure, the tail of the pancreas rarely can be seen with the patient in the supine position. Figure 4.27 is an unusual case because of the large left lobe of the liver. When the patient is in the prone position, the left kidney (fig. 4.28), is used as an ultrasonic window. The pancreas is seen just caudal to the splenic artery and the splenic vein. We must be careful not to determine that a mass is anterior to the left kidney when it is actually secondary to the proximal jejunum. The jejunum often will given an ill-defined echogenicity anterior to the left kidney which we now recognize on CAT scans. It is important to attempt to identify the splenic artery and splenic vein in the prone position in order to be certain of the location of the tail of the pancreas. If this is not done, the proximal jejunum mistakenly may be called a mass in the tail of the pancreas.

A	=	Aorta
CA	=	Celiac axis
Cr	=	Crus of the diaphragm
Du	=	Duodenum
EGJ	=	Esophagogastric junction
F	=	Foot
H	=	Head
HV	=	Hepatic vein
J	=	Jejunum
LGA	=	Left gastric artery
Li	=	Liver
LK	=	Left kidney
LRV	=	Left renal vein
P	=	Pancreas
S	=	Spleen
SA	=	Splenic artery
SMA	=	Superior mesenteric artery
St	=	Stomach
SV	=	Splenic vein

Left-Sided Pancreas and Acute Pancreatitis

Occasionally we see the pancreas more to the left of the midline than is usual. In figure 4.29, the head of the pancreas is anterior to the aorta, and the body and tail of the pancreas are even more to the left side than expected. The echo amplitude level of the pancreas is slightly greater than that seen in the liver.

The diagnosis of pancreatitis by ultrasound is a difficult one. Whenever the echoes arising from the pancreas are of less amplitude than those noted in the liver, the diagnosis of acute pancreatitis is suggested. Figure 4.30 is a scan of a 39-year-old man who entered the hospital for a head trauma and was noted to have an elevated amylase. He gave a suggestive history of alcoholic abuse. During his hospital stay, the diagnosis of acute pancreatitis was determined by the elevated amylase. The ultrasonic findings in figure 4.30 demonstrate a pancreas with echoes that are less echogenic than those within the liver. The major drawback of this diagnostic technique is that the liver echogenicity is used as a standard for comparing the pancreas. If the liver had an increased echogenicity, as seen in cirrhosis or fatty infiltration, then the pancreas would appear much more lucent than usual.

Figures 4.31 and 4.32 represent another case of acute pancreatitis. The echoes arising from the pancreas are somewhat coarser than those usually seen and also less echogenic than the liver. This is best noted on longitudinal scan (fig. 4.32). It is important to compare the echogenicity in the liver at approximately the same depth as we are looking at the pancreas. Normal body attenuation within the liver can give rise to varying amplitude echoes in the liver when we compare the anterior to the posterior echoes of the liver. This is especially true if the time gain compensation curve is incorrectly set.

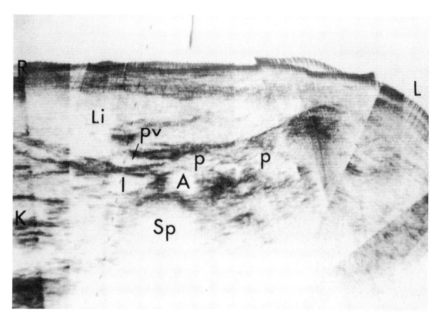

Fig. 4.29

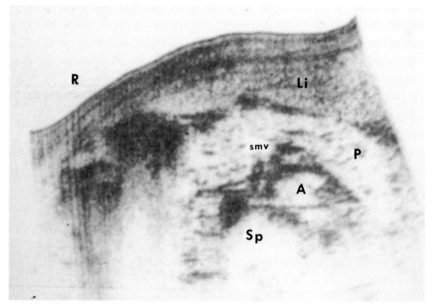

Fig. 4.30

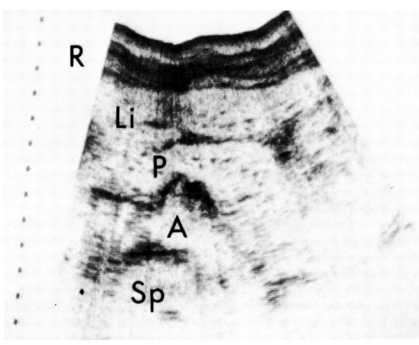

A   = Aorta
EGJ = Esophagogasatric junction
H   = Head
I   = Inferior vena cava
K   = Kidney
L   = Left
Li = Liver
P   = Pancreas
p   = Pancreas
pv = Portal vein
R   = Right
smv = Superior mesenteric vein
Sp = Spine
St = Stomach

Fig. 4.31

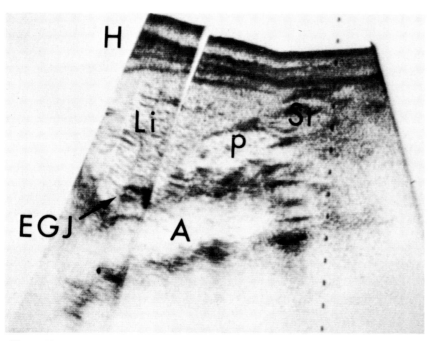

Fig. 4.32

Chronic Pancreatitis ; Cystic Fibrosis

With increasing fibrosis, the pancreas manifests increased echogenicity. Patients with chronic pancreatitis have an even higher amplitude echo arising from the pancreas. This can be so high that the pancreas will be lost in the highly echogenic fibrofatty retroperitoneum. Figures 4.33 and 4.34 are examples of chronic pancreatitis in which the pancreas is extremely echogenic. Identification of the pancreas is confirmed by the surrounding anatomy. In figure 4.33 the pancreas is seen lateral to the superior mesenteric vein. The liver echoes are much less echogenic than the echoes arising from the pancreatic head. On the longitudinal scans (fig. 4.34), the head of the pancreas is markedly increased in echogenicity when compared with the echoes arising from the liver. The fluid-filled mass anterior to the pancreatic head represents fluid in the stomach. Elderly patients also can demonstrate increased echogenicity of the pancreas which probably is part of the aging process and which causes increased fibrosis to the pancreatic parenchyma.

Increased echogenicity arising from the pancreas also has been noted in patients with cystic fibrosis. Figures 4.35 and 4.36 represent scans obtained from a 19-year-old patient with severe cystic fibrosis. Figure 4.35 is a longitudinal scan through the head of the pancreas which has a markedly increased echogenicity when compared to the adjacent liver parenchyma. Figure 4.36 is a longitudinal scan through the body of the pancreas anterior to the superior mesenteric vein and the superior mesenteric artery. The pancreas is extremely echogenic when compared to the liver parenchyma. It can be lost, however, in the highly echogenic fibrofatty retroperitoneal echoes.

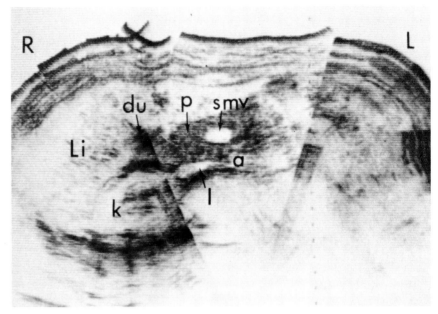

Fig. 4.33

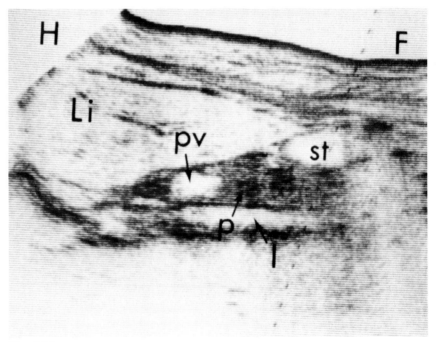

Fig. 4.34

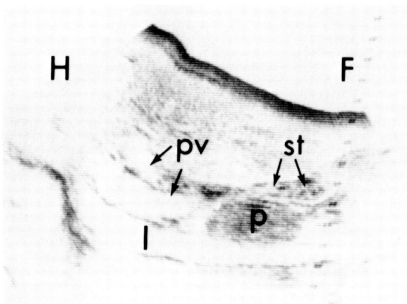

Fig. 4.35

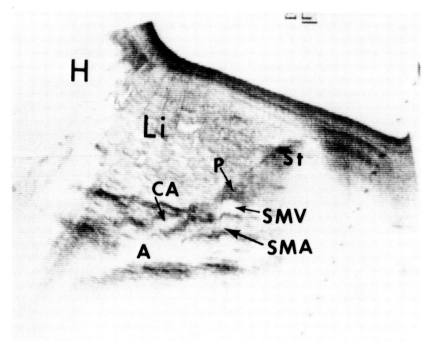

Fig. 4.36

A	= Aorta
a	= Aorta
CA	= Celiac axis
du	= Duodenum
F	= Foot
H	= Head
I	= Inferior vena cava
k	= Kidney
L	= Left
Li	= Liver
P	= Pancreas
p	= Pancreas
pv	= Portal vein
R	= Right
SMA	= Superior mesenteric artery
SMV	= Superior mesenteric vein
smv	= Superior mesenteric vein
St	= Stomach

Chronic Pancreatitis with Calcification

When chronic pancreatitis progresses, calcification will eventually involve the region of the pancreatic bed. The ultrasonic findings of a calcified pancreas produce an extremely high-amplitude echo to the surrounding pancreatic bed. Often, the calcification will be large enough to cause shadowing. A markedly calcified pancreas can be extremely difficult to diagnose in some instances, since it can be confused with bowel air. Figures 4.37–4.39 are scans of a 40-year-old man with a long history of ethanol abuse. The patient had had previous alcoholic hepatitis. He was admitted with a two-month history of nausea and abdominal pain. The scans in figures 4.37 and 4.38 demonstrate a markedly enlarged pancreas (arrows). The central portion of the pancreatic bed is highly echogenic; this is consistent with calcification. The periphery is less echogenic, indicating the surrounding pancreatic tissue. Figure 4.39 is an X-ray of the same patient demonstrating the calcifications best seen to the right of midline.

Figure 4.40 is a transverse scan of a 45-year-old man whose first episode of alcholic pancreatitis was noted 11 years earlier. The present examination demonstrates a highly echogenic pancreatic bed. We are unable to see the area posterior to the pancreatic bed because of shadowing arising from the calcification within the pancreas. It is evident, however, that the pancreas can easily be confused with bowel air. It is the nodular irregular appearance of the high-level echoes that gives the clue that calcification is present within the pancreatic bed.

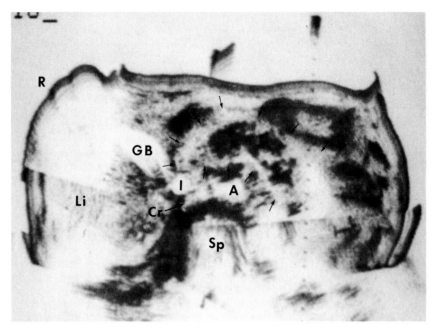

Fig. 4.37

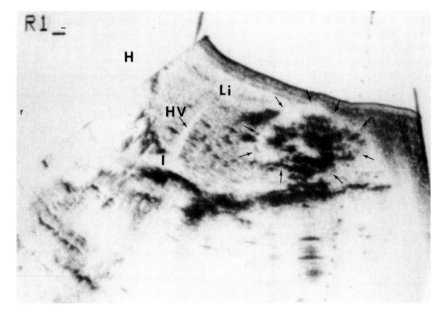

Fig. 4.38

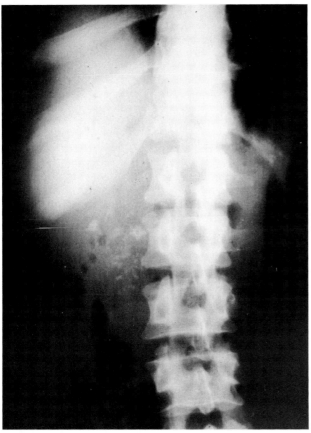

Fig. 4.39

A   = Aorta
Arrows = Outline the pancreatic bed
Cr   = Crus of the diaphragm
GB   = Gallbladder
H   = Head
HV   = Hepatic vein
I   = Inferior vena cava
K   = Kidney
Li   = Liver
P   = Pancreatic bed
R   = Right
Sh   = Shadow from the calcified
            pancreas
Sp   = Spine

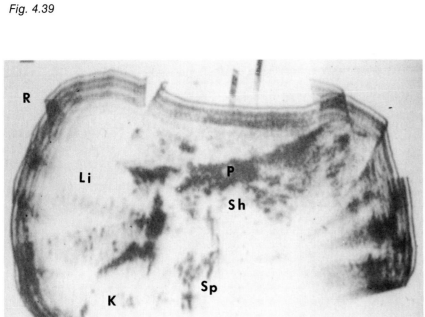

Fig. 4.40

Chronic Pancreatitis versus Neoplasm

Often, chronic pancreatitis leads to a pancreatic mass that is difficult to distinguish from carcinoma of the pancreas. Figures 4.41–4.45 represent such a case. This patient was a 25-year-old woman with complaints indicating jaundice of approximately 2–3 months' duration. Viral hepatitis was suspected, and she underwent ultrasound examination. Figure 4.41 is a transverse section through the liver and demonstrates both a dilated biliary tree (arrows) and a dilated common bile duct. Transverse scans through the head of the pancreas (fig. 4.42) demonstrate a pancreatic mass. The borders are somewhat irregular, and the mass is less echogenic than the liver. A longitudinal scan through the head of the pancreas (fig. 4.43) again demonstrates the dilated biliary tree (arrows) and the dilated common bile duct. Some indentation is noted on the inferior vena cava due to this pancreatic mass. The findings are highly suggestive of a pancreatic tumor within the head. An upper gastrointestinal series (fig. 4.44) demonstrates enlargement of the C loop with effacement of the second portion of the duodenum. A transhepatic cholangiogram (fig. 4.45) shows dilatation of the biliary tree with narrowing of the distal common bile duct.

The patient underwent laparotomy, and biopsy demonstrated chronic pancreatitis. There was no evidence of neoplasm. The common bile duct was obstructed and choledochojejunostomy was performed. This ultrasound study illustrates the fact that severe chronic pancreatitis can present as a mass that cannot be distinguished from a neoplasm.

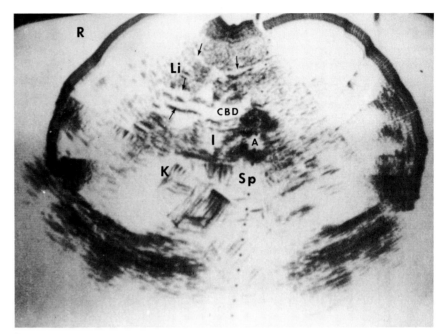

Fig. 4.41

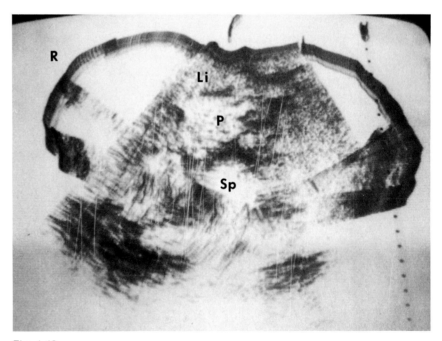

Fig. 4.42

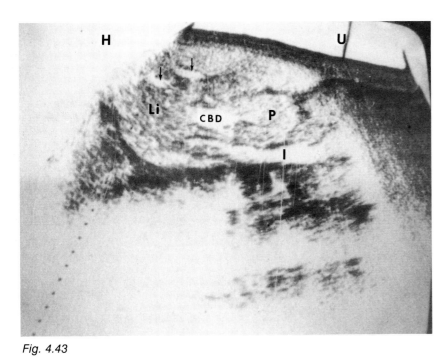

A	= Aorta
Arrows	= Dilated biliary tree
CBD	= Common bile duct
H	= Head
I	= Inferior vena cava
K	= Kidney
Li	= Liver
P	= Pancreas
R	= Right
Sp	= Spine
U	= Umbilical level

Fig. 4.43

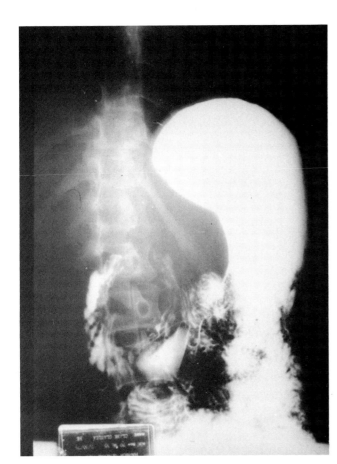

Fig. 4.44

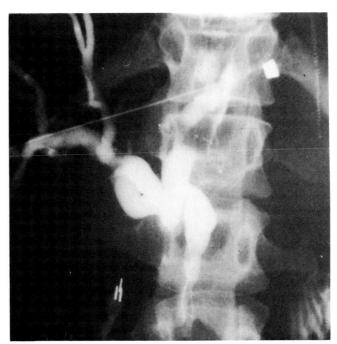

Fig. 4.45

Pancreatic Abscess

This 31-year-old man experienced a sudden onset of a sharp midepigastric pain. He had a long history of chronic ethanol abuse. His white blood count and amylase were elevated. Figures 4.46 and 4.47 are scans obtained by ultrasound examination. Figure 4.46 is a transverse section of the midepigastric region. Two large sonolucent masses are present with fairly thick walls. These represent pancreatic abscesses. A longitudinal scan (fig. 4.47) demonstrates a sonolucent mass in the pancreatic bed anterior to the aorta and crus of the diaphragm. The pancreatic abscess would be difficult to distinguish from a pseudocyst or severe edema of the pancreas, as it is present in a pancreatic phlegmon. Figure 4.48 is an X-ray of the upper abdomen obtained several days later. Air is noted in the pancreatic abscess just to the left of T12.

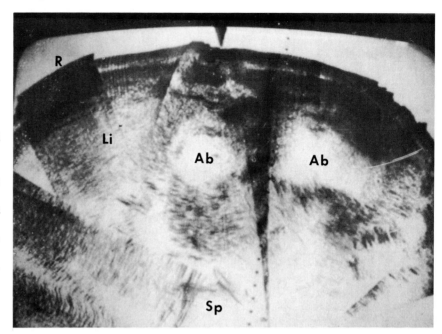

Fig. 4.46

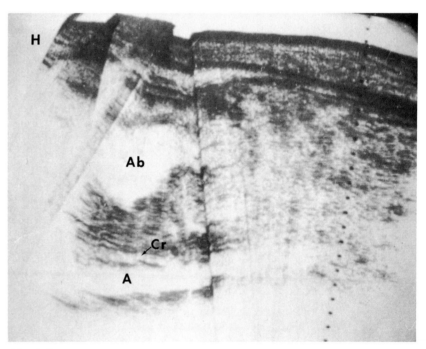

Fig. 4.47

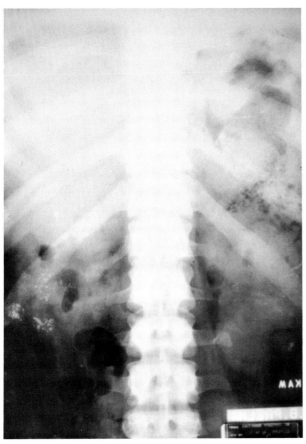

Fig. 4.48

A   = Aorta
Ab = Pancreatic abscess
Cr = Crus of the diaphragm
H   = Head
Li = Liver
R   = Right
Sp = Spine

Unilocular Pancreatic Pseudocyst with Spontaneous Resolution

Ultrasound plays an important role in the diagnosis of pancreatic pseudo-cysts. Since fluid can easily be detected by ultrasound, it is the imaging modality of choice in their differential diagnosis. Pseudocysts may be unilocular or multi-loculated. Figures 4.49–4.52 are scans of a unilocular pseudocyst. The patient was a 52-year-old woman who had a long history of alcoholic pancreatitis. She was admitted with epigastric pain and was noted to have a sonolucent mass posterior to the left lobe of the liver which was felt to be a pseudocyst (figs. 4.49 and 4.50). She was scheduled for surgery and followed serially by ultrasound. Just prior to surgery the pseudocyst began to decrease in size (fig. 4.51). Surgery was postponed, and follow-up examination eventually demonstrated complete disappearance of the pseudocyst (fig. 4.52).

This case demonstrates the dynamic nature of pancreatic pseudocysts. Many patients do drain spontaneously without any marked side effects. Ultrasound should be used to serially follow all patients with pseudocysts who do not go on to surgery.

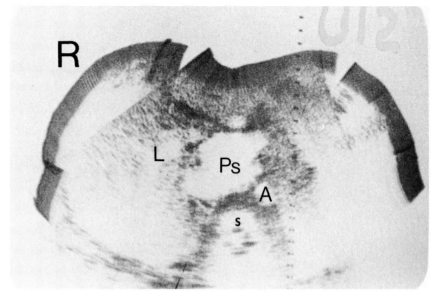

Fig. 4.49

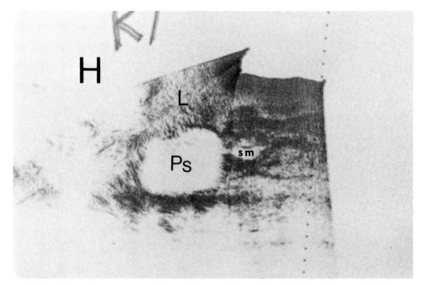

Fig. 4.50

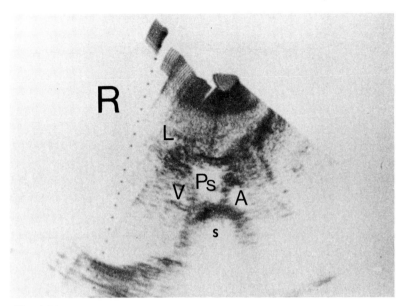

A = Aorta
H = Head
L = Liver
Ps = Pseudocyst
R = Right
S = Spine
sm = Superior mesenteric vein
V = Inferior vena cava

Fig. 4.51

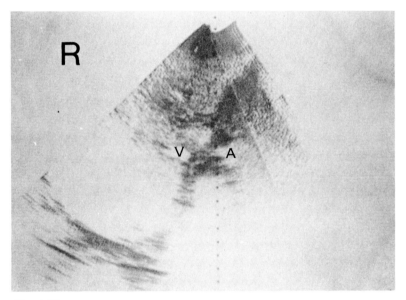

Fig. 4.52

Rapid Development of a Pancreatic Pseudocyst

Pancreatic pseudocysts may arise quite rapidly. Ultrasound is an excellent means of following a patient with acute pancreatitis. A change in the clinical symptoms such as acute pain indicates that ultrasound should be ordered to detect whether or not a pseudocyst has developed. The case in figures 4.53–4.56 is an excellent example of the rapid development of a pancreatic pseudocyst. This 33-year-old man with a long history of ethanol abuse was in the hospital for several months and underwent serial ultrasound examinations. The patient had somehow managed to continue drinking during his hospitalization and while on hyperalimentation. Figures 4.53 and 4.54 demonstrate a relatively normal pancreas (arrows) with no mass noted anteriorly. Figures 4.55 and 4.56, approximately one week later, followed an episode of acute abdominal pain. A large sonolucent mass secondary to a pancreatic pseudocyst is now visible. Subsequent surgery documented the presence of a pancreatic pseudocyst anterior to the body of the pancreas.

This case demonstrates the rapid development of a pancreatic pseudocyst which can be followed best by ultrasound examination.

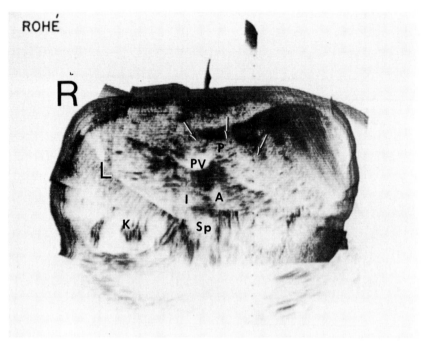

Fig. 4.53

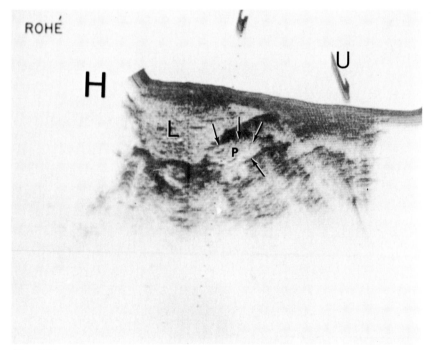

Fig. 4.54

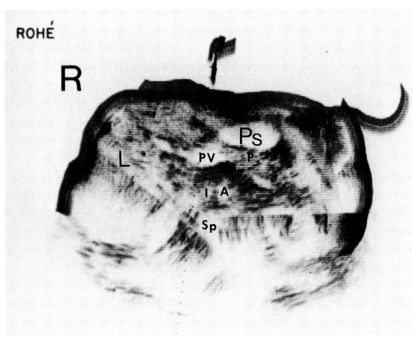

Fig. 4.55

A	= Aorta
H	= Head
I	= Inferior vena cava
K	= Kidney
L	= Liver
P	= Pancreas
Ps	= Pseudocyst
PV	= Portal vein
R	= Right
SA	= Splenic artery
Sp	= Spine
SV	= Splenic vein
U	= Umbilical level

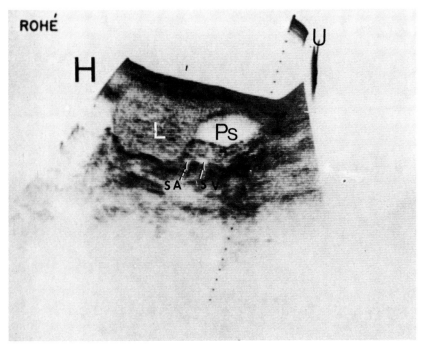

Fig. 4.56

Pseudocyst of the Uncinate Process

The smallest pathological entity of the pancreas can best be diagnosed in the area of the uncinate process. This is due to excellent vascular anatomy which can delineate small masses. Figures 4.57 and 4.58 are from an ultrasound examination of a patient with chronic alcoholism and continual abdominal pain. The head of the pancreas is slightly enlarged, but no masses are noted in figure 4.57. Figure 4.58 demonstrates the superior mesenteric vein to have a straight course.

Follow-up exam two months later demonstrates a small pseudocyst in the uncinate process of the pancreas (fig. 4.59). Figure 4.60 is a longitudinal scan which demonstrates an altered course to the superior mesenteric vein which is now draped over the small pseudocyst in the uncinate process of the pancreas.

This case illustrates the excellent anatomy about the head of the pancreas, especially the uncinate process, which it is possible to demonstrate with ultrasound. It is also an example of the development of a pancreatic pseudocyst over a short period of time.

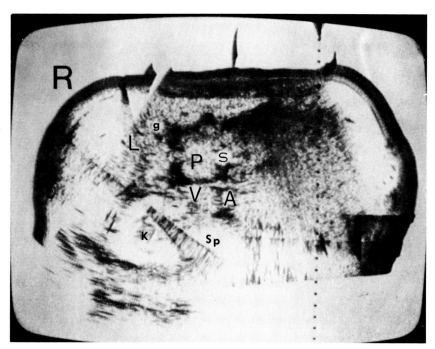

Fig. 4.57

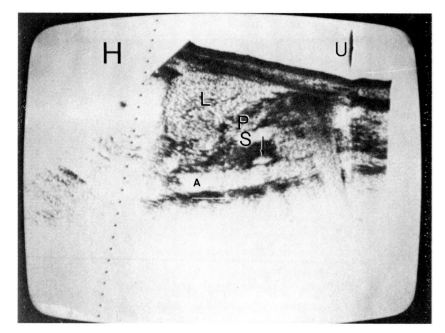

Fig. 4.58

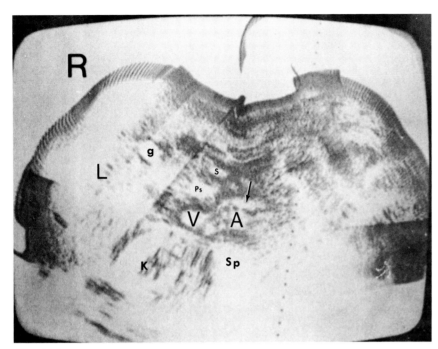

Fig. 4.59

A   = Aorta
Arrow   = Left renal vein
G   = Gallbladder
H   = Head
K   = Kidney
L   = Liver
P   = Pancreas
Ps   = Pseudocyst
R   = Right
S   = Superior mesenteric vein
Sp   = Spine
U   = Umbilical level
V   = Inferior Vena cava

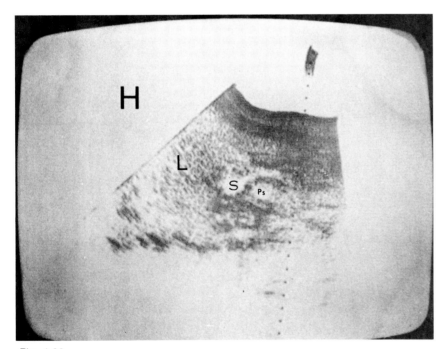

Fig. 4.60

Multiloculated Pseudocysts

Pseudocysts may be multiloculated lucent masses around the pancreatic bed. Curvilinear echoes can be present within the pseudocyst, indicating septation. There can also be debris on the posterior wall. Figures 4.61–4.63 represent a multiloculated pseudocyst. Figures 4.61 and 4.62 are ultrasound examinations of a large sonolucent pseudocyst in the epigastric region posterior to the left lobe of the liver. Some curvilinear echoes are present within the pseudocyst (arrows) and represent septations. The walls are somewhat irregular. Figure 4.63 is a CAT scan demonstrating the pseudocyst posterior to the left lobe of the liver and effacing the posterior aspect of the stomach.

Figure 4.64 is a multiloculated pseudocyst with many more septations than were noted in the previous case. The patient was a 19-year-old woman who was referred because of the recurrence of a pancreatic pseudocyst. She had previous surgery with supposed drainage of the pseudocyst, but the mass did not disappear. It is not unusual for a multiloculated pseudocyst not to disappear completely following surgery; all of the chambers may not have been drained. It is important to notify the surgeon specifically that a multiloculated pseudocyst is present. Figure 4.64 demonstrates the multiloculated pseudocyst in the right abdomen. It has numerous small circular sonolucencies which explain the difficulty in obtaining adequate surgical drainage.

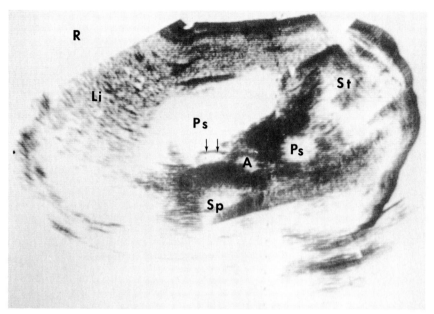

Fig. 4.61

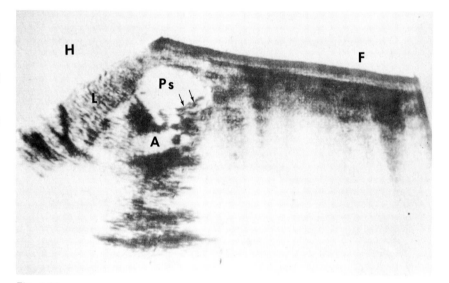

Fig. 4.62

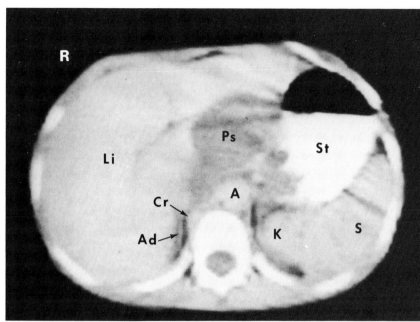

Fig. 4.63

A	=	Aorta
ad	=	Adrenal gland
Arrows	=	Septations
Cr	=	Crus of the diaphragm
F	=	Foot
H	=	Head
K	=	Kidney
L	=	Left
Li	=	Liver
M	=	Multiloculated pseudocyst
Ps	=	Pseudocyst
R	=	Right
S	=	Spleen
Sp	=	Spine
St	=	Stomach
SV	=	Splenic vein

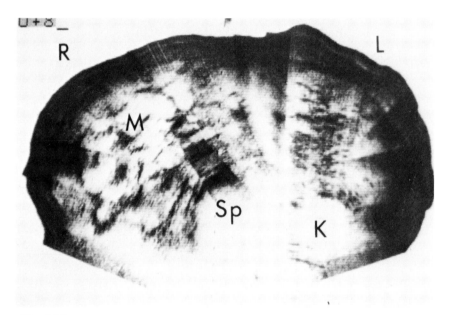

Fig. 4.64

Other Sonolucent Masses near the Pancreas

Any time we see a fluid-filled mass in the upper abdomen, a pseudocyst is usually considered in the differential diagnosis. Other entities must, however, be ruled out before the diagnosis can be made. The most common error in the diagnostic interpretation is visualization of a fluid-filled loop of bowel. Figure 4.65 is an example of a fluid-filled stomach with echoes noted posteriorly due to food in the posterior aspect of the stomach. It is important to repeat the examination the next day with the patient having had no oral intake. If a similarly shaped sonolucency is present in the same location, the diagnosis of a pancreatic pseudocyst is quite likely.

The patient in figures 4.66–4.68 is an excellent serial examination of what a fluid-filled loop of bowel can look like. In figure 4.66 the duodenum is air-filled as it lies between the gallbladder and the pancreas. The patient was given a small amount of water, and the duodenum became partially fluid-filled (fig. 4.67). There is now some enhanced through transmission posterior to the duodenum and adjacent to the head of the pancreas. A portion of fluid-filled stomach is also seen to the left of the body of the pancreas. The patient was given more water, and the duodenum was noted to enlarge (fig. 4.68). The duodenum now presents as a larger sonolucent mass with through transmission between the gallbladder and the pancreas. If this fluid-filled mass had been present initially, the diagnosis of a pseudocyst would most likely have been made. It is always necessary to reexamine the patient the following day. We have used nasogastric suction on inpatients to rule out a fluid-filled loop of bowel. An outpatient should be requested to remain without oral intake after midnight prior to the day of exam. Real time examination may be used to detect peristalsis.

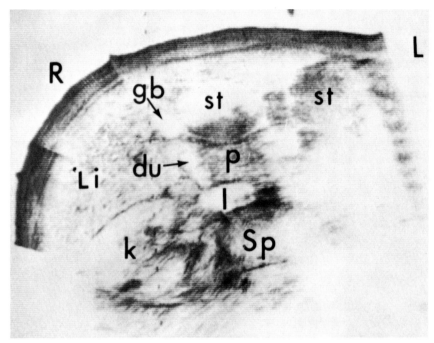

Fig. 4.65

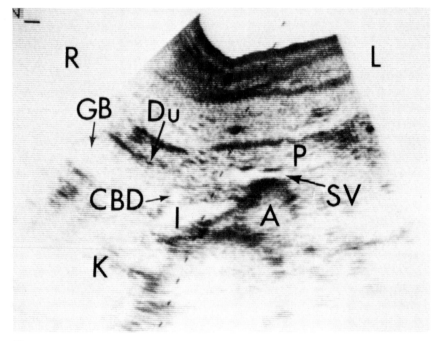

Fig. 4.66

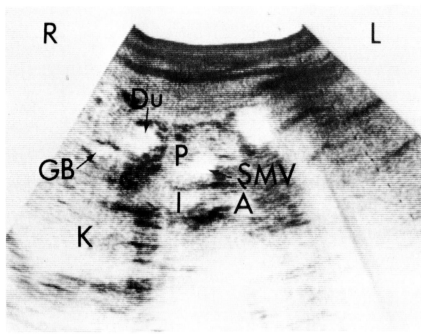

Fig. 4.67

A   = Aorta
CBD = Common bile duct
Du = Duodenum
du = Duodenum
GB = Gallbladder
gb = Gallbladder
I   = Inferior vena cava
K   = Kidney
k   = Kidney
L   = Left
Li = Liver
P   = Pancreas
p   = Pancreas
R   = Right
SMV = Superior mesenteric vein
Sp = Spine
St = Stomach
SV = Splenic vein

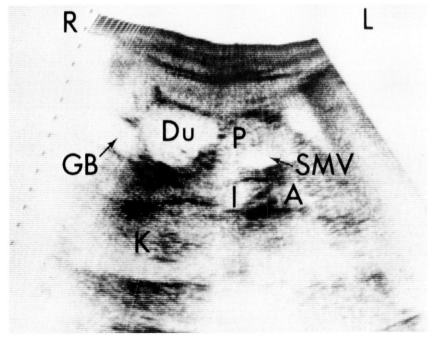

Fig. 4.68

Other Sonolucent Masses near the Pancreas

Another cause of a fluid-filled mass in the upper abdomen can be loculated ascites. The lesser sac is a common spot for a pancreatic pseudocyst to occur. We have, however, seen ascites present in unusual locations and shapes, and the lesser sac can be the site of loculated ascites. Figures 4.69 and 4.70 are scans of a 40-year-old woman with a diagnosis of ovarian carcinoma. She had a fluid-filled area noted in the region of the lesser sac anterior to the pancreas. Figure 4.69 demonstrates a large sonolucency anterior to the pancreas and secondary to loculated ascites. A longitudinal scan shows the ascites anterior to the body of the pancreas (fig. 4.70). The patient underwent laparotomy, and poorly differentiated diffuse carcinoma of the pelvis was noted along with loculated ascites.

Occasionally, large dilated vessels may present as fluid-filled masses in the upper abdomen. Very prominent portal and splenic veins are quite commonly seen. Figures 4.71 and 4.72 demonstrate an unusual aneurysm of the celiac axis. Figure 4.71 is a transverse section of the upper abdomen in which the celiac axis presents as a sonolucency anterior to the aorta. On longitudinal scans the communication between the celiac artery aneurysm and the celiac artery can be identified as it takes off from the aorta. Any time we see a sonolucent mass in the upper abdomen, it is important to attempt to determine whether or not it communicates with any of the vessels in the area. If this communication can be demonstrated, the diagnosis of an aneurysm or a dilated venous structure can be made. If it cannot be shown, the possibility of a small pseudocyst must be considered.

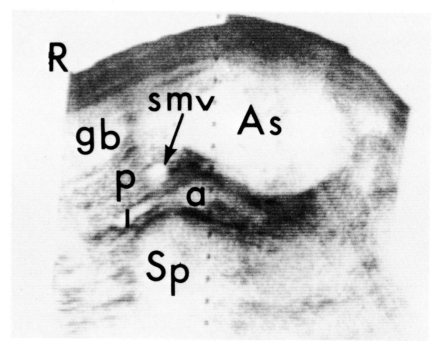

Fig. 4.69

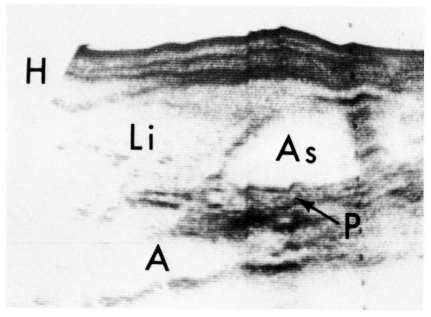

Fig. 4.70

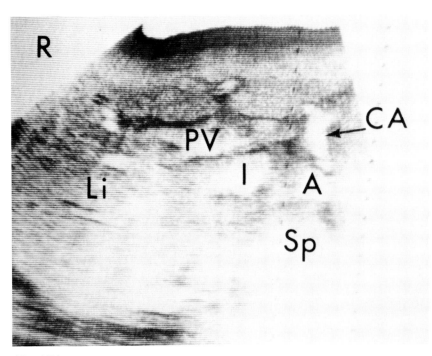

A   = Aorta
a   = Aorta
As = Ascites
CA = Celiac artery aneurysm
F   = Foot
gb = Gallbladder
H   = Head
I   = Inferior vena cava
Li = Liver
P   = Pancreas
p   = Pancreas
PV = Portal vein
R   = Right
SA = Splenic artery
smv = Superior mesenteric vein
Sp = Spine
SV = Splenic vein

Fig. 4.71

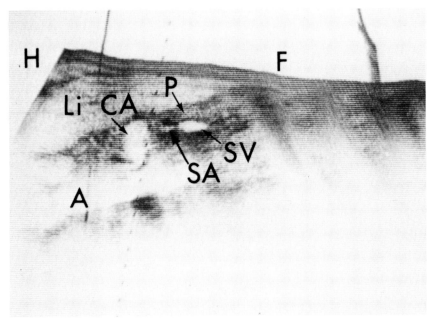

Fig. 4.72

Pancreatic Carcinoma

Tumors of the pancreas usually present on ultrasound examination as slightly less echogenic masses with irregular borders. They appear solid with diffuse echoes throughout. Often, they are less echogenic than the normal liver. The borders are somewhat irregular or ill-defined. The even echo pattern seen in the normal pancreas is not present in carcinoma. This even echo pattern has been called "cobblestoning." The patient in figures 4.73–4.76 is a 47-year-old man with progressive weight loss. An upper GI examination demonstrated anterior displacement of the stomach. The ultrasound examination showed a large echogenic mass in the head of the pancreas. The borders are somewhat irregular, and the splenic vein is displaced anteriorly along with the superior mesenteric vein. In figure 4.74 the superior mesenteric artery is in a fairly normal position, but the superior mesenteric vein is displaced anteriorly. The longitudinal examination (fig. 4.75) demonstrates the mass anterior to the aorta, displacing the superior mesenteric vein anteriorly. This represents a mass in the head of the pancreas, and of the uncinate process, that is displacing the superior mesenteric vein in an anterior position.

The biliary tree is obstructed as numerous tubular structures are noted within the liver (arrows). A longitudinal scan through the lateral aspect of the liver again demonstrates fairly diffuse biliary tree distention (fig. 4.76).

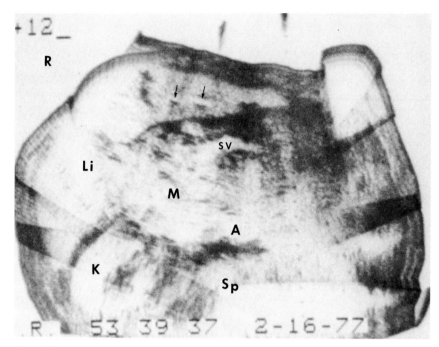

Fig. 4.73

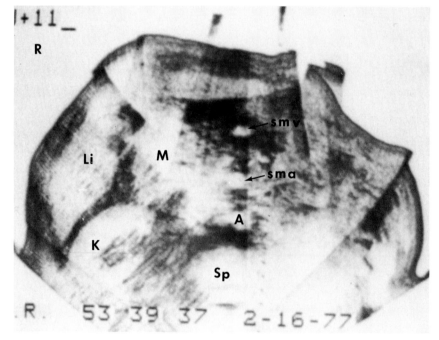

Fig. 4.74

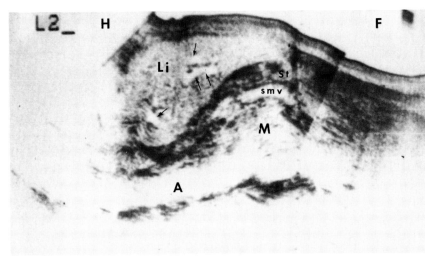

Fig. 4.75

A	=	Aorta
Arrows	=	Dilated biliary tree
D	=	Diaphragm
F	=	Foot
H	=	Head
K	=	Kidney
Li	=	Liver
M	=	Carcinoma of the head of the pancreas
R	=	Right
sma	=	Superior mesenteric artery
smv	=	Superior mesenteric vein
Sp	=	Spine
St	=	Stomach
SV	=	Splenic vein

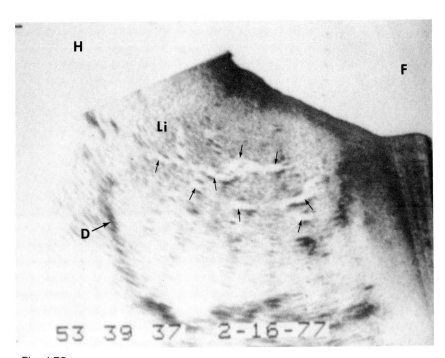

Fig. 4.76

Insulinoma and Cystadenoma

As mentioned earlier, detection of a small mass is easiest in the uncinate process of the pancreas, because of the surrounding vascular anatomy. Figures 4.77 and 4.78 represent a 1.5-cm insulinoma of the uncinate process of the pancreas. The transverse section in figure 4.77 demonstrates a relatively sonolucent solid mass in the uncinate process of the pancreas, just posterior to the superior mesenteric vein. The mass is medial to the common bile duct. In a longitudinal section (fig. 4.78) the insulinoma appears as a relatively less echogenic region in the posterior aspect of the pancreas.

A cystadenocarcinoma usually presents as a sonolucent mass with multiple septations (figs. 4.79 and 4.80). The mass is often confused with a multiloculated pseudocyst of the pancreas. Figure 4.79 is an ultrasound examination in the transverse plane with a mass in the region of the body and tail of the pancreas. There are some linear echoes and some wall thickening to the lateral aspect of the mass. Figure 4.80 is a CAT scan of approximately the same area, demonstrating a large mass anterior to the left kidney and medial to the spleen. The mass is less dense centrally with some increased density representing the septations (arrow).

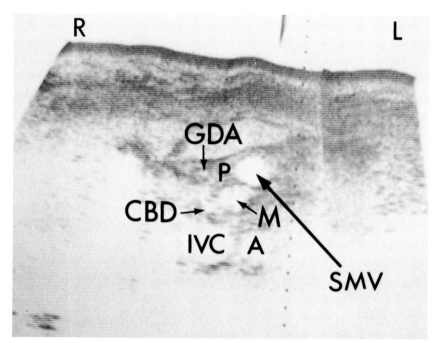

Fig. 4.77

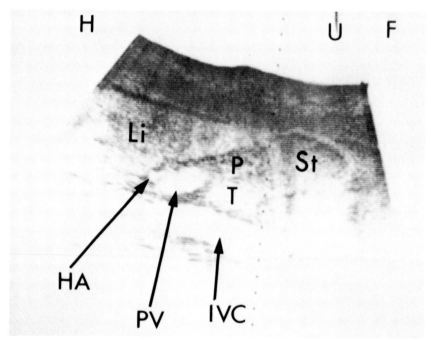

Fig. 4.78

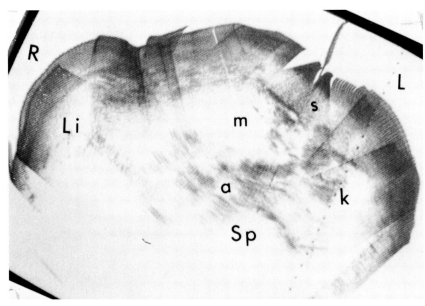

Fig. 4.79

A	=	Aorta
a	=	Aorta
Arrows	=	Septations within cystadenoma
CBD	=	Common bile duct
Du	=	Duodenum
F	=	Foot
GDA	=	Gastroduodenal artery
H	=	Head
HA	=	Hepatic artery
I	=	Inferior vena cava
IVC	=	Inferior vena cava
k	=	Kidney
L	=	Left
Li	=	Liver
M	=	Insulinoma
m	=	Cystadenocarcinoma
P	=	Pancreas
PV	=	Portal vein
R	=	Right
s	=	Spleen
SMV	=	Superior mesenteric vein
Sp	=	Spine
St	=	Stomach
T	=	Insulinoma tumor
U	=	Umbilical level

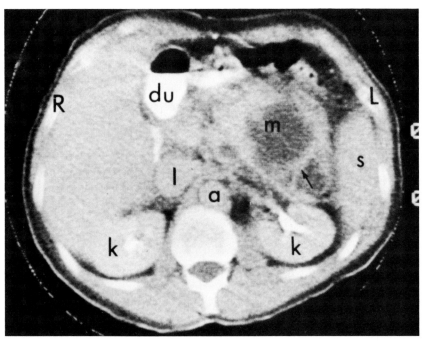

Fig. 4.80

Pancreatic Carcinoma and Duodenal Diverticulum

This 76-year-old woman entered the hospital with a history of guaiac-positive stools and progressive weight loss. Ultrasound examination demonstrated two masses in the pancreatic region. Transverse section (fig. 4.81) demonstrates a pancreatic carcinoma (arrows) in the region of the head of the pancreas. Figure 4.82 is a transverse section, slightly lower, that demonstrates a mass posterior to the body of the pancreas and secondary to a duodenal diverticulum arising from the third portion of the duodenum. This scan also demonstrates dilatation of the biliary tree (arrows) and common bile duct. Figure 4.83 is a longitudinal scan through the carcinoma of the head of the pancreas which shows the markedly dilated common bile duct ending abruptly at the site of the tumor. This represents a solid mass of the head of the pancreas obstructing the biliary tree. An X-ray (fig. 4.84) of the C loop of the duodenum shows the duodenal diverticulum arising from the third portion of the duodenum which is the mass posterior to the pancreas (fig. 4.83). The X-ray also demonstrates the marked irregular mucosa to the lateral aspect of the duodenum (fig. 4.84), where the mass in the head of the pancreas is invading the duodenum.

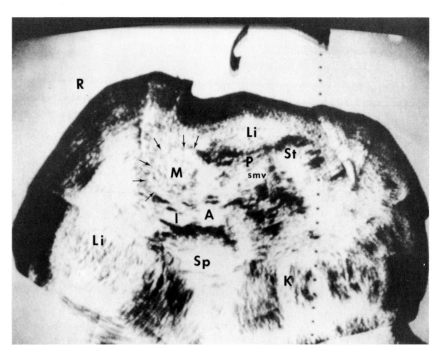

Fig. 4.81

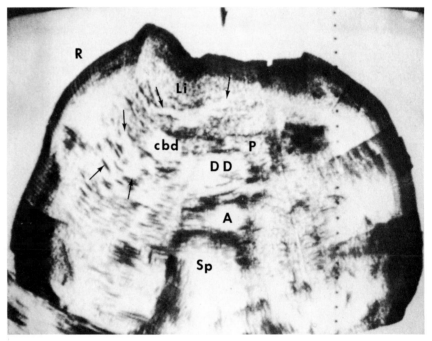

Fig. 4.82

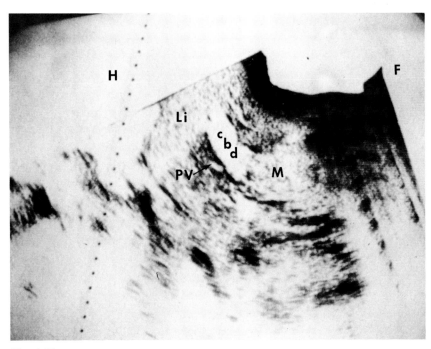

Fig. 4.83

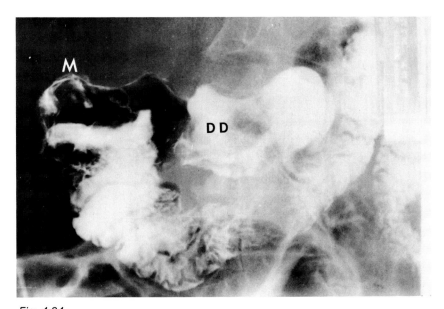

Fig. 4.84

A	=	Aorta
Arrows	=	Dilated biliary tree
cbd	=	Common bile duct
DD	=	Duodenal diverticulum
F	=	Foot
H	=	Head
I	=	Inferior vena cava
K	=	Kidney
Li	=	Liver
M and arrows	=	Carcinoma of the head of the pancreas
P	=	Pancreas
PV	=	Portal vein
R	=	Right
smv	=	Superior mesenteric vein
Sp	=	Spine
St	=	Stomach

Pancreatic Carcinoma of the Tail

As already mentioned in this chapter, examination of the tail of the pancreas is best performed with the patient in the prone position. The left kidney is used as an ultrasonic window. Figure 4.85 is an intravenous pyelogram of a patient with marked distortion and deformity of the upper pole collecting system of the left kidney caused by a mass suspected of being a hypernephroma. Ultrasound examination of the patient was performed in the prone position. Figure 4.86 is a longitudinal scan through the long axis of the kidney. The mass is markedly anterior to the kidney, more in the region of the tail of the pancreas. There is loss of the renal contour adjacent to the mass, indicating invasion. This turned out to be a carcinoma of the tail of the pancreas that also invaded the kidney.

A similar case (figs. 4.87 and 4.88), from M. D. Anderson Hospital in Houston, Texas, represents a carcinoma of the tail of the pancreas. A transverse section (fig. 4.87) through the left kidney demonstrates the mass anterior to the left kidney. Again, the anterior border of the kidney is invaded by the tumor. A longitudinal scan through the left kidney (fig. 4.88) shows the mass situated anterior to the kidney. These findings indicate a solid lesion of the tail of the pancreas.

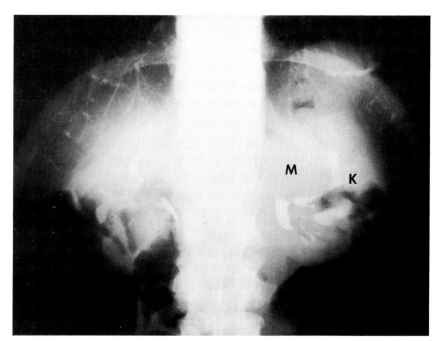

Fig. 4.85

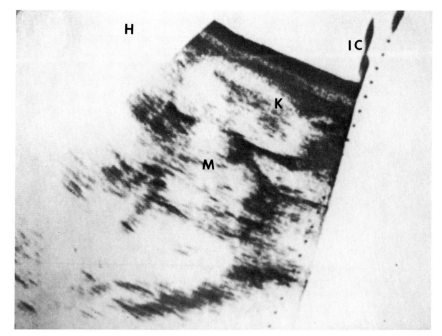

Fig. 4.86

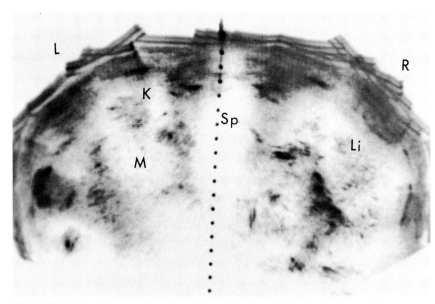

Fig. 4.87

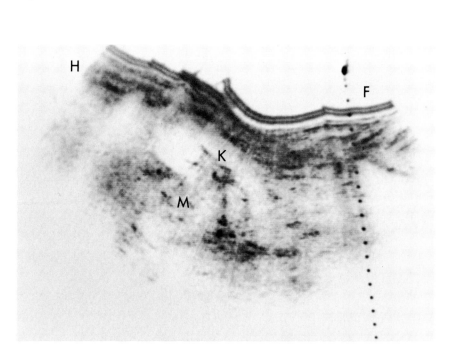

Fig. 4.88

F = Foot
H = Head
IC = Level of the iliac crest
K = Kidney
L = Left
Li = Liver
M = Carcinoma of the tail of the pancreas
R = Right
Sp = Spine

Dilated Pancreatic Duct

This patient with ampullary carcinoma demonstrated dilatation of the common bile duct and the pancreatic duct. Figures 4.89 and 4.90 are transverse sections at different levels through the pancreas. Figure 4.89 is close to the level of the splenic vein. Anterior to the splenic vein is another tubular structure representing a dilated pancreatic duct. We can also see a dilated common bile duct. A transverse section (fig. 4.90), slightly lower, at the level of the superior mesenteric vein, demonstrates the uncinate process of the pancreas posterior to the superior mesenteric vein. The dilated pancreatic duct is seen to approach the common bile duct.

Figures 4.91 and 4.92 are longitudinal scans showing the dilated common bile duct of the same patient. The dilated pancreatic duct (fig. 4.91) is seen coursing caudally, just anterior to the dilated common bile duct. Finally, figure 4.92 shows the region close to the ampulla where the dilated common bile duct and proximal portion of the pancreatic duct near the ampulla can be seen. The head of the pancreas, anterior to the common bile duct and cephalad to the stomach, is also visible. Dilated bile ducts are noted also within the liver. These scans manifest the finding of dilatation of the pancreatic duct normally seen as a strong linear echo, not as a tubular structure within the pancreas.

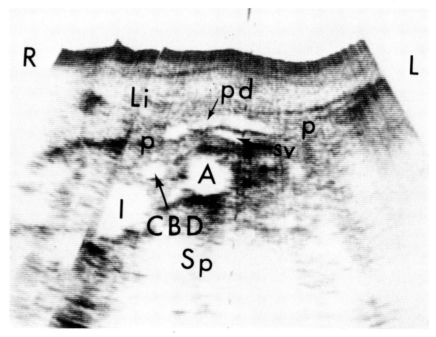

Fig. 4.89

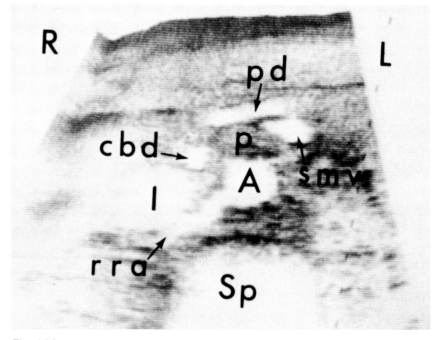

Fig. 4.90

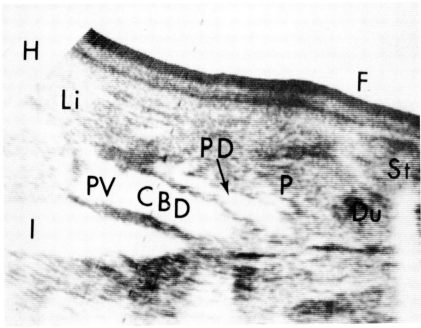

A   = Aorta
BD = Dilated bile duct
CBD = Common bile duct
cbd = Common bile duct
Du = Duodenum
F   = Foot
H   = Head
ha = Hepatic artery
hv = Hepatic vein
I   = Inferior vena cava
L   = Left
Li = Liver
P   = Pancreas
p   = Pancreas
PD = Pancreatic duct
pd = Pancreatic duct
PV = Portal vein
pv = Portal vein
R   = Right
rra = Right renal artery
smv = Superior mesenteric vein
Sp = Spine
St = Stomach
sv = Splenic vein

Fig. 4.91

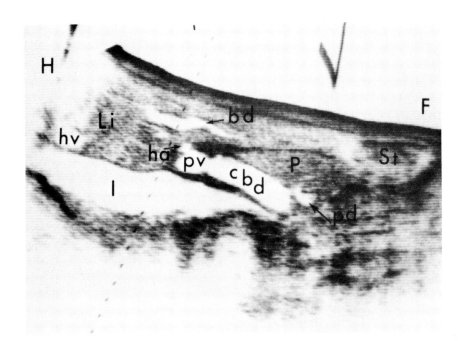

Fig. 4.92

Dilated Pancreatic Duct

Figures 4.93 and 4.94 represent another case of a dilated pancreatic duct. The patient was a 28-year-old woman who had a perforated duodenal ulcer. The perforation and surgery in the area caused stricture around the ampulla of Vater. This, in turn, led to dilatation of the pancreatic duct. A transverse section (fig. 4.93) demonstrates the dilated pancreatic duct anterior to the splenic vein. It is important to identify the splenic vein so as not to confuse it with a dilated pancreatic duct. Longitudinal section of this patient (fig. 4.94) shows the pancreatic duct again anterior to the splenic vein. The celiac axis and the superior mesenteric artery arising from the aorta are also seen.

Another case (figs. 4.95 and 4.96) demonstrates a dilatation of the pancreatic duct, secondary to ampullary carcinoma. In a transverse section through the pancreas (fig. 4.95), pancreatic tissue is well seen on both sides of this slightly dilated pancreatic duct. Figure 4.96 is a longitudinal scan through the body of the pancreas at the region of the superior mesenteric vein. We again see a small circular sonolucency representing the pancreatic duct situated in the central portion of the body of the pancreas.

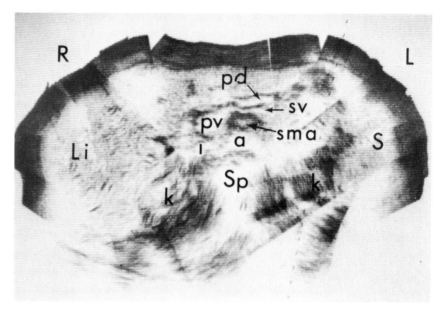

Fig. 4.93

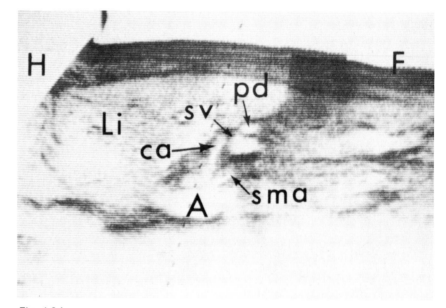

Fig. 4.94

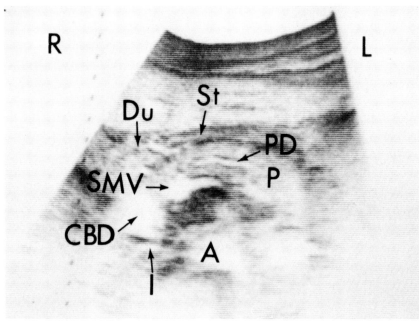

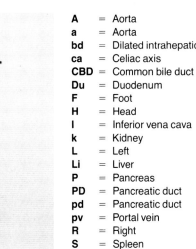

A = Aorta
a = Aorta
bd = Dilated intrahepatic bile ducts
ca = Celiac axis
CBD = Common bile duct
Du = Duodenum
F = Foot
H = Head
I = Inferior vena cava
k = Kidney
L = Left
Li = Liver
P = Pancreas
PD = Pancreatic duct
pd = Pancreatic duct
pv = Portal vein
R = Right
S = Spleen
sma = Superior mesenteric artery
SMV = Superior mesenteric vein
smv = Superior mesenteric vein
Sp = Spine
St = Stomach
sv = Splenic vein

Fig. 4.95

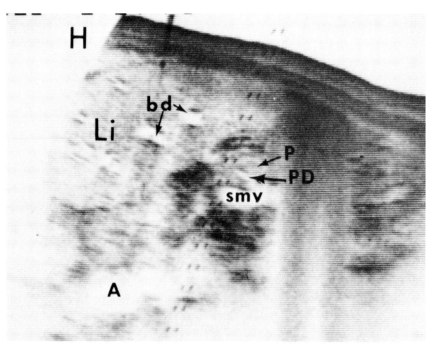

Fig. 4.96

5.
Ultrasonography of the Abdominal Aorta

Michael M. Raskin, M.D.

Ultrasound Technique

The abdominal aorta frequently is visualized during routine study of the abdomen. Special techniques are necessary in order to study adequately the entire extent of the abdominal aorta and its major branches.

Supine transverse scans are usually first obtained by starting at the level of the xiphoid process and continuing caudally at 2-cm intervals to below the umbilicus. An attempt is made to visualize the bifurcation of the distal abdominal aorta into the common iliac arteries. While performing the transverse scans, a general idea of the longitudinal course of the abdominal aorta can be obtained. Occasionally, with an extremely tortuous or dilated abdominal aorta, it may be necessary to mark its lateral borders on the patient's skin to obtain proper longitudinal scans.

Longitudinal scans are performed with the transducer path aligned parallel to the long axis of the abdominal aorta. Scans are obtained at 5-mm intervals, covering the entire width of the abdominal aorta. If considerable tortuosity of the abdominal aorta is noted, real-time ultrasound may be of value in more accurately determining its course (Mulder et al. 1973; Winsberg, Cole-Beuglet, and Mulder 1974).

One of the major disadvantages of this technique is that gas or barium within the bowel, interposed between the transducer and the aorta, often will preclude its adequate visualization. This can be minimized by having the patient fast for 12 hours prior to the examination and insuring that no barium studies have been performed for at least two days prior to the examination. Still, bowel gas may occasionally obscure the abdominal aorta, but gentle pressure with the transducer can often displace it away, permitting an adequate study. (See p. 230 for additional comments on examination technique.)

Anatomy of the Abdominal Aorta

The abdominal aorta appears as a circular sonolucency on transverse scans. It is situated anteriorly and slightly to the left of the vertebral bodies. More caudally the distal abdominal aorta decreases slightly in diameter and is situated more toward the midline. At the level of the umbilicus, the distal abdominal aorta bifurcates into the common iliac arteries. The normal abdominal aorta on longitudinal scan is a sonolucent tubular structure anterior to the vertebral bodies and slightly to the left of midline. Differentiation from the inferior vena cava is fairly easy; the inferior vena cava lies to the right of the abdominal aorta. In addition, near the level of the diaphragm, the inferior vena cava courses more anteriorly than the abdominal aorta as it enters the right atrium. It also changes size dramatically during deep inspiration.

The first major branch of the abdominal aorta is the celiac artery which originates from the ventral surface of the superior level of the first lumbar vertebral body. Classically, the celiac axis divides close to its origin into three major subdivisions: the splenic artery, the common hepatic artery, and the left gastric artery.

The superior mesenteric artery arises 1–2 cm below the celiac axis on the ventral aspect of the aorta at the lower level of the first lumbar vertebral body. The renal arteries arise approximately opposite each other at the level of the lower first lumbar vertebral body or upper second lumbar vertebral body, about 2 cm below the superior mesenteric artery, along the anterolateral aspect of the aorta. It should be noted that multiple renal arteries occur in approximately 20% of patients. Most frequently, they arise from the aorta below the main renal artery (Rogoff and Lipchik 1971).

Pathology of the Abdominal Aorta

Tortuosity of the Abdominal Aorta

With advancing age, the abdominal aorta becomes dilated, elongated, and less elastic. In addition, there are plaque formation and calcification of the aortic wall. The aorta may become quite tortuous and may even extend to the right of the midline. Although the overall dimension may not exceed 3 cm, the course of the aorta can be so serpiginous that transverse ultrasound scans may exaggerate the true dimension and be misread as an aneurysm.

Due to loss of normal elasticity, some dilatation of the distal abdominal aorta may be present and still not represent an aneurysm. Normally, the maximum external diameter of the aorta is at the level of the celiac axis with a gradual tapering distally. Dilatation of the distal abdominal aorta may exist if there is a lack of normal tapering distally, particularly if the infrarenal abdominal aorta is at least the same diameter or larger than the aorta at the level of the celiac axis. If this dilatation is greater than 3 cm in diameter, however, an aneurysm of the abdominal aorta is said to exist.

Aortic Aneurysm

Abdominal aortic aneurysms are usually arteriosclerotic in etiology and fusiform in shape; sacular aneurysms of the abdominal aorta are rare. Loss of elasticity results in weakening of the media of the wall of the aorta. Fusiform abdominal aortic aneurysms will most often project anteriorly and to the left of midline, as this is the path of least resistance. Laminar blood flow is no longer present in the expanded portion, and eddy currents increase the likelihood of thrombus formation. Therefore, intraluminal thrombus formation is more commonly seen anteriorly in a fusiform abdominal aortic aneurysm.

A measurement of > 3.0 cm in either the anteroposterior or transverse dimension of the abdominal aorta should be considered suspicious for aneurysm (Maloney et al. 1977). It should be noted, however, that the anteroposterior diameter is more accurate, for it can be measured in both the longitudinal and transverse scans; whereas the transverse diameter can only be measured in the transverse scan. This results in inherently better accuracy in the anteroposterior diameter which is based predominantly on the axial resolution of the system. The transverse diameter is partially determined from tangentially reflected sound waves, with a corresponding decrease in lateral resolution. The accuracy of ultrasound in identifying an abdominal aortic aneurysm is greater than 95% (Maloney et al. 1977). Not only can ultrasound identify the presence of an abdominal aortic aneurysm, but ultrasound can measure accurately the external diameter of the aneurysm as well as determine the presence of a mural thrombus (Raskin et al. 1977). For patients who are poor surgical risks or who refuse surgical resection, ultrasound provides a totally noninvasive method for following the external diameter of the aneurysm, as well as possible progressive obliteration of the true lumen, by increasing thrombus formation.

The likelihood of rupture of an abdominal aortic aneurysm is most dependent upon the external diameter of the aneurysm (Darling et al. 1977). Many studies have shown that the propensity for an abdominal aortic aneurysm to rupture was directly dependent upon the size of the aneurysm (Darling et al. 1977; Filly and Goldberg 1977; Wheeler, Beachley, and Ranniger 1976). However, it has been appreciated that small aneurysms do indeed rupture. Approximately one-third of 473 nonresected abdominal aortic aneurysms that ruptured were 5 cm or less in diameter (Darling et al. 1977). In addition, the incidence of rupture for aneurysms 4.1–7.0 cm in size is similar. Not until the aneurysm exceeds 7 cm in diameter, does the incidence of rupture greatly increase. Since the mortality of ruptured abdominal aortic aneurysms is 40–60% and the mortality of elective resection is 2–5%, abdominal aortic aneurysms as small as 4 cm may be considered for resection (Darling et al. 1977).

Aortography is the only reliable way of determining the relationship of an abdominal aortic aneurysm to the renal arteries or its extension into the common iliac arteries. Information about the renal and common iliac arteries may aid in planning the appropriate surgery, but it does not significantly alter the basic surgical procedure. The major factors that determine the surgical repair of an aneurysm are the size of the aneurysm, the presence of symptoms, and the patient's medical condition, rather than possible renal or iliac artery involvement. Since less than 4% of abdominal aortic aneurysms involve the renal arteries, and since most surgeons decide which type of graft to use after direct observation at laparotomy, aortography to determine the presence of renal artery involvement usually is not justified.

Occasionally, the renal arteries, particularly the right renal artery, may be visualized by ultrasound (Filly and Goldberg 1977). An indirect method of determining renal artery involvement is to locate the more readily identifiable origin of the superior mesenteric artery. Since the renal arteries usually originate below the level of the superior mesenteric artery, an aneurysm which extends proximally, to the level of the superior mesenteric artery, is likely to involve the renal arteries. If an abdominal aortic aneurysm is seen to extend considerably above the level of the renal arteries, the possibility of an abdominal aortic extension of a thoracic aortic aneurysm should be considered.

Aneurysms of the common iliac arteries are often well visualized by ultrasound. Common iliac artery aneurysms are usually seen in conjunction with aneurysms of the distal abdominal aorta.

Aortic Dissection

A dissecting aneurysm of the abdominal aorta is almost always the result of a dissecting thoracic aortic aneurysm. Dilatation of the abdominal aorta with a double lumen frequently may be present. The most character-istic finding of an aortic dissection is the demonstration of an intimal flap within the diffusely dilated abdominal aorta (Filly and Goldberg 1977). Real time or slow B-scan examination will demonstrate pulsations of the intimal flap.

Grafts

Abdominal aortic grafts are usually readily visible with ultrasound. Most synthetic graft materials are made of Dacron and produce strong, well-defined echoes. Because the synthetic material has transverse ribbing, the ultrasonic appearance is that of accordioned echoes conforming to the graft contour.

A Comparison of Ultrasound with Other Methods of Examination

Physical Examination

A pulsatile mass may be palpated by physical examination. Extremely thin patients, however, may normally have a palpable abdominal aorta and not have an aneurysm. Or, the examiner may be unable to palpate an aneurysm in an obese patient or a patient with a tense abdomen. When an abdominal aortic aneurysm can be palpated, the physical examination usually overestimates the size by 20% (Brewster et al. 1977).

Plain Film Radiographs

Evaluation of the size of the abdominal aortic aneurysm by plain film radiography is highly dependent upon the visualization of calcium within the wall of the aneurysm. This can only be seen in a little more than half of the abdominal aortic aneurysms. The accuracy, however, is somewhat greater on a lateral radiograph, because there is difficulty in visualizing calcification in the medial wall of the aneurysm on a conventional anteroposterior radiograph due to superimposition of the lumbar spine. Also, it should be noted that plain film radiography will consistently overestimate the size of the abdominal aortic aneurysm. This is due to X-ray magnification of up to 15% (Maloney et al. 1977).

Aortography

As the size of the aneurysm increases, so does the presence of mural thrombus. Aortography only opacifies the true lumen and may underestimate the external diameter of the aneurysm due to the presence of a mural thrombus (Brewster et al. 1977). Consequently, aortography is of limited value in the diagnosis and determination of the size of an abdominal aortic aneurysm.

Computed Tomography

Computed tomography is equally effective in measuring the external diameter of an abdominal aortic aneurysm (Raskin et al. 1977). It is not, however, as accurate as ultrasound in determining the presence of a mural thrombus.

References

Brewster, D. C.; Darling, R. C.; Raines, J. K.; Sarno, R.; O'Donnell, T. F.; Expeleta, M.; and Arthanasoulis, C. Assessment of abdominal aortic aneurysm size. *Circulation* 56(II):164–169, September 1977.

Darling, R. C.; Messina, C. R.; Brewster, D. C.; and Ottinger, L. W. Autopsy study of unoperated abdominal aortic aneurysm—The case for early resection. *Circulation* 56(II):161–164, September 1977.

Filly, R. A., and Goldberg, B. B. Abnormal vessels. Pp. 63–101 in *Abdominal gray scale ultrasonography*, ed. B. B. Goldberg. New York: John Wiley & Sons, 1977.

Lee, K. R.; Walls, W. J.; Martin, N. L.; and Templeton, A. W. A practical approach to the diagnosis of abdominal aortic aneurysms. *Surgery* 78:195–201, August 1975.

Maloney, J. D.; Pairolero, P. C.; Smith, B. E.; Hattery, R. R.; Brakke, D. M.; and Spittell, J. A. Ultrasound evaluation of abdominal aortic aneurysms. *Circulation* 56(II):80–85, September 1977.

Mulder, D. S.; Winsberg, F.; Cole, C. M.; Blundell, P. E.; Scott, H. J. Ultrasound "B" scanning of abdominal aneurysms. *Ann. Thorac. Surg.* 16:361–367, October 1973.

Raskin, M. M.; Cunningham, J. B.; Vining, P.; Salter, J.; and Syer, K. Abdominal aortic aneurysms: ultrasound versus computed tomography. Pp. 531–532 in *Ultrasound in medicine*, eds. D. White and R. E. Brown. New York: Plenum Publishing Corporation, 1977.

Rogoff, S. M., and Lipchik, E. O. The normal lumbar aortogram. Pp. 732–733 in *Angiography*, ed. H. L. Abrams. Boston: Little, Brown and Company, 1971.

Wheeler, W. E.; Beachley, M. C.; and Ranniger, K. Angiography and ultrasonography. *Am. J. Roentgenol.* 126:95–100, January 1976.

Winsberg, F.; Cole–Beuglet, C.; and Mulder, D. S. Continuous ultrasound "B" scanning of abdominal aortic aneurysms. *Am. J. Roentgenol.* 121:626–633, July 1974.

CASES
Dennis A. Sarti, M.D.
W. Frederick Sample, M.D.

Technique for Abdominal Aortic Examination

Scans of the abdominal aorta are obtained with the patient in the supine position. Transverse scans are obtained at 1-cm intervals (fig. 5.1). It is very helpful to map the medial and lateral borders of the aorta while performing the transverse scans. This makes the longitudinal scans much easier and more accurate. Figure 5.2 is a longitudinal scan in which the borders of the aorta are well outlined. The transducer scanning plane can be aligned parallel to the long axis of the aorta. Longitudinal scans should be obtained at 5-mm intervals and cover the entire width of the aorta. By mapping the medial and lateral borders of the aorta on the patient's skin, we can detect tortuosity or aneurysmal dilatation during the course of the transverse scans. Sometimes the distal aorta will be difficult to see because of overlying bowel air. Gentle pressure with the transducer on the abdomen may displace some of the bowel air. Very often this gentle pressure can yield an adequate examination which was initially thought to be nondiagnostic due to air. Very often transverse scans will yield visualization of the aorta only from the lateral aspect. In this instance, longitudinal scans that parallel the aorta but angle in through the ultrasonic window, detected on the transverse scans, may have to be obtained.

Figure 5.3 is a transverse scan of the upper abdomen through the major portion of the liver. The large sonolucent structure to the right of the spine is the inferior vena cava. The aorta is seen slightly to the left of the spine. Its borders are often not as sharp as those of a distended inferior vena cava. We also see the crus of the diaphragm draping over the abdominal aorta at this level. The abdominal aorta usually can be visualized high in the abdomen, because the liver acts as an ultrasonic window. As we continue lower in the abdomen,

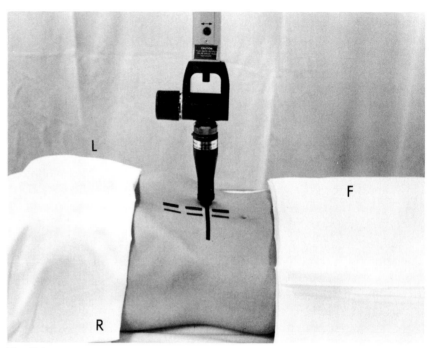

Fig. 5.1

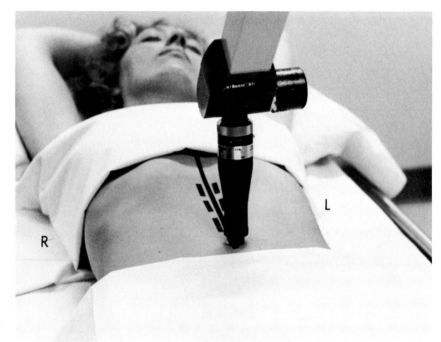

Fig. 5.2

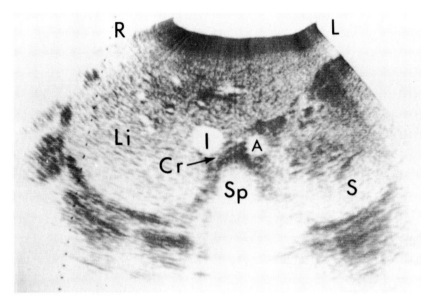

Fig. 5.3

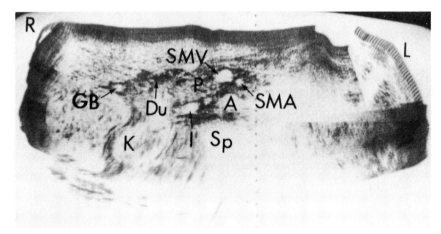

Fig. 5.4

bowel air is found very often to obscure visualization of the aorta. Figure 5.4 is a transverse scan in which we can see the aorta anterior to the spine. We are at the level of the pancreas which can also act as an ultrasonic window for visualizing the aorta. Anterior to the aorta in this scan are the superior mesenteric artery and the superior mesenteric vein.

A   = Aorta
cr = Crus of the diaphragm
Du = Duodenum
F   = Foot
GB = Contracted gallbladder following eating
I   = Inferior vena cava
K   = Kidney
L   = Left
Li = Liver
P   = Pancreas
R   = Right
S   = Spleen
SMA = Superior mesenteric artery
SMV = Superior mesenteric vein
Sp = Spine

Normal Aorta

Numerous circular structures are present anterior to the spine on transverse scans. It is important to understand the anatomy in order to determine accurately which circular sonolucency is represented by the various structures. Figure 5.5 is a transverse scan in which the aorta is directly anterior to the spine. Very often the circular sonolucency of the aorta is displaced slightly to the left of the spine. The inferior vena cava is situated on the right side of the aorta. It can have a variable appearance, depending upon the phase of respiration and whether or not a Valsalva maneuver is present. A large circular sonolucency will often be seen anterior to the aorta; this is due to the superior mesenteric vein. It can reach quite a large size and even be nearly as large as the aorta itself (fig. 5.5). The superior mesenteric vein is often the largest sonolucent circle anterior to the aorta. The superior mesenteric artery is not anywhere near the size of the superior mesenteric vein. Figure 5.5 also yields several circular sonolucencies just anterior to the inferior vena cava; these are secondary to the common bile duct and the gastroduodenal artery. Because of their small size, they present no difficulties.

Longitudinal scans of the abdominal aorta are usually obtained close to the midline. Figures 5.6–5.8 are examples of normal abdominal aortic ultrasound examinations in the longitudinal plane. Very often, the inferior vena cava gives a confusing picture and may be misinterpreted as the aorta. The inferior vena cava, however, courses anteriorly to empty into the right atrium as it goes through the hemidiaphragm. The tubular lucency of the aorta continues straight back as it goes through the left hemidiaphragm. The aorta will also appear to have a steplike posterior border (figs. 5.6 and 5.7). Since the aorta is very often situated directly anterior to the spine, we are actually able to see the vertebral bodies on its posterior aspect. These will present as strong steplike echoes intermixed with decreased echoes, representing the disk space. The disk spaces (arrows) are delineated quite easily in figure 5.6 and more cau-

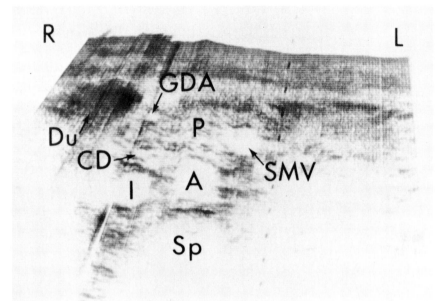

Fig. 5.5

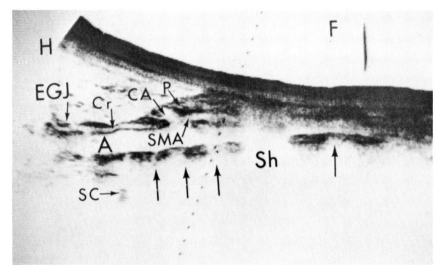

Fig. 5.6

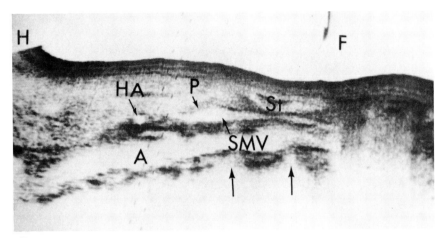

Fig. 5.7

dally near the umbilical region in figure 5.7. Often, we actually can penetrate through the disk spaces to view the spinal canal (fig. 5.6). We are sending sound waves through the cartilaginous disk structure to visualize the canal, but the vertebral bodies cannot be penetrated on the longitudinal scan. Numerous structures, such as the superior mesenteric artery and the celiac axis, arise from the aorta. If bowel air is present, the aorta cannot be seen, due to shadowing. In an airless abdomen it may be seen from the diaphragm to the umbilical level. The range of normal aortic diameter is 2.5 cm in women and 3.0 in men.

A	=	Aorta
Arrows	=	Intervertebral disk spaces
CA	=	Celiac axis
CD	=	Common duct
Co	=	Colon
Cr	=	Crus of the diaphragm
Du	=	Duodenum
EGJ	=	Esophagogastric junction
F	=	Foot
GDA	=	Gastroduodenal artery
H	=	Head
HA	=	Hepatic artery
I	=	Inferior vena cava
L	=	Left
P	=	Pancreas
R	=	Right
SC	=	Spinal canal
Sh	=	Shadowing
SMA	=	Superior mesenteric artery
SMV	=	Superior mesenteric vein
Sp	=	Spine
St	=	Stomach

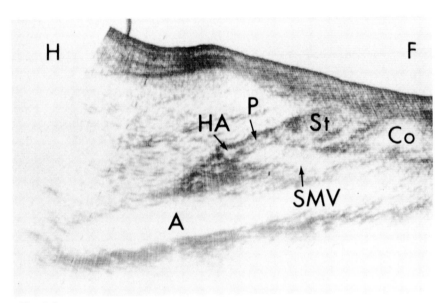

Fig. 5.8

Abdominal Aortic Aneurysms

Figures 5.9–5.11 are of a 63-year-old man admitted because of a palpable mass in the midabdomen. Ultrasound examination demonstrated a 4.5–5 cm aneurysm of the distal aorta. A longitudinal scan of the aorta (fig. 5.9) demonstrates the aneurysm in its distal half. The size of the proximal aorta is within normal limits. A transverse scan through the normal proximal portion (fig. 5.10) shows the aorta to be normal in size and just posterior to the superior mesenteric artery and the splenic vein. Figure 5.9 demonstrates elevation of the superior mesenteric artery and the superior mesenteric vein over the aneurysm in the lower abdomen. The origin of the superior mesenteric artery in figure 5.9 is not, however, involved with dilatation of the abdominal aorta at that site. A transverse section (fig. 5.11), more caudally, over the level of the aneurysm delineates the enlarged aorta adjacent to the much smaller inferior vena cava. An angiogram confirmed the presence of a 5-cm aneurysm in this region. The ultrasound did not show any large thrombus, and no thrombus was evident on angiogram.

Figure 5.12 is a longitudinal scan of a 55-year-old man with a large calcified abdominal aortic aneurysm. It demonstrates a normally sized aorta posterior to the liver. Distal to the take-off of the celiac axis, however, is a large aneurysm measuring 7 cm in diameter and 12 cm in length. This is an excellent example of an extremely large aneurysm originating below the level of the celiac axis. Again, no thrombus is evident with the aneurysm.

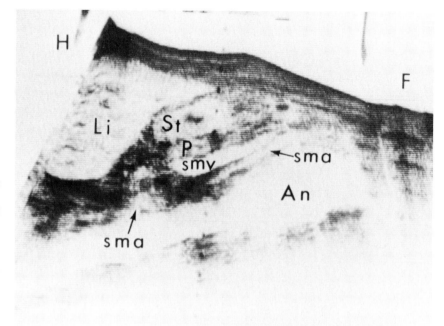

Fig. 5.9

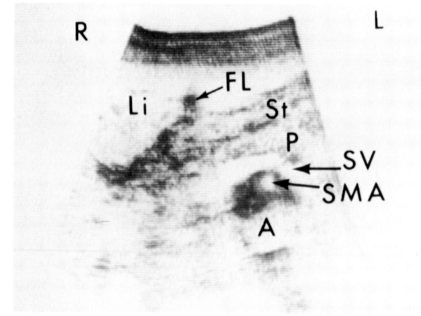

Fig. 5.10

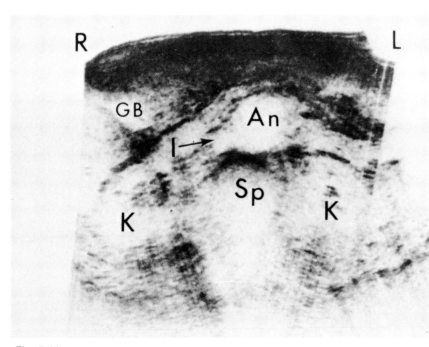

Fig. 5.11

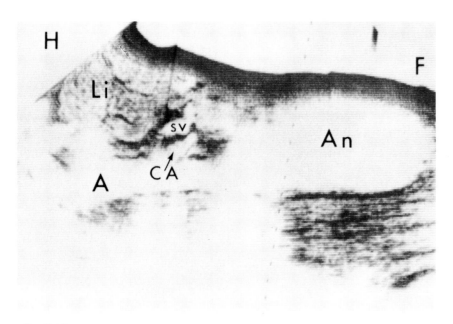

Fig. 5.12

A = Normal aorta
An = Aneurysm
CA = Celiac axis
F = Foot
FL = Falciform ligament
GB = Gallbladder
H = Head
I = Inferior vena cava
K = Kidney
L = Left
Li = Liver
P = Pancreas
R = Right
SMA = Superior mesenteric artery
sma = Superior mesenteric artery
SMV = Superior mesenteric vein
Sp = Spine
St = Stomach
SV = Splenic vein

Abdominal Aortic Aneurysms

The abdominal aorta tends to become smaller in diameter as it approaches the iliac arteries. Aortic dilatation of greater than 3 cm in men is considered aneurysmal. The main advantage of ultrasound over angiography is that we can see the thrombus along with the lumen of the aorta, as figures 5.13 and 5.14 illustrate. These two figures were obtained from a 61-year-old man who had a chief complaint of continual aching pain in the abdomen. A palpable mass was noted over the mid abdomen. Ultrasound examination just above the umbilical level demonstrated a large aortic aneurysm (fig. 5.13). The aortic lumen is approximately one-third the size of the actual diameter of the aorta, including the thrombus.

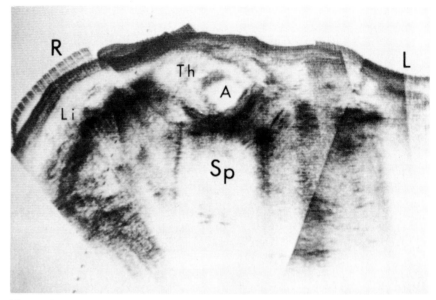

Fig. 5.13

Figure 5.14 is a longitudinal scan of the same patient; the thrombus is localized to the lower abdominal aorta. The lumen is quite visible and sonolucent, as compared with the echogenicity present within the thrombus. There was protuberance over the anterior abdominal wall (arrows) secondary to the palpable mass.

Figures 5.15 and 5.16 are transverse scans from two different patients who also had abdominal aortic aneurysms of the lower abdominal aorta. In figure 5.15 the lumen of the aorta is somewhat eccentrically located, as compared with the entire thrombus. Figure 5.16 is an example of a centrally situated lumen. Here the thrombus is fairly even in thickness and completely surrounds the aortic lumen. In these instances an angiogram would only show the size of the abdominal aorta to be that of the lumen. Ultrasound is necessary to determine the exact extent of an abdominal aortic aneurysm. If calcification is present in the wall of the aorta, an angiogram or an abdominal X-ray will give the accurate dimensions of an abdominal aortic aneurysm.

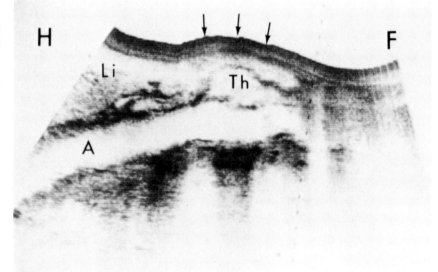

Fig. 5.14

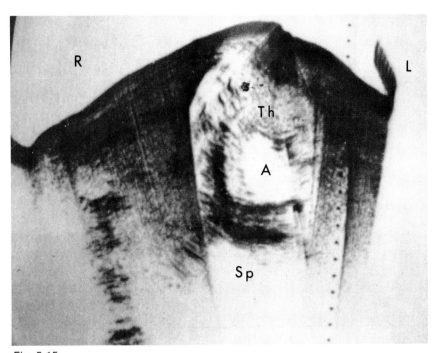

A	=	Aortic lumen
Arrows	=	Protuberant abdomen
		secondary to an aortic aneurysm
F	=	Foot
H	=	Head
I	=	Inferior vena cava
L	=	Left
Li	=	Liver
R	=	Right
Sp	=	Spine
Th	=	Aortic aneurysm thrombus

Fig. 5.15

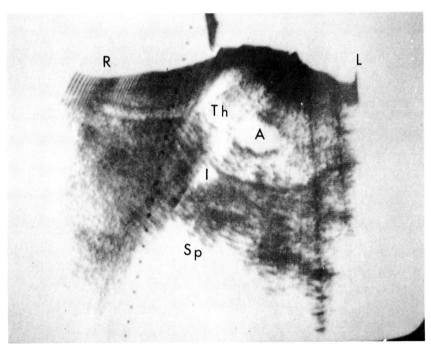

Fig. 5.16

Abdominal Aortic Aneurysms; Atherosclerosis

Figure 5.17 is a longitudinal scan in the midline of the abdomen over the abdominal aorta. It demonstrates a large aortic aneurysm with thrombus noted peripherally. This aneurysm involves nearly all of the abdominal aorta. It is situated from the umbilical level to well under the left lobe of the liver. There is a sharp bend (arrow) noted in the mid portion of the abdominal aorta. The lumen of the aorta is well defined, since it is quite sonolucent. The solid thrombus is echogenic on ultrasound.

Figure 5.18 is a transverse abdominal scan of a 73-year-old man who was having rather severe abdominal pain. An aortic aneurysm is seen over the midabdomen. A large mass is noted on the right side of the aneurysm and is quite echogenic. At surgery, this turned out to be a large hematoma. The aortic aneurysm had ruptured into the right posterior retroperitoneum.

Usually the walls of the aorta are fairly sharp and smooth. In cases of severe atherosclerosis, however, they can appear quite irregular. Figures 5.19 and 5.20 are of a 63-year-old woman with fairly severe atherosclerotic disease. The longitudinal scan (fig. 5.19) shows the aorta to have a marked irregular border, especially in the posterior aspect. Here we see numerous atheromatous plaques (arrows) indenting the aortic lumen on its posterior aspect. A transverse section of the aorta (fig. 5.20) demonstrates marked irregularity of the aortic lumen which usually is not seen. The findings are compatible with severe atherosclerotic disease.

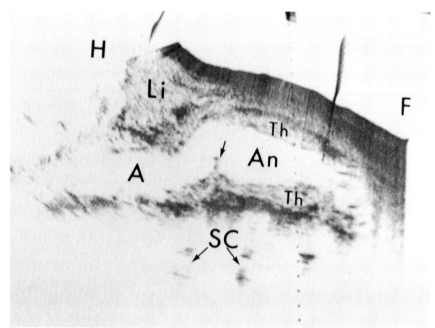

Fig. 5.17

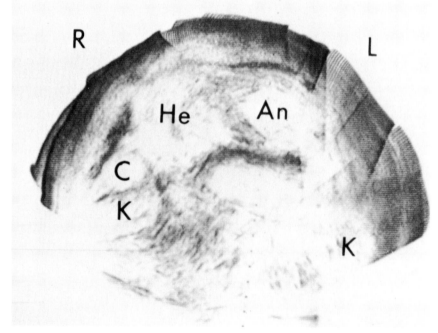

Fig. 5.18

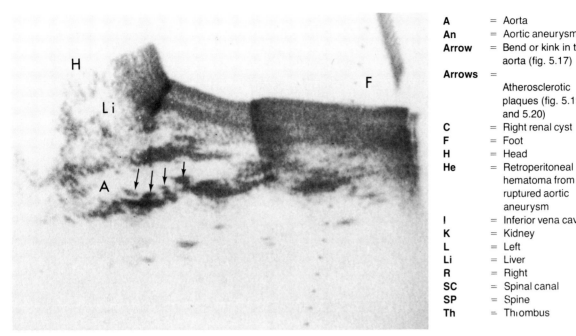

Fig. 5.19

A	=	Aorta
An	=	Aortic aneurysm
Arrow	=	Bend or kink in the aorta (fig. 5.17)
Arrows	=	Atherosclerotic plaques (fig. 5.19 and 5.20)
C	=	Right renal cyst
F	=	Foot
H	=	Head
He	=	Retroperitoneal hematoma from a ruptured aortic aneurysm
I	=	Inferior vena cava
K	=	Kidney
L	=	Left
Li	=	Liver
R	=	Right
SC	=	Spinal canal
SP	=	Spine
Th	=	Thrombus

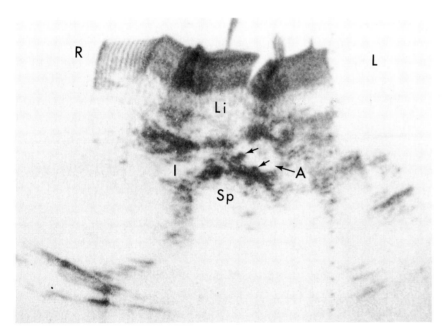

Fig. 5.20

Infected Aortic Graft

Figures 5.21–5.24 were obtained from a middle-aged woman who had recently undergone surgery with the placement of an aortic graft. She had had recent onset of abdominal pain with fever and elevated white blood cell count. Figures 5.21 and 5.22 are transverse and longitudinal sections of the abdomen which demonstrate a mass surrounding the aorta. The mass is quite circumferential. It would be compatible with an aortic aneurysm, but the patient had a graft in place at this site. In fact, the extremely strong echoes of the distal aorta (fig. 5.22, arrows) are fairly characteristic of those echoes arising from the graft. It is evident from figure 5.22 that the mass is surrounding the site of the graft.

Because of the ultrasonic findings, an angiogram was performed (fig. 5.23). The distal aorta is narrowed (arrows) in the same area where the mass was noted on ultrasound. The patient was taken to the operating room, and an infected aortic graft was found. An abscess surrounding the distal aorta was over the region of the graft. Figure 5.24 is a contrast examination of the abscess cavity performed at the time of surgery. The filling defect of the distal aorta is seen in the superior aspect of the abscess cavity. The findings at the time of surgery corresponded to the previous ultrasound examinations.

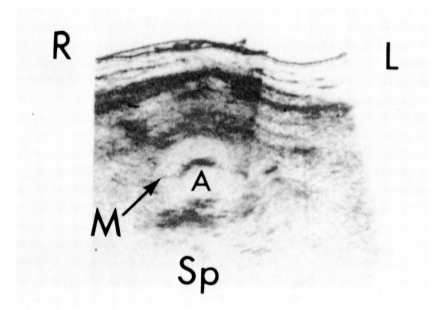

Fig. 5.21

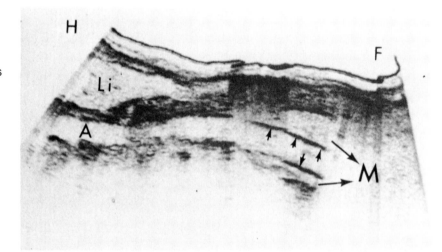

Fig. 5.22

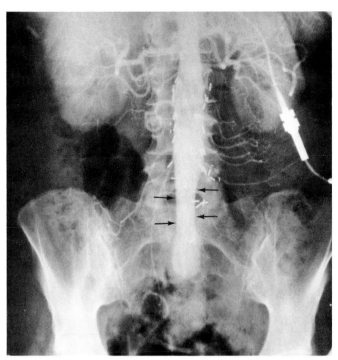

Fig. 5.23

A   = Aorta
Arrows   = Strong echoes arising
             from the aortic graft
             (fig. 5.22)
Arrows   = Indentation from the
             abscess on the aortic
             lumen (fig. 5.23)
F   = Foot
H   = Head
L   = Left
Li   = Liver
M   = Abscess surrounding
             the aortic graft
R   = Right
Sp   = Spine

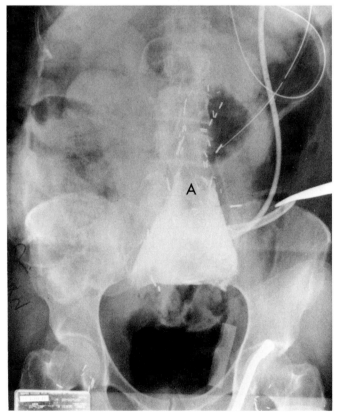

Fig. 5.24

Dissecting Abdominal Aortic Aneurysm

Figures 5.25–5.28 are ultrasound examinations obtained from a 45-year-old man with known cystic medial necrosis. Just prior to his last hospital admission, he noted the sudden onset of back pain which was not relieved by positional changes. He also noted abdominal pain with nausea and vomiting. An abdominal ultrasound was performed to evaluate the abdominal pain. Figure 5.25 is a transverse scan of the initial portion of the study. At first, the study appears unremarkable. A close look at the lateral posterior right border of the aorta, however, elicits a strong echo (arrow) within the lumen of the aorta. This unusual finding prompted closer scrutiny of the abdominal aorta.

Figure 5.26 is a transverse scan performed with an extremely slow scanning speed over the abdominal aorta. A definite internal echo which has cardiac pulsations can now be seen within the lumen of the aorta. This turned out to be a dissecting aneurysm. The slow scanning speed over the aorta is demonstrated by the arrows within the liver. The scanning speed over the aorta took approximately 3–4 seconds. Once this finding was noted, an attempt was made to visualize the dissection in a longitudinal scan.

Figures 5.27 and 5.28 are examples of longitudinal scans at extremely slow scanning speeds over the abdominal aorta. The dissection is quite nicely seen within the lumen of the aorta. Cardiac pulsations are easily evident as the dissecting flap moves anteriorly and posteriorly with each cardiac cycle. Figure 5.28 demonstrates the slow scanning speed as the linear lines through the liver and irregular border to the skin echo come into view. Since the aorta was not dilated, the ultrasound findings were the first confirmatory evidence of the diagnosis of a dissecting aneurysm in this patient.

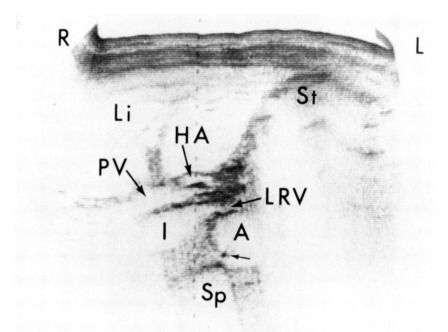

Fig. 5.25

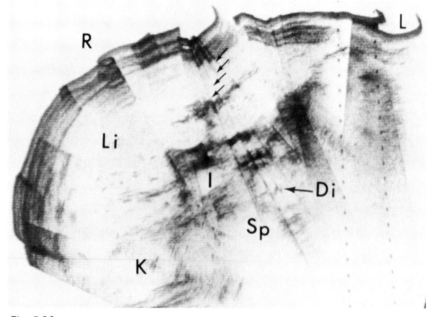

Fig. 5.26

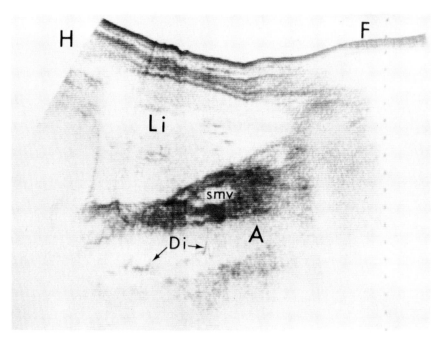

Fig. 5.27

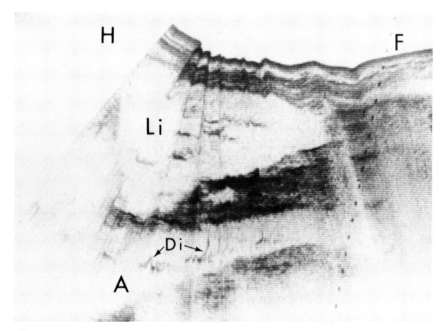

Fig. 5.28

6.
Ultrasonography of the Spleen

Peter Cooperberg, M.D.

Ultrasound can frequently be useful in the evaluation of abnormalities of the spleen. Although the normal spleen may be difficult to visualize ultrasonographically, most pathological processes involving the spleen cause splenic enlargement, and therefore, the ultrasound examination can be clinically useful when splenic pathology is suspected.

Examination Technique

All routine abdominal sonograms include an attempt to demonstrate the spleen, both on transverse and longitudinal sections, with the patient in the supine position. If the spleen is enlarged, this presents no problem, and pathological processes may be easily demonstrated. The normal spleen may be demonstrated on transverse section with the patient supine by moving the transducer as far posteriorly as possible on the left side and angling anteromedially. Longitudinal scanning generally will not, however, show the normal spleen, because of gas in the stomach or splenic flexure. In routine abdominal scanning, the demonstration of a normally sized spleen on the transverse scan should be adequate. If the spleen is not enlarged, but the demonstration of an abnormality of the spleen is requested, supplementary techniques may be used to show the longitudinal axis of the spleen.

The simplest maneuver is to have the patient roll the left side up to an oblique position and to angle the scanning arm medially. Or the patient can be rolled into a lateral decubitus position with the left side up or, if necessary, into the prone position. The spleen can frequently be visualized superior and lateral to the left kidney in these sections. The air-filled lung in the left costophrenic sulcus and the lower left ribs may hinder good visualization.

Deep inspiration frequently displaces the spleen inferiorly, and this is helpful, but it may displace the spleen medially, and this is not helpful. Varying degrees of inspiration should be attempted to determine which affords the best visualization of the spleen. When there is a left pleural effusion, the diaphragm can be visualized along with the upper portion of the spleen, which is usually obscured by the air-filled lung. To overcome rib artifacts, the intercostal spaces are used as windows, and the transducer should be moved in a sector motion. Another technique for visualizing the spleen is to arc the transducer obliquely along the intercostal space. Although this may be helpful in demonstrating the spleen, the unusual plane of section can cause difficulty in recognizing the relationships between spleen and splenic size. Usually, the supine position is used for the transverse scans, and the left side up decubitus position, with intercostal sectoring, is used for the longitudinal sections.

Generally, the same technical setting of gain, time gain compensation, and amplification are used for the examination of the spleen as for other organs of the upper abdomen. Since the spleen is a superficial structure, and since there is generally little absorption of the sound within the spleen, a frequency of 3.5 MHz and a medium-internally focused transducer are recommended. Although both 19 mm and 13 mm diameter transducers are acceptable, the smaller-faced crystals are easier to use from the smaller "windows" of the intercostal spaces.

Examination of the Normal Spleen

The shape of the normal spleen is variable. The spleen can be seen to have two components joined at the hilum, a superior and medial component, and an inferior and lateral component. On transverse scanning, the spleen will have a crescentic appearance usually with a considerable medial component. As the scanning plane is moved inferiorly, the medial component is lost, and only the lateral component is visualized. On longitudinal scanning from the left side of the patient, the superior component is noted to extend more medially than the inferior component. It is this irregular nature of the spleen that makes it difficult to assess accurately mild degrees of splenic enlargement.

It is important to recognize the normal structures related anatomically to the spleen. The diaphragm is posterior, lateral, and superior to the spleen. The fundus of the stomach and lesser sac are medial and anterior to the splenic hilum. The tail of the pancreas lies posterior to the stomach and lesser sac and also approaches the hilum of the spleen from the medial aspect. The left kidney generally lies inferior and medial to the spleen, but the medial component may extend anterior to the left kidney (Gooding 1978). A useful landmark in identifying the spleen and the splenic hilum is the splenic vein which generally can be demonstrated, especially in splenic enlargement.

The splenic parenchyma is extremely homogeneous, and therefore, the textural appearance of the spleen on gray scale ultrasonography generally shows a diffuse homogenous low-level echo pattern. In large patients, especially those with broad flat ribs, and therefore with small intercostal spaces, the low-level echoes from the spleen may be difficult to demonstrate. This is especially true unless great care is taken in adjusting the near gain. Every attempt must be made to demonstrate the low-level echoes in the spleen and therefore to differentiate the normal spleen from a left pleural effusion, ascities, or rarely, from a left adrenal or renal cyst. (See p.248 for additional comments on splenic examination technique.)

Pathological Conditions

Splenomegaly

As is well known, the differential diagnosis of splenomegaly is a lengthy one, and unfortunately, ultrasound is not generally useful in establishing its etiology. Several exceptions will be discussed here. Frequently, the question is whether or not there is splenomegaly. This again can be a difficult decision to make on the sonographic study if only mild enlargement is present. One proposed rule of thumb is that if the anterior margin of the spleen extends more anteriorly than the anterior wall of the abdominal aorta on the transverse section, and the patient is in the supine position, then this represents splenomegaly (Leopold and Asher 1975). Mild splenomegaly certainly is sometimes present, however, without the spleen extending anteriorly, and in a very thin patient, the spleen may extend more anteriorly than the anterior wall of the aorta, without being pathologically enlarged. Techniques have been described to measure serial sections of the spleen by planimetry and to add the product of the areas and the thickness of the section (Holm et al. 1975; Koga and Morikawa 1975; Rasmussen et al. 1973). This technique is unfortunately cumbersome and hampered by the same problems encountered when examining the ribs and left lung. It does not enjoy widespread use. The "eyeball" technique is the method most commonly applied; if it looks big, it is big. This, unfortunately, takes considerably more experience than is necessary with other imaging techniques.

Plain radiography of the abdomen and radionuclide

spleen scans with Tc^{99m} are alternate methods of evaluating splenic size. These techniques, however, suffer similarly from the inability to evaluate accurately mild degrees of splenic enlargement. Isotope studies are, however, superior to ultrasound for evaluation of splenomegaly.

The spleen is capable of growing to an enormous size. It may extend inferiorly into the left iliac fossa. When the spleen is moderately to grossly enlarged, it is easier to demonstrate sonographically, and its size may be more accurately determined. In most situations in which the spleen is enlarged, an increased echogenicity may be as high as the echogenicity of the normal liver. In a study by Taylor and Milan (1976), an attempt was made to correlate the degree of echogenicity with the etiology of splenomegaly. Generally, however, the sonographic appearance of the splenic parenchyma is not distinctive enough to diagnose the etiology of the splenomegaly (Hunter and Haber 1977).

Occasionally, a mass is palpable in the left upper quadrant. The clinical dilemma is whether this is an enlarged spleen or an extrinsic mass located against the spleen. It can be helpful if the spleen is demonstrated separately from the mass. Another helpful feature is the demonstration of the splenic vein entering the splenic hilum. This indicates the mass is, in fact, an enlarged spleen.

Splenic Cysts

The etiology of splenic cysts is unclear (Bhimji et al. 1977). They may be related to trauma. As elsewhere in the body, splenic cysts characteristically appear as echo-free areas with smooth, sharp borders and enhancement of the echoes deep to the lesion. When small, they may be demonstrated to be within the outline of the spleen. Frequently, these cysts attain a very large size. In these cases, compressed splenic tissue may be seen peripheral to the cyst. Because these patients present as splenomegaly, and ultrasound can easily and noninvasively make the definitive diagnosis, it is suggested than an ultrasound study be a component of all undiagnosed cases of gross splenomegaly. This is especially true in young, adult female patients. Radionuclide spleen scans also will demonstrate a "cold" area within the spleen, but will not differentiate between a cystic and solid lesion.

Neoplasm.

In the vast majority of cases, where an enlarged spleen is associated with lymphoma or chronic leukemia, the consistency of the splenic parenchyma appears unremarkable. We have, however, seen one case in which two large echogenic structures were noted within the spleen. Other retroperitoneal masses were demonstrated, and the patient subsequently proved to have lymphoma. In another patient with Hodgkin's disease, a large solid mass was seen arising from the spleen. The mass subsequently disappeared after chemotherapy and radiation therapy. These were rare presentations of lymphoma in the spleen. Metastases from other primary sources are equally rare in the spleen.

Splenic Trauma

The spleen is frequently involved in blunt abdominal trauma. Two possible abnormalities ensue. If the capsule remains intact, a subcapsular hematoma may result, or the capsule may rupture and lead to retroperitoneal or intraperitoneal hematoma (Asher et al. 1978; Ayala 1974; Kristensen, Buemann, and Kuhl 1971). In the latter situations, it might be possible to demonstrate a fluid space separate from the spleen in the left upper quadrant. It is frequently difficult to demonstrate the hematoma and the spleen separately. This is especially true for trauma, which causes associated left lower rib fractures and contusions, and the patient may experience pain as the transducer comes into contact with the ribs. Usually, only a irregularly echogenic mass is larger than we would expect with a normal spleen. The differentiation of incidental splenomegaly from a retroperitoneal splenic hematoma may be difficult. If the rupture is intraperitoneal, the sonogram may demonstrate free fluid in the flanks, between the right lobe of the liver and the right kidney and posterior to the bladder. These findings in a patient who has suffered blunt trauma should alert the referring physician to the possibility of splenic rupture, and arteriography should be performed to confirm the diagnosis.

Aside from splenic rupture, there may be internal damage to the spleen with an intact splenic capsule. This results in a subcapsular hematoma of the spleen which may be demonstrated as a relatively cystic structure arising peripherally in the splenic substance. The subcapsular hematoma may persist or, with time, may gradually decrease in size. Surgeons differ in estimating the danger of nonintervention in such situations, since the possibility exists that a subcapsular hematoma may eventually rupture.

Congenital Anomalies

Congenital absence of the spleen may be difficult to diagnose, since occasionally, a normal size spleen is impossible to visualize. The diagnosis of agenesis of the spleen, however, can be ruled out by the demonstration of the spleen. Accessory spleens may be demonstrated as masses near the splenic hilum or remote from the spleen. It is difficult, if not impossible, to suggest the origin of these masses on the sonogram alone.

References

Asher, W. M.; Parvin, S; Virgilio, R. W.; and Haber, K. Echographic evaluation of splenic injury after blunt trauma. *Radiology* 118:411–415, 1978.

Ayala, L. A.; Williams, L. R.; and Widrich, W. C. Occult rupture of the spleen: the chronic form of splenic rupture. *Ann. Surg.* 179:4:472–478, 1974.

Bhimji, S. D.; Cooperberg, P. L.; Naimon, S.; Morrison, R. T.; and Shergill, P. S. Ultrasound diagnosis of the splenic cysts. *Radiology* 122:787–789, 1977.

Gooding, G. The ultrasonic and computed tomographic appearance of splenic lobulations: a consideration in the ultrasonic differential of masses adjacent to the left kidney. *Radiology* 126:719–729, 1978.

Holm, H. H.; Kristensen, J. K.; Petersen, J. F.; Rasmussen, S. N.; and Hancke, S. P. 159 in *Abdominal ultrasound*, University Park Press, 1975.

Hunter, T. B., and Haber, K. Unusual sonographic appearance of the spleen in a case of myelofibrosis. *Am. J. Roentgenol.* 128:138–139, January 1977.

Koga, T., and Morikawa, Y. Ultrasonographic determination of the splenic size and its clinical usefulness in various liver diseases. *Radiology* 115:157–161, April 1975.

Kristensen, J. K.; Buemann, B.; and Kuhl, E. Ultrasonic scanning in the diagnosis of splenic hematomas. *Acta Chir. Scand.* 137:653–657, 1971.

Leopold, G. R., and Asher, W. M. P. 77 in *Fundamentals of abdominal and pelvic ultrasonography*, Philadelphia: W. B. Saunders Co., 1975.

Miller, E. Wandering spleen and pregnancy: case report. *J. Clin. Ultrasound* 3:281–282, 1975.

Rasmussen, S. N.; Christensen, B. E.; Holm, H. H.; Kardel, T.; Stigsby, B.; and Larsen, M. Spleen volume determination by ultrasonic scanning. *Scand. J. Haemat.* 10:298–304, 1973.

Taylor, K. J. W., and Milan, J. Differential diagnosis of chronic splenomegaly by gray-scale ultrasonography: clinical observations and digital A-scan analysis. *Br. J. Radiol.* 49:519–525, 1976.

CASES
Dennis A. Sarti, M.D.
W. Frederick Sample, M.D.

Technique for Splenic Examination

Examination of the spleen is quite difficult because of its anatomic location in the left upper quadrant. Two air-containing structures obscure visualization of the spleen in many instances. These are the fundus of the stomach and the splenic flexure. The spleen may be well seen, however, if we scan through the intercostal spaces on the left side.

In figure 6.1, with the patient in the supine position, we are scanning the spleen in a transverse plane while rocking through the intercostal spaces, demonstrated by the dark lines on the patient's skin. The patient can be examined in the supine position or in the decubitus position with the left side up.

Figure 6.2 is a scan of the patient in the decubitus position with a transverse scan obtained through the intercostal spaces (dark lines). By rocking or sector scanning within the intercostal spaces, we can obtain excellent visualization of the splenic parenchyma. It is also important to have the patient take a deep breath to drive the spleen down as caudally as possible.

Figure 6.3 is a longitudinal scan of the spleen with the patient in the decubitus position with the left side up. Here we see a longitudinal scan paralleling the mid axillary line (dark lines). By scanning below the costal margin and then through the intercostal spaces, we can obtain longitudinal scans of the spleen.

Scanning through the ribs often will cause numerous artifacts. It will sometimes be difficult to evaluate the splenic parenchyma. In order to get good visualization of the splenic parenchyma, we can scan through the intercostal spaces as is demonstrated in figure 6.4 where the patient is in a decubitus position with the left side up. The scanning plane is parallel to the lower intercostal spaces, with the transducer actually tracking between the ribs. This scan gives excellent visualization of the splenic parenchyma and the organ can be evaluated without rib artifacts.

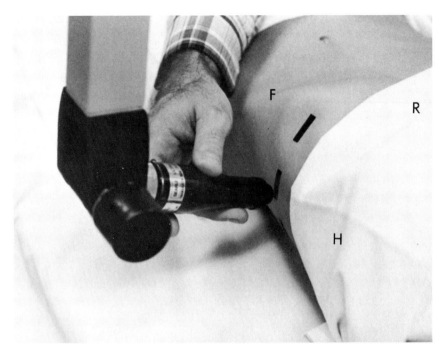

Fig. 6.1

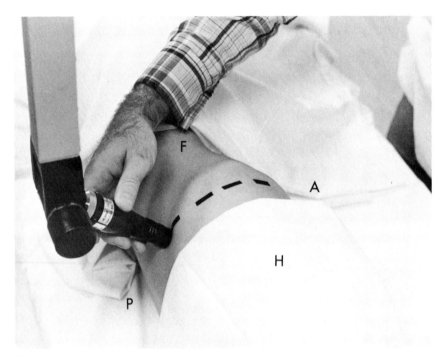

Fig. 6.2

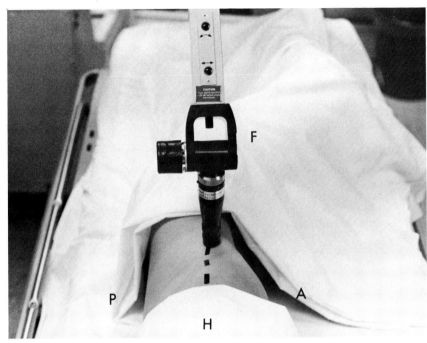

A = Anterior
F = Foot
H = Head
P = Posterior
R = Right

Fig. 6.3

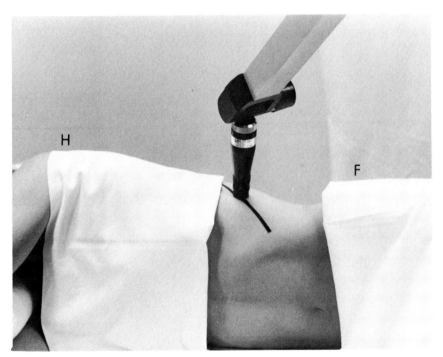

Fig. 6.4

Normal Spleen

Figures 6.5 and 6.6 are transverse scans of a normal spleen. In figure 6.5 the spleen is visualized through the intercostal spaces, laterally on the left side. Because of the collapsed and airless stomach, however, the spleen can be seen from an anterior projection. Here we are scanning through the left lobe of the liver and the collapsed stomach to visualize the spleen. Figure 6.6 is a transverse scan of the spleen through the intercostal spaces, laterally on the left. Most of the information comes from the scans obtained through the intercostal spaces, rather than from the scans obtained from an anterior location. The spleen may be horizontal in orientation and difficult to visualize by ultrasound because of air in the stomach or the splenic flexure. Spleens with a lateral orientation are visualized best (fig. 6.6).

Longitudinal scans of the spleen are best obtained with the patient in a decubitus position with the left side up. Scans are then obtained in the mid axillary line beneath the costal margin and in the intercostal spaces.

Figures 6.7 and 6.8 are longitudinal scans of the spleen with the patient in the decubitus position. They demonstrate excellent splenic parenchyma. The spleen is situated cephalad to the left kidney and caudal to the left hemidiaphragm. By sector scanning through the intercostal space, we can get an excellent visualization of the splenic parenchyma. The aorta is seen deep to the spleen, because the patient is in a decubitus position. By varying the patient's respiration, the spleen can be moved into an optimal position, with excellent visualization.

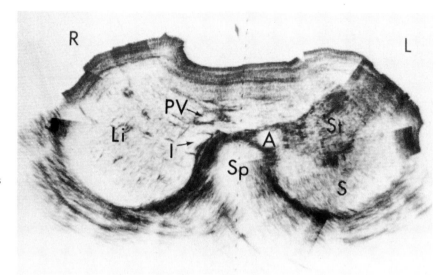

Fig. 6.5

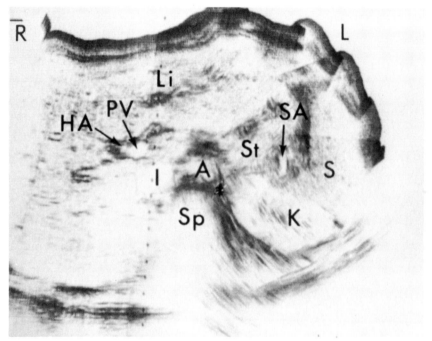

Fig. 6.6

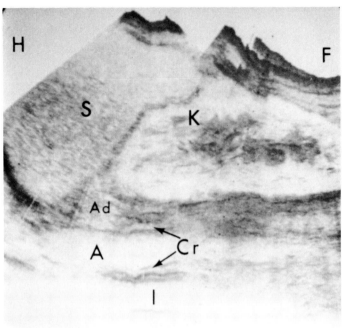

Fig. 6.7

A	=	Aorta
Ad	=	Left adrenal gland
Cr	=	Crus of the diaphragm
D	=	Left hemidiaphragm
F	=	Foot
H	=	Head
HA	=	Hepatic artery
I	=	Inferior vena cava
K	=	Left kidney
L	=	Left
Li	=	Liver
PV	=	Portal vein
R	=	Right
S	=	Spleen
SA	=	Splenic artery
Sp	=	Spine
St	=	Stomach

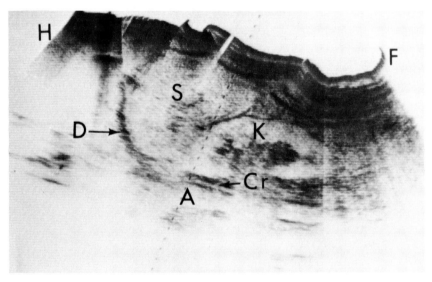

Fig. 6.8

Mild Splenomegaly

Figures 6.9 and 6.10 are of a 76-year-old woman with a history of breast carcinoma. She entered the hospital with a palpable left upper quadrant mass which was felt to be due to splenic enlargement. A transverse ultrasound examination (fig. 6.9) demonstrated enlargement of the spleen in the left upper quadrant. There is a fairly even parenchymagram to the spleen. A CAT scan was also performed (fig. 6.10). This again demonstrated splenomegaly. A rule of thumb in diagnosing splenomegaly is to find the spleen situated anterior to the aorta. In this case, it was situated quite anterior to the abdominal aorta. Also seen in figure 6.9 is cholelithiasis in the right upper quadrant.

Figure 6.11 is another example of splenomegaly. This is a transverse scan with marked enlargement of the spleen, which is situated in the anterior abdomen and markedly anterior to the abdominal aorta.

Figure 6.12 is an example of splenomegaly due to chronic alcoholism. Ascites is visualized surrounding the liver and the spleen. When splenomegaly is present, there is usually little difficulty in visualizing the spleen with ultrasound. The reason for this is that the spleen is very often situated below the left costal margin, which gives ready access to the transducer.

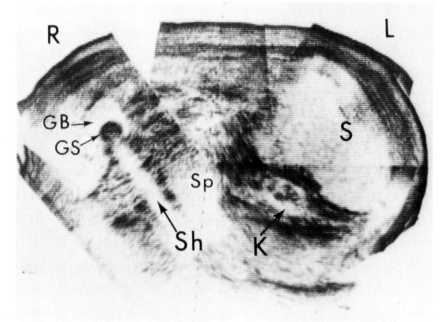

Fig. 6.9

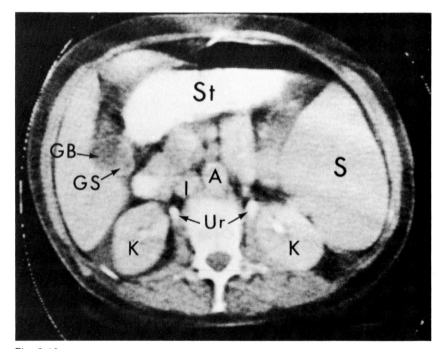

Fig. 6.10

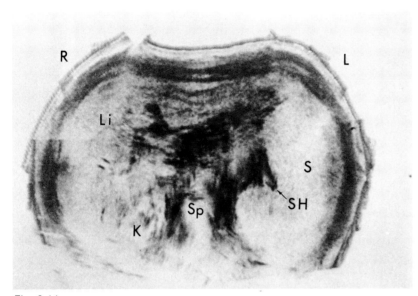

Fig. 6.11

Source: Figures 6.11 and 6.12 are obtained through the courtesy of Dr. Peter Cooperberg, University of British Columbia, Vancouver, British Columbia, Canada.

A	= Aorta
As	= Ascites
GB	= Gallbladder
Gs	= Gallstone
I	= Inferior vena cava
K	= Kidney
L	= Left
Li	= Liver
R	= Right
S	= Spleen
SH	= Splenic hylum
Sh	= Shadowing from the gallstone
Sp	= Spine
St	= Stomach
Ur	= Ureters

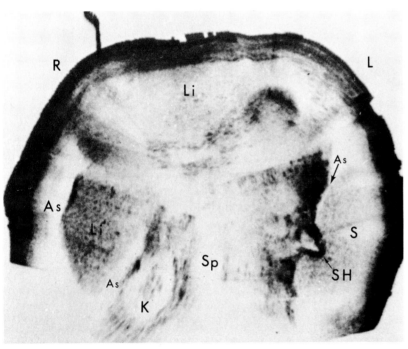

Fig. 6.12

Massive Splenomegaly

Figures 6.13–6.16 were obtained from a patient with chronic myelogenous leukemia. Here we see massive splenomegaly.

Figure 6.13 is a transverse scan high up in the abdomen in which we see the spleen as large as the liver. As we move more caudally in figure 6.14, we see that the spleen is involving the entire abdomen across the midline and to the right side. At this point, the liver is quite small over its caudal portion.

Figure 6.15 is a longitudinal scan on the left side. The spleen is seen displacing the left kidney somewhat caudally. Another longitudinal scan (fig. 6.16) demonstrates massive splenomegaly well below the umbilical level. The spleen is seen anterior to the pancreas. It has continued to enlarge to the point where it is visualized below the bifurcation of the aorta.

Figure 6.13 is an example of a false mass created by the sector scanning through the left lateral aspect of the patient. Thus, the sonolucent mass appears, due to technical factors rather than any real mass within the spleen.

Evaluation of the splenic parenchyma is best obtained on longitudinal scans. Transverse scans obtained through the intercostal spaces very often will have numerous artifacts. This case shows massive splenomegaly in which the spleen is seen across the midline and below the umbilical level.

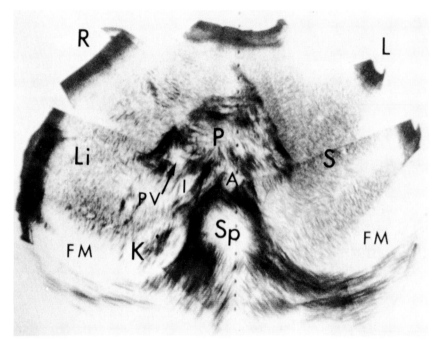

Fig. 6.13

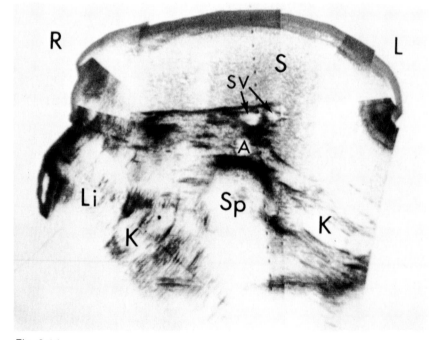

Fig. 6.14

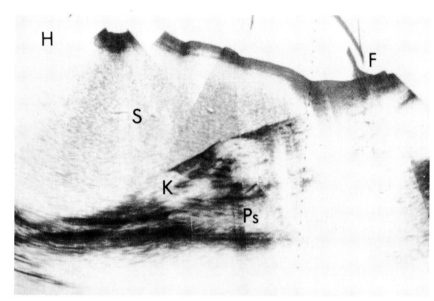

Fig. 6.15

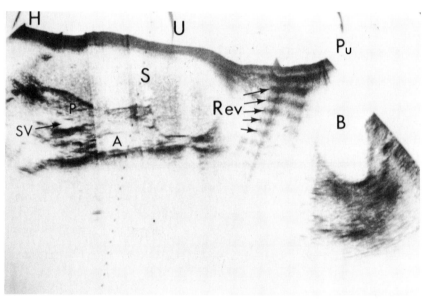

Fig. 6.16

Lymphoma ; Lymphosarcoma

Figure 6.17 is a transverse scan of a patient with lymphoma with a large mass in the left upper quadrant. A longitudinal scan (fig. 6.18) shows the mass situated caudal and anterior to the spleen. This mass, arising from the spleen, was secondary to a lymphomatous lesion in the spleen. It completely disappeared with radiation and chemotherapy. Usually, splenic enlargement secondary to lymphoma or chronic leukemia gives a fairly even splenic parenchymagram. It is not easy to distinguish the lymphomatous infiltrate from the normal splenic echoes. This case, however, shows a very discrete mass arising from the spleen.

Figures 6.19 and 6.20 are of a patient with lymphosarcoma of the spleen. An isotope study (fig. 6.19) demonstrates large filling defects within the enlarged spleen. A longitudinal ultrasound scan of the spleen shows a highly echogenic central mass (arrows) which is markedly different from the surrounding less echogenic splenic tissue. The discrete lesions within the spleen were secondary to lymphosarcoma.

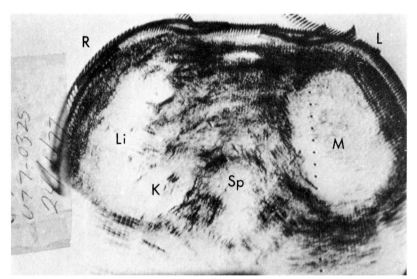

Fig. 6.17

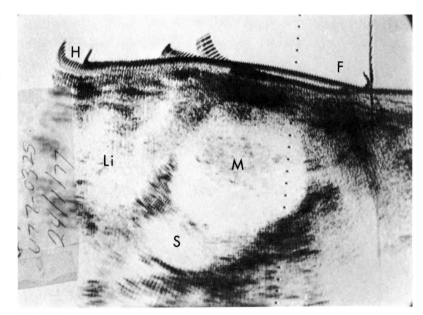

Fig. 6.18

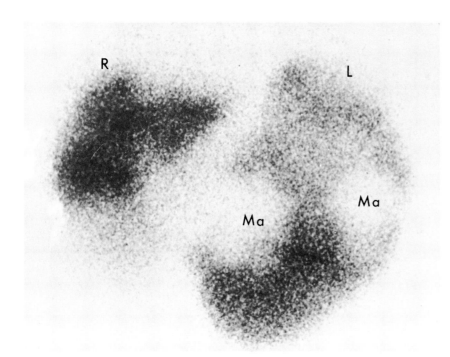

Fig. 6.19

SOURCE: The cases for figures 6.17–6.20 were provided through the courtesy of Dr. Peter Cooperberg, University of British Columbia, Vancouver, British Columbia, Canada.

Arrows	=	Lymphosarcomatous lesion within the spleen
F	=	Foot
H	=	Head
K	=	Kidney
L	=	Left
Li	=	Liver
M	=	Mass
R	=	Right
S	=	Spleen
Sp	=	Spine

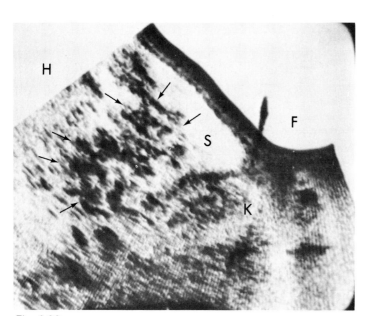

Fig. 6.20

Small Splenic Cysts

Figure 6.21 is an isotope study of the spleen with a filling defect in the medial aspect of its lower portion. As with a liver examination, ultrasound is an excellent means for detecting the nature of defects noted on isotope study. A transverse scan of the same patient (fig. 6.22) demonstrates a large, fluid-filled mass anterior to the spleen. This represents a small splenic cyst.

A longitudinal scan (fig. 6.23) shows the cyst as a sonolucent mass with sharp borders within the spleen. Deep to the cyst are increased splenic echos due to through transmission; this confirms the fluid nature of the splenic mass.

Figure 6.24 is an isotope study of a spleen with a large filling defect. Ultrasound is an excellent means for determining the nature of such defects. The case shown in figure 6.24 follows (figs. 6.25–6.28).

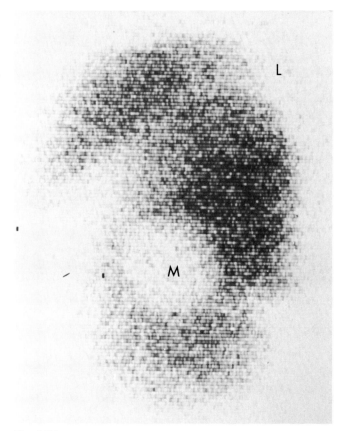

Fig. 6.21

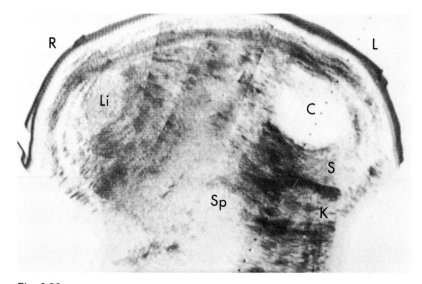

Fig. 6.22

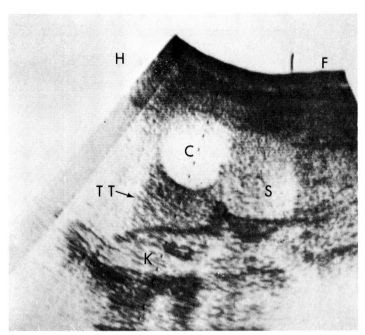

Fig. 6.23

SOURCE: The cases for figures 6.21–6.24 are provided through the courtesy of Dr. Peter Cooperberg, University of British Columbia, Vancouver, British Columbia, Canada.

C	=	Small splenic cyst
F	=	Foot
H	=	Head
K	=	Kidney
L	=	Left
Li	=	Liver
M	=	Mass noted on isotope study of the spleen
R	=	Right
S	=	Spleen
Sp	=	Spine
TT	=	Through transmission behind the cyst

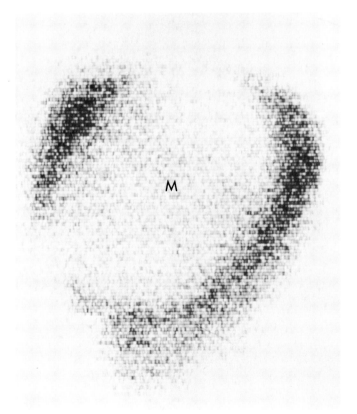

Fig. 6.24

Large Splenic Cyst

Figures 6.25–6.27 are ultrasound examinations of the spleen (fig. 6.24) with a large sonolucent mass in the anterior aspect of the left upper quadrant. This mass was found to be a large splenic cyst. The fluid-filled mass is situated anterior to the spleen in figures 6.25 and 6.26. The excellent through transmission and fairly sharp borders indicate the fluid-filled nature of the mass.

A prone scan (fig. 6.27) indicates the cyst situated anterior to the left kidney. The upper pole of the left kidney is compressed by this large splenic cyst. Figure 6.28 is an angiogram of the same patient. A large avascular mass is seen in the left upper quadrant with splaying and stretching of the vessels from the splenic artery.

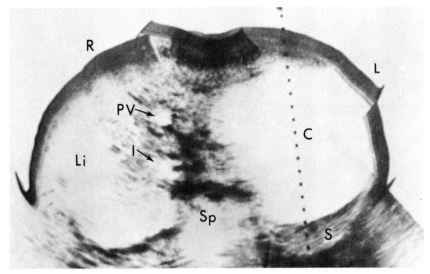

Fig. 6.25

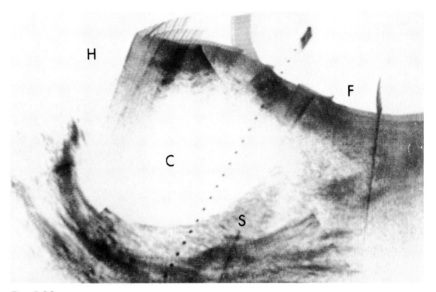

Fig. 6.26

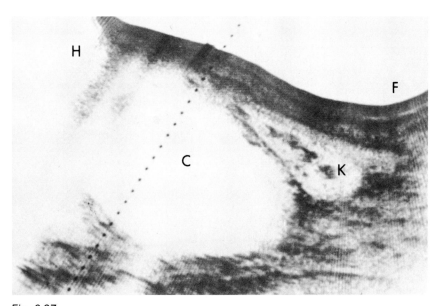

Fig. 6.27

SOURCE: The case for figures 6.25–6.28 were provided through the courtesy of Dr. Peter Cooperberg, University of British Columbia, Vancouver, British Columbia, Canada.

C = Large splenic cyst
F = Foot
H = Head
I = Inferior vena cava
K = Left kidney
L = Left
Li = Liver
PV = Portal vein
R = Right
S = Spleen
Sp = Spine

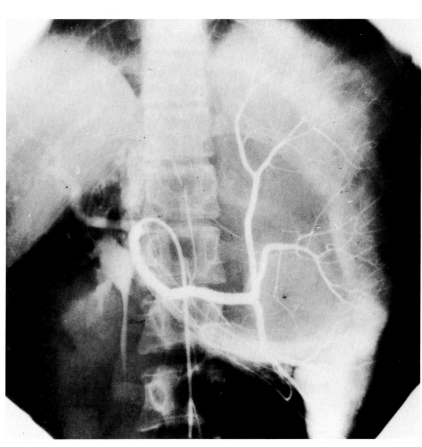

Fig. 6.28

Splenic Hematomas

Figures 6.29 and 6.30 are of a patient with a left-sided empyema. Multiple attempts at thoracentesis were performed, but were unsuccessful because of the loculated empyema. A few hours after the thoracentesis attempts, the patient became hypotensive, and the hematocrit dropped. A sonolucent mass representing a splenic hematoma within the surrounding parenchyma of the spleen is seen. Splenic hematomas may be within the splenic parenchyma, as in this case, or they may be extracapsular in the peritoneal cavity. This patient was taken to surgery, where a large splenic hematoma near the hilum of the spleen was identified. The sonolucent mass within the mid portion of the spleen is consistent with a hematoma. The possibility of a splenic cyst could not be ruled out, although the walls were not as sharp as in the previous cases of splenic cysts.

The ultrasound scans in figures 6.31 and 6.32 are of a patient who suffered recent trauma to the left upper quadrant. A large sonolucent mass is seen in the left upper quadrant secondary to a splenic hematoma. Figure 6.31 is an excellent example of a transverse scan with the splenic capsule (arrows) displaced away from the lateral abdominal wall due to the left upper quadrant hematoma. The spleen is displaced toward the midline by this large mass.

A longitudinal scan (fig. 6.32) demonstrates the hematoma anterior to the splenic echoes. This case is a fairly classic example of an extracapsular hematoma in which we see the capsule (arrows) quite well between the spleen and the hematoma. Ascites can be ruled out because of the linear echoes noted within the hematoma. This finding is more characteristic of a hematoma or an abscess.

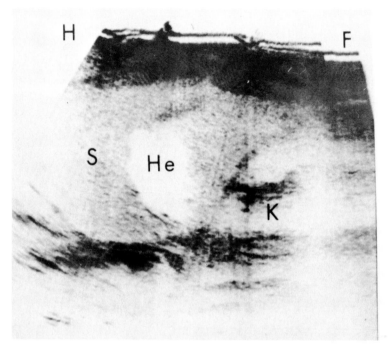

Fig. 6.29

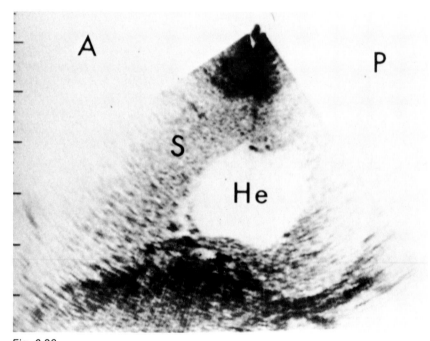

Fig. 6.30

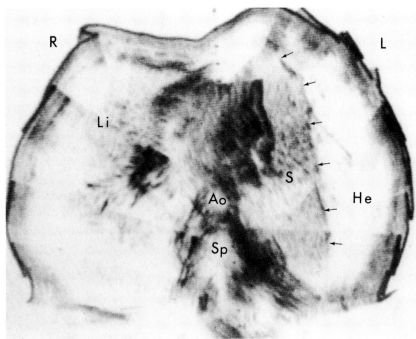

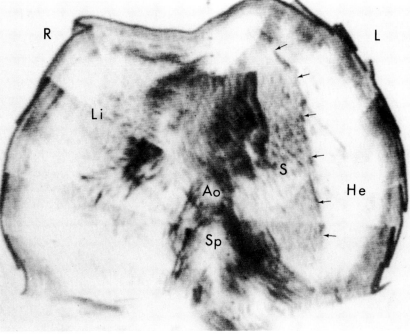

A	=	Aorta
An	=	Anterior
Arrows	=	Splenic capsule displaced away from the abdominal wall by the splenic hematoma
F	=	Foot
H	=	Head
He	=	Splenic hematoma
K	=	Kidney
L	=	Left
Li	=	Liver
P	=	Posterior
R	=	Right
S	=	Spleen
Sp	=	Spine

Fig. 6.31

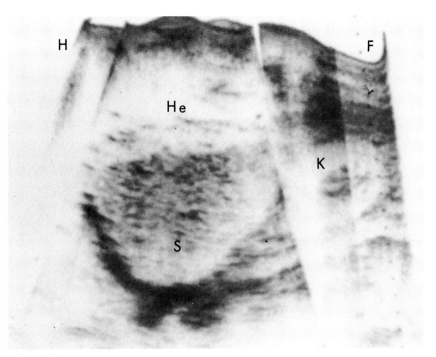

Fig. 6.32

Splenic Hematoma;
Left Subphrenic Abscess

Frequently, blunt abdominal trauma leads to splenic rupture, and fluid is found in the abdominal cavity secondary to hematoma. Figures 6.33 and 6.34 are scans obtained from a patient with blunt abdominal trauma with intraperitoneal hemorrhage. In the transverse scan (fig. 6.33), fluid is noted posterior to the liver and anterior to the right kidney. A longitudinal scan (fig. 6.34) over this site, shows the hematoma in the hepatorenal angle, on the right side. The spleen in figure 6.33 was not markedly enlarged, but rupture of the spleen led to hemorrhage into the peritoneal cavity. Another usual site for the collection of blood is in the pelvis, just superior to the urinary bladder.

A longitudinal scan (fig. 6.35) of another patient with a splenic hematoma demonstrates a sonolucent mass superior to the spleen in the left upper quadrant. This hematoma was loculated in the left upper quadrant and did not spread into the peritoneal cavity.

Figure 6.36 is an example of a mass, in the left upper quadrant, which was secondary to a left subphrenic abscess. It is extremely difficult to distinguish an abscess from a hematoma, for they can have a similar appearance on ultrasound. The clinical history, however, will contribute to the correct diagnosis. Figure 6.36 is also an excellent example of fluid both above and below the left hemidiaphragm. There is a left pleural effusion in the left pleural space, cephalad to the diaphragm. Below the diaphragm is an abscess in the left upper quadrant, which is superior to the spleen.

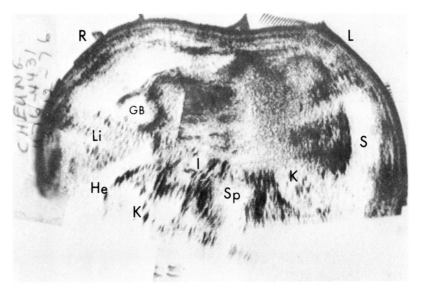

Fig. 6.33

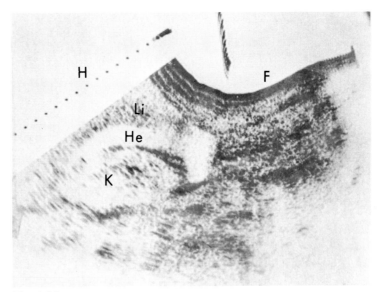

Fig. 6.34

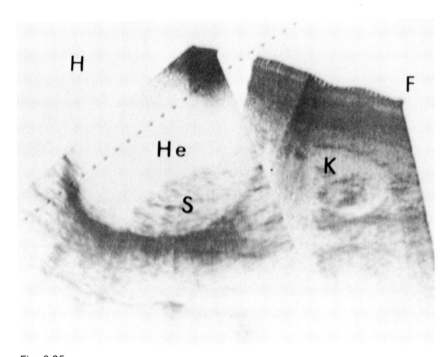

Fig. 6.35

SOURCE: The cases for figures 6.33, 6.34, and 6.36 are provided through the courtesy of Dr. Peter Cooperberg, University of British Columbia, Vancouver, British Columbia, Canada.

Ab	=	Left subphrenic abscess
D	=	Left hemidiaphragm
F	=	Foot
GB	=	Gallbladder
H	=	Head
He	=	Hematoma
I	=	Inferior vena cava
K	=	Kidney
L	=	Left
Li	=	Liver
PE	=	Left pleural effusion
R	=	Right
S	=	Spleen
Sp	=	Spine

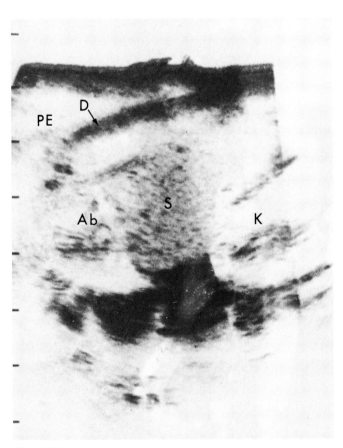

Fig. 6.36

Splenic Calcification; Markedly Enlarged Splenic Vein

Occasionally very strong circular echoes can be visualized within the splenic parenchyma. Ultrasound scans (figs. 6.37 and 6.38) obtained from a patient with splenic calcifications noted on X-ray demonstrate strong circular echoes within the spleen. These are secondary to calcific areas. In figure 6.38, we can see shadowing behind the calcific areas.

Often, large circular sonolucencies are noted adjacent to the splenic hilum. This may raise difficulties in distinguishing among ascites, hematomas, or abscesses. The problem may, however, be due to massive enlargement of the splenic vein.

Figures 6.39 and 6.40 are scans obtained from a 38-year-old man with a long history of ethanol abuse. He had mild splenomegaly. The large circular sonolucencies near the splenic hilum are secondary to a massively dilated splenic vein. Also noted is some fluid surrounding the spleen in figure 6.39, due to ascites. The large circular sonolucencies in the splenic hilum, in this case, are secondary to a dilated splenic vein. Although hematomas, abscesses, and other fluid collections may be confused for the sonolucencies, a dilated tortuous splenic vein gives a characteristic tubular appearance.

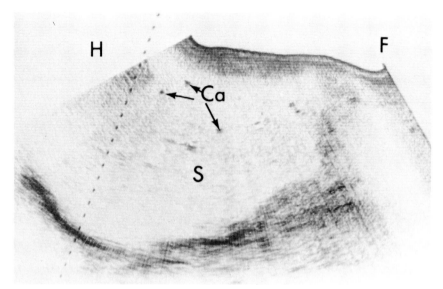

Fig. 6.37

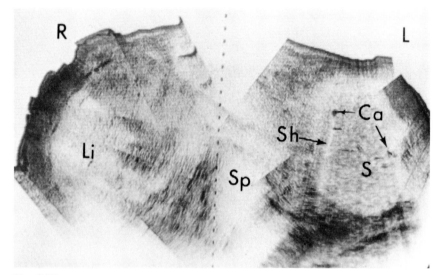

Fig. 6.38

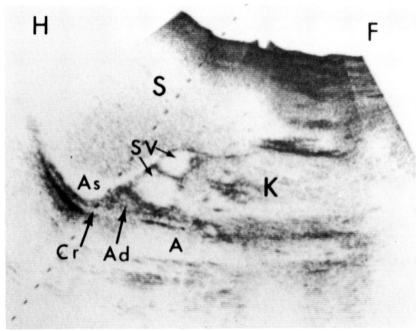

Fig. 6.39

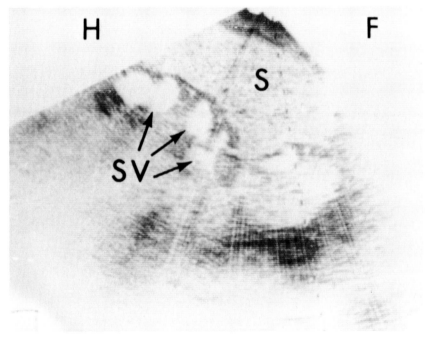

Fig. 6.40

7.
Renal, Adrenal, Retroperitoneal, and Scrotal Ultrasonography

W. Frederick Sample, M.D.

Since the retroperitoneum contains numerous structures, any discussion requires that its various components be arbitrarily segmented. In this chapter, the anatomy and pathology of the retroperitoneum in general will be discussed, and primary and secondary neoplasms, fluid collections, and chronic inflammatory states will also be included. In addition, the anatomy and pathology of the kidney and adrenal glands will be covered. Finally, the scrotum will be included in this chapter, since the remaining urological applications of ultrasound have been discussed in other chapters.

Renal Anatomy

The position of the kidneys is variable, but normally they are located between the iliac crest and lower ribs. For proper identification, as many of the surrounding structures as possible should be identified. On the right, the liver, gallbladder, second portion of the duodenum, adrenal gland, inferior vena cava, crus of the diaphragm, psoas muscle, and quadratis lumborum muscle should be recognized, depending on the scanning plane. Similarly on the left, the spleen, pancreas, adrenal, fourth portion of the duodenum, aorta, crus of the diaphragm, psoas muscle, and quadratus lumborum muscle represent potentially identifiable boundary structures.

The renal veins are visualized routinely. The right renal vein has a shorter course from the inferior vena cava to the renal hilus. The longer left renal vein passes between the superior mesenteric artery and the aorta. The renal arteries are visualized less frequently than the veins, and care must be exercised in distinguishing them from the crura of the diaphragm. The right renal artery may be seen passing anterior to the caudal extension of the right crus and posterior to the inferior vena cava; it often causes an indentation in the latter.

With the newer gray scale systems, an increasing amount of renal architecture has been appreciable (Cook, Rosenfield, and Taylor 1977; Rosenfield et al. 1978; Sample, Gyepes, and Ehrlich 1977; Sanders and Conrad 1977). At a minimum, the lower-amplitude reflections of the parenchyma can be separated from the more reflective renal sinus. The normal renal parenchyma is less echogenic than the normal liver. In some patients, the renal cortex can be distinguished from the renal pyramids, and occasionally even the arcuate vessels identified at the corticomedullary junction. It is common to resolve the normal renal pelvis, especially when it is extrarenal in location.

Renal Scanning Techniques

Transverse and longitudinal scans performed in the prone position traditionally have been used to study the kidneys. Although renal size and many lesions can be detected with this approach, the thick paraspinous muscles and bony impediments frequently prevent visualization of the upper poles and optimal renal architecture. Furthermore, the prevertebral and renal vessels cannot be visualized. As a result, a complete renal study should include transverse and longitudinal scans with the patient in both the decubitis and supine positions (Cook, Rosenfield, and Taylor 1977; Rosenfield et al. 1978; Sample, Gyepes, and Ehrlich 1977).

Regardless of the scanning position, transverse scans should be performed first, to determine the oblique plane to be used in the longitudinal scans of the kidney. Using all of these approaches, single sector or linear scans and suspended respiration should insure optimal visualization of renal architecture and relationships.

Other than good general hydration, no special patient preparation is required. When an intravenous urogram has already been performed, it should be reviewed to help guide the ultrasound study. (See p. 280 for additional comments on renal scanning technique.)

General Signs of Renal Disease

Focal renal disease is usually detected as a mass effect with associated change in the renal architecture or ultrasonic texture. Changes in transmission of the sound through the area of concern may add differential information. In regions where the normal renal contours are altered, or the renal sinus texture is dislocated or diffused, simple scans attempting to delineate alterations in texture will differentiate pseudotumors from true pathology (Maklad et al. 1977). In some focal and most diffuse diseases of the kidney, the relative echogenicity of the various portions of the kidney may be altered.

Indications for Renal Ultrasound Examination

In most patient groups, the intravenous urogram is the screening procedure for renal disease. The ultrasonogram is used to evaluate further a suspected or definite lesion, based on the intravenous urographic findings, such as a mass, renal axis deviation, or poor or non-renal function, for example. Ultrasonography is, however, being used primarily to screen obstetrical patients, patients who are allergic to iodinated contrast agents, and children with abdominal masses (Bearman, Hine, and Sanders 1976; Sample, Gyepes, and Ehrlich 1977; Skolnik 1977; Teele 1977). In addition, families of patients with known adult polycystic disease are primarily evaluated with ultrasound (Kelsey and Bowie 1977). Finally, ultrasound can serve as a guide for aspiration or biopsy of known renal lesions.

Renal Pathology

Congenital Anomalies

Since the kidneys migrate cephalad to the upper abdomen, a variety of malpositions can result if the migration is altered during the gestational period. Malpositions range from simple ptosis to a pelvic kidney. Usually the ultrasonic features of normal renal tissue identify the renal origin of a mass suspected clinically. Pelvic kidneys may, however, be hypoplastic with a distorted renal architecture. When no kidney is seen in the renal fossa on an ultrasound study, then the lower abdomen and pelvis should be examined. Similarly, if a mass is discovered in the lower abdomen or pelvis with any semblance of a renoform configuration, the flanks should be examined.

One or both kidneys may be hypoplastic. Hypoplastic kidneys are usually small and function poorly on intravenous urography. On ultrasonograms, the configuration, accentuated lobulation, and architecture may be distorted (Sample, Gyepes, and Ehrlich 1977). As a result, differentiation from a chronically diseased kidney may be difficult although the latter frequently generates increased parenchymal echoes. Hypoplasia may also be difficult to distinguish from true agenesis, since in the latter condition the renal fossa may be filled with bowel simulating a hypoplastic kidney (Toomey et al. 1977). Furthermore, in both entities, compensatory hypertrophy of the contralateral kidney may occur.

Duplication of the kidney may range from an incomplete duplication, involving only the collecting system, to complete separation of the kidney and collecting system into two components (Mascatello et al. 1977; Sample, Gyepes, and Ehrlich 1977). In the milder form where the intrarenal collecting system only is duplicated, the normally continuous echogenic hilar echoes will be indented or completely separated in the mid portions by a band of normal cortex. Careful scanning will show that this area has an acoustic texture similar to normal renal parenchyma.

When a complete duplication is present, the upper pole ureter is often ectopically inserted onto the bladder with a dilatation known as an ureterocele which leads to obstruction and variable degrees of hydronephrosis. Furthermore, the ureter to the lower portions of the kidney may insert abnormally into the bladder, leading to reflux and chronic pyelonephritis. Scanning of the renal and pelvic areas may delineate any of these possibilities (Sample, Gyepes, and Ehrlich 1977).

A variety of fusions can affect the kidneys. The most common fusion abnormality is the horseshoe kidney where the fusion usually occurs at the inferior poles of the kidneys. In this condition, the kidneys are more medially and anteriorly situated and are connected by a solid mass of tissue across the midline, simulating a retroperitoneal mass (Mindell and Kupic 1977).

Cystic Disease

By far the most common renal abnormality in adults is the simple renal cyst which accounts for 95% of masses seen on intravenous urography. Renal cysts conform to the general criteria of cysts on ultrasonograms. Because tumors may form in the wall of cysts, however, and because more ominous pathological processes may contain significant fluid areas, the strictest criteria for a simple cyst must be adhered to before the workup is terminated after the ultrasonogram. In cases of doubt, or when the entire cyst cannot be seen, aspiration should be performed.

Multicystic kidney represents a severe form of usually unilateral renal dysplasia whereby the ureter is atretic, and the kidney is a multicystic mass with minimal to no functioning tissue. The fluid areas do not communicate, thereby distinguishing this entity from most cases of hydronephrosis (Bearman, Hine, and Sanders 1976; Sample, Gyepes, and Ehrlich 1977). However, when a single large cyst is present, the configuration may be similar to long-standing hydronephrosis. Multicystic kidney is most frequently encountered in the neonate.

Polycystic kidneys are bilateral genetic abnormalities. In the infantile form, a spectrum of hepatic fibrosis and tubular ectasia occurs. The kidneys are large, and the renal sinus architecture is distorted (Rosenfield et al. 1977; Sample, Gyepes, and Ehrlich 1977). In the adult form, hypertension and renal failure present in middle age. The kidneys are enlarged and contain multiple resolvable cysts of varying size in both the parenchymal and renal sinus regions. Associated cystic disease is frequently present in the liver and less often in the pancreas or spleen.

Hydronephrosis

Hydronephrosis usually implies obstruction of the urinary system, most commonly at the ureteropelvic junction, the ureterovesical junction, or the bladder outlet. Although pelvocalyceal dilatation can be detected with ultrasound, it does not necessarily imply obstruction, which must be further determined in many cases by correlation with intravenous urography or scintigraphic evaluation (Ellenbogen 1978; Rosenfield et al. 1978; Sanders and Conrad 1977). Furthermore, segmental hydronephrosis can be confused with other intrarenal fluid pathologies.

The pelvocalyceal dilatation takes many forms on ultrasonograms, ranging from minimal separation of the normal echogenic renal sinus by an oval fluid collection to a saclike fluid collection with no surrounding renal parenchyma. The major cystic area, however, tends to bulge anteromedially. A dilated ureter may be visualized near the kidney or in the pelvis, and the site or cause of obstruction can sometimes be ascertained (Pollack et al. 1978; Zegal and Edell 1978).

Solid Renal Masses

A number of benign and malignant solid masses affect the kidney. Although the solid nature can be determined by sonograms, histological differential diagnosis seldom is possible. Pelvic fibrolipomatosis consists of excessive fat in the renal sinus. It may occur as a replacement process in renal atrophy or simply reflect obesity. On sonograms, the renal sinus may be prominent without any alteration in acoustic texture, or it may be separated by a solid hypoechoic mass (Yeh, Mitty, and Wolf, 1977). Differentiation of the latter pattern from that of a transitional cell carcinoma is impossible.

Angiomyolipoma is a benign renal tumor which may

appear as a discrete mass or as an overall enlarged kidney. The fatty components are hyperechoic. In addition, the sound may be severely scattered, leading to high attenuation.

Hypernephromas are the most common form of malignant renal tumors and have a variety of ultrasonic patterns (Maklad et al. 1977). The prevalence of solid masses with acoustic texture greater or less than normal renal parenchyma is the commonest finding. However, areas of calcification, necrosis, or cystic degeneration will cause alterations in this general pattern, which can mimic other benign processes. Since many of the acoustic patterns for benign and malignant masses overlap, scanning for secondary signs of malignancy is mandatory when a renal mass is encountered. The liver, retroperitoneum, and adrenals should be scanned for metastases. In addition, the possibility of malignant extension into the renal veins or inferior vena cava should be investigated (Goldstein, Green, and Weaver Jr. 1978).

Infectious Diseases

Acute pyelonephritis may go undetected on ultrasonograms. A slightly enlarged kidney with a prominent renal pelvis secondary to reflex atony and a hypoechoic renal parenchyma may, however, be confirmatory. Usually, ultrasonography is requested to search for complications of renal infection, such as pyonephrosis, renal carbuncle, or perinephric abscess (Goldman et al. 1977; Schneider et al. 1976). In pyonephrosis the dilated pelvocalyceal system frequently demonstrates debris. In renal carbuncles, localized, hypoechoic, solid, or irregular fluid areas are found within the kidney. In perinephric abscesses, a similar ultrasonic pattern is seen in conjunction with a loss of the external renal contour and an extrarenal mass.

Diffuse Renal Diseases

A number of medical diseases diffusely affect the kidneys and lead to altered renal function. With the increasing renal architecture now visible on sonograms, some of these diseases are being recognized by not only a change in renal size but an alteration in the cortico-medullary-renal sinus acoustic textures (Rosenfield et al. 1978). In general, diseases associated with vascular congestion and edema, such as renal vein thrombosis, lead to reduced cortical echogenicity. Diseases associated with collagen deposition, for example, glomerulonephritis, lead to a generalized increase in cortical echogenicity. Considerably more experience will be necessary to determine the specificity of the patterns now being described.

Renal Transplants

The role of ultrasound in the evaluation of the failing transplanted kidney is evolving (Bartrum et al. 1976; Cahill, Cochran, and Sample 1977). Transplant volume can be determined from sonograms, and the normally slow increase in volume representing compensatory hypertrophy has been documented. Similarly, the acute increase in renal size associated with transplant rejection has been detectable. The relative predictive value of renal transplant volume, however, changes over other signs of rejection awaits further evaluation.

By far, the most important contribution of ultrasound to the management of renal transplant patients is in the detection of obstruction and peritransplant fluid collections. Hydronephrosis, abscesses, hematomas, urinomas, and lymphoceles may have symptoms and signs indistinguishable from those of transplant rejection. They are often accompanied by deterioration of renal function and frequently are not palpable. Although the ultrasound patterns of the different types of peritransplant fluid collections are not specific, sonographic examination can detect the presence and size of the fluid collection and whether or not associated obstructive uropathy is present. Aspiration of the fluid for diagnostic or therapeutic purposes can also be performed under ultrasound guidance.

Anatomical Considerations of the Adrenal Glands

Delineating the adrenal gland always has been a challenge for the ultrasonographer, since the gland is small, triangular, and within the confines of the lower rib cage. The right adrenal gland is suprarenal and situated between the liver, inferior vena cava, and right crus of the diaphragm. One limb may extend along the medial aspect of the kidney. In either the transaxial or longitudinal planes, the right adrenal gland normally has a linear, coma, or elongated triangular shape.

The left adrenal gland is intimately related to the left crus of the diaphragm, the anterosuperomedial aspect of the left kidney, and the tail of the pancreas. In addition, the esophagogastric junction is cephalad, and the fourth portion of the duodenum is caudal to the gland. The left adrenal gland tends to be more triangular in shape but may have one limb extend linearly along the medial aspect of the left kidney.

Adrenal Scanning Techniques

Although larger adrenal masses can be imaged with conventional transverse and longitudinal scans with the patient in the supine and prone positions, small masses and normal adrenal glands are best imaged in the decubitis positions with special alignment procedures (Sample 1977; Sample 1978). On the right, the liver is used as an acoustic window. On transverse scans, the transducer should be aimed perpendicular to the planes of the medial border of the liver, the adrenal gland, and the crus of the diaphragm. The liver-adrenal interface is usually the most difficult to resolve.

A longitudinal view of the right adrenal gland can be obtained from several approaches. If the left lobe of the liver crosses the midline, a plane through the left lobe of the liver and inferior vena cava may delineate the adrenal gland. Alternatively, a plane through the right lobe of the liver perpendicular to the right crus can be used. Finally, if the liver is diseased, or if the colon is interposed anteriorly, the right kidney can be used as an acoustic window.

The left adrenal gland can infrequently be seen on transverse scans, even with the patient in the decubitis position, since air in the stomach blocks the sound. However, a coronal approach through the spleen and the kidney has been successful in a good percentage of patients, but it requires a specific alignment. Transverse scans are performed in the decubitis position, and the line passing through the aorta and kidney is marked on the patient in the lower, middle, and upper pole regions. The resultant longitudinal scanning plane is coronal and oblique in orientation. With this approach, the left adrenal gland normally has a triangular configuration with straight or concave margins.

The major indication of adrenal abnormality on sonograms is adrenal enlargement (Bernardino, Goldstein, and Green 1978; Forsythe, Gosink, and Leopold 1977; Sample 1977; Yeh et al. 1978a; Yeh et al. 1978b). This may take the subtle form of convex margins. Larger abnormalities usually convert the gland to a round mass. Changes in acoustic texture without enlargement has not been a reliable sign. Areas of calcification or fluid are detectable using the standard criteria.

Indications for Adrenal Ultrasonography

A variety of clinical syndromes are associated with adrenal abnormality. From the clinical picture, as well as the sophisticated laboratory tests, it is usually possible to determine the potential adrenal pathology. The main role of sonography is to determine whether one or both glands are involved. The choice between ultrasonography and other imaging procedures such as computed tomography and scintigraphy will depend on the clinical syndrome, the laboratory findings, the age of the patient, and whether such circumstances as pregnancy prevent the use of X-ray (Berger, Kuhn, and Munschauer 1978; Sample and Sarti 1978). Clearly, ultrasound has been most effective in children, thinner adults, and disease processes which cause tumorous enlargement of the gland rather than nontumorous hyperplasia.

Adrenal Pathology

Cystic Disease

Adrenal cystic disease may present in children or adults. In adults, nonfunctioning pseudocystic masses are most common and must be distinguished anatomically from renal, pancreatic, and splenic cystic disease. In children, this entity takes the form of neonatal hemorrhage and must be distinguished from neuroblastoma and hydronephrosis. Adrenal hemorrhage has a variety of sonographic patterns, depending on the stage of clot organization (Lawson and Teele 1978). Usually a sonolucent mass is seen, but solid components and even calcification can be present.

Neuroblastoma

Neuroblastoma occurs in later childhood and usually is a bulky mass which must be differentiated from Wilm's tumor of the kidney and hydronephrosis. Neuroblastoma is predominately solid and may have hyperechoic areas related to calcification or, less frequently, hypoechoic areas related to necrosis (Berger, Kuhn, and Munschauer 1978). The liver and retroperitoneum should be scanned for secondary extension of this pathology.

Adenocarcinoma

Adenocarcinoma of the adrenal gland can occur in children or adults. Since these tumors may not be functional, and since they present as large masses, ultrasound is used primarily to assign the proper organ of origin to the mass and to detect evidence of metastases, chiefly to the liver.

Functional Abnormalities

The functional abnormalities of the adrenal gland may be secondary to nontumerous hyperplasia, multinodular hyperplasia, adenoma, or carcinoma. Often, the chemical tests will suggest the nature of the process. Ultrasound has been most effective in detecting adenomas and carcinomas. Since aldosteronomas may be quite small, and phechromocytomas may be in aberrant locations and difficult to reach by ultrasound, negative sonograms of the adrenal areas may be unreliable.

Pitfalls in the Diagnosis of Adrenal Disease

The major problem in adrenal scanning is proper localization of the gland (Sample and Sarti 1978). On the right, the crus of the diaphragm can be mistaken for the adrenal gland and must be specifically identified. The second portion of the duodenum also can be mistaken for a right adrenal mass.

On the left, the esophagogastric junction, antrum of the stomach, body of the pancreas, and medial lobulations of the spleen all can mimic adrenal masses (Gooding 1978).

In older patients, tortuous splenic vessels and prominent left renovascular bundles can cause confusion. If attempts are made to identify as many of the surrounding anatomic structures as possible, fewer errors will occur.

Anatomical Considerations of the Retroperitoneum

The retroperitoneum is that portion of the abdomen bounded by the parietal peritoneum and the transversalis fascia. The retroperitoneum is largest posteriorly but continues anteriorly as the properitoneal fat. Superficial to the transversalis fascia is the retrofascial space which predominently contains muscles. Although the retrofascial space is, strictly speaking, not part of the retroperitoneum, pathological processes in the region can mimic retroperitoneal abnormalities and will be included in the discussion.

The retroperitoneum is divided into a number of compartments by several fascial planes (Meyers 1976). The anterior and posterior renal fasciae (Gerota's fasciae) envelope the kidney and adrenal gland creating the perirenal space. The anterior and posterior renal fasciae fuse laterally to become the lateroconal fascia which extends behind the colon and ends at the paracolic gutters of the peritoneal cavity. The anterior renal fascia fuses medially with the dense fibrous tissue anterior to the prevertebral vessels (aorta and inferior vena cava). The posterior renal fascia fuses medially with the fascial coverings of the psoas muscle. Although the prevertebral vessels are included in the perirenal space, communication across the midline does not exist. Inferiorly, the renal fascial layers fuse weakly or blend with the ilias fasciae. Superiorly, the renal fascial layers fuse strongly at the apex of the crus of the diaphragm.

The anterior pararenal space is bounded by the parietal peritoneum, the lateroconal fascia, and the anterior renal fascia. The space contains the ascending and descending colon, the duodenal loop, the pancreas, and the mesenteric vessels. The space potentially communicates across the midline, although only pancreatic or lymph node abnormalities usually affect the space bilaterally.

The posterior pararenal space is invested by the transversalis fascia, the lateroconal fascia, and the posterior renal fascia. No organs are contained within the space. This space is continuous with the properitoneal spaces anterolaterally and in the pelvis.

Although the various fascial planes subdividing the retroperitoneum cannot usually be distinguished with ultrasound, a knowledge of the boundaries of the various compartments may allow the proper localization of a pathological process. A distinction between the retrofascial space and the retroperitoneum, however, can sometimes be made on sonograms.

Retroperitoneal Scanning Techniques

Ultrasonic visualization of the retroperitoneal structures is variably hindered by bowel gas, bone, and, in some patients, thick musculature and fatty layers. The thin, relatively gasless patient is most ideally suited for an ultrasound study. Because of the natural impediments to the sound beam, an extremely flexible approach to the retroperitoneum is necessary.

Transverse and longitudinal scans performed with the patient in the supine position usually outline the major organs and determine where the troublesome gas pockets are located. The high retroperitoneum frequently can be well visualized, since the liver and spleen serve as acoustic windows. Adequate penetration should be confirmed by delineation of the crus of the diaphragm and the prevertebral vessels. In the mid abdomen, the pancreas, kidneys, duodenal sweep, prevertebral vessels, and psoas muscles should be identified. In the lower abdomen the prevertebral vessels, the ileopsoas muscle, and the quadratus lumborum muscle should be delineated for diagnostic scans.

In order to avoid or redistribute the bowel contents, transverse and longitudinal scans performed in the decubitis or prone positions are necessary. Other retroperitoneal structures such as the kidney can then serve as ultrasonic windows. Segments of the prevertebral vessels not seen on supine scans may be visualized with these additional views. Oblique scans, progressing from the midline laterally to the groin, may also give optimal views of the ileopsoas muscles.

Patient preparation for retroperitoneal ultrasound examination is minimal. Withholding oral intake for 12 hours prior to the study may diminish gas. Attempts at pharmacological reduction of gas have not been beneficial enough to be used routinely. The examination of patients with recent barium studies generally should be delayed. Similarly, patients tend to be gaseous immediately following an intravenous urogram.

Signs of Retroperitoneal Disease

The most common sign of retroperitoneal disease is the presence of a mass (Filly, Marglin, and Castellino 1976). Careful delineation of the boundaries and the manner in which normal organs and vasculature are displaced sometimes will indicate the organ of origin and, rarely, the retroperitoneal compartment involved.

Masses should be further identified as to their cystic, complex, or solid nature by the usual criteria of wall characteristics, texture, and through transmission. Through transmission can be difficult to evaluate since the boundaries may be bone. Evaluation of enhanced through transmission is not possible at a bone or air interface (see chapter 1). Finally, both the echo-amplitude information denoted by the gray scale and the presence of shadowing caused by solid components may provide additional differential information.

The abnormal displacement of normal structures may indicate retroperitoneal pathology. Displacement of the aorta away from the spine or indentations of the inferior vena cava may be the first indications of an infiltrative process or of a mass (Spirt et al. 1974). Carefully performed scans directed at the anticipated boundaries of the mass may outline the abnormality.

On the other hand, the asymmetry of normal bilateral structures may be the only clue to a retroperitoneal abnormality (Kaftori et al. 1977). This sign is especially important when the muscles of the retrofascial space are evaluated. Careful questioning of the patient usually will determine whether muscle asymmetry is related to neuromuscular abnormalities, skeletal abnormalities, or differential use.

Finally, the loss of the normal retroperitoneal detail may indicate abnormality (Sanders et al. 1977). We must be certain that technical factors or poor penetration related to body habitus are not accounting for this finding. If these sources of error are excluded, disease can be suspected, and other studies such as computed tomography or nuclear scanning can be recommended.

Indications for Retroperitoneal Sonography

Ultrasonography has become an important noninvasive imaging modality for evaluating the retroperitoneum. When compared to other imaging procedures, such as computed tomography and gallium scanning, ultrasound may be the general procedure of choice in very thin patients, very ill patients, and the pediatric age group. In these groups, ultrasound can be used to find occult malignacies, to stage known neoplasms, and to detect hematomas and abscesses (Brascho, Durant, and Green 1977; Bree and Green 1978; Doust, Quiroz, and Stewart 1977; Laing and Jacobs 1977; McCullough and Leopold 1976; Rochester et al. 1977; Tyrrell et al. 1977).

Ultrasound also should be considered in the appropriate patient with a fever of unknown origin. Other imaging procedures may indirectly suggest a retroperitoneal mass. Ultrasound should be considered in the confirmation of the abnormality and in the assessment of its origin, extent, and differential diagnosis. Finally, ultrasound can serve as a guide for the aspiration or biopsy of known masses and aid in the treatment planning or follow-up (Gronvall, Gronvall, and Hegedus 1977; Holm et al. 1972; Smith and Bartrum 1974).

Retroperitoneal Pathology

Lymphadenopathy

On ultrasonograms, lymphadenopathy may have several configurations (Brascho, Durant, and Green 1977; Filly, Marglin, and Castellino 1976; Rochester, Bowie, Kunzmann, and Lester 1977; Tyrrell et al. 1977). A mantle-shaped mass bridging the prevertebral vessels may be observed. The fluid nature of the embedded vessels is usually discernible. Alternatively, separate dominant transonic masses around the prevertebral vessels can be delineated. Another pattern is simply psoas muscle asymmetry. In general, the solid nature of the process will be indicated by the standard criteria. Adenopathy secondary to lymphoma, however, is frequently sonolucent, and particular attention must be paid to the sound transmission. Adenopathy secondary to metastatic disease tends to have more internal texture, making the solid characterization easier. After therapy, enlarged nodes may become more echogenic or develop cystic areas presumably related to necrosis.

In spite of the fact that portions of the retroperitoneum may be obscured on sonograms, the detection of lymph adenopathy with ultrasound has been good (Filly, Marglin, and Castellino 1976; Rochester et al. 1977; Tyrrell et al. 1977). In scanning patients for adenopathy, it is important to examine the renal, hepatic, and splenic hili as well as the retrocrural area, since these regions are not evaluated with lymphangiography and are accessible to the sound beam.

Primary Neoplasms

Primary retroperitoneal tumors are rare and usually represent mesenchymal sarcomas (Bree and Green 1978).

Since these tumors are frequently large and outgrow their blood supply, they can have a variable ultrasonic appearance. Solid hypoechoic and hyperechoic masses have been described. In addition, large fluid areas may be present. No distinguishing ultrasonic patterns have been seen, and the diagnosis can be suggested only by the location and perhaps the presence of a large necrotic component. Since the masses tend to be large and infiltrative, it even may be difficult to determine the organ of origin of the mass.

Fluid Collection

A variety of fluid collections can occur in the retroperitoneum including hematomas, abscesses, urinomas, and lymphoceals. In general the ultrasonic patterns are similar with round or oval fluid collections having irregular and slightly thickened walls (Doust, Quiroz, and Stewart 1977; Laing and Jacobs 1977; McCullough and Leopold 1976). Fresh hematomas may, however, appear homogenously solid. Furthermore, as liquifaction and clot retraction progress, hyperechoic areas can develop. Similarly, abscesses which contain microairbubbles may be hyperechoic. Any of these sources of fluid can contain septations, solid debris, or fluid-solid interfaces which change with gravity. Usually, clinical or laboratory correlation will suggest the etiology of the fluid. Aspiration under ultrasonic guidance, however, often will establish the diagnosis and direct therapy.

Retroperitoneal Fibrosis

Retroperitoneal fibrosis may be idiopathic, secondary to certain drugs, or related to infiltrative tumor (metastatic breast carcinoma). On sonography a mass may be seen enveloping the distal prevertebral vessels and extending down the sacral promontory (Sanders et al. 1977). The aorta may not be elevated off the spine. Unilateral or bilateral hydronephrosis usually is present. This entity may mimic aortic aneurysms, lymphoma, or small retroperitoneal hemorrhages. As a result, the diagnosis usually can be suggested only after clinical correlation.

Pitfalls in the Diagnosis of Retroperitoneal Disease

The most serious error in retroperitoneal sonography is

mistaking the aberrant location of a normal organ for a pathological process. Ptosis and congenital variants of the kidney and the low-lying pancreas in the elderly patient account for the most frequent errors. Similarly, fluid pockets in the retroperitoneal portions of the colon and duodenum can mimic pathological fluid collections. Positional changes in the fluid, peristalsis, and real-time examination sometimes can eliminate this error. Finally, considerable overlap in the appearance of solid and fluid masses from a variety of pathological processes prevents specific differential diagnosis.

Anatomical Considerations of the Scrotum

The testis is covered by a number of tissue layers which, in total, are called the scrotum. The various layers represent extensions of the abdominal wall layers and include the skin, dartos tunic, external spermatic fascia, and internal spermatic fascia (tunica vaginalis).

The glandular elements of the testis drain into tubules which unite in the upper-pole region to form the efferent ductules (rete testis) which lead to the head of the epididymis. The body and tail of the epididymis extend to the lower pole of the testis and are continuous with the ductus deferens. The epididymis descends posterolaterally, whereas the ductus ascends posteromedially to the testis.

The appendix testis is a vestigial remnant of the mullerian duct and lies beneath the head of the epididymis. The appendix epididymis represents a detached efferent duct. The epididymis normally is strongly attached to the posterolateral aspect of the testis and the scrotum.

Scrotal Scanning Techniques

The scrotum can be scanned immersed in water, covered by a water bath, or by direct contact depending on the equipment used. Since the scrotum has an inherent symmetry, transverse and longitudinal scans are performed, and the sides are compared at appropriate levels. Attempts should be made to obtain longitudinal scans of each side with the testis lined up with the epididymis. Transducers with frequencies of 5 MHz or greater can be used to scan the superficial scrotum.

Signs of Scrotal Disease

The glandular elements of the testis normally have a granular texture of medium echogenicity (Sample, Gottesman, Skinner, and Ehrlich 1978; Winston, Handler, and Pritchard 1978). The epididymal area is more echogenic than the testis, and occasionally the epididymis or ductus deferens can be resolved. The appendix epididymis, the appendix testis, and the rete testis area normally are not resolved.

The major criteria for abnormality is the presence of an extratesticular or testicular mass. Some testicular abnormalities are detected only by subtle alterations in acoustic texture which require careful comparison of the two sides. Masses are characterized further as to their cystic or solid nature and general configuration for differentially diagnostic purposes.

Indications for Ultrasonography of the Scrotum

Ultrasound can aid in the differential diagnosis of the acutely enlarged scrotum and the chronic scrotal mass (Sample, Gottesman, Skinner, and Ehrlich 1978; Winston, Handler, and Pritchard 1978). In these instances, the extratesticular, testicular, or combined involvement is the key determination necessary. Many extratesticular abnormalities can be handled medically, whereas most testicular and combined abnormalities must be approached surgically. Ultrasound has also proved very effective in the evaluation of the clinically negative scrotum for occult neoplasm (Sample, Gottesman, Skinner, and Ehrlich 1978).

Pathology of the Scrotum

Epididymitis

Uncomplicated acute epididymitis is recognized on sonograms by delineating an enlarged hypoechoic epididymis in the epididymal region. The testicular texture usually is unaltered unless focal orchitis, usually in the rete testis area, is present. Focal orchitis cannot be distinguished from an occult testicular neoplasm except on serial exam, whereby the former will resolve.

A reactive hydrocele in the presence of epididymitis cannot always be distinguished from a peritesticular, or even sometimes a testicular, abscess. The findings, however, will indicate that the epididymitis is not simple.

Torsion of the Testis

Torsion of the testis is distinguishable from uncomplicated epididymitis, since the testis is abnormal. Acutely, the testis is enlarged and may have increased or decreased echogenicity, depending on whether it is just congested or necrotic.

Chronic Masses

Chronic scrotal masses can be differentiated as to their origin in 80% of cases. The configuration and location of simple extratesticular fluid areas will usually indicate whether the process is a hydrocele, a spermatocele, or a varicocele. The patterns of benign and malignant testicular masses overlap in such a fashion that this differentiation cannot be made.

Because of the rich normal acoustic texture of the testis, very small occult neoplasms can be resolved. Most tumors have been hypoechoic and have demonstrated striking attenuation.

Pitfalls in the Diagnosis of Testicular Disease

The main error in scrotal scanning is not adhering to strict criteria for testicular involvement. If we are not certain whether the testis is involved, then the primary care physician should be alerted that the abnormality could require surgery.

References

Bartrum, R. J.; Smith, E. H.; D'Orsi, C. J.; Tilney, N. L.; and Dantono, J. Evaluation of renal transplants with ultrasound. *Radiology* 118:405–410, February 1976.

Bearman, S. B.; Hine, P. L.; and Sanders, R. C. Multicystic kidney: a sonographic pattern. *Radiology* 118:685–688, March 1976.

Berger, P. E.; Kuhn, J. P.; and Munschauer, R. W. Computed tomography and ultrasound in the diagnosis and management of neuroblastoma. *Radiology* 128:663–667, September 1978.

Bernardino, M. E.; Goldstein, H. M.; and Green, B. Gray scale ultrasonography of adrenal neoplasms. *Am. J. Roentgenol.* 130:741–744, April 1978.

Brascho, D. J.; Durant, J. R.; and Green, L. E. The accuracy of retroperitoneal ultrasonography in Hodgkin's disease and non-Hodgkin's lymphoma. *Radiology* 125:485–487, November 1977.

Bree, R. L., and Green, B. The gray scale sonographic appearance of intra-abdominal mesenchymal sarcomas. *Radiology* 128:193–197, July 1978.

Cahill, P. J.; Cochran, S.; and Sample, W. F. Conventional radiographic and ultrasonic imaging in renal transplantation. *Urology* 10:33–42, July 1977.

Cook, J. H.; Rosenfield, A. T.; and Taylor, K. J. W. Ultrasonic demonstration of intrarenal anatomy. *Am. J. Roentgenol.* 129:831–835, November 1977.

Doust, B. D.; Quiroz, F.; and Stewart, J. M. Ultrasonic distinction of abscesses from other intra-abdominal fluid collections. *Radiology* 125:213–218, October 1977.

Ellenbogen, P. H.; Scheible, F. W.; Talner, L. B.; and Leopold, G. R. Sensitivity of gray scale ultrasound in detecting urinary tract obstruction. *Am. J. Roentgenol.* 130:731–733, April 1978.

Filly, R. A.; Marglin, S.; and Castellino, R. A. The ultrasonographic spectrum of abdominal and pelvic Hodgkin's disease and non-Hodgkin's lymphoma. *Cancer* 38:2143–2148, November 1976.

Forsythe, J. R.; Gosink, B. B.; and Leopold, G. R. Ultrasound in the evaluation of adrenal metastases. *J. Clin. Ultrasound* 5:31–34, February 1977.

Goldman, S. M.; Minkin, S. D.; Naraval, D. C.; Diamond, A. B.; Pion, S. J.; Meringoff, B. N.; Sidh, S. M.; Sanders, R. C.; and Cohen, S. P. Renal carbuncle: the use of ultrasound in its diagnosis and treatment. *J. Urol.* 118:525–528, October 1977.

Goldstein, H. M.; Green, B.; and Weaver, R. M., Jr. Ultrasonic detection of renal tumor extension into the inferior vena cava. *Am. J. Roentgenol.* 130:1083–1085, June 1978.

Gooding, G. A. W. The ultrasonic and computed tomographic appearance of splenic lobulations: a consideration in the ultrasonic differential of masses adjacent to the left kidney. *Radiology* 126:719–720, March 1978.

Gronvall, J.; Gronvall, S.; and Hegedus, V. Ultrasound-guided drainage of fluid-containing masses using angiographic catheterization techniques. *Am. J. Roentgenol.* 129:997–1002, December 1977.

Holm, H. H.; Kristensen, J. K.; Rasmussen, S. N.; Northeved, A.; and Barledo, H. Ultrasound as a guide in percutaneous puncture technique. *Ultrasonics* 10:83–86, 1972.

Kaftori, J. K.; Rosenberger, A.; Pollack, S.; and Fish, J. H. Rectus sheath hematoma: ultrasonographic diagnosis. *Am. J. Roentgenol.* 128:283–285, February 1977.

Kelsey, J. A., and Bowie, J. D. Gray scale ultrasonography in the diagnosis of polycystic kidney disease. *Radiology* 122:791–795, March 1977.

Laing, F. C., and Jacobs, R. P. Value of ultrasonography in the detection of retroperitoneal inflammatory masses. *Radiology* 123:169–172, April 1977.

Lawson, E. E., and Teele, R. Diagnosis of adrenal hemorrhage by ultrasound. *J. Pediatr.* 92:423–426, March 1978.

Maklad, W. F.; Chuang, V. P.; Doust, B. D.; Cho, K. J.; and Curran, J. E. Ultrasonic characterization of solid renal lesions: echogenic, angiographic and pathologic correlation. *Radiology* 123:733–739, January 1977.

Mascatello, J. J.; Smith, E. H.; Carrera, G. F.; Berger, M.; and Teele, R. L. Ultrasonic evaluation of the obstructed duplex kidney. *Am. J. Roentgenol.* 129:113–120, July 1977.

McCullough, D. L., and Leopold, G. R. Diagnosis of retroperitoneal fluid collections by ultrasonography: a series of surgically proved cases. *J. Urol.* 115:656–659, June 1976.

Meyers, A. M. *Dynamic radiology of the abdomen: normal and pathologic anatomy*, pp. 113–194. New York: Springer-Verlag, 1976.

Mindell, H. J., and Kupic, E. A. Horseshoe kidney: ultrasonic demonstration. *Am. J. Roentgenol.* 129:526–527, September 1977.

Pollack, H. M.; Arger, P. H.; Goldberg, B. B.; and Mulholland, S. G. Ultrasonic Detection of non-opaque renal calculi. *Radiology* 127:233–237, April 1978.

Rochester, D.; Bowie, J. D.; Kunzmann, A.; and Lester, E. Ultrasound in the staging of lymphoma. *Radiology* 124:483–487, August 1977.

Rosenfield, A. T.; Siegel, N. J.; Kappelman, N. B.; and Taylor, K. J. W. Gray scale ultrasonography in medullary cystic disease of the kidney and congenital hepatic fibrosis with tubular ectasia: new observations. *Am. J. Roentgenol.* 129:297–303, August 1977.

Rosenfield, A. T.; Taylor, K. J. W.; Cosade, M.; and de Graaf, C. S. Anatomy and pathology of the kidney by gray scale ultrasound. *Radiology* 128:737–744, September 1978.

Sample, W. F.; Gyepes, M. T.; and Ehrlich, R. M. Gray scale ultrasound in pediatric urology. *J. Urol.* 117:518–526, April 1977.

Sample, W. F. Adrenal ultrasonography. *Radiology* 127:462–466, May 1977a.

Sample, W. F. A new technique for the evaluation of the adrenal gland with gray scale ultrasonography. *Radiology* 124:463–469, August 1977b.

Sample, W. F.; Gottesman, J. E.; Skinner, D. G.; and Ehrlich, R. M. Gray scale ultrasound of the scrotum. *Radiology* 127:225–228, April 1978.

Sample, W. F., and Sarti, D. A. Computed tomography and gray scale ultrasonography of the adrenal gland: a comparative study. *Radiology* 128:377–383, August 1978.

Sanders, R. C.; Duffy, T.; McLaughlin, M. G.; and Walsh, P. C. Sonography in the diagnosis of retroperitoneal fibrosis. *J. Urol.* 118.944–946, December 1977.

Sanders, R. C., and Conrad, M. R. The ultrasonic characteristics of the renal pelvicalyceal echo complex. *J. Clin. Ultrasound* 5:372–377, December 1977.

Schneider, M.; Becker, J. A.; Staiano, S.; and Campos, E. Sonographic radiographic correlation of renal and perirenal infections. *Am. J. Roentgenol.* 127:1007–1014, 1976.

Skolnik, A. B-mode ultrasound and the nonvisualizing kidney in pediatrics. *Am. J. Roentgenol.* 128:121–125, January 1977.

Smith, E. H., and Bartrum, R. J. Ultrasonically-guided percutaneous aspiration of abscesses. *Am. J. Roentgenol.* 122:308–312, October 1974.

Spirt, B. A.; Skolnick, M. L.; Carsky, E. W.; and Ticen, K. Anterior displacement of the abdominal aorta: a radiographic and sonographic study. *Radiology* 111:

399–403, May 1974.

Teele, R. L. Ultrasonography of the genitourinary tract in children. *Radiol. Clin. North Am.* 15:109–128, April 1977.

Toomey, F. B.; Fritzsche, P.; Carlsen, E.; Caggiano, H.; Vyhmeister, N.; and Kullman, V. Application of aortography and ultrasound in evaluation of renal agenesis. *Pediatr. Radiol.* 6:168–171, October 1977.

Tyrrell, C. J.; Cosgrove, D. O.; McReady, V. R.; and Peckham, M. J. The role of ultrasound in the assessment and treatment of abdominal metasases from testicular tumours. *Clin. Radiol.* 28:475–481, September 1977.

Winston, M. A.; Handler, S. J.; and Pritchard, J. H. Ultrasonography of the testes: correlation with radio-

tracer perfusion. *J. Nucl. Biol. Med.* 19:615–618, June 1978.

Yeh, H. C.; Mitty, H. A.; and Wolf, B. S. Ultrasonography of renal sinus lipomatosis. *Radiology* 124:799–801, September 1977.

Yeh, H. C.; Mitty, H. A.; Rose, J.; Wolf, B. S.; and Gabrilove, J. L. Ultrasonography of adrenal masses: usual features. *Radiology* 127:467–474, May 1978a.

Yeh, H. C.; Mitty, H. A.; Rose, J.; Wolf, B. S.; and Gabrilove, J. L. Ultrasonography of adrenal masses: unusual manifestations. *Radiology* 127:475–483, May 1978b.

Zegel, H., and Edell, S. Ultrasonic evaluation of renal calculi. *Am. J. Roentgenol.* 130:261–263, February 1978.

CASES
Dennis A. Sarti, M.D.
W. Frederick Sample, M.D.

Technique for Renal Examinations

A renal examination can be performed with the patient in the prone or decubitus position. Figure 7.1 is an example of a transverse scan obtained with the patient in the prone position. Each kidney can be scanned individually, or both kidneys can be scanned together. While performing a transverse scan it is often very helpful to have the patient in deep inspiration. This will place the kidney more caudally and allow better visualization below the twelfth rib. The major difficulty of a renal ultrasound examination in the prone position is that the eleventh and twelfth ribs are over the upper pole of the kidney. It is also quite helpful to draw the medial and lateral borders of each kidney on the patient's skin with a marking pencil. This will facilitate the longitudinal scans.

For longitudinal prone scans, it is best to align the transducer parallel to the long axis of the kidney as is shown in figure 7.2 with the right kidney. This is extremely important when attempting to obtain an accurate measurement of the renal length. If the scans are parallel to the patient's spine a falsely low reading for the renal length will be obtained. By scanning parallel to the renal axis the kidney can be covered in its entirety and accurate measurements secured. Therefore, the right kidney should be aligned first. The alignment can then be changed on the longitudinal scans while working on the left side. Mapping the renal borders on the patient's skin helps to concentrate on certain areas which may be of major interest. For example, if the intravenous pyelogram demonstrates a questionable mass in the lateral midportion of the right kidney, mapping on the patient's skin will facilitate concentration of the examination in this area.

Coronal examinations of the kidney also can be extremely helpful. Often the prone examinations are suboptimal because of overlying ribs or other renal

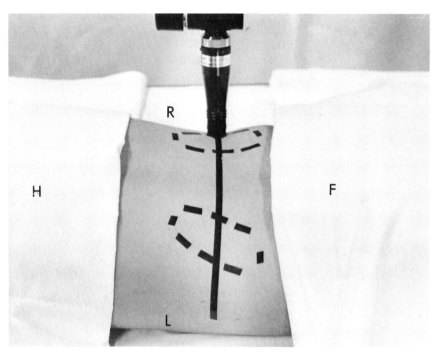

Fig. 7.1

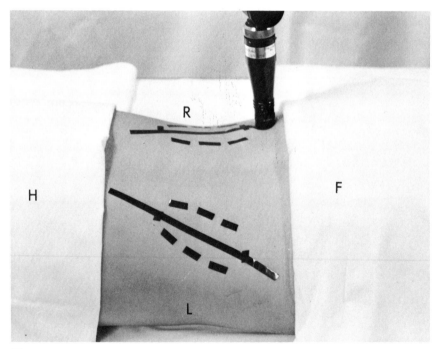

Fig. 7.2

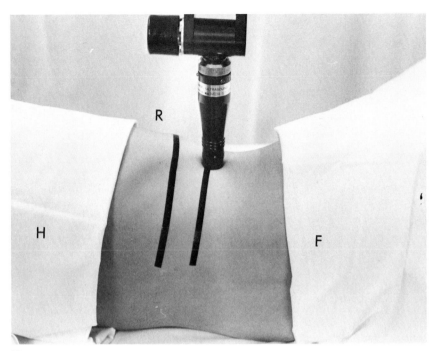

Fig. 7.3

positional problems. The patient can be placed in the decubitus position and the kidneys examined in transverse and coronal planes. Figure 7.3 is a transverse scan of the right kidney with the patient in the decubitus position with the right side up. After scanning the kidney from posterior and anterior to determine the best ultrasonic window, longitudinal coronal scans of the kidney should be obtained. In the coronal scan of the right kidney (fig. 7.4), with the patient in the decubitus position, the scanning plane is along the mid axillary line with the transducer angled perpendicular to the patient's skin. This allows excellent visualization of the kidney. For an analysis of the lateral aspect of the kidney, this scanning plane probably is the best available.

F = Foot
H = Head
L = Left
R = Right

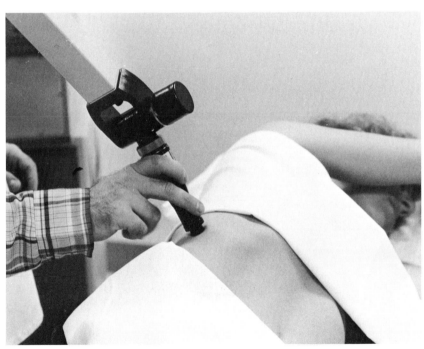

Fig. 7.4

Normal Renal Scans

Figure 7.5 is a transverse scan of both kidneys with the patient in the prone position. The characteristic appearance of the kidneys, with strong central echoes surrounded by the relatively lucent renal parenchyma, can be seen. The normal kidney borders are usually easily visualized since the strong echoes of Gerota's fascia and the renal capsule stand out against the renal parenchyma. Just medial to the kidneys is the psoas muscle parallel to the sonolucent spine. The muscle bundle posterior to the kidney is the quadratus lumborum. Anterior to the right kidney are echoes arising from the liver. The renal contour and size is usually fairly symmetrical. The left kidney will most often have a more cephalad position than the right.

Figure 7.6 is a longitudinal oblique scan obtained through the right kidney with the patient in the prone position. We can see the normal contour and shape of the right kidney with the strong central echoes surrounded by the lucent renal parenchyma. A small amount of fluid is noted in the collecting systems of the upper pole (arrow), which represents a small extrarenal duplex pelvis. Superior and anterior to the kidney is the liver, which is not very echogenic, since the unit has been adjusted to echo in the kidney rather than the deeper structures of the liver.

A longitudinal scan (fig. 7.7) demonstrates the left kidney just caudal to the spleen. Deep to the left kidney, with the patient in the prone position, the echogenic tail of the pancreas can be seen. These longitudinal oblique scans not only detail the renal architecture, but also give important measurements as to the length and depth of both kidneys.

It is extremely important to evaluate the renal echogenicity in comparison with other organs. This is best performed using the liver as a standard. A routine comparison is made between the liver and pancreas when trying to decide whether or not pancreatic pathology is present. The same can be done with a comparison of the liver with the right kidney. Figure 7.8 is a transverse scan with the patient in the supine position. Scanning through the liver and

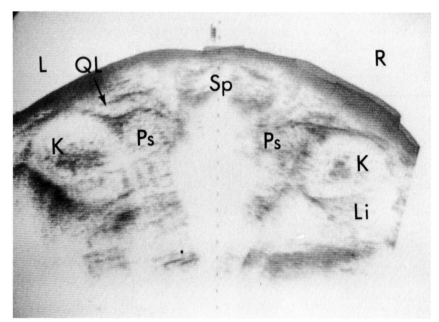

Fig. 7.5

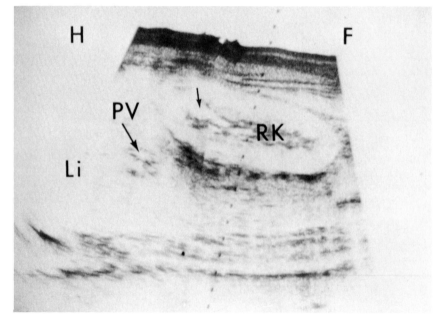

Fig. 7.6

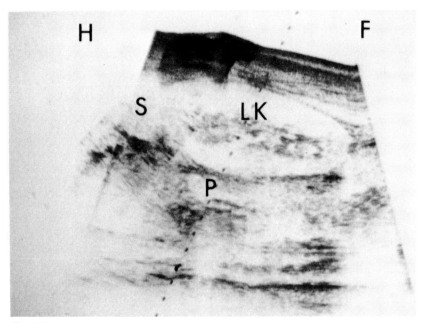

Fig. 7.7

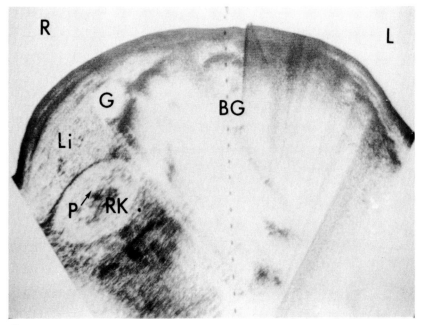

Fig. 7.8

right kidney usually shows the kidney to be less echogenic in amplitude than the liver. The parenchyma of the right kidney (fig. 7.8) is slightly less echogenic than the liver. A lucent area is noted in the renal cortex and medulla and is secondary to renal pyramids.

The echogenic amplitude relationship among the three organs of the upper abdomen is important and must be remembered. The pancreas usually has a higher-echo amplitude than the liver, which is usually higher than the kidney. If this normal relationship is not present, then all three organs must be examined to determine which one is abnormal.

Arrow	=	Slight dilation of the collecting system of the right upper pole
BG	=	Bowel gas
F	=	Foot
G	=	Gallbladder
H	=	Head
K	=	Kidney
L	=	Left
Li	=	Liver
LK	=	Left kidney
P	=	Pancreas
P arrow	=	Renal pyramid
Ps	=	Psoas muscle
PV	=	Portal vein
QL	=	Quadratus lumborum
R	=	Right
RK	=	Right kidney
S	=	Spleen
Sp	=	Spine

Normal Renal Scans

The right kidney often can be examined with the patient in the supine position if the right lobe of the liver is large enough. Figure 7.9 is a longitudinal supine scan of the kidney. The renal outline is seen deep to the right lobe of the liver. In the renal parenchyma are several lucent areas representing the renal pyramids. The borders of these pyramids contain a very soft linear echo (arrows) which is felt to be secondary to the arcuate vessels within the kidney. This longitudinal scan through the right lobe of the liver can be very helpful in evaluating the kidney, especially in the upper pole region. Often, the upper pole of the kidney is difficult to visualize with the patient in the prone position because of the overlying ribs. For any attempt to visualize the upper pole of the right kidney, the patient should be in a supine position. Again, the normal echo relationship in which the liver is more echogenic than the right kidney is seen.

Usually we are unable to visualize the left kidney in the supine position because of the overlying air in the stomach and splenic flexure. When there is marked enlargement of the left lobe of the liver, however, this structure can be used as an ultrasonic window to visualize the left kidney. A longitudinal scan (fig. 7.10) in the supine position uses the left lobe of the liver to visualize the kidney. The pancreas is seen between the left lobe of the liver and the left kidney. A "bull's-eye"-appearing mass is present just cephalad to the left kidney; this represents the fundus of the stomach. It should not be confused for a mass within the liver, kidney, or adrenal gland. There is also an ill-defined structure present just caudal to the lower pole of the kidney, secondary to the fourth portion of the duodenum.

As already mentioned, a coronal scan is very helpful in evaluating kidneys which are difficult to examine in the prone position. It also provides excellent visualization of the lateral border of the kidney when evaluating a mass in that region. Figure 7.11 is a longitudinal coronal scan of the left kidney which is situated caudal to the spleen. Deep to the left kidney is a tubular structure

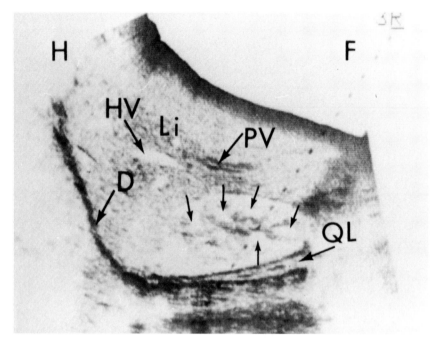

Fig. 7.9

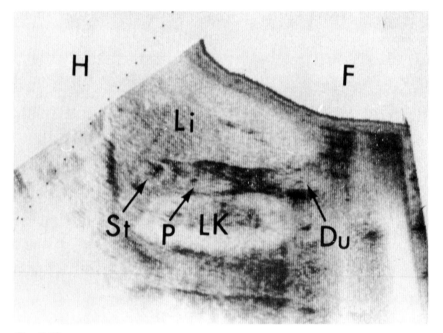

Fig. 7.10

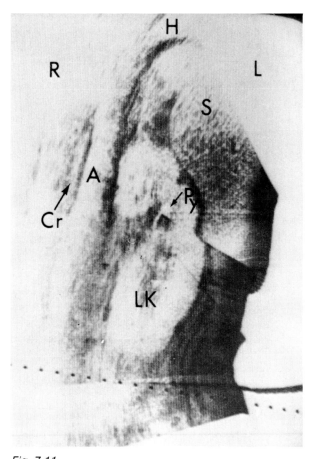

Fig. 7.11

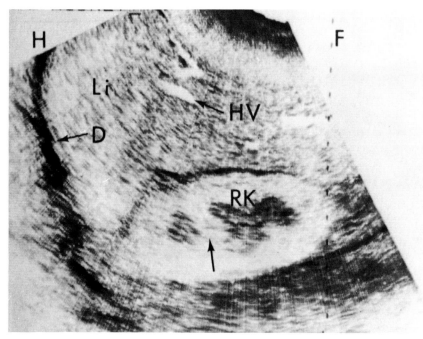

Fig. 7.12

which represents the aorta. We are also able to visualize the crus of the diaphragm. With this coronal section, an excellent visualization of the lateral border of the kidney, and also the splenic indentation on this border, is obtained. A lucent region within the kidney, secondary to a renal pyramid (arrow) is seen.

A longitudinal supine scan of the right kidney through the right lobe of the liver (fig. 7.12) demonstrates the normal echogenic relationship between the liver and the right kidney. This scan was obtained to demonstrate a normal variant of a duplex collecting system on the right side. The strong central echoes of the right kidney are not continuous as is usually seen. There is a larger central collection situated caudal with a smaller collection situated cephalad, with renal parenchyma (arrow) separating the two central echoes. This is the characteristic ultrasound appearance of a duplex collecting system.

A	= Aorta
Arrow	= Renal parenchyma separating a duplex collecting system (fig. 7.12)
Cr	= Crus of the diaphragm
D	= Diaphragm
Du	= Duodenum
F	= Foot
H	= Head
HV	= Hepatic vein
L	= Left
Li	= Liver
LK	= Left kidney
P	= Pancreas
PV	= Portal vein
Py	= Renal pyramid
QL	= Quadratus lumborum muscle
R	= Right
RK	= Right kidney
S	= Spleen
Small arrows	= Arcuate arteries (fig. 7.9)
St	= Stomach

Normal Renal Vascular Anatomy

Understanding the renal vascular anatomy can be extremely helpful in ruling out certain lesions and in identifying the many tubular structures situated around the retroperitoneal area. Figure 7.13 is a transverse supine scan of a tubular structure arising from the inferior vena cava and coursing posteriorly to the right kidney. When communication with the inferior vena cava is demonstrated the right renal vein is visualized.

Figure 7.14 is a longitudinal oblique scan with the transducer on the left side of the abdomen, angled toward the right posterior aspect of the patient. This results in scanning down the long axis of the right renal vein. The inferior vena cava is seen as a tubular structure coursing through the liver. Coming off the right posterior aspect of the inferior vena cava is the right renal vein. Evaluation of the right renal vein can become important when we are attempting to rule out tumor invasion. Also the right renal vein often may reach a large size in patients with congestive heart failure and be confused with a cystic or sonolucent mass.

The right renal vein can be confused for a renal cyst, when scanning the right kidney near its medial aspect, just as the right renal vein is entering the renal hilum (fig. 7.15). It is sonolucent and quite large and could be misdiagnosed as a renal cyst. Figure 7.16 demonstrates the right renal vein as it enters the renal hilum. We can see some dilatation of the right renal vein at this point that could be misdiagnosed as a peripelvic cyst.

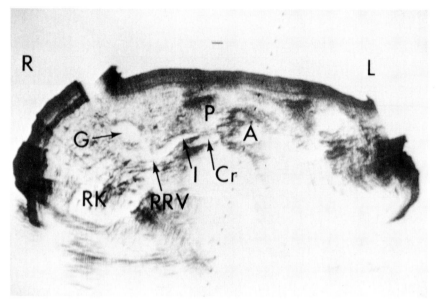

Fig. 7.13

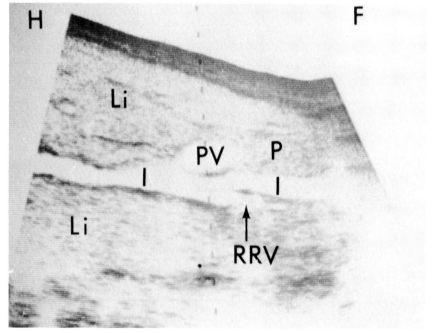

Fig. 7.14

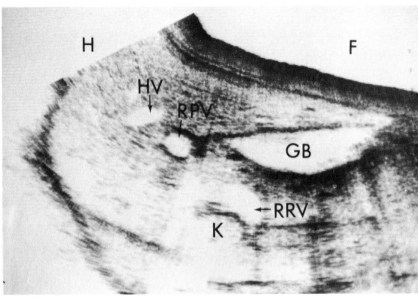

Fig. 7.15

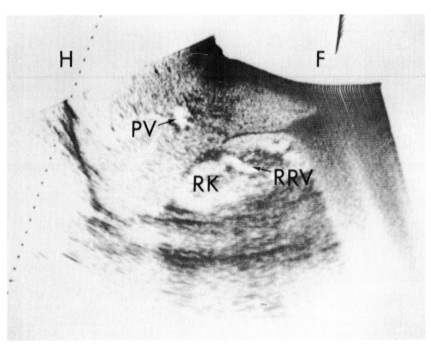

Fig. 7.16

A	=	Aorta
Cr	=	Crus of the diaphragm
F	=	Foot
G	=	Gallbladder
GB	=	Gallbladder
H	=	Head
HV	=	Hepatic vein
I	=	Inferior vena cava
K	=	Kidney
L	=	Left
Li	=	Liver
P	=	Pancreas
PV	=	Portal vein
R	=	Right
RK	=	Right kidney
RPV	=	Right portal vein
RRV	=	Right renal vein

Normal Renal Vascular Anatomy

Many times when evaluating the retroperitoneal area the crus of the diaphragm is misdiagnosed as the right renal artery. The crus of the diaphragm can attain a fairly large size. It is situated adjacent to the aorta, and it may be difficult to separate the crus completely from the aorta. It is important to visualize the tubular structure of the right renal artery entering the right lateral aspect of the aorta. Figure 7.17 is a transverse scan which gives an excellent visualization of the right renal artery and aorta. There is no doubt that the vessel is arising from the aorta. Situated posterior to the right renal artery is the crus of the diaphragm. Anterior to the right renal artery is the inferior vena cava which appears pointed on its left lateral aspect. The entrance of the left renal vein can be seen at this site. The right renal artery courses posterior to the inferior vena cava.

Figure 7.18 is a transverse scan of the left renal artery as it arises from the aorta. It arises off the more posterior aspect of the aorta while the right renal artery is more anterior. Situated anterior to the left renal artery in this instance is the left renal vein which drapes over the aorta and empties into the inferior vena cava. Another C-shaped lucency situated anterior to the left renal vein is the splenic vein. The splenic vein is situated anterior to the superior mesenteric artery which is the structure helping best to determine whether we are visualizing the splenic vein or the left renal vein. The splenic vein courses anterior to the superior mesenteric artery, while the left renal vein is posterior to the superior mesenteric artery.

A longitudinal scan (fig. 7.19) demonstrates the position of the right renal artery in relationship to the inferior vena cava. The inferior vena cava is a tubular structure coursing posterior to the liver. Deep to the inferior vena cava are two circular structures which represent the right renal arteries. We usually see a singular circular structure deep to the inferior vena cava. This case is an example of two arteries supplying the right kidney, and it is not an unusual finding.

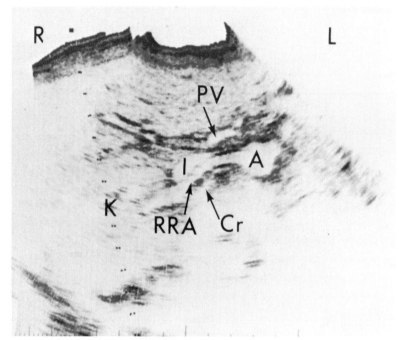

Fig. 7.17

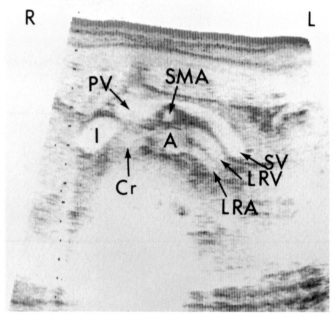

Fig. 7.18

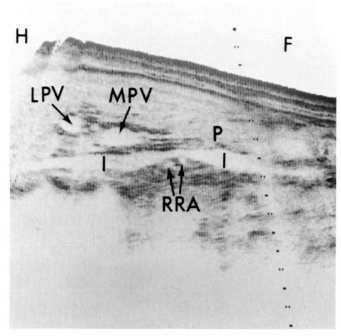

Fig. 7.19

The circular structures situated within the liver represent the main portal vein and the left portal vein.

Often when scanning the left upper quadrant in a longitudinal plane, numerous circular structures are encountered. In a fairly large lobe of the liver (fig. 7.20), the pancreas is seen deep to the left lobe. Numerous circular sonolucencies are noted in the left upper quadrant; they supply and drain the organs of the area. Just posterior to the pancreas the splenic artery and splenic vein are seen. Deep to the splenic vascular structures are the left renal vein and left renal artery. A reexamination of the transverse scan in figure 7.18 will provide a good comparison with the anatomy on the longitudinal scan (fig. 7.20).

A = Aorta
Cr = Crus of the diaphragm
Du = Duodenum
EGJ = Esophagogastric junction
F = Foot
H = Head
I = Inferior vena cava
K = Kidney
L = Left
Li = Liver
LPV = Left portal vein
LRA = Left renal artery
LRV = Left renal vein
MPV = Main portal vein
P = Pancreas
PV = Portal vein
R = Right
RRA = Right renal artery
SA = Splenic artery
SMA = Superior mesenteric artery
St = Stomach
SV = Splenic vein

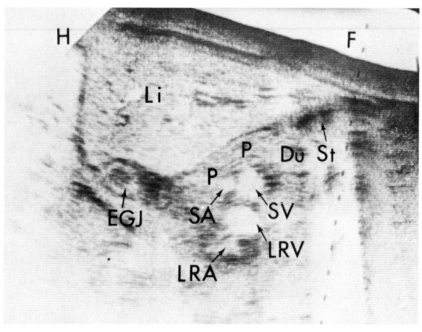

Fig. 7.20

Low-lying Kidney; Hypoplastic Kidney

A patient is referred often for ultrasound examination because of a palpable right abdominal mass. This has been shown to be the lower pole of the right kidney in many instances. This is especially true in thinner patients. Figure 7.21 is a longitudinal scan of a patient with a palpable mass in the right abdomen. By simultaneously examining the patient and performing ultrasound, the etiology of the palpable mass usually can be determined. In this scan, the right kidney is situated below the right lobe of the liver. The lower pole of the right kidney, approximately 1 cm beneath the patient's skin, could be palpated. This is not an unusual occurrence and can be an extremely helpful diagnosis to the referring clinician.

Figures 7.22 and 7.23 show another example of a low-lying kidney with palpable masses. A transverse scan over the right mid abdomen demonstrates the kidney in a longitudinal plane (fig. 7.22). It is not only low in position, but it lies in an unusual way.

Figure 7.23 is a longitudinal scan of the same patient. The right kidney is situated below the right lobe of the liver. The inferior vena cava and portal vein can be seen on this scan also. The kidney is not only low in position but it has a horizontal orientation.

Frequently, we are asked to evaluate the kidneys with ultrasound because one kidney cannot be seen on the intravenous pyelogram. Ultrasound can provide very important information in this instance. First, we can determine whether or not a kidney is present in its normal location. Second, if a kidney is present we can obtain information about its architecture. It may be small or difficult to visualize; it may be obstructed and hydronephrotic; or it may be extremely large and edematous.

Figure 7.24 is a transverse scan in which a normal right kidney is seen in its usual position although there is marked difficulty in visualizing the left kidney. Here we see a hypoplastic kidney that is markedly smaller than the normal right. Another diagnostic possibility in this in-

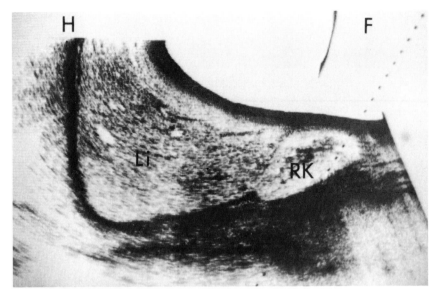

Fig. 7.21

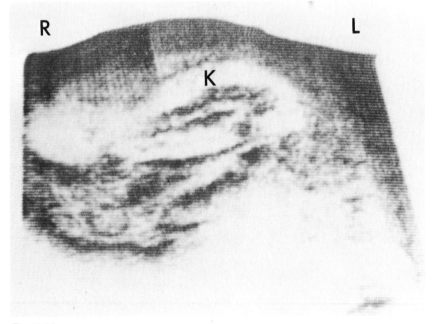

Fig. 7.22

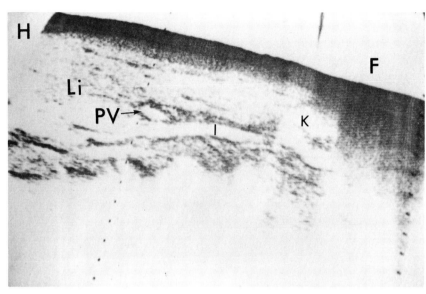

Fig. 7.23

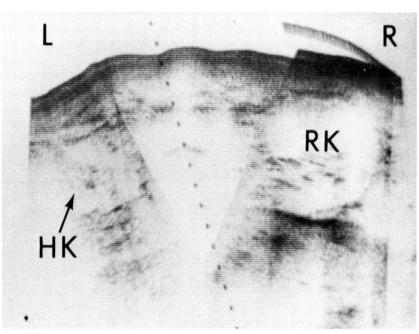

Fig. 7.24

stance would be severe renal inflammatory disease such as unilateral chronic
pyelonephritis.

F	=	Foot
H	=	Head
HK	=	Hypoplastic kidney
I	=	Inferior vena cava
K	=	Right kidney situated below the right lobe of the liver
L	=	Left
Li	=	Liver
LK	=	Left kidney
PV	=	Portal vein
R	=	Right
RK	=	Right kidney

Pelvic Kidney and Horseshoe Kidney

As already mentioned, ultrasound can play an important role in evaluating a patient with unilateral visualization on the intravenous pyelogram. The retro-peritoneal region should be examined to determine whether or not a kidney is present. If no kidney is present, the possibility of agenesis or ectopy should be raised. After the routine renal scan, the pelvis should be evaluated to rule out a pelvic kidney. Figure 7.25 illustrates a nonvisualization of the right kidney. A pelvic examination demonstrated a pelvic kidney superior to the uterus and urinary bladder. Since ultrasound methods do not need renal function and are not hindered by the bony structures of the sacrum, visualization of a pelvic kidney is quite possible. A pelvic kidney, however, is often confused for bowel gas, since bowel can give a strong central echo with surrounding lucent periphery.

Figures 7.26–7.28 are scans of a patient with a horseshoe kidney. Figure 7.26 is a transverse scan over the mid abdomen. The central collecting system is surrounded by the renal parenchyma. As mentioned earlier, this can be confused for transverse colon or other bowel loops. A longitudinal scan, however, (fig. 7.27) demonstrates the isthmus of the horseshoe kidney which courses anterior to the aorta. The isthmus is seen just superior to the umbilical level. A CAT scan (fig. 7.28) confirms the diagnosis of a horseshoe kidney. With computed tomographic techniques, we have relatively little difficulty in distinguishing a horseshoe or ectopic kidney from bowel.

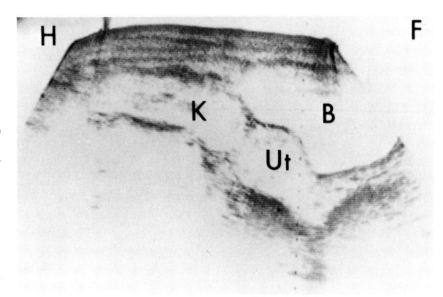

Fig. 7.25

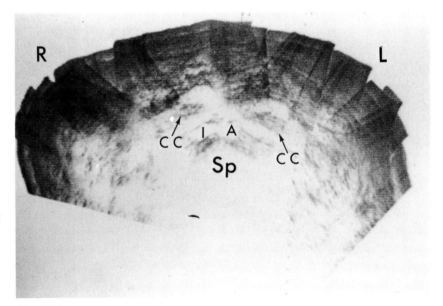

Fig. 7.26

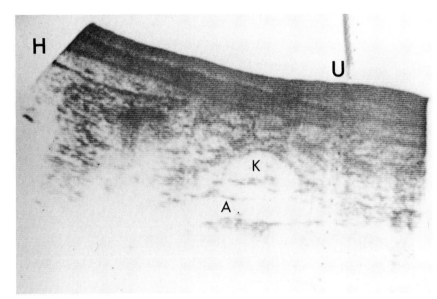

A	=	Aorta
B	=	Urinary bladder
CC	=	Central collecting systems
F	=	Foot
H	=	Head
I	=	Inferior vena cava
K	=	Kidney
L	=	Left
R	=	Right
Sp	=	Spine
U	=	Umbilical level
Ut	=	Uterus

Fig. 7.27

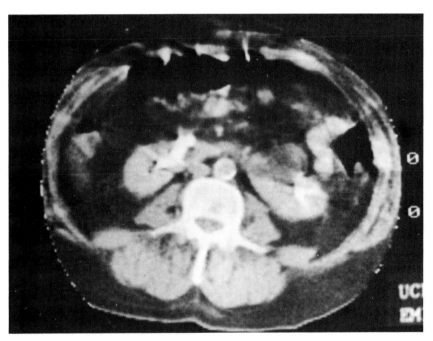

Fig. 7.28

Renal Cyst

One of the most common reasons for ultrasonic renal examination is to evaluate a renal mass detected on the intravenous pyelogram. If the ultrasonographer can provide information that determines that the mass is a simple cyst, angiography is unnecessary. A cyst puncture can be performed to establish the diagnosis. If the patient is quite elderly, and the diagnosis of a simple cyst is confirmed, nothing further need be done.

Some of the problems arising in evaluation of a renal cyst are due to its location. Some are caused by artifacts due to overlying ribs. A cyst arising in the lower pole can be evaluated more easily than one arising in the upper pole. Upper pole cysts are more difficult to define because of the overlying eleventh and twelfth ribs. Figure 7.29 is a longitudinal supine scan demonstrating a lower pole cyst of the right kidney. The walls are quite sharp. We can notice through transmission here, and this is an important sign in the evaluation of a sonolucent mass. Through transmission indicates the fluid-filled nature of the mass.

A supine scan through the right kidney (fig. 7.30) shows a sonolucent mass situated in the anterior renal parenchyma. When examining a cyst in this region, it is always important to know where the gallbladder is situated. It can be confused with a renal cyst, if it is situated adjacent to the kidney.

Figure 7.31 is a larger cyst of the right lower pole in which we again see a sonolucent mass with through transmission.

The most difficult cysts to evaluate are those arising from the upper pole of either kidney. A longitudinal prone scan of the left kidney (fig. 7.32) illustrates a cyst in the posterosuperior aspect of the kidney. Through transmission is present. However, echoes are noted on the near wall of the cyst (arrows). As discussed in chapter one, these represent reverberation artifacts off a cystic structure found in the urinary bladder or in any other fluid-filled masses. If there is any doubt as to whether or not this represents artifacts, it is necessary to examine the cyst in different positions to rule out the possibility of internal echoes.

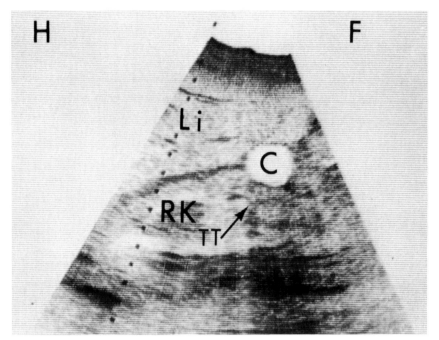

Fig. 7.29

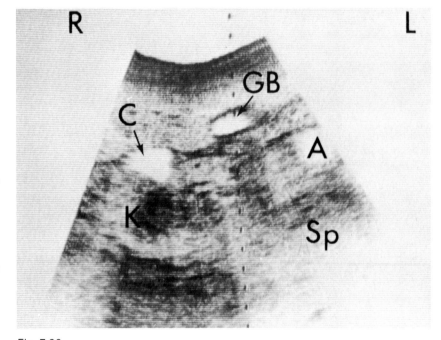

Fig. 7.30

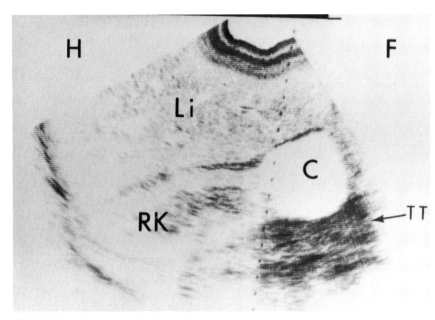

A	=	Aorta
Arrow	=	Reverberation artifact (fig. 7.32)
C	=	Renal cyst
F	=	Foot
GB	=	Gallbladder
H	=	Head
K	=	Kidney
L	=	Left
Li	=	Liver
LK	=	Left kidney
R	=	Right
RK	=	Right kidney
S	=	Spleen
Sp	=	Spine
TT	=	Through transmission

Fig. 7.31

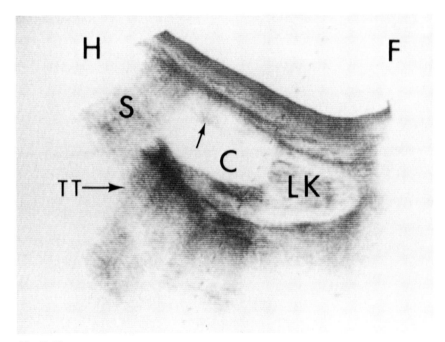

Fig. 7.32

Renal Cyst

As mentioned earlier, evaluation of upper pole masses is the most difficult. A longitudinal scan (fig. 7.33) was obtained with the patient in the supine position. Adequate visualization of the upper pole mass was impossible with the patient in the prone position because of the overlying ribs. In figure 7.33 we see the right kidney situated deep to the liver. A sonolucent mass is noted in the upper pole; this was felt to be a renal cyst. Although the mass was sonolucent, the borders were not extremely sharp, and there was a suggestion of soft echoes within it. This turned out to be secondary to artifact. The cyst was situated so deeply in the abdomen that the output of the ultrasound unit was high enough to cause these artifacts. A simple cyst of the upper pole was found. Ultrasound could not completely clear the borders of the cyst, and a cyst puncture had to be performed.

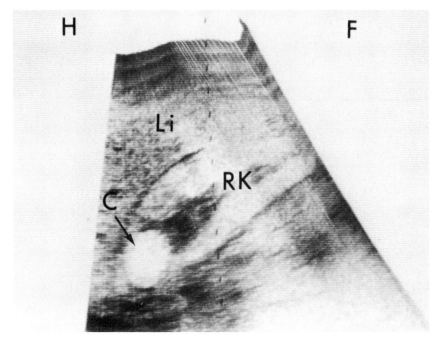

Fig. 7.33

A longitudinal scan (fig. 7.34) of the right kidney demonstrates a peripelvic cyst splaying the highly echogenic central echoes of the right kidney. Peripelvic cysts can present a confusing picture as they can be difficult to distinguish from hydronephrosis. Usually, they give circular to oval borders in all dimensions. The lucent portion of a hydronephrosis continues toward the midline as it drains into a proximal dilated ureter.

Figure 7.35 is a fluid-filled extrarenal pelvis. It could be confused for a peripelvic cyst. One of the important differentiating points between a renal pelvis and a peripelvic cyst is the fact that the renal pelvis is oriented more toward the midline. In many instances, however, distinction between the two will be impossible.

Figure 7.36 is a transverse scan of an unusual renal cyst which could have been confused for the gallbladder had we not visualized the latter elsewhere during the course of the study. The cyst is situated quite laterally and appears to be completely separate from the right kidney.

We were fortunate to visualize the gallbladder more medially. Within the gallbladder is an echogenic region consistent with cholelithiasis.

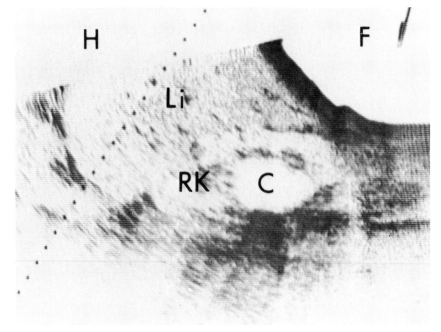

Fig. 7.34

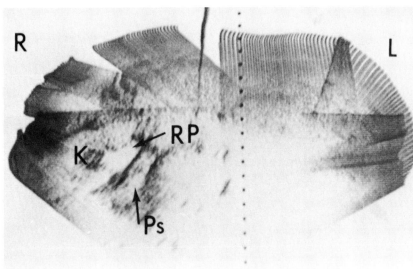

C   = Renal cyst
F   = Foot
GS = Gallstone
H   = Head
K   = Kidney
L   = Left
Li = Liver
Ps = Psoas muscle
R   = Right
RK = Kidney
RP = Renal pelvis

Fig. 7.35

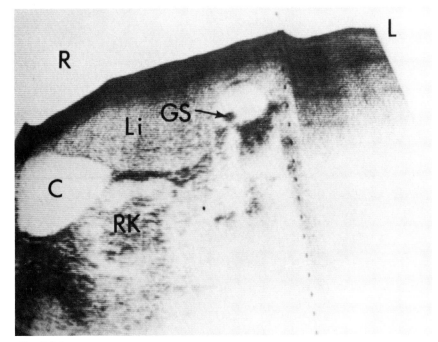

Fig. 7.36

Septated and Bilobed Renal Cysts

It is important to evaluate the walls and lumen of a renal cyst to rule out any internal echoes. Figure 7.37 demonstrates a septated cyst with a linear echo arising from a septum within the renal cyst. There is through transmission present behind the cyst, but diagnosis of a simple cyst is impossible with the linear echo noted within the cyst. Another example (fig. 7.38) shows a small septum situated within the renal cyst. Cyst puncture with the injection of contrast material confirmed a septated renal cyst in both instances.

This transverse scan (fig. 7.39) shows a renal cyst which is not characteristically oval or circular in shape. We can see what appears to be two compartments to the cyst; these represent a bilobed renal cyst. The renal cyst demonstrates through transmission and has a smaller compartment (arrows) situated laterally.

Figure 7.40 makes an important diagnostic point in the evaluation of renal cysts. Frequently, the portion of a renal cyst that is in contact with the renal parenchyma will show an irregular border. This scan shows how the entire borders of the renal cyst were cleared except for that portion which was in contact with the renal parenchyma (arrows). This most likely means that the renal cyst is not markedly distended and is somewhat collapsible when it is adjacent to renal parenchyma. Although this represented a simple cyst, we could not completely clear it as such because of the suggestion of indentation on this portion of the kidney. We must be very concerned about the border of a cyst which shows this type of finding. Even though it is secondary to normal parenchymal compression, the diagnosis of an uncomplicated simple cyst cannot be made, and cyst puncture is indicated.

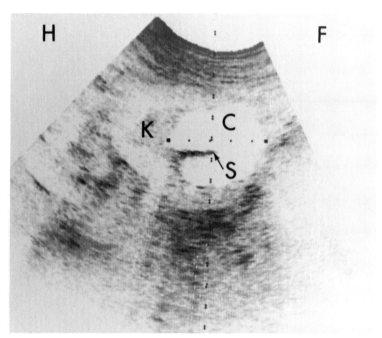

Fig. 7.37

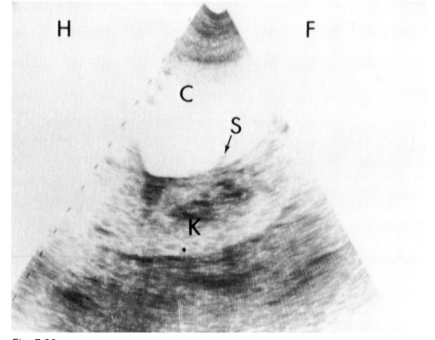

Fig. 7.38

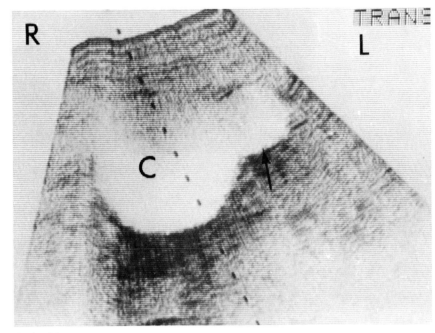

Fig. 7.39

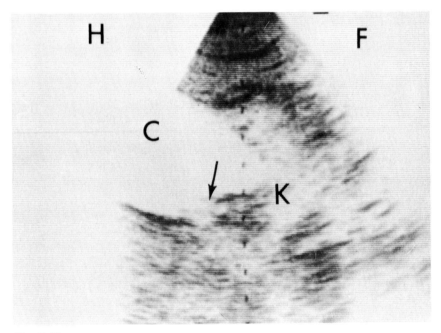

Fig. 7.40

Arrow	=	Bilobed renal cyst (fig. 7.39)
Arrow	=	Compression of the renal cyst by renal parenchyma (fig. 7.40)
C	=	Renal cyst
F	=	Foot
H	=	Head
K	=	Kidney
L	=	Left
R	=	Right
S	=	Septum

Multicystic Kidneys; Polycystic Kidneys

Ultrasound examination of the newborn is usually requested after palpation of an abdominal mass. Figures 7.41 and 7.42 are examples of a palpable right abdominal mass which turned out to be a multicystic kidney. This often appears as a highly echogenic region since numerous extremely small cysts are present. Sometimes, very large sonolucent masses are seen by ultrasound in these multicystic kidneys, because a cyst can attain a large size. In figure 7.41, a longitudinal supine scan, a multicystic kidney is seen as a large septated appearing mass in the right abdomen.

Figure 7.42 is a transverse prone scan with a normal left kidney and a large fluid-filled multicystic kidney on the right side. It would be difficult to distinguish this multicystic kidney from hydronephrosis in the newborn. The cysts in this kidney are so large that hydronephrosis would not be ruled out. This is a common difficulty.

Ultrasound is an excellent means of diagnosing polycystic disease in the adult. Usually polycystic disease is not diagnosed on an intravenous pyelogram until the patients are in their 30s or 40s. Ultrasound can, however, demonstrate multiple renal cysts much earlier than can an intravenous pyelogram. Figure 7.43 is a transverse supine scan of a patient with severe polycystic disease. Here we visualize numerous sonolucent masses within both flanks; these are separated by multiple curvilinear echoes. This finding was indicative of severe polycystic disease. Figure 7.44 is a longitudinal supine scan with the right polycystic kidney situated below the liver.

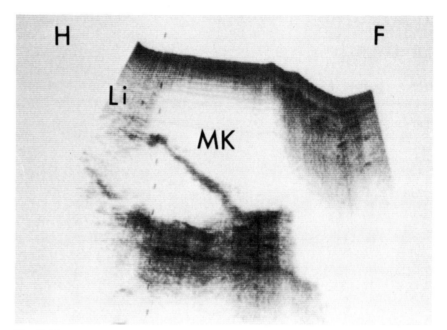

Fig. 7.41

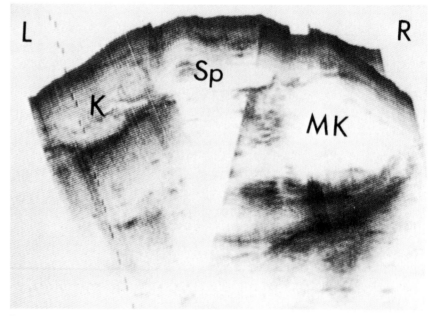

Fig. 7.42

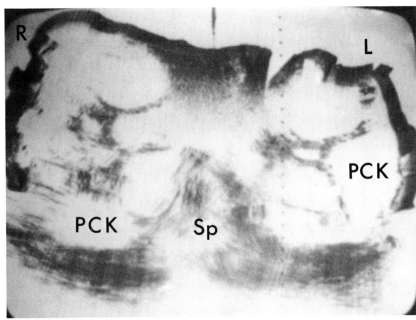

F	=	Foot
H	=	Head
K	=	Left kidney
L	=	Left
Li	=	Liver
MK	=	Multicystic kidney
PCK	=	Polycystic kidney
R	=	Right
Sp	=	Spine

Fig. 7.43

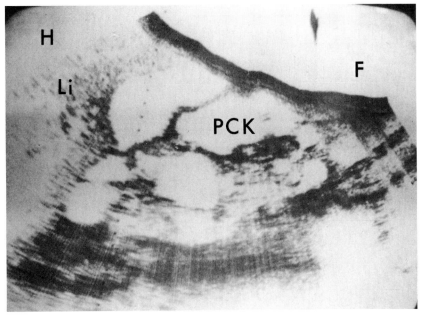

Fig. 7.44

Polycystic Disease with Complications

When examining polycystic kidneys, the possibility of other diagnoses should not be forgotten. Figure 7.45 is a longitudinal scan of a polycystic kidney with the characteristic multiple sonolucent masses throughout the renal bed. Very little renal parenchyma is noted. In figure 7.46, however, we not only see evidence of a polycystic kidney, but also a soft tissue echo with a fluid level (arrow) situated in one of the cysts. Such a finding should raise concern, since the majority of polycystic kidneys are mainly fluid-filled. This eventually was discovered to be hemorrhage within a polycystic kidney.

Figures 7.47 and 7.48 are scans of a patient with polycystic kidneys associated with a renal cell carcinoma in the right kidney. Figure 7.47 is a longitudinal scan of the right kidney demonstrating multiple sonolucent cysts indicative of polycystic disease. An area of high echogenicity (arrows) is situated deep to the cyst. This corresponded to calcifications on the abdominal X-ray film. Figure 7.48 is another longitudinal scan which was slightly more lateral. A solid mass is seen in the lower pole of this polycystic kidney. This was discovered to be renal cell carcinoma involving a polycystic kidney.

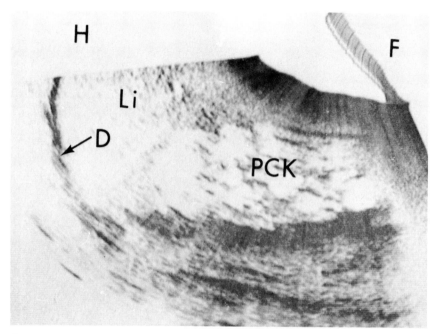

Fig. 7.45

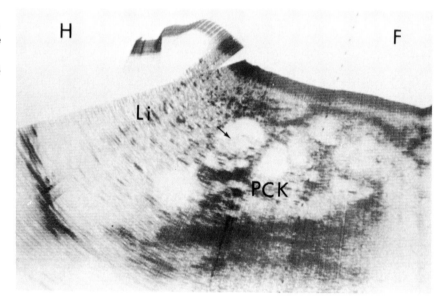

Fig. 7.46

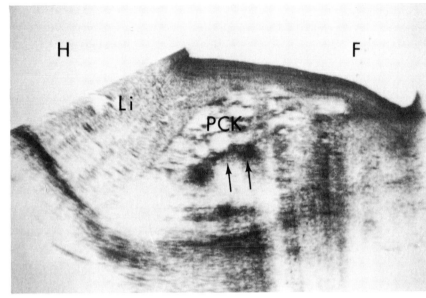

Fig. 7.47

Arrow   = Hemorrhage within a
            cyst (fig. 7.48)
Arrows = Areas of calcification
            (fig. 7.47)
D   = Diaphragm
F   = Foot
G   = Gallbladder
H   = Head
Li   = Liver
M   = Renal cell carcinoma
            in a polycystic kidney
PCK   = Polycystic kidney

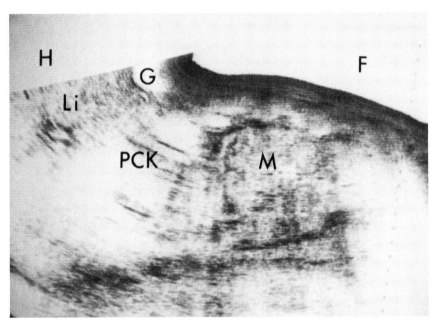

Fig. 7.48

Duplex Collecting System

Various degrees of duplication of the renal collecting system can be visualized with ultrasound. A longitudinal coronal scan (fig. 7.49) shows a slight splaying of the upper pole central collecting systems by fluid. This finding would be compatible with either a mild extrarenal pelvis or a minimal hydronephrosis of the upper pole collecting system. Another longitudinal coronal scan of the left kidney (fig. 7.50) demonstrates a sonolucent mass in the upper pole collecting systems which is showing a moderate degree of obstruction. This hydronephronic duplex system in the upper pole of the left kidney could be confused for an upper pole cyst. An intravenous pyelogram, however, confirmed the suspected ultrasonic diagnosis of an obstructed upper-pole-collecting system.

In another longitudinal coronal scan of the left kidney (fig. 7.51), an extremely large sonolucent mass is seen in its superior portion, displacing the lower pole. This also turned out to be a severe hydronephrosis of the upper-pole-collecting system on the left side. A transverse scan of the pelvis (fig. 7.52) suggested a mass within the bladder; this was found to be an ectopic ureterocele.

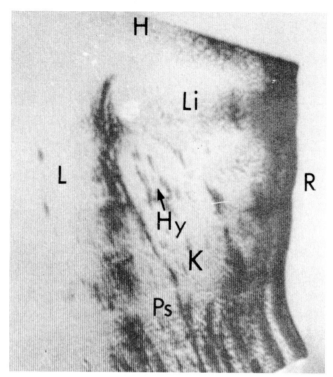

Fig. 7.49

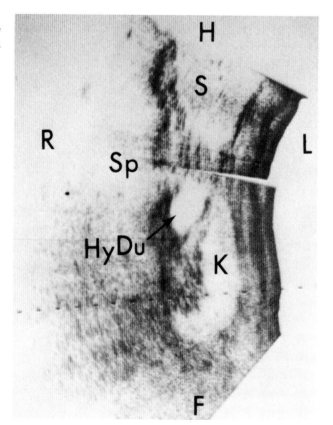

Fig. 7.50

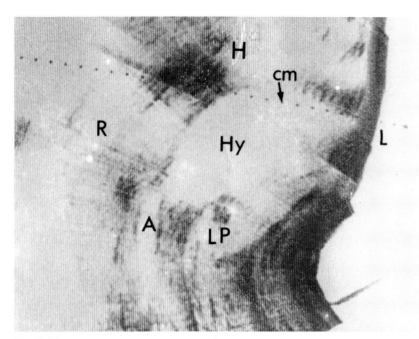

A	=	Aorta
B	=	Urinary bladder
cm	=	Centimeter markers
EU	=	Ectopic ureterocele
F	=	Foot
H	=	Head
Hy	=	Hydronephrosis of a duplex collecting system
Hydu	=	Hydronephrosis of a duplex collecting system
IP	=	Iliopsoas muscle
K	=	Kidney
L	=	Left
Li	=	Liver
LP	=	Lower pole of left kidney
OI	=	Obturator internus muscle
Ps	=	Psoas muscle
R	=	Right
S	=	Spleen
Sp	=	Spine
Ut	=	Uterus

Fig. 7.51

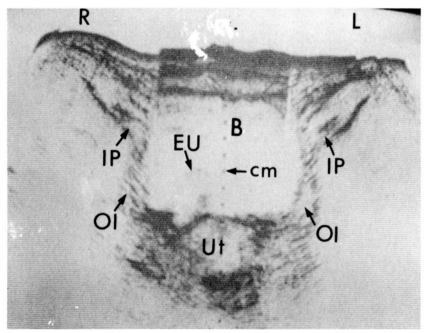

Fig. 7.52

Hydronephrosis

Ultrasonic evaluation of a nonfunctioning kidney can yield a diagnosis of hydronephrosis by the visualization of fluid within the renal pelvis. Figure 7.53 is a coronal section of the right kidney in which we see marked fluid instead of strong central echoes within the central portion of the kidney. The fluid extends out into the calyceal area. This hydronephrosis has not yet caused a marked decrease in the renal parenchyma.

Frequently, it is difficult to distinguish hydronephrosis from a peripelvic cyst, and we should look for extension of the sonolucent mass toward the midline and anterior to the spine. Figure 7.54 is a transverse scan of the right kidney with a hydronephrotic sac extending toward the midline and anterior to the inferior vena cava.

Visualization of the medial extension of the sonolucency is extremely helpful in distinguishing peripelvic cysts from hydronephrosis. Figure 7.55 is a longitudinal coronal scan which again demonstrates marked fluid in the central portion of the kidney secondary to hydronephrosis. A portion of the fluid can be visualized in the caudal direction as part of a dilated ureter.

A transverse scan (fig. 7.56) resolves a normal right kidney and a large fluid-filled sac in the region of the left kidney. The hydronephrotic sac again extends medially, somewhat anterior to the spine. This finding helps to establish a diagnosis of hydronephrosis as opposed to cystic lesions. A marked paucity of renal parenchyma, compared to the previous studies, is also noted. In the previous three scans, a normal amount of renal parenchyma is present, indicating recent hydronephrosis. In figure 7.56, practically no renal parenchyma is evident; this is more consistent with a long-standing hydronephrotic change.

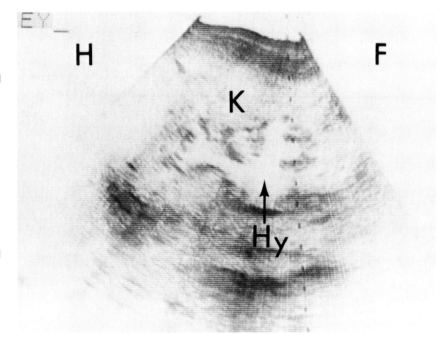

Fig. 7.53

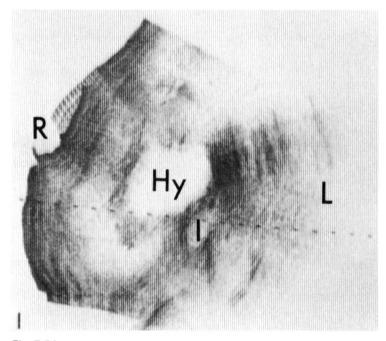

Fig. 7.54

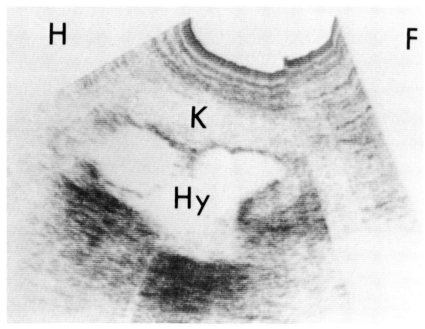

Fig. 7.55

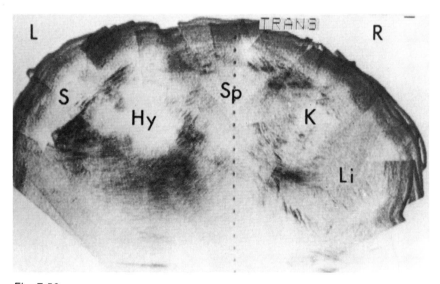

Fig. 7.56

F   = Foot
H   = Head
Hy = Hydronephrosis
I   = Inferior vena cava
K   = Kidney
L   = Left
Li = Liver
R   = Right
S   = Spleen
Sp = Spine

Hydroureter ; Pyonephrosis

It can be extremely helpful to the clinician to localize the level of obstruction when making the ultrasonic diagnosis of hydronephrosis. A dilated ureter over the mid abdomen usually cannot be visualized with the patient in the supine position; this is because of the overlying bowel air. It can be extremely informative to perform a pelvic ultrasound examination when a hydronephrosis is seen. By distending the urinary bladder a dilated ureter posterior to the urinary bladder can be visualized.

Figures 7.57 and 7.58 are scans of a 14-year-old girl who had a ureteral reimplantation approximately 10 years earlier. A recent intravenous pyelogram demonstrated that the left kidney could not be identified. A longitudinal prone scan (fig. 7.57) demonstrates a hydronephrotic sac in the central portion of the left kidney. A decreased amount of renal parenchyma is evident. Because of the finding of hydronephrosis, a pelvic examination was carried out with the urinary bladder filled. Figure 7.58 is a longitudinal scan of the pelvis with the transducer angled to the left side in order to better visualize the left ureter. The urinary bladder is situated anteriorly. Posteriorly, a dilated J-shaped tubular structure is seen which represents the dilated distal ureter. The ultrasonic findings were able to demonstrate a hydroureter with a ureterovesicular junction obstruction.

Frequently, a long-standing hydronephrosis will yield soft internal echoes on the dependent portion. Figure 7.59 is an example of hydronephrosis with debris (arrow) on the dependent portion of the hydronephrotic sac. With this ultrasonic finding, hemorrhage or abscess could not be ruled out. Figure 7.60 is an example of pyonephrosis in which we see a sonolucent mass in the superior portion of the left kidney. Again, soft echoes (arrows) are noted on the dependent portion. The distinction between pyonephrosis and hydronephrosis with debris could not be made in these two instances.

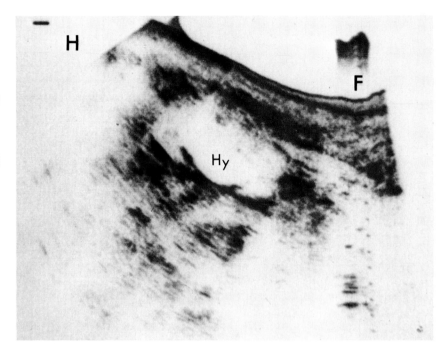

Fig. 7.57

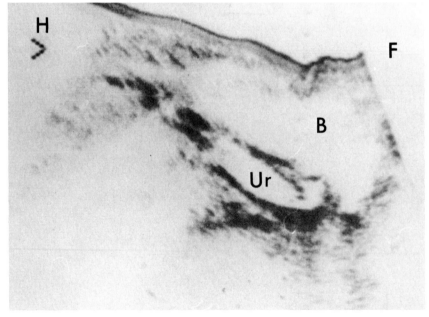

Fig. 7.58

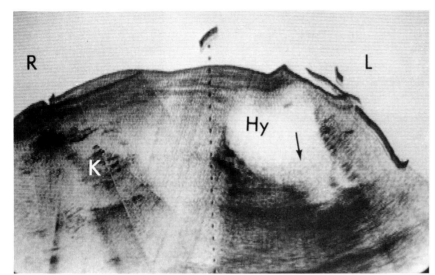

Fig. 7.59

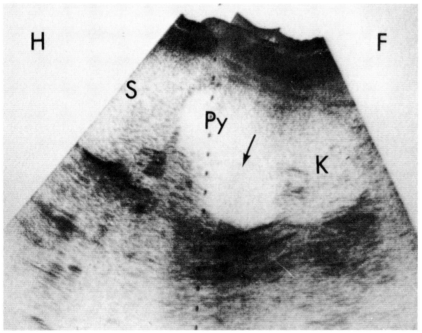

Fig. 7.60

Arrow	=	Debris in hydro-nephrosis (fig. 7.59)
Arrow	=	Pyonephrosis (fig. 7.60)
B	=	Urinary bladder
F	=	Foot
H	=	Head
Hy	=	Hydronephrosis
K	=	Kidney
L	=	Left
Py	=	Pyelonephrosis
R	=	Right
S	=	Spleen
Ur	=	Dilated ureter

Renal Calculi;
Carbuncles

Renal calculi are best diagnosed with abdominal films and intravenous pyelogram. Ultrasound is certainly not the diagnostic test of choice, although ultrasonic examinations are performed often on patients with renal stones. Figure 7.61 is a longitudinal supine scan of the right kidney with multiple strong echoes (arrows) within the renal pelvis. Some of these echoes are large enough to cause shadowing. With this type of finding, the diagnosis of renal calculi can be made with ultrasound.

Figure 7.62 is a longitudinal scan with a renal carbuncle (arrow) in the upper pole of the right kidney in a patient suspected of having a perinephric abscess. The area was extremely difficult to visualize with the patient in the prone position because of the overlying ribs. Therefore, the patient was turned to the supine position and the liver used as an ultrasonic window to visualize the upper pole of the right kidney. The area of the renal carbuncle is less echogenic than the surrounding renal parenchyma. A galium scan demonstrated increased uptake in this region and confirmed the diagnosis of a renal carbuncle.

Figures 7.63 and 7.64 were obtained from another patient sent to us to rule out a perinephric abscess. We can see marked asymmetry in the size of the kidneys, with the left kidney much larger than the right (fig. 7.63). The lateral portion of the left kidney is much less echogenic than the medial portion. Also, the large left kidney (arrows) has an inhomogeneous echo pattern to it. Figure 7.64 is a coronal scan with an uneven echo pattern throughout the left kidney. The large sonolucent area (arrows) in the periphery of the kidney established the ultrasonic diagnosis of renal abscesses. The patient was taken to surgery where numerous renal abscesses were found.

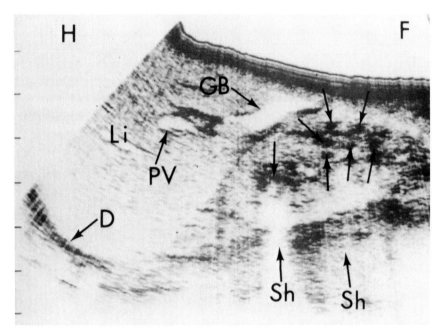

Fig. 7.61

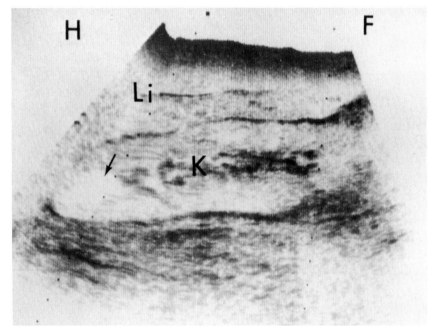

Fig. 7.62

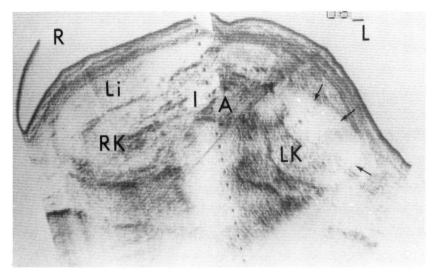

Fig. 7.63

<table>
<tr><td>A</td><td>=</td><td>Aorta</td></tr>
<tr><td>Arrows</td><td>=</td><td>Renal stones (fig. 7.61)</td></tr>
<tr><td>Arrow</td><td>=</td><td>Upper-pole renal carbuncle (fig. 7.62)</td></tr>
<tr><td>Arrows</td><td>=</td><td>Large left kidney (fig. 7.63)</td></tr>
<tr><td>Arrows</td><td>=</td><td>Multiple renal carbuncles (fig. 7.64)</td></tr>
<tr><td>D</td><td>=</td><td>Diaphragm</td></tr>
<tr><td>F</td><td>=</td><td>Foot</td></tr>
<tr><td>GB</td><td>=</td><td>Gallbladder</td></tr>
<tr><td>H</td><td>=</td><td>Head</td></tr>
<tr><td>I</td><td>=</td><td>Inferior vena cava</td></tr>
<tr><td>K</td><td>=</td><td>Kidney</td></tr>
<tr><td>L</td><td>=</td><td>Left</td></tr>
<tr><td>Li</td><td>=</td><td>Liver</td></tr>
<tr><td>LK</td><td>=</td><td>Left kidney</td></tr>
<tr><td>PV</td><td>=</td><td>Portal vein</td></tr>
<tr><td>R</td><td>=</td><td>Right</td></tr>
<tr><td>RK</td><td>=</td><td>Right kidney</td></tr>
<tr><td>Sh</td><td>=</td><td>Shadowing</td></tr>
</table>

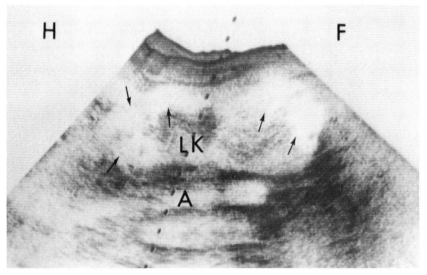

Fig. 7.64

Acute Pyelonephritis;
Renal Vein Thrombosis

The inability to visualize one kidney on intravenous pyelogram can be related to numerous factors. Ultrasound examination of the kidneys often will assist in narrowing the differential diagnosis. If no kidney is seen in the renal bed, the possibility of agenesis or ectopy should be considered. If a small shrunken kidney can be resolved, chronic infection or possible arterial disease should be considered. There will be instances in which the unseen kidney will be larger than the one on the normal side. Figures 7.65 and 7.66 are examples of a markedly enlarged left kidney compared to a normal right kidney. This turned out to be a case of acute pyelonephritis with the left kidney markedly swollen and nonfunctioning. Figure 7.66 is a longitudinal decubitus scan of the kidney; it appears more edematous and lucent than the normal right side.

Another cause of a nonvisualized large kidney is renal vein thrombosis. Figures 7.67 and 7.68 are scans obtained from a 23-year-old man who had been in a recent automobile accident. An intravenous pyelogram demonstrated nonfunctioning of the left kidney several days after the accident. In a prone transverse scan (fig. 7.67) the left kidney is approximately 2–3 times the size of the normal right kidney. In a longitudinal scan through the large left kidney (fig. 7.68) the pancreas is situated deep to it. A venogram demonstrated right-renal vein thrombosis. These entities should be considered when an ultrasound examination demonstrates a large unilateral kidney which is not functioning.

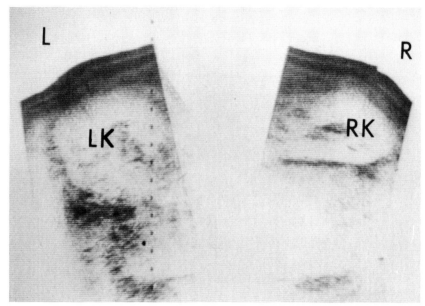

Fig. 7.65

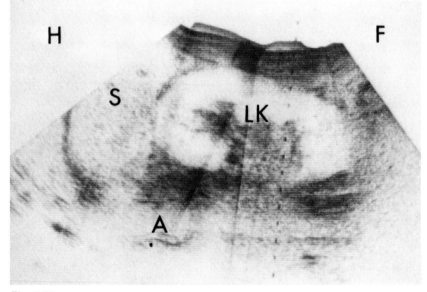

Fig. 7.66

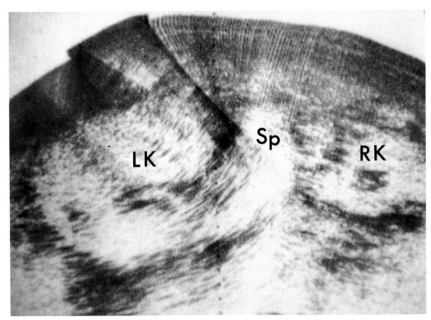

Fig. 7.67

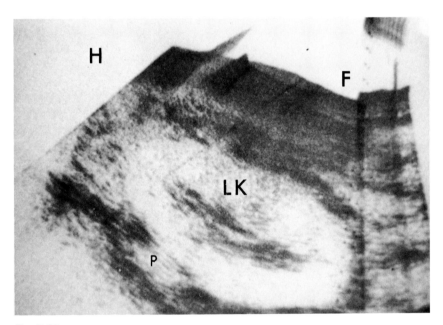

Fig. 7.68

A	=	Aorta
F	=	Foot
H	=	Head
L	=	Left
LK	=	Left kidney
P	=	Pancreas
R	=	Right
RK	=	Right kidney
S	=	Spleen
Sp	=	Spine

Chronic Renal Disease

An intravenous pyelogram usually is performed before an ultrasonic examination. It is still the best screening tool for renal pathology. Ultrasound is a tomographic study which is time-consuming and not as valuable as a screening procedure. Some patients, however, have marked creatinine elevation in which an intravenous pyelogram would not be fruitful. Therefore, ultrasound becomes an excellent means of initially examining these patients. For example, we can easily rule out bilateral hydronephrosis as seen in previous examples.

Figure 7.69 is a longitudinal supine scan of the right kidney. It is a fairly classic example of the ultrasound findings in chronic renal disease. The renal parenchyma is normally less echogenic than the liver.

In figure 7.69 we have a reversal of the usual relationship between the liver and kidney. The kidney is much more echogenic than the liver. Gallstones are present and block the view of the lower pole of the kidney. However, the mid portion and upper pole of the kidney are well seen and of extremely high amplitude in echogenicity.

Another example of chronic renal disease is seen in figure 7.70. The right kidney is a higher-amplitude echo than the liver. It is extremely important to evaluate the right kidney through the liver when making this determination. If the right kidney is scanned through the gallbladder, the kidney will be increased in echogenicity secondary to the through transmission of the gallbladder. (This point is explained further in chapter 1.) Since chronic renal disease is bilateral, we are able to evaluate the right kidney in relationship to the liver. The left kidney is not used, since we do not have an adequate organ for comparison. Usually, the spleen is too cephalad in location to give a comparison to the left kidney. Therefore, an important reason for diagnosing chronic renal disease is a comparison of the right kidney to the liver.

Occasionally while scanning the renal areas, we find small shrunken kidneys which are extremely difficult to identify

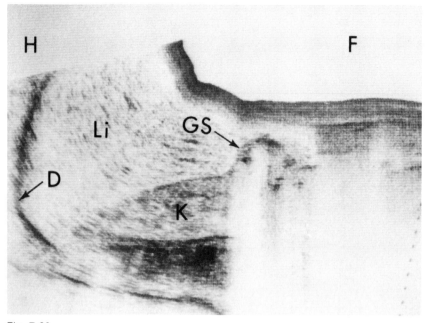

Fig. 7.69

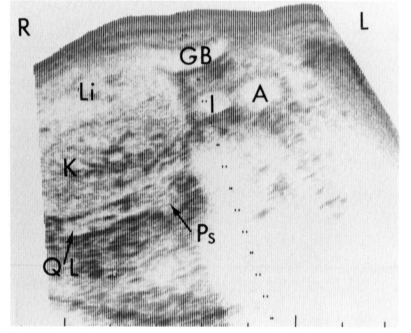

Fig. 7.70

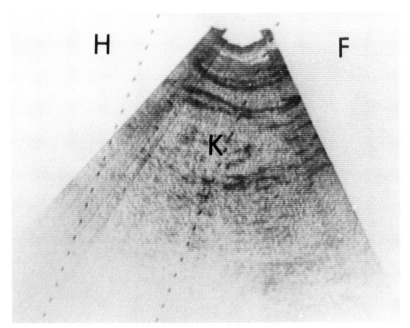

Fig. 7.71

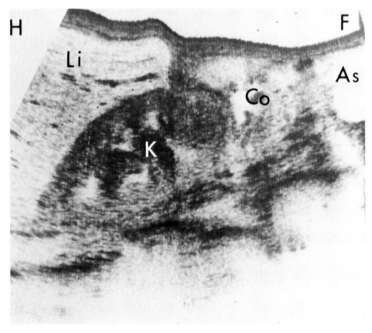

Fig. 7.72

on an ultrasound examination. Figure 7.71 is a longitudinal prone scan of the left kidney. It is very difficult to distinguish the renal borders. The echogenicity of the kidney is also highly consistent with chronic renal disease. When there is difficulty in seeing the renal borders, chronic pyelonephritis is to be suspected. The irregular outer surface of the kidney scatters the echoes which do not return to the transducer. Therefore, we find extremely poor visualization of the renal borders.

Figure 7.72 is the most severe example of increased echogenicity that we have seen. The right kidney is of extremely high amplitude compared with the echogenicity of the liver. The confusing thing about this case was that the kidneys were not decreased in size. If anything, they have a normal-to-increased size. The patient went to autopsy approximately two weeks after the ultrasound examination, and severe amyloid of the kidneys was found.

A	=	Aorta
As	=	Ascites
Co	=	Colon
D	=	Diaphragm
F	=	Foot
GB	=	Gallbladder
GS	=	Gallstone
H	=	Head
I	=	Inferior vena cava
K	=	Kidney
L	=	Left
Li	=	Liver
Ps	=	Psoas muscle
QL	=	Quadratus lumborum
R	=	Right

Chronic Renal Disease

When examining a patient with chronic renal disease, it is important to remember that asssociated pathology may be identified. Figures 7.73 and 7.74 are transverse and longitudinal scans of a patient with severe chronic renal disease. This is easily recognized because of the high echogenicity to the right kidney when compared to the normal echogenicity of the liver. A sonolucent central region is, however, noted in the kidney, indicating concomitant hydronephrosis. Figure 7.73 is a transverse scan which indicates that the hydronephrosis is continuing medially; this is a fairly characteristic sign. Figure 7.74 is a longitudinal scan obtained more peripherally in the kidney, in which we see areas of dilated calyces.

Chronic renal disease with a renal cyst is seen in figure 7.75. The renal echogenicity is slightly greater than in the liver. Some lucencies within the renal parenchyma, secondary to renal pyramids (arrows), can be seen. The large sonolucency noted anteriorly is a fluid-filled mass representing a renal cyst.

Figure 7.76 is an unusual case, demonstrating irregular areas of decreased echogenicity (arrows) in the lateral and posterior aspect of the right kidney. The patient was found to have severe vasculitis with hemorrhage of the right kidney in the areas of sonolucency noted on ultrasound. This case is somewhat similar in appearance to the cases of renal carbuncles.

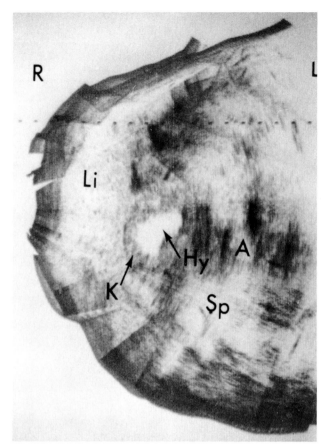

Fig. 7.73

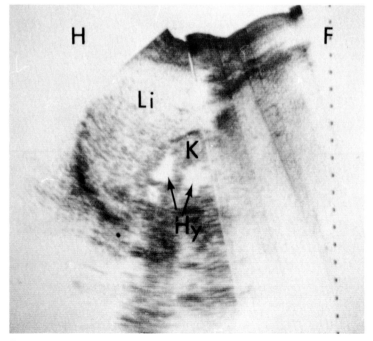

Fig. 7.74

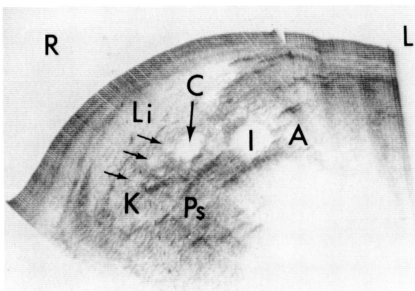

A	=	Aorta
Arrows	=	Renal pyramids (fig. 7.75)
Arrows	=	Renal hemorrhage secondary to vasculitis (fig. 7.76)
C	=	Renal cysts
F	=	Foot
GB	=	Gallbladder
H	=	Head
Hy	=	Hydronephrosis
I	=	Inferior vena cava
K	=	Kidney
L	=	Left
Li	=	Liver
Ps	=	Psoas muscle
R	=	Right
Sp	=	Spine

Fig. 7.75

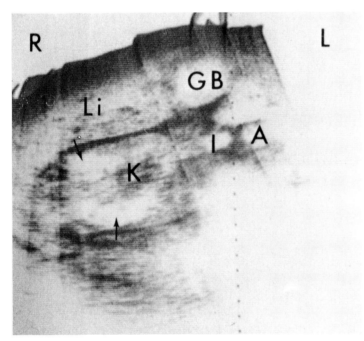

Fig. 7.76

Sinus Lipomatosis

Fat is an extremely perplexing tissue to evaluate. It can present as either lucent or echogenic material on ultrasound examination, depending upon its location, and sometimes, its composition. There is great confusion as to how adipose tissue presents ultrasonographically. Figure 7.77 is an X ray of the kidneys following the injection of contrast material. The characteristic appearance of sinus lipomatosis on the left kidney is seen. The left kidney demonstrates a spider-like appearance to the collecting systems when compared with the right side. This is characteristic of sinus lipomatosis. A transverse prone scan of the same patient (fig. 7.78) shows a sonolucent central collection of tissue in the left kidney. The normally appearing central echoes of the right kidney can be seen. The possibility of hydronephrosis arises. Figure 7.79, a longitudinal scan of the left kidney, also shows the central sonolucency. This case is a good demonstration of the sonolucent appearance to sinus lipomatosis which occurs in some patients.

Sinus lipomatosis can also be echogenic. Figure 7.80 is a longitudinal supine scan of the right kidney in another patient who had a similar radiographic appearance of sinus lipomatosis. Central echoes that are extremely echogenic are seen. It may be that a different amount of fibrotic tissue in certain cases will give an increased echogenicity. To date, however, there is no satisfactory answer as to why adipose tissue provides such a large spectrum of echogenic appearances. Therefore, sinus lipomatosis can occur anywhere on the spectrum, from extremely lucent to extremely echogenic.

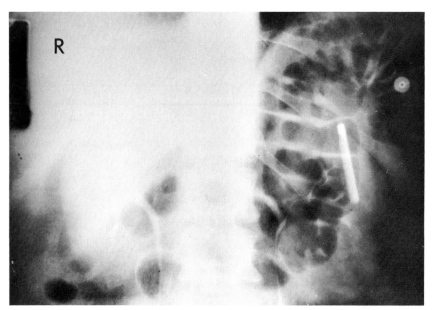

Fig. 7.77

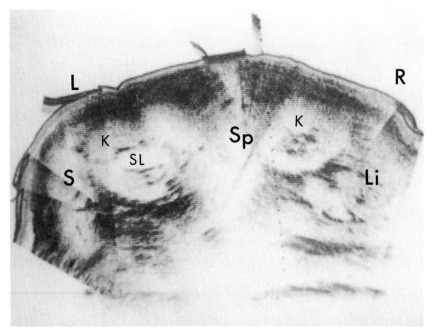

Fig. 7.78

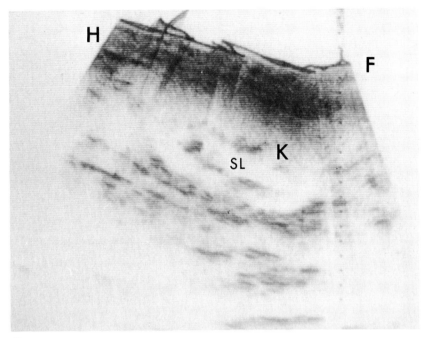

Fig. 7.79

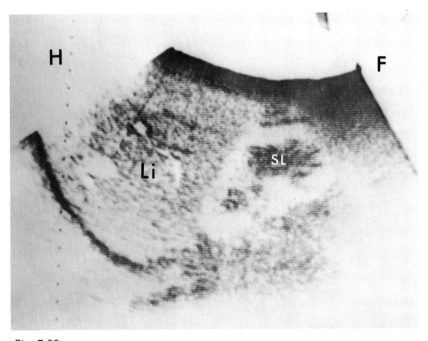

Fig. 7.80

F = Foot
H = Head
K = Kidney
L = Left
Li = Liver
R = Right
S = Spleen
SL = Sinus lipomatosis
Sp = Spine

Angiomyolipoma

Figure 7.81 is a longitudinal coronal scan of the left kidney which demonstrates a highly echogenic central portion with attenuation (arrows). The ultrasonic appearance of this mass could be consistent with calcification within the kidney. It is, however, an angiomyolipoma. Angiomyolipomas often yield highly echogenic masses that distort the renal architecture and parenchyma. When such a mass is visualized, a CAT scan should be performed. It will yield valuable information which will rule out a renal carcinoma versus an angiomyolipoma. A CAT scan of the same patient (fig. 7.82) indicates the angiomyolipoma on the left side (arrows), displacing the collecting system posteriorly. Bilateral angiomyolipomas were diagnosed. On the right side, hemorrhage is present in the mass, and the collecting systems are displaced medially and anteriorly. A small residual portion of the fatty tissue (arrows) has been displaced laterally and anteriorly.

Another example of an angiomyolipoma presenting as a highly echogenic mass is seen in figure 7.83. Only a small portion of normal renal tissue can be seen. Marked attenuation distal to the angiomyolipoma (arrows) is noted. Fatty tissue attenuates ultrasound quite dramatically.

A CAT scan of the patient (fig. 7.84) demonstrates the large fatty angiomyolipomas. The renal parenchyma is situated posterior to this large fatty mass.

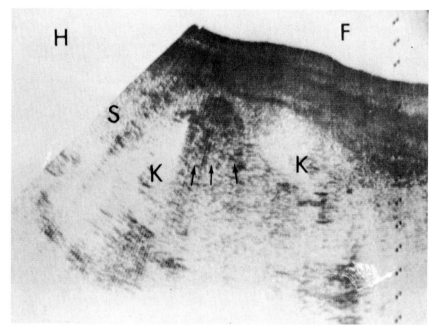

Fig. 7.81

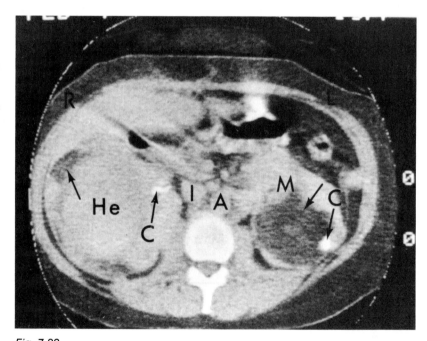

Fig. 7.82

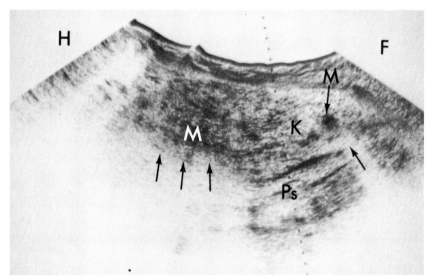

Fig. 7.83

A	=	Aorta
Arrows	=	Marked attenuation posterior to the angiomyolipoma (fig. 7.81)
Arrows	=	Fat density of the angiomyolipoma (fig. 7.82)
Arrows	=	Attenuation from the angiomyolipoma (fig. 7.83)
Arrows	=	Gerota's fascia (fig.7.84)
C	=	Renal-collecting systems
Co	=	Colon
Du	=	Duodenum
F	=	Foot
H	=	Head
He	=	Hemorrhage in right angiomyolipoma
I	=	Inferior vena cava
K	=	Kidney
L	=	Left
M	=	Angiomyolipoma
Ps	=	Psoas muscle
R	=	Right
S	=	Spleen

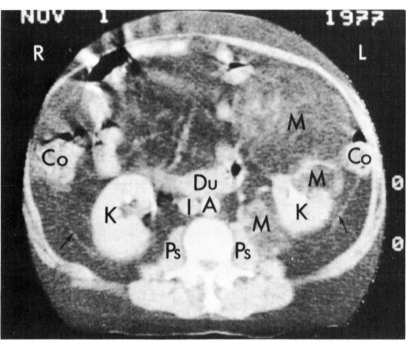

Fig. 7.84

Renal Lymphoma

Figure 7.85 is a tomogram of an intravenous pyelogram which demonstrates large kidneys with stretching and splaying of the renal collecting systems. This is one of several cases sent to us to rule out polycystic disease. Polycystic disease is well diagnosed by ultrasound technique. Numerous fluid-filled masses, disbursed throughout the renal parenchyma, are seen. Figures 7.86 and 7.87 are longitudinal scans of the kidneys obtained from the same patient. Here we find no evidence of any fluid-filled masses throughout the renal parenchyma. Instead, the kidneys are diffusely echogenic. The collecting systems are difficult to see and consistent with the splayed appearance on intravenous pyelogram. The areas of the kidneys are completely filled with soft tissue masses. This patient was found to have diffuse lymphoma of the kidneys bilaterally. Figure 7.88 is a CAT scan which demonstrates the soft tissue density of the kidneys. It confirmed the fact that polycystic disease was not present. Ultrasound provided an excellent means for ruling out polycystic disease in this case, as it has in several others.

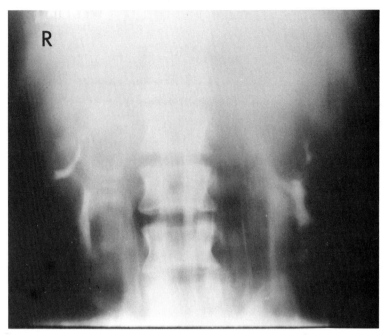

Fig. 7.85

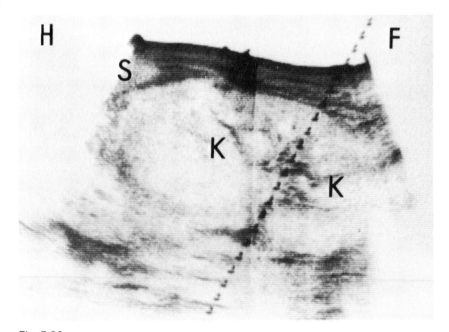

Fig. 7.86

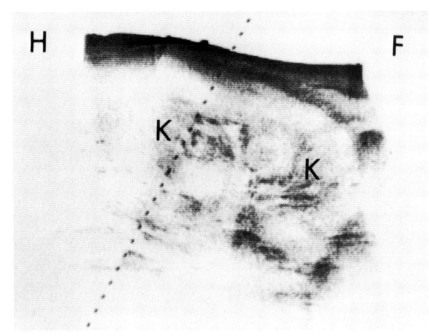

A = Aorta
Du = Duodenum
F = Foot
H = Head
I = Inferior vena cava
K = Kidney
L = Left
Ps = Psoas muscle
R = Right
S = Spleen

Fig. 7.87

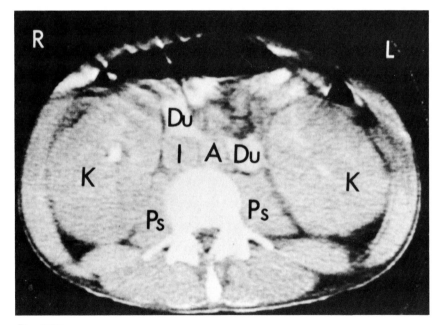

Fig. 7.88

Echogenic Renal Carcinoma

Ultrasonic evaluation of renal masses found on intravenous pyelogram can be extremely helpful in determining whether or not an angiogram should be performed. If a simple cyst is present on ultrasonic examination, then a cyst puncture can be done instead of an angiogram. If ultrasound demonstrates an echogenic or solid mass, however, an angiogram is the next diagnostic step. Renal cell carcinomas can present with a variety of ultrasonic appearances. They may be extremely echogenic, relatively sonolucent, or fluid-filled, in the case of necrotic tumors. Figure 7.89 is a longitudinal scan of the right kidney of a patient with recent hematuria. The upper pole was hydronephrotic, secondary to obstruction by a large lower-pole tumor. The renal mass is echogenic and consistent with a solid lesion of the lower pole of the kidney. A portion of the kidney is not visible; this is due to overlying bowel gas in the hepatic flexure. Examination of the liver was normal at the time of the initial diagnosis of renal cell carcinoma. The patient was operated upon, and a large tumor of the right kidney was removed. At the time of surgery the liver was felt to be normal.

A transverse scan of the liver (fig. 7.90) was performed approximately one year after the initial ultrasonic examination. The liver now contains several highly echogenic masses consistent with vascular metastatic lesions. Chapter 2 demonstrates numerous highly echogenic metastatic lesions similar to this case. The left renal fossa was found to be empty of tumor. Numerous metastatic lesions, however, were noted in the liver.

Figure 7.91 is an example of a small hyperechotic tumor of the lower pole of the right kidney. An increased echogenic region in the lower pole, which measures approximately 2 cm in diameter, is seen. The remainder of the renal parenchyma is relatively sonolucent. The output and sensitivity were intentionally set up to make it extremely sonolucent. This technique brought out the marked discrepancy between the lower-pole echo-

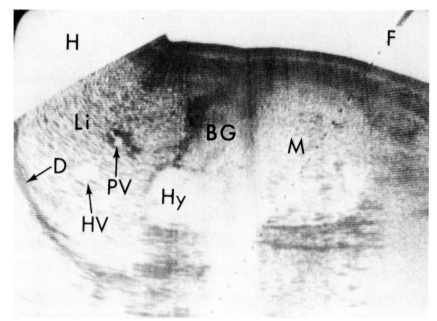

Fig. 7.89

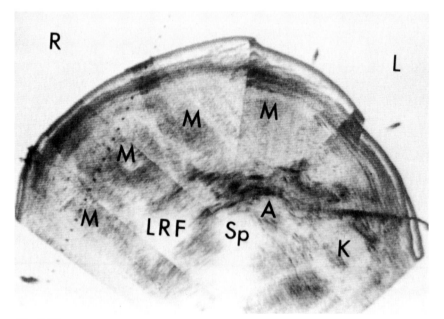

Fig. 7.90

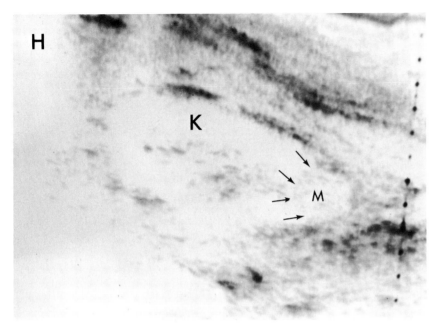

Fig. 7.91

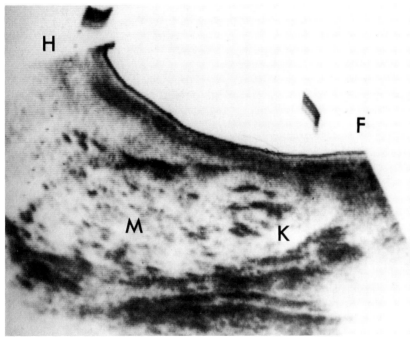

Fig. 7.92

genicity and the remainder of the normal renal parenchyma.

Figure 7.92 is an example of a hyper-echotic neoplasm of the right upper pole. This is an extremely large mass which involves the majority of the right upper pole and extends beneath the liver. Extremely vascular renal lesions will appear as highly echogenic lesions on ultrasound.

A	= Aorta
BG	= Bowel gas
D	= Diaphragm
F	= Foot
H	= Head
HV	= Hepatic vein
Hy	= Hydronephrotic upper pole
K	= Left kidney
L	= Left
Li	= Liver
LRF	= Left renal fossa
M (fig. 7.89)	= Hypernephroma of the right lower pole
M (fig. 7.90)	= Metastatic lesions to the liver
M (fig. 7.91)	= Right lower pole hypernephrotic mass
M (fig. 7.92)	= Hypernephroma of the right upper pole
PV	= Portal vein
R	= Right
Sp	= Spine

Hypoechotic Renal Neoplasms

Renal masses may also be decreased in echogenicity. This is usually true of hypovascular tumors. Close scrutiny of the central echoes on ultrasound is important in the evaluation of the kidney. A longitudinal scan of a left kidney (fig. 7.93) demonstrates marked distortion of the lower pole central echoes. The normal highly echogenic central region is disrupted by a relatively lucent mass. The borders of this mass are irregular and are distorting the central echoes. This is a transitional cell carcinoma of the lower pole. Figure 7.94, another transverse scan of a left kidney, indicates distortion of the central echoes by an anterior mass. The mass is relatively hypoechogenic, as compared with the renal parenchyma. It was found to be a renal cell carcinoma and was somewhat hypovascular.

Figure 7.95, a longitudinal coronal scan of the left kidney, demonstrates a mass (arrows) situated on the lateral aspect of the kidney. Again, the important finding is distortion of the central echoes. Not only the architecture of the renal capsule and outline but also the central echoes must be closely examined during the course of an ultrasound study. The only clue to renal pathology may be distortion of the central echoes, as these cases demonstrate.

Figure 7.96 is a longitudinal scan of the right kidney with a hypovascular mass adjacent to its upper pole. This mass could not be completely separated from the right upper pole. This is an extremely difficult area to evaluate because it is impossible to place the transmitted beam perpendicular to interfaces in this region. Several diagnostic possibilities, such as renal carcinoma or an adrenal lesion, exist. At surgery, it was found to be a benign renal adenoma arising from the upper pole of the right kidney.

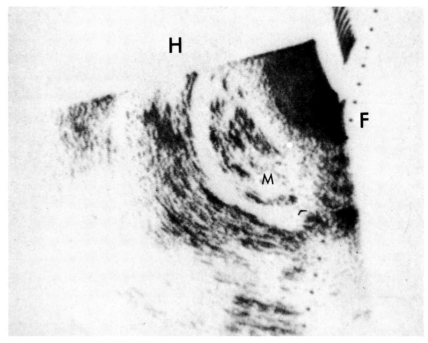

Fig. 7.93

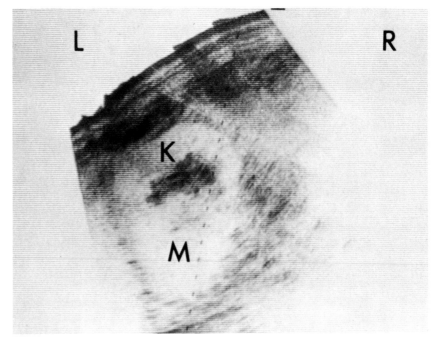

Fig. 7.94

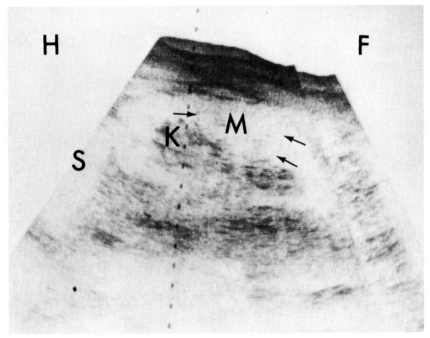

Fig. 7.95

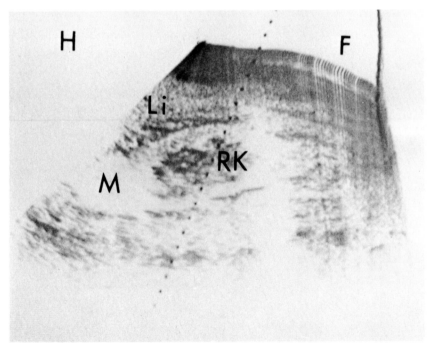

Fig. 7.96

Hypernephroma

Figures 7.97 and 7.98 are scans of a patient with renal cell carcinoma of the left kidney. The longitudinal scan of the left kidney (fig. 7.97) demonstrates marked distortion of the normal renal architecture. Visualization of the central echoes, as we see in the normal kidney, is not apparent. There are areas of increased echogenicity along with areas of decreased echogenicity (small arrows) noted throughout the kidney. This entire left kidney was filled with tumor. A longitudinal scan of the inferior vena cava of the same patient (fig. 7.98) delineates a large tumor within the lumen of the inferior vena cava. The inferior vena cava is markedly dilated due to partial obstruction by the tumor. There is also evidence of a tumor posterior to the inferior vena cava. The tumor mass extending from the left kidney is also seen in the caudal portion of the scan.

Figure 7.99 is a longitudinal scan in the midline of another patient with an unusual vascular finding. It demonstrates the aorta with the celiac axis and superior mesenteric artery arising from it. A marked abnormal angulation to the superior mesenteric artery is noted. This is secondary to a massively dilated left renal vein. The patient has a large hypernephroma of the left kidney with marked arteriovenous shunting. The dramatically dilated left renal vein is secondary to increased blood flow. It is stretching and elevating the superior mesenteric artery.

Figure 7.100 is a transverse supine scan of the right kidney of another patient with a large tumor in the right renal bed. The tumor extends through the right renal vein to the inferior vena cava. The right renal vein is completely echo-filled; this is consistent with tumor deposits within it.

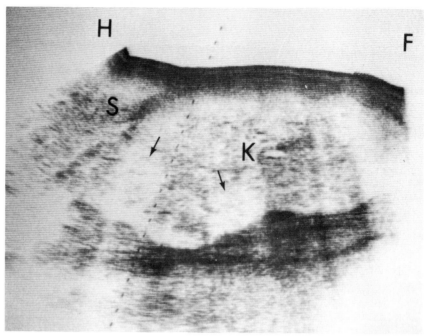

Fig. 7.97

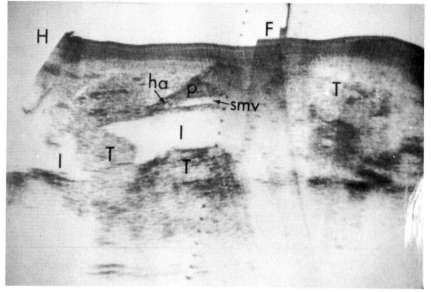

Fig. 7.98

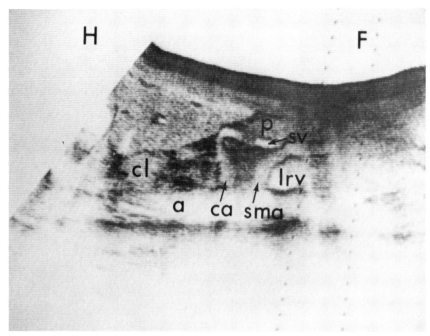

Fig. 7.99

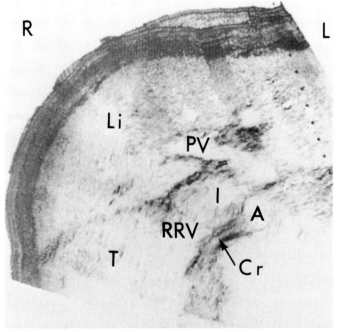

Fig. 7.100

A	= Aorta
a	= Aorta
Arrows	= Hypoechogenic region of the tumor, hypogenic regions of the hypernephroma (fig. 7.97)
CA	= Celiac axis
CL	= Caudate lobe
Cr	= Crus
F	= Foot
H	= Head
HA	= Hepatic artery
I	= Inferior vena cava
K	= Kidney
L	= Left
Li	= Liver
LRV	= Left renal vein
P	= Pancreas
PV	= Portal vein
R	= Right
RRV	= Tumor in the right renal vein
S	= Spleen
SMA	= Superior mesenteric artery
SMV	= Superior mesenteric vein
SV	= Splenic vein
T	= Tumor in the inferior vena cava and abdomen
t	= Hypernephroma of the right kidney (fig. 7.100)

Renal Transplants

A longitudinal scan of a renal transplant in the right lower quadrant is seen in figure 7.101. The strong central echoes are surrounded by the less echogenic renal parenchyma. A relatively lucent area is present within the renal parenchyma, secondary to a renal pyramid. The patient's right kidney is much more echogenic than the liver. This finding is consistent with chronic renal disease and warranted the renal transplant.

Figure 7.102 is an oblique longitudinal scan of a transplanted kidney suffering rejection. Here we have difficulty visualizing the central echoes. The kidney is larger and thicker than is usually seen. It is also somewhat less echogenic than normal. Renal transplants will enlarge in size when undergoing rejection.

Figure 7.103 is an example of a renal transplant that has developed hydronephrosis. Hydronephrosis of a renal transplant is similar to that of a normally positioned kidney. We see a central sonolucency separating the central echoes. In this instance, the hydronephrosis extends into the calyceal region.

Figure 7.104 is another scan of a transplanted kidney in which we see mild hydronephrosis. The cause of the hydronephrosis, a renal stone, is visualized. Deep to the stone is acoustic shadowing.

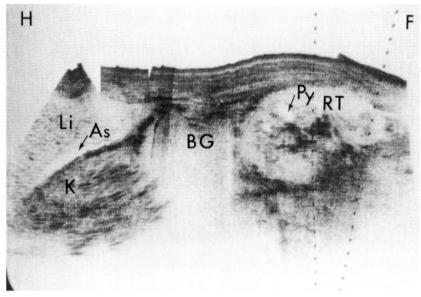

Fig. 7.101

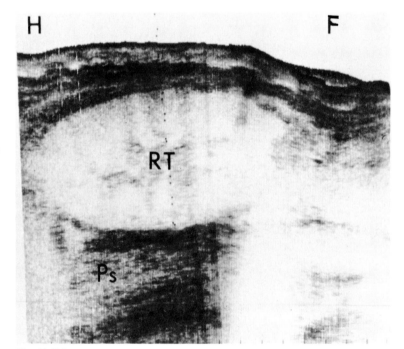

Fig. 7.102

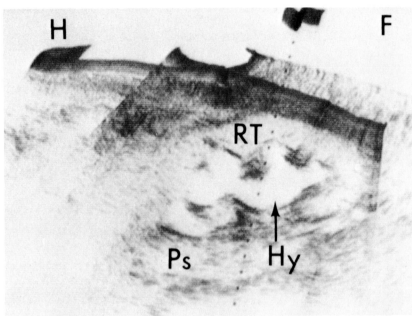

Fig. 7.103

As = Ascites
BG = Bowel gas
F = Foot
H = Head
Hy = Hydronephrosis
K = Right kidney with chronic renal disease
Li = Liver
Ps = Psoas muscle
Py = Pyramid
RT = Renal transplant
RT = Renal transplant rejection (fig. 7.102)
Sh = Shadowing
St = Renal stone

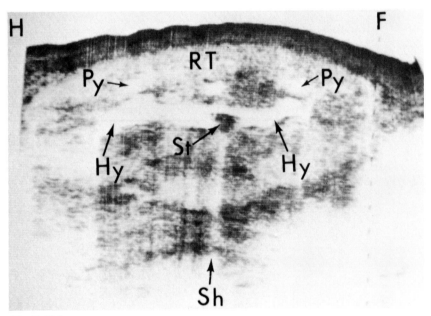

Fig. 7.104

Renal Transplant Associated with Abscess and Urinoma

When examining a renal transplant, we can easily evaluate the perinephric region with ultrasound examination. An attempt should be made to visualize fluid collections around the transplanted kidney to rule out the possibility of abscesses, lymphoceles, hematomas, or urinomas. In a transverse section of a transplanted kidney (fig. 7.105), we see a relatively lucent mass on the lateral aspect of the kidney. This eventually was found to be a perinephric abscess (arrows). It was quite localized, and its expansion can be seen indenting the renal border.

Figure 7.106 is a scan of the transplanted kidney of another patient. It demonstrates a large fluid collection surrounding both the upper and lower poles of the transplanted kidney. The fluid collection is not specific for any etiology, and at surgery it was found to be a large perinephric abscess that completely surrounded the transplanted kidney.

Figures 7.107 and 7.108 are scans from two different patients who also had fluid collections surrounding transplanted kidneys. In figure 7.107, the fluid collection has some internal echoes within it. These could represent abscess, hematoma, urinoma with debris, or lymphocele with debris. At surgery, a urinoma was found. In figure 7.108, a longitudinal scan of the abdomen demonstrates a transplanted kidney cephalad to a fluid-filled mass. Within the mass is a septum. This was also urinoma.

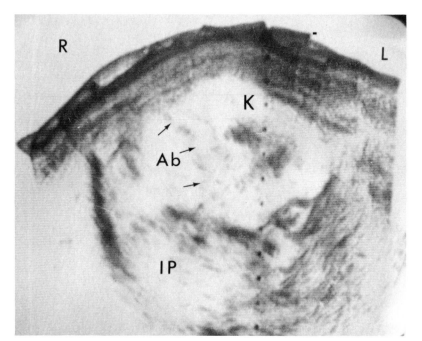

Fig. 7.105

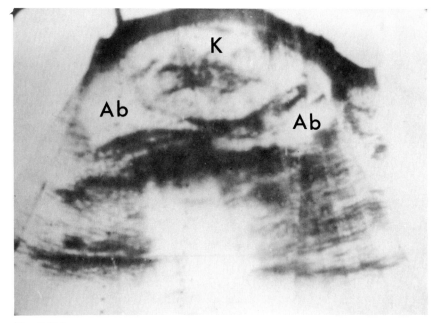

Fig. 7.106

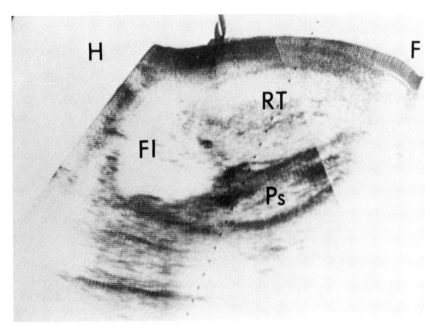

Ab	= Perinephric abscess
Arrows	= Abscess
B	= Urinary bladder
F	= Foot
FI	= Urinoma
H	= Head
IP	= Iliopsoas muscle
K	= Kidney
L	= Left
Ps	= Psoas muscle
R	= Right
RT	= Renal transplant
S	= Septum in a urinoma

Fig. 7.107

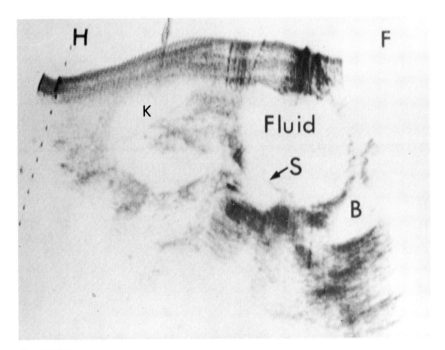

Fig. 7.108

Normal Right Adrenal Gland

Although the normal right adrenal gland sometimes can be visualized on routine transverse scans performed in the supine position (fig. 7.109), its orientation and important surrounding interfaces are parallel to the sound beam with this approach. As a result, the laterally resolving capabilities of the beam, even with well focused transducers, frequently are insufficient to distinctly delineate the gland. By having the patient move onto the left side, in the decubitus position and by scanning through the intercostal spaces, the sound beam can be directed perpendicular to the major interfaces. Depending upon the body habitus of the patient, a variable amount of retroperitoneal fibrofatty tissue will surround the gland and separate it from the medial aspect of the right lobe of the liver and the crus of the diaphragm. The interface between the medial aspect of the liver and the right adrenal gland is frequently the most difficult to resolve (fig. 7.110).

During the preliminary scans in the left lateral decubitus position, the precise orientation of these interfaces for each patient can be determined and a transducer scanning motion can be designed which will keep the beam perpendicular to the various interfaces throughout the entire scanning motion. Since most of these interfaces represent specular reflectors, when the proper scanning motion is achieved they will be visualized with the better axial resolution of the system (figs. 7.111 and 7.112). The proper scanning motion usually is a small sector scan performed in one of the intercostal spaces. The right adrenal gland is usually linear or curvilinear in configuration and runs parallel to the right crus of the diaphragm. The surrounding fibrofatty tissue provides a highly reflective background. Usually, only one limb of the right adrenal gland is seen on any one scanning plane, since the limbs run along the cephalocaudal plane rather than the right-to-left plane. The acoustic texture of the adrenal gland is usually quite similar to the crus of the diaphragm.

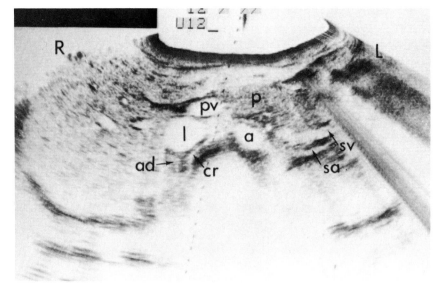

Fig. 7.109

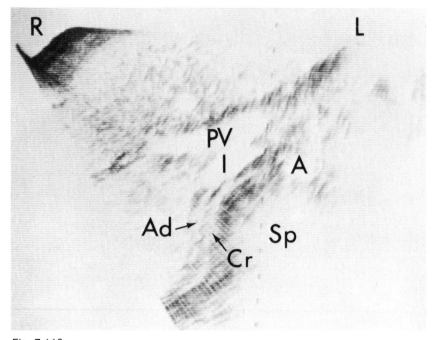

Fig. 7.110

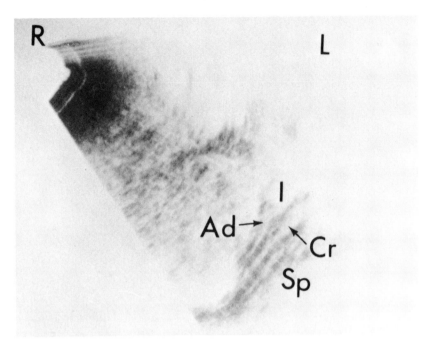

Fig. 7.111

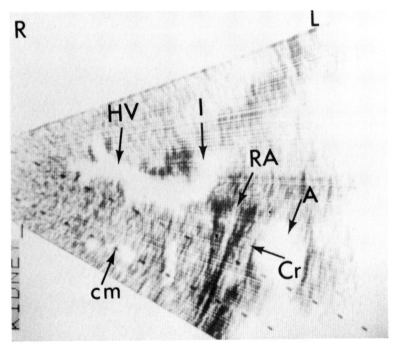

Fig. 7.112

The exact degree of rotation into the decubitus position varies with each patient. As the amount of fibrofatty tissue surrounding the adrenal gland increases with the more obese patients, it becomes more difficult to achieve adequate resolution to visualize the right adrenal gland. Furthermore, if there is marked attenuation within the liver due to superimposed disease, penetration may not be adequate. With this technique, however, the right adrenal gland can be visualized in approximately 90% of patients.

A	=	Aorta
a	=	Aorta
Ad	=	Adrenal gland
ad	=	Adrenal gland
cm	=	Centimeter marker
Cr	=	Crus of the diaphragm
cr	=	Crus of the diaphragm
HV	=	Hepatic vein
I	=	Inferior vena cava
L	=	Left
P	=	Pancreas
p	=	Pancreas
PV	=	Portal vein
pv	=	Portal vein
R	=	Right
RA	=	Right adrenal gland
SA	=	Splenic artery
sa	=	Splenic artery
Sp	=	Spine
SV	=	Splenic vein
sv	=	Splenic vein

Normal Right Adrenal Gland

Since the liver usually serves as an acoustic window to the right adrenal area, the right adrenal gland can be visualized by a number of potential longitudinal approaches. When the left lobe of the liver extends across the midline, a scanning plane through the left lobe of the liver and the inferior vena cava (approach no. 1 in figure 7.113) can be performed. With this scanning plane, the right adrenal gland will be seen immediately beneath the inferior vena cava, caudal to the diaphragmatic hiatus (fig. 7.114). The main danger with this plane is the inability to define precisely the crus of the diaphragm which is parallel but somewhat posterior in position to the adrenal gland. If scanning plane no. 2 (fig. 7.113) is inadvertently performed, the right crus of the diaphragm can be mistaken for the adrenal gland beneath the inferior vena cava (fig. 7.115). The right crus of the diaphragm is usually visualized several centimeters below the diaphragmatic hiatus for the inferior vena cava. Because of this potential danger, scanning plane no. 3 (fig. 7.113) is fraught with fewer hazards. With this scanning plane, the beam again passes perpendicular to both the right adrenal gland and the right crus of the diaphragm. As a result, both structures can be specifically identified (fig. 7.116). The orientation of the right adrenal gland determines whether it is seen as a linear or slightly triangular structure. The upper pole of the right kidney also may be seen on the same section (fig. 7.116).

Scanning plane no. 3 frequently is best achieved again with the patient in the left lateral decubitus position. The degree to which the patient is rolled into the decubitus position will vary with the body habitus and the configuration and mobility of the liver.

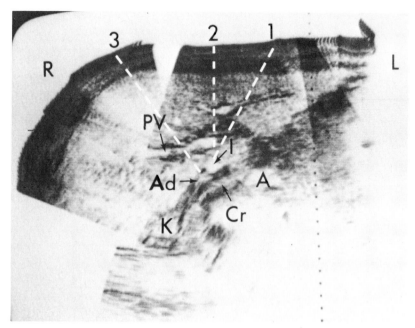

Fig. 7.113

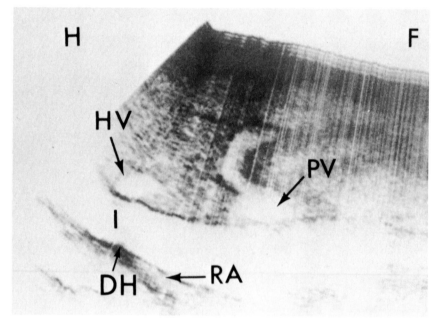

Fig. 7.114

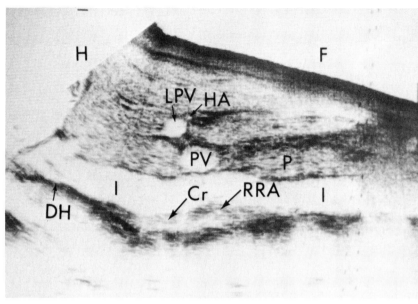

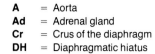

A   = Aorta
Ad   = Adrenal gland
Cr   = Crus of the diaphragm
DH   = Diaphragmatic hiatus
F   = Feet
H   = Head
HA   = Hepatic artery
I   = Inferior vena cava
K   = Kidney
L   = Left
LPV = Left portal vein
P   = Pancreas
PV   = Portal vein
R   = Right
RA   = Right adrenal gland
RRA = Right renal artery

Fig. 7.115

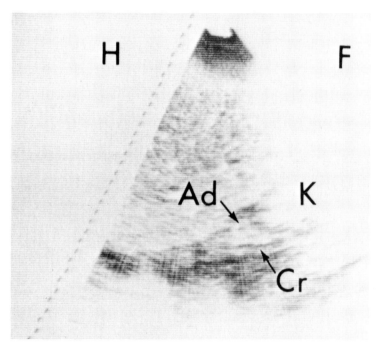

Fig. 7.116

Normal Right Adrenal Gland

In patients whose livers are so diseased that high attenuation of the sound beam occurs, the only approach to the right adrenal gland may be through the right kidney. Scanning may be performed in the left lateral decubitus position. Initially, transverse scans are performed to determine the exact orientation of the right kidney to the prevertebral vessels (fig. 7.117). Where the imaginary line connecting the right kidney and the prevertebral vessels cross the skin surface, an X is placed on the patient. This maneuver is performed in the lower, mid, and upper pole regions of the kidney, and the resulting 3 Xs represent the oblique coronal longitudinal plane for the final scans (fig. 7.118). The scanning plane must, however, be performed at an angle from the perpendicular (figs. 7.117 and 7.118) in order to achieve the proper alignment. The resulting image is very similar to that of a nephrotomogram, with a large segment of the kidney visualized along its long axis. Normally, a triangular shaped adrenal gland can be seen superior to the kidney and medial to the liver (fig. 7.119). In some scans, the cephalic portions of the psoas muscle, as well as the right crus of the diaphragm, can be seen (fig. 7.119). Occasionally, the right adrenal gland will be situated more anteromedially to the upper pole of the right kidney, in which case the inferior vena cava may also be visualized (fig. 7.120). In this location, the gland frequently has a more curvilinear configuration.

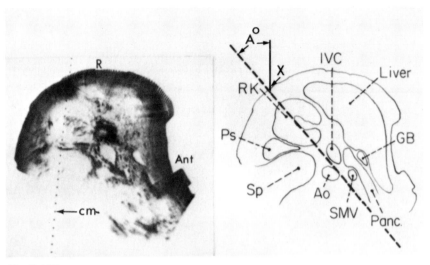

Fig. 7.117

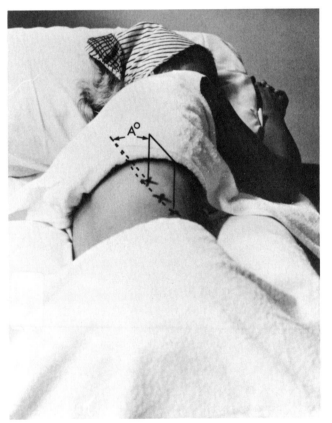

Fig. 7.118

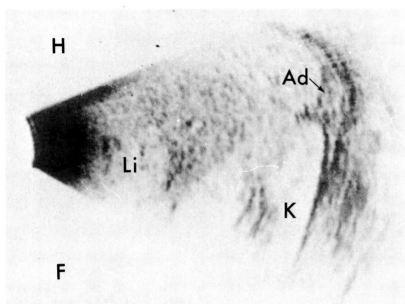

Fig. 7.119

A°	=	Angle of inclination
Ad	=	Adrenal gland
Ant	=	Anterior
Ao	=	Aorta
cm	=	Centimeter marker
Cr	=	Right crus of the diaphragm
F	=	Foot
GB	=	Gallbladder
H	=	Head
I	=	Inferior vena cava
IVC	=	Inferior vena cava
K	=	Kidney
L	=	Left
Li	=	Liver
P	=	Pancreas
Ps	=	Psoas muscle
R	=	Right
RK	=	Right kidney
SMV	=	Superior mesenteric vein
Sp	=	Spine
X	=	Mark on patient's skin

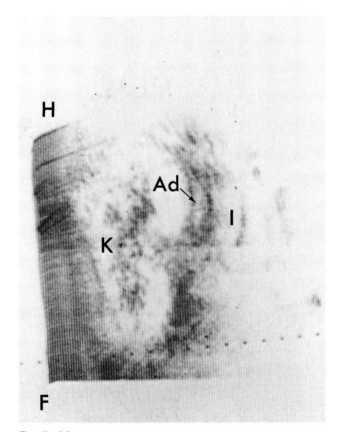

Fig. 7.120

Normal Left Adrenal Gland

Only rarely can the left adrenal gland be visualized in routine transverse and longitudinal scans performed in the supine position (figs. 7.121 and 7.122). Usually, the patient has a prominent left lobe of the liver which either collapses the stomach or deviates it to the left so that the sound beam is not totally reflected by gas. Nevertheless, when visualized in these planes, the close relationship of the left adrenal gland to the left crus of the diaphragm, aorta, kidney, splenic vessels, pancreas, stomach, and duodenum can be appreciated. The most important anatomic consideration is the number of structures that lie at the same depth in the left upper quadrant which can be confused with the left adrenal gland. Moving from a cranial to a caudal position they include the cardia of the stomach, splenic vessels, pancreas, left renal vessels, and fourth portion of the duodenum (fig. 7.122).

In the majority of patients, the gastric air bubble prevents adequate visualization of the left adrenal gland from the supine position. Patients are best studied in the right lateral decubitus position, using the kidney and the spleen as acoustic windows. In order to avoid confusion with the surrounding structures, advantage is taken of the fact that the left adrenal gland is attached at its apex to Gerota's fascia next to the left crus of the diaphragm and the aorta. As a result, a specific scanning plane is mapped out initially using transverse scans (fig. 7.123). An imaginary line passing through the aorta and left kidney is marked on the patient's skin with an X. Marks are obtained with this alignment in the lower-, mid-, and upper-pole regions of the kidney (fig. 7.124). The three Xs will designate the proper longitudinal, oblique, coronal plane. Furthermore, since the proper scanning plane is not perpendicular to the patient's skin surface, it must, in addition, be properly inclined.

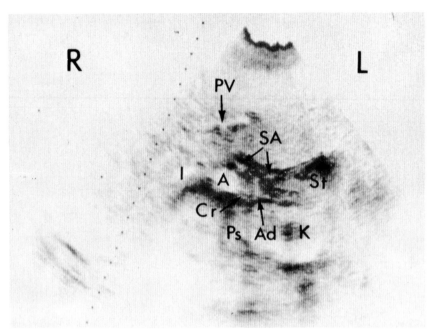

Fig. 7.121

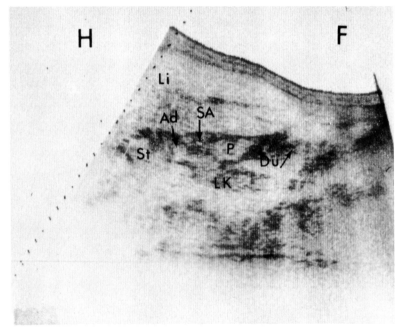

Fig. 7.122

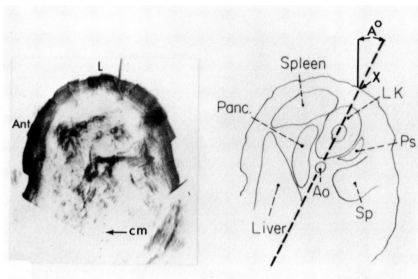

Fig. 7.123

A	=	Aorta
A°	=	Angle of inclination
Ad	=	Adrenal gland
Ant	=	Anterior
Ao	=	Aorta
cm	=	Centimeter marker
Cr	=	Crus of the diaphragm
Du	=	Duodenum
F	=	Feet
H	=	Head
I	=	Inferior vena cava
K	=	Kidney
L	=	Left
Li	=	Liver
LK	=	Left kidney
P	=	Pancreas
Panc.	=	Pancreas
Ps	=	Psoas muscle
PV	=	Portal vein
R	=	Right
SA	=	Splenic artery
Sp	=	Spine
St	=	Stomach
X	=	Mark on patient's skin

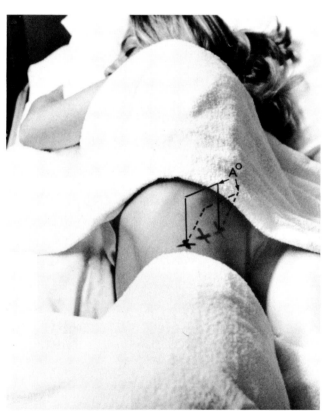

Fig. 7.124

Normal Left Adrenal Gland

The longitudinal oblique coronal scanning planes (figs. 7.125–7.128) demonstrate the detailed anatomy of the left
adrenal gland in a high percentage of
patients. Visualization of the necessary
anatomical landmarks, however, greatly
depends upon the body habitus of the
patient. Sufficient detail may not be obtained in obese patients. Therefore, true
visualization of the left adrenal can be
achieved in only approximately 80% of
patients. The critical landmarks for the
adrenal area are the left crus of the diaphragm, the medial aspect of the
spleen, and the upper pole of the left
kidney (fig. 7.125). With this approach,
the normal adrenal gland has a triangular shape with straight to concave margins. The echogenic texture is similar to
that of the crus, but it may be somewhat
variable. Since the adrenal gland may
contain considerable fat, it may be difficult to distinguish it from the suprarenal
fat pad bounded by Gerota's fascia (fig.
7.126). Nevertheless, with small gain
changes, the subtle differences in echogenicity frequently can be moved into a
portion of the gray scale which can be
separated visually.

The left adrenal gland is frequently
more variable in position in terms of its
superior versus medial location near the
kidney. Depending upon the amount of
perirenal fat, as well as the exact configuration of the spleen, it may be completely suprarenal in position or more
perirenal in position, along the medial
aspect of the upper pole (fig. 7.128).
Occasionally, both limbs of the adrenal
gland can be distinguished separately
(figs. 7.126 & 7.127). In addition, the
anterior medial limb of the adrenal gland
frequently extends for some distance
caudally along the anterior medial aspect of the kidney (figs. 7.125 & 7.127).

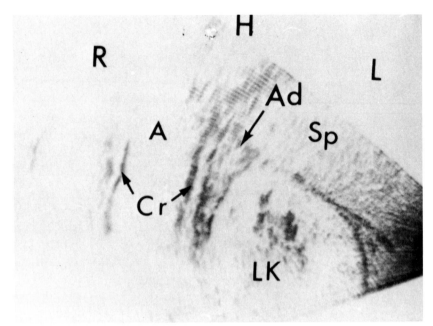

Fig. 7.125

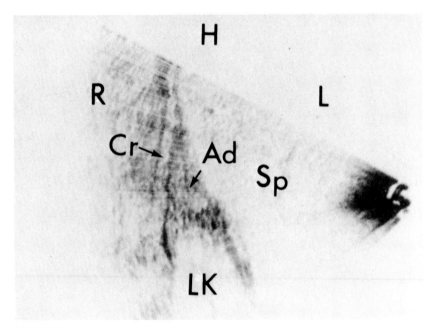

Fig. 7.126

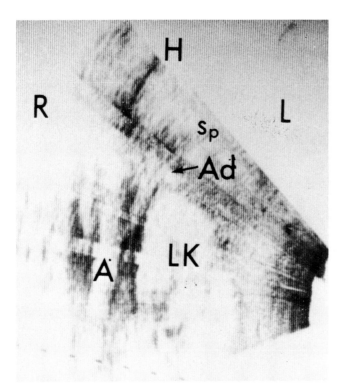

Fig. 7.127

A   = Aorta
A   = Adrenal gland (fig. 1.128)
Ad = Adrenal gland
Cr = Crus of the diaphragm
H   = Head
L   = Left
LK = Left kidney
R   = Right
Sp = Spleen

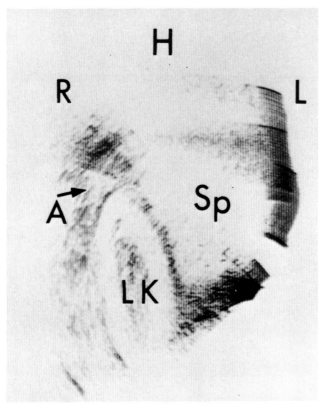

Fig. 7.128

Pitfalls in the Localization of the Left Adrenal Gland

One of the potential problems in the localization of the left adrenal gland is caused by the esophagogastric junction and the cardia of the stomach. As the esophagogastric junction forms at the diaphragmatic hiatus, it presents as a rounded mass anterior and to the left of the aorta. On routine transverse scans in the supine position, if the left lobe of the liver extends across the midline, this junctional zone can be seen (fig. 7.129). Since the esophagogastric junction is usually collapsed with fasting patients, the more echogenic lining mucosa may not be demonstrated. Scans obtained slightly caudal to the esophageal hiatus may demonstrate the cardia and fundus of the stomach, which even in the collapsed state frequently demonstrates the echogenic mucosal lining (fig. 7.130).

Longitudinal oblique coronal scans used to demonstrate the left adrenal gland may demonstrate the cardia of the stomach cephalad to the adrenal gland and medial to the spleen, particularly if the central echogenic mucosal pattern can be recorded (fig. 7.131). Since the cardia of the stomach is at the same anteroposterior depth in the abdomen as the adrenal gland, if all of the landmarks are not appreciated, this structure can mimic a mass in the suprarenal region (fig. 7.132). Consequently, to scan the left adrenal gland, all approaches should be used in an attempt to identify the cardia of the stomach. Additional techniques include having the patient swallow water and noting a change in a questionable mass in this region. Alternatively, real-time examination of the area during ingestion of water may demonstrate the presence of air bubbles in the region.

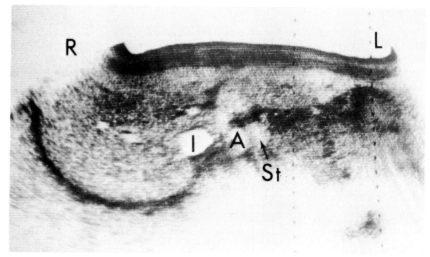

Fig. 7.129

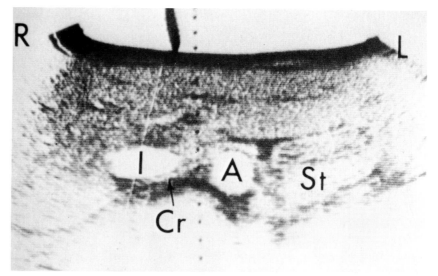

Fig. 7.130

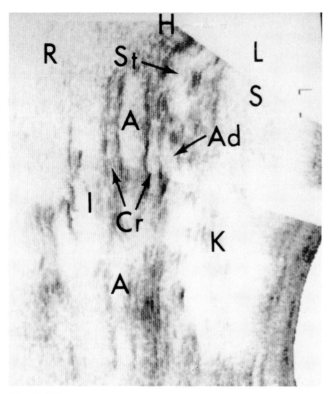

Fig. 7.131

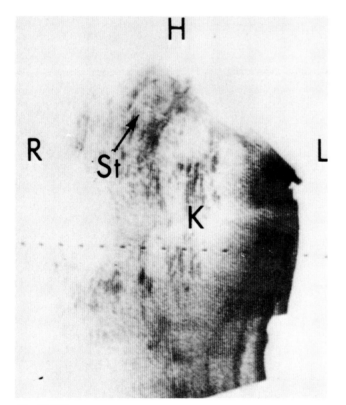

Fig. 7.132

A	=	Aorta
Ad	=	Left adrenal gland
Cr	=	Crus of the diaphragm
H	=	Head
I	=	Inferior vena cava
K	=	Kidney
L	=	Left
R	=	Right
S	=	Spleen
St	=	Stomach

Pitfalls in the Localization of the Left Adrenal Gland

Previous experience with nephrotomography has demonstrated that medial lobulations of the spleen can mimic suprarenal masses. The medial extent of some spleens can be appreciated on transverse sonograms performed in the supine position, again when the left lobe of the liver extends across the midline (fig. 7.133). These medial lobulations occur at the same anteroposterior level as the adrenal gland. In the longitudinal coronal oblique scans, the medial projection of the spleen also may be appreciated (figs. 7.134 and 7.135). In order to bring out the detailed anatomy, however, adequate sector scans in the appropriate intercostal space are necessary to delineate the crus of the diaphragm extending superiorly around the spleen and the adrenal gland. In obese patients particularly, all the anatomy may not be visualized, and a medial lobulation of the spleen, or an accessory spleen, may mimic a suprarenal mass (fig. 7.136). Again, all approaches to the suprarenal region should be used to try to determine the medial extent of the spleen. When the spleen extends medially, the left adrenal gland is frequently situated along the anterior medial aspect of the kidney rather than in a true suprarenal position.

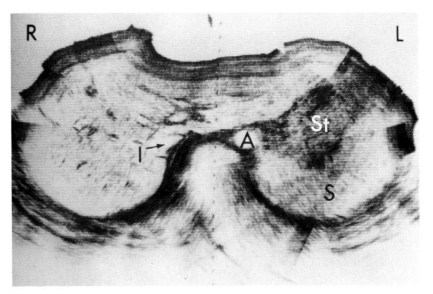

Fig. 7.133

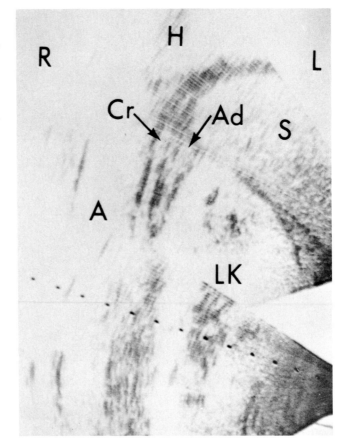

Fig. 7.134

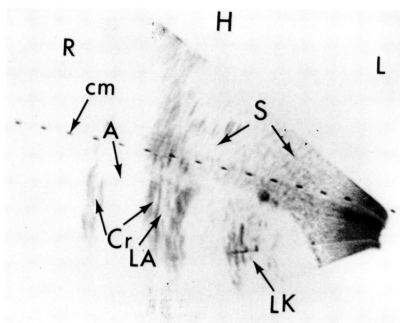

A = Aorta
Ad = Left adrenal gland
cm = Centimeter marker
Cr = Crus of the diaphragm
H = Head
I = Inferior vena cava
K = Kidney
L = Left
LA = Left adrenal gland
LK = Left kidney
M? = Splenic lobulation
R = Right
S = Spleen
St = Stomach

Fig. 7.135

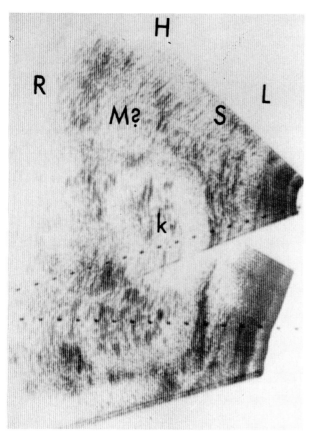

Fig. 7.136

Pitfalls in the Normal Localization of the Left Adrenal Gland

The splenic vasculature represents another obstacle in the left suprarenal region. On transverse scans performed in the supine position, the close relationship of the splenic artery and vein to the left adrenal gland can be appreciated (figs. 7.137 and 7.138). Particularly in older patients, the splenic artery can be very tortuous and prominent. If this variation is not recognized it may cause a bulge in the adrenal gland and give the appearance of a mass.

On longitudinal coronal oblique scans, the splenic vessels usually are visualized between the lateral border of the left kidney and the spleen (fig. 7.139). In those patients with portal hypertension (fig. 7.140) or with aneurysmal dilatation of the splenic artery, however, the vessels may appear as fluid areas in the suprarenal region. Only if the left adrenal gland can be identified separately can this interpretation be avoided.

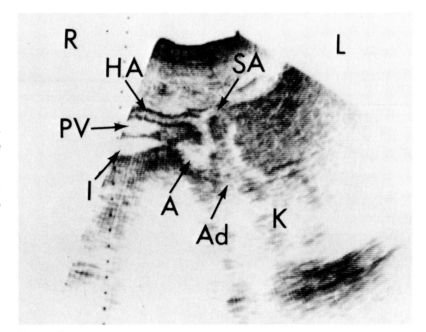

Fig. 7.137

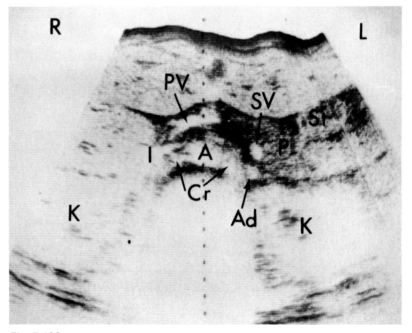

Fig. 7.138

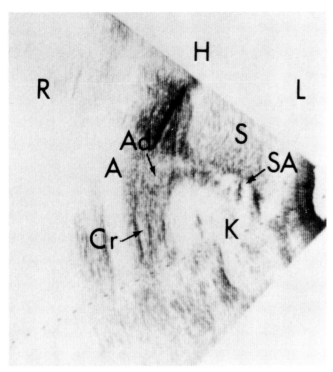

Fig. 7.139

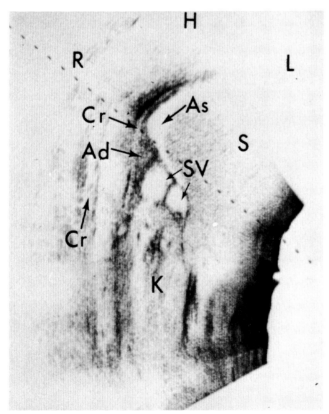

Fig. 7.140

A   = Aorta
Ad = Left adrenal gland
As = Ascites
Cr = Crus of the diaphragm
H   = Head
HA = Hepatic artery
I   = Inferior vena cava
K   = Kidney
L   = Left
P   = Pancreas
PV = Portal vein
R   = Right
S   = Spleen
SA = Splenic artery
St = Stomach
SV = Splenic vein

Pitfalls in the Localization of the Normal Adrenal Gland

Two other structures are in close proximity to the left adrenal gland. The left renal vascular bundle, which may be very prominent in some patients, usually passes at the same anteroposterior level as the adrenal gland, but somewhat more caudally (fig. 7.141). The vascular nature of the mass can be recognized on real time by the pulsations. Nevertheless, during the breath-holding process, the left renal vein may be pinched between the aorta and the superior mesenteric artery, leading to temporary obstruction and dilatation.

Another potential pitfall in the localization of the adrenal gland is caused by the course of the fourth portion of the duodenum (fig. 7.142) which also lies at the same anteroposterior level as the left adrenal gland, but again, somewhat more caudally. Although the central echogenic mucosa pattern often can be recognized specifically identifying the bowel, this region is collapsed in many patients, and it cannot be recognized. As a result, a mass effect is created lateral to the aorta. These problems occur most frequently in the search for a pheochromocytoma whereby the tumor may reside in an extraadrenal location, frequently near the left renal hilus.

A final difficulty in the localization of either adrenal gland occurs when the nearby kidney is located more caudally, either due to ptosis, hepatomegaly, splenomegaly, or a congenital variation. Since the adrenal glands are attached at their apex to Gerota's fascia, they will remain adjacent to either the aorta or the inferior vena cava some distance away from the kidney (figs. 7.143 and 7.144). In these situations, it may be more difficult to differentiate the adrenal gland from the more abundant, surrounding perirenal fat.

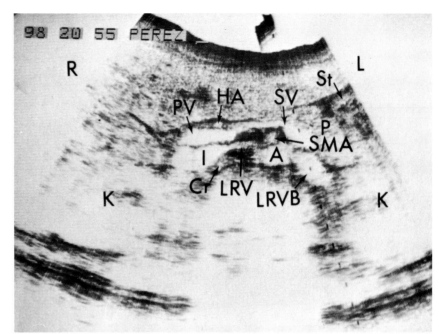

Fig. 7.141

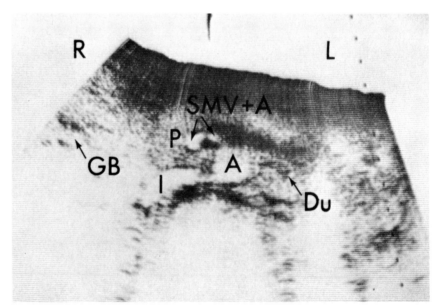

Fig. 7.142

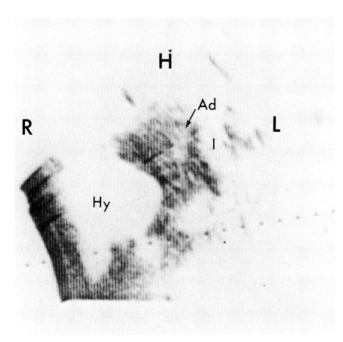

Fig. 7.143

A	= Aorta
Ad	= Left adrenal gland
Cr	= Crus of the diaphragm
Du	= Fourth portion of the duodenum
GB	= Gallbladder
H	= Head
HA	= Hepatic artery
Hy	= Hydronephrosis
I	= Inferior vena cava
K	= Kidney
L	= Left
LK	= Left kidney
LRV	= Left renal vein
LRVB	= Left-renal vascular bundle
P	= Pancreas
PV	= Portal vein
R	= Right
SMA	= Superior mesenteric artery
SMV+A	= Superior mesenteric vein and artery
Sp	= Spleen
St	= Stomach
SV	= Splenic vein

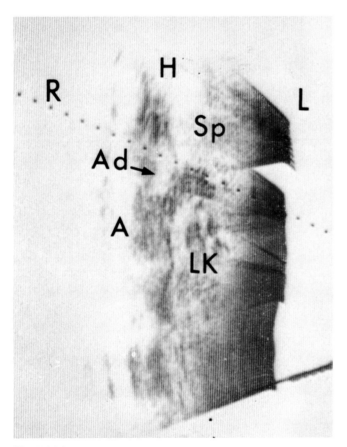

Fig. 7.144

Adrenal Cysts; Adenomas

Pseudocysts of the adrenal gland are the most common type of adrenal cystic disease. They are usually the result of hemorrhage into, or around, the adrenal gland. They may be either secondary to trauma, or in many cases idiopathic. Alternatively, pseudocysts may form secondary to hemorrhage or necrosis into a tumor. A common form of pseudocyst occurs during the neonatal period and is related to adrenal hemorrhage into the gland or the juxtaglandular tissue. Pseudocysts appear as rounded, fluid-containing areas and usually demonstrate all the features of a fluid mass (fig. 7.145). In some cases, however, regions of calcification or a dense clot retraction may persist and give some substance to the cyst wall or account for a solid projection within the fluid (fig. 7.146). In these cases, the presence of a necrotic tumor cannot be excluded, and often a cyst puncture demonstrating cholesterol crystals is necessary. Ultrasound can, however, serve as a guidance procedure for the puncture.

The functioning adenomas causing Cushing's syndrome may vary in size but usually are greater than 2 cm in diameter. With careful scanning techniques, using multiple approaches to identify as much of the surrounding anatomy as possible, very small adrenal adenomas can be demonstrated (fig. 7.147). In cases of larger adenomas, the major task is an exercise in anatomy to demonstrate the organ of origin of the process. To localize the mass to the posterior retroperitoneal area, we must demonstrate a location posterior to the splenic vein and either anterior or superior to the left renal vein (fig. 7.148). In the larger masses, further tissue characterization into cystic, solid, and calcified components can be made on the ultrasonogram (fig. 7.148).

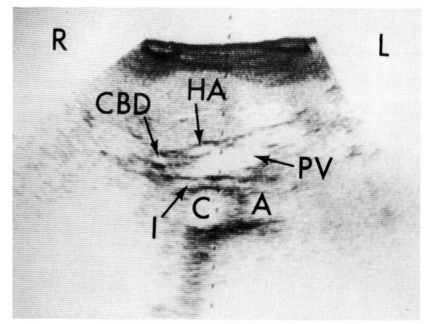

Fig. 7.145

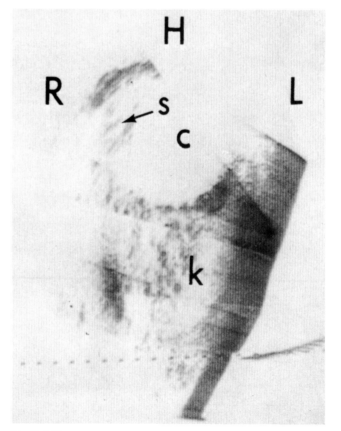

Fig. 7.146

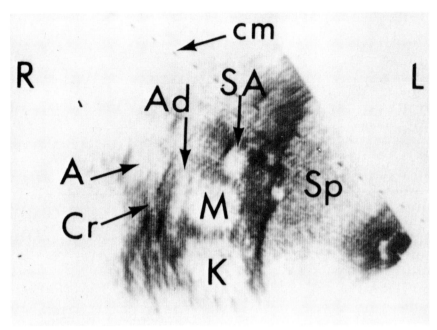

Fig. 7.147

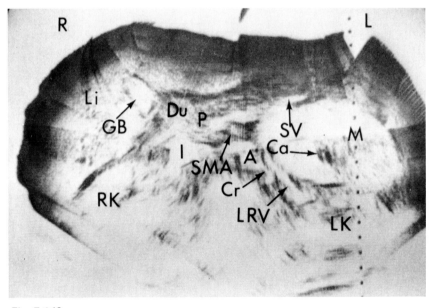

Fig. 7.148

A	=	Aorta
Ad	=	Adrenal adenoma
C	=	Adrenal cyst
Ca	=	Calcium
CBD	=	Common bile duct
cm	=	Centimeter marker
Cr	=	Crus of the diaphragm
Du	=	Duodenum
GB	=	Gallbladder
H	=	Head
HA	=	Hepatic artery
I	=	Inferior vena cava
K	=	Kidney
k	=	Kidney
L	=	Left
Li	=	Liver
LK	=	Left kidney
LRV	=	Left renal vein
M	=	Mass
P	=	Pancreas
PV	=	Portal vein
R	=	Right
RK	=	Right kidney
S	=	Solid elements
SA	=	Splenic artery
SMA	=	Superior mesenteric artery
Sp	=	Spleen
SV	=	Splenic vein

Adrenal Hyperplasia; Pheochromocytoma

Nontumorous hyperplasia of the adrenal glands is one of the more difficult diagnoses to make on ultrasound examination. In Cushing's syndrome, the adrenal glands or contours may not be abnormal in a significant percentage of patients. Nevertheless, in many patients subtle enlargements of the gland can be appreciated by noting the loss of a straight or concave contour to the margins of the gland (figs. 7.149 and 7.150). However, normally sized and contoured adrenal glands in the presence of Cushing's syndrome on ultrasonograms should lead to further evaluation either with adrenal scintigraphy, adrenal angiography, and/or adrenal venous sampling.

Pheochromocytomas are generally medium-sized tumors, usually over 2 cm in diameter. Because of their size, they are usually readily visualized on ultrasonograms when they occur in the adrenal or perirenal regions. The smaller tumors usually appear as rounded masses with a low level of echogenicity (figs. 7.151 and 7.152). Since pheochromocytomas may occur bilaterally in 10% of patients, both adrenal areas must be scanned carefully, even if a mass is already discovered on one side.

Pheochromocytomas may occur in extraadrenal locations such as the periaortic region in either the chest or the abdomen or near the origin of the inferior mesenteric artery in the region of the organ of Zuckerkandl. These latter locations are frequently not well visualized on sonograms due to overlying gas. For this reason, computed tomography is often preferred over ultrasound in the evaluation of pheochromocytomas except among children or pregnant women.

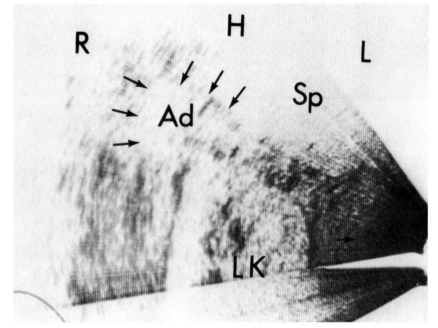

Fig. 7.149

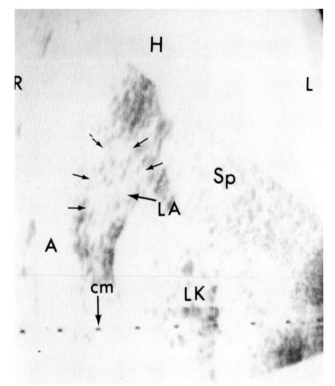

Fig. 7.150

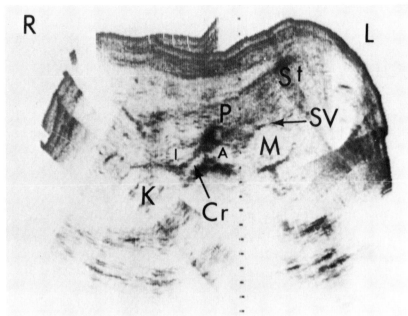

Fig. 7.151

A	=	Aorta
Ad	=	Adrenal gland
Arrows	=	Abnormal adrenal contours
cm	=	Centimeter marker
Cr	=	Crus of the diaphragm
Du	=	Duodenum
F	=	Foot
H	=	Head
I	=	Inferior vena cava
K	=	Kidney
L	=	Left
LA	=	Left adrenal gland
LK	=	Left kidney
M	=	Mass
P	=	Pancreas
R	=	Right
Sp	=	Spleen
St	=	Stomach
SV	=	Splenic vein

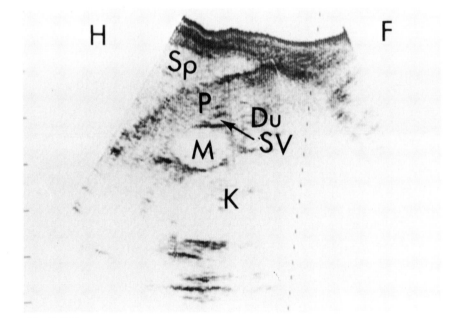

Fig. 7.152

Pheochromocytoma

Pheochromocytomas may be large, bulky tumors. They may demonstrate a number of different consistencies, including solid, cystic, and calcified components. In addition, when they are large, the organ of origin may be difficult to determine, particularly if the clinical syndrome of pheochromocytoma is not appreciated. Nevertheless, close attention to anatomical detail usually will demonstrate the posterior retroperitoneal origin of the process. In the present case (figs. 7.153–7.156), the characteristic elevation of the inferior vena cava, the posteroinferior depression of the kidney with a clean margin between the mass and the right kidney, and the draping of the right renal vein anteriorly over the mass properly localize the process to the right posterior retroperitoneum. Unless this kind of detailed anatomy is identified, the renal, adrenal, or hepatic origin of such a large mass may not be appreciated.

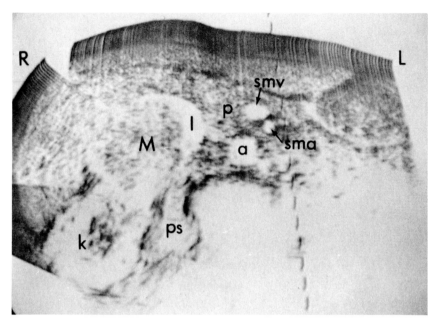

Fig. 7.153

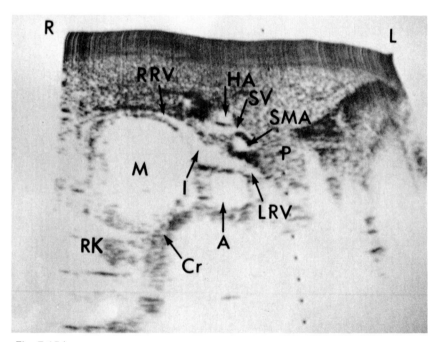

Fig. 7.154

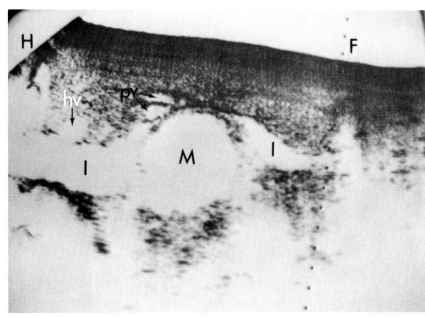

Fig. 7.155

A	=	Aorta
a	=	Aorta
Arrows	=	Borders of the pheochromocytoma
Ca⁺⁺	=	Calcification
Cr	=	Crus of the diaphragm
D	=	Diaphragm
F	=	Foot
H	=	Head
HA	=	Hepatic artery
hv	=	Hepatic vein
I	=	Inferior vena cava
k	=	Kidney
L	=	Left
LRV	=	Left renal vein
M	=	Mass
P	=	Pancreas
p	=	Pancreas
ps	=	Psoas muscle
PV	=	Portal vein
pv	=	Portal vein
R	=	Right
RK	=	Right kidney
RRV	=	Right renal vein
SMA	=	Superior mesenteric artery
sma	=	Superior mesenteric artery
smv	=	Superior mesenteric vein
SV	=	Splenic vein

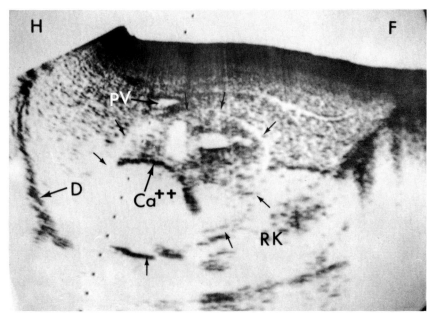

Fig. 7.156

Adrenal Aldosteronoma

Aldosteronomas tend to be small tumors and thereby represent a challenge for both ultrasound and computed body tomography. Furthermore, the clinical syndrome can be secondary to nontumorous hyperplasia or a nodular form of hyperplasia. If the clinical syndrome is caused by a single adenoma, careful scanning in the adrenal areas with close attention to the nearby anatomy can detect a rounded mass frequently only 1.5–2.0 cm in diameter (figs. 7.157–7.160). Since adenomas may be multiple and bilateral, careful scanning of both adrenal glands is necessary. Furthermore, since the adenomas may be very small, even though a mass is discovered on one side and the other side is normal, it may be provident to proceed to venous sampling to ensure that the hypersecretion is unilateral. Finally, since these tumors may be small, it is possible to identify one limb of the adrenal gland as normal with the tumor residing in the other limb (figs. 7.159 and 7.160).

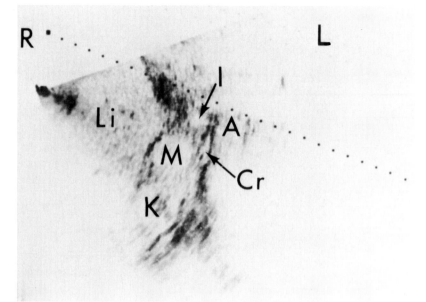

Fig. 7.157

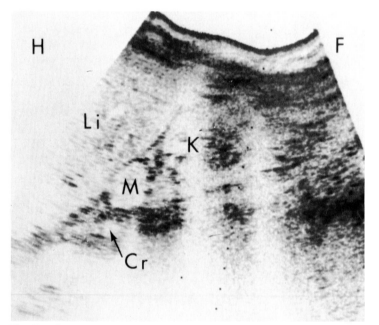

Fig. 7.158

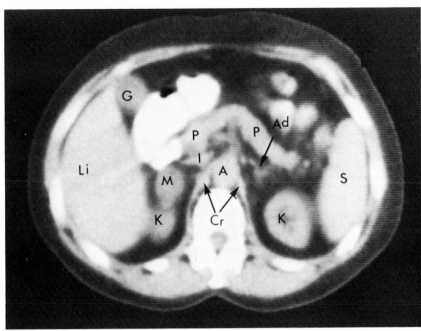

Fig. 7.159

A	=	Aorta
Ad	=	Adrenal gland
Cr	=	Crus of the diaphragm
F	=	Foot
G	=	Gallbladder
H	=	Head
I	=	Inferior vena cava
K	=	Kidney
L	=	Left
Li	=	Liver
M	=	Mass
P	=	Pancreas
R	=	Right
S	=	Spleen

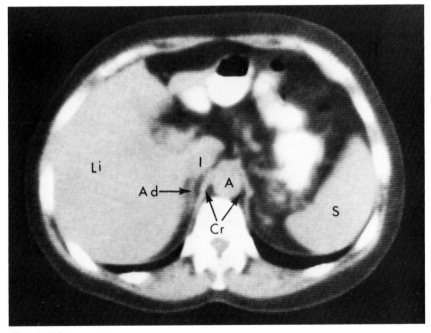

Fig. 7.160

Adrenal Carcinoma and Metastases

Most adrenal carcinomas are not functional; they may, however, account for Cushing's syndrome or hyperaldosteronemia. The major task of the ultrasonographer is to determine the organ of origin of the process. Careful attention to the displacement of vessels, especially the anterior displacement of the splenic vein on the left (fig. 7.161) and the inferior vena cava on the right will usually determine the proper organ of origin. In addition, careful scanning to bring out the specular reflector planes between the surrounding organs will usually minimize any confusion (fig. 7.162).

Adrenal metastases are a relatively common lesion encountered in ultrasonography. They vary substantially in size and echogenicity. Frequently, central necrosis will be present, leading to the development of central fluid areas. The main task for the ultrasonographer, again, is to delineate as much of the surrounding anatomy as possible for proper localization of the origin of the mass (fig. 7.163). Often, metastases in other nearby organs can be identified (fig. 7.164).

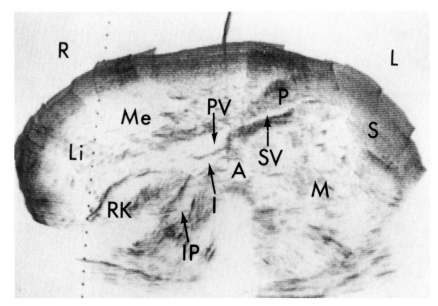

Fig. 7.161

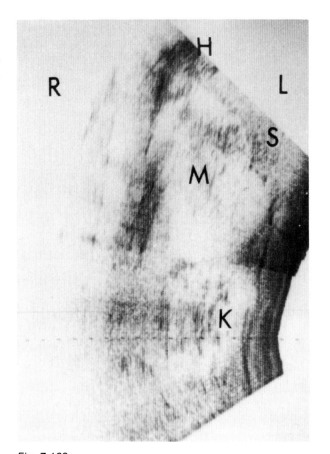

Fig. 7.162

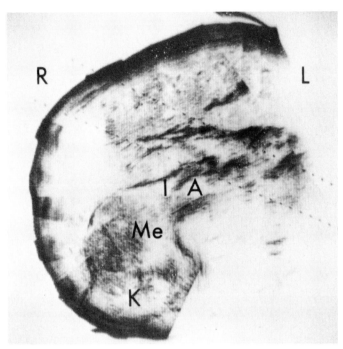

Fig. 7.163

A	=	Aorta
H	=	Head
I	=	Inferior vena cava
IP	=	Iliopsoas muscle
K	=	Kidney
L	=	Left
Li	=	Liver
M	=	Mass
Me	=	Metastases
P	=	Pancreas
PV	=	Portal vein
R	=	Right
RK	=	Right kidney
S	=	Spleen
SV	=	Splenic vein

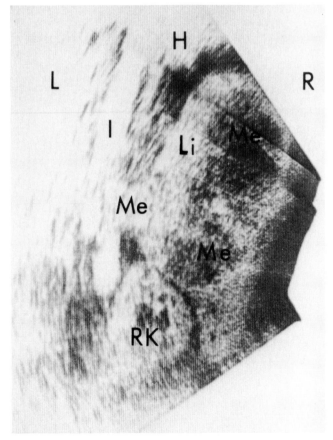

Fig. 7.164

Adrenal Neuroblastoma

Neuroblastoma is the adrenal malignancy of childhood, the second most common tumor of infancy. Approximately 50% of cases originate in the adrenal medulla but also may be found in extra-adrenal locations related to the sympathetic ganglia. Although the children are frequently a symptomatic, neuroblastoma may present as a palpable abdominal mass and must be differentiated from neonatal adrenal hemorrhage and hydronephrosis. The tendency toward microscopic calcification in neuroblastoma usually leads to a relatively solid-appearing echogenic mass that is easily differentiated from adrenal hemorrhage and hydronephrosis (fig. 7.165). The tumors are frequently large and spread by extension to the lymph nodes. In addition, early metastases are frequent to the bones and liver. The latter may be demonstrated on routine sonograms. One of the most important functions of ultrasound in these cases is not only to demonstrate the location of the primary tumor, but also its extension to the retroperitoneal nodes (figs. 7.166–7.168). According to the extent of the primary tumor and local metastases, different forms of therapy may be instituted.

Careful scanning of the high retroperitoneum is necessary to demonstrate displacement of the prevertebral vessels and central retroperitoneal organs. Extension across the midline or bilateral adrenal involvement is important to delineate (fig. 7.168). Ultrasound also may be used to follow the response of the disease to the various types of therapy.

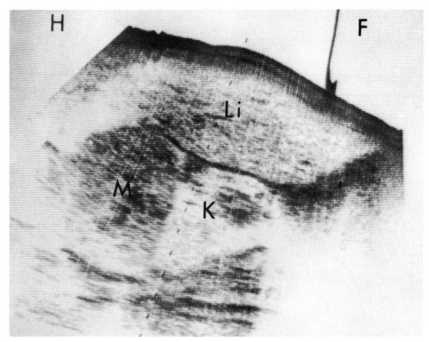

Fig. 7.165

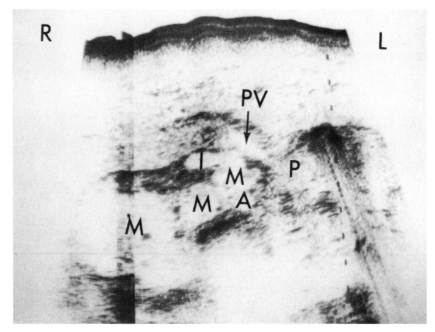

Fig. 7.166

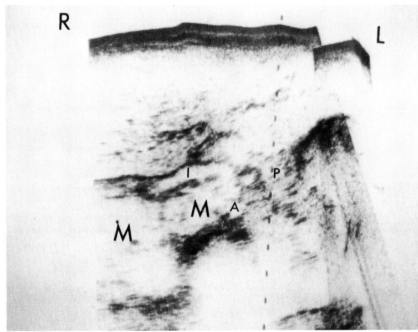

Fig. 7.167

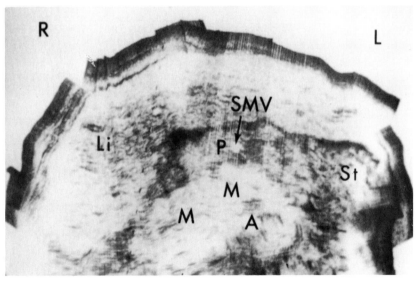

Fig. 7.168

A	=	Aorta
F	=	Foot
H	=	Head
I	=	Inferior vena cava
K	=	Kidney
L	=	Left
Li	=	Liver
M	=	Mass
P	=	Pancreas
PV	=	Portal vein
R	=	Right
SMV	=	Superior mesenteric vein
St	=	Stomach

Normal Retroperitoneum

When evaluating the retroperitoneum, it is extremely important to have a good understanding of its normal anatomy so as not to misdiagnose masses for normal structures. Figure 7.169 is a transverse scan of the retroperitoneum demonstrating the characteristic sonolucencies of the aorta and inferior vena cava. Anterior to the right kidney is a fluid-filled duodenum. This should not be mistaken for a retroperitoneal mass. The head of the pancreas is situated anterior to the inferior vena cava. It gives a fairly characteristic echo pattern which will not be confused for any pathological entity. Often, the fourth portion of the duodenum, situated to the left of the aorta, can be mistaken for a solid mass of the retroperitoneum. The patient may be given fluid or asked to change position in order to make the diagnosis of the duodenum.

Figure 7.170, another transverse scan of the high retroperitoneum, shows the aorta and the inferior vena cava in characteristic locations. There is an area of shadowing situated deep to the falciform ligament within the liver. In this example we see the fourth portion of the duodenum presenting as a circular echogenic mass which could be easily confused for a retroperitoneal or adrenal tumor. Figure 7.171 is a transverse scan in which the inferior vena cava presents as an extremely large sonolucent mass in the retroperitoneum. Deep to the inferior vena cava is the right renal artery draping over an extremely thickened crus of the diaphragm. The crus of the diaphragm often is misdiagnosed as lymphadenopathy. Figure 7.172 is a transverse scan of the abdomen, a little lower than the previous studies. In this scan we see two large paraspinous masses secondary to the iliopsoas muscles. The left iliopsoas is larger than the right and could be mistakenly diagnosed for lymphadenopathy. The orientation of the spine in this case is, however, somewhat unusual. The patient has scoliosis. This explains the marked asymmetry of the iliopsoas muscles.

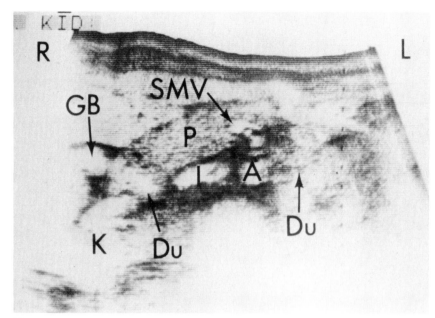

Fig. 7.169

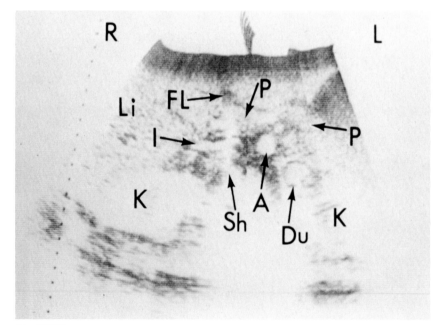

Fig. 7.170

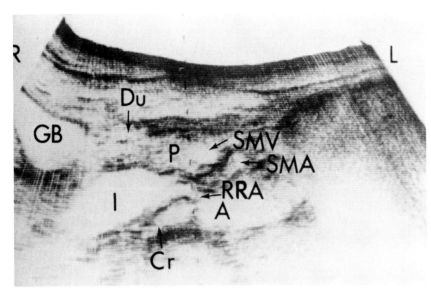

Fig. 7.171

A	=	Aorta
Cr	=	Crus of the diaphragm
Du	=	Duodenum
FL	=	Falciform ligament
GB	=	Gallbladder
I	=	Inferior vena cava
IP	=	Iliopsoas muscle
K	=	Kidney
L	=	Left
Li	=	Liver
P	=	Pancreas
QL	=	Quadratus lumborum muscle
R	=	Right
RRA	=	Right renal artery
Sh	=	Shadowing
SMA	=	Superior mesenteric artery
SMV	=	Superior mesenteric vein
Sp	=	Spine

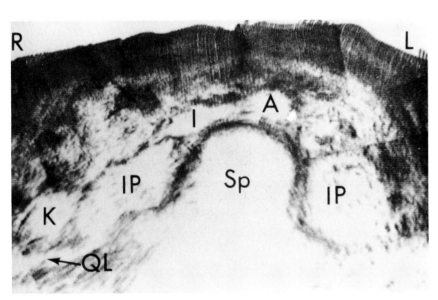

Fig. 7.172

Normal Retroperitoneum

A longitudinal scan of the retroperitoneal region (fig. 7.173) demonstrates a fairly dilated inferior vena cava. Anterior to the inferior vena cava we see the main portal vein and the left portal vein. The sonolucency draining into the inferior vena cava near the superior portion of the liver is secondary to an hepatic vein. The lower portion of the inferior vena cava is extremely close to the skin surface. Near the umbilical level the inferior vena cava is only 2 cm deep.

Figure 7.174 is another longitudinal scan over the inferior vena cava indicating an indentation on its posterior aspect. This is secondary to the right renal artery. The echogenic region deep to the inferior vena cava is secondary to the iliopsoas muscle. The pancreas is seen as an echogenic region anterior to the inferior vena cava.

A longitudinal scan of the retroperitoneum over the aortic region (fig. 7.175) demonstrates a common origin to the celiac artery and superior mesenteric artery. The tubular sonolucency noted anterior to the high abdominal aorta is secondary to the crus of the diaphragm. This is a normal finding and should not be confused for lymphadenopathy. A portion of the aorta is obscured by bowel gas which is common in an abdominal examination. The more caudal portion of the abdominal aorta is well visualized and only 2 cm beneath the skin surface.

Figure 7.176 is another scan of the abdominal aorta in which we see the duodenum and stomach presenting as echogenic masses anterior to the aorta. These should not be confused for lymphadenopathy.

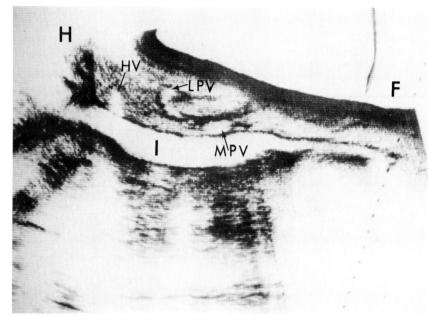

Fig. 7.173

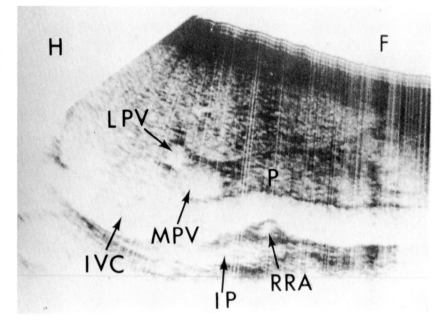

Fig. 7.174

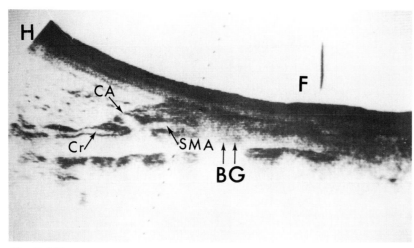

A	= Aorta
BG	= Bowel gas
CA	= Celiac axis
Cr	= Crus of the diaphragm
Du	= Duodenum
F	= Foot
H	= Head
HA	= Hepatic artery
HV	= Hepatic vein
I	= Inferior vena cava
LPV	= Left portal vein
MPV	= Main portal vein
P	= Pancreas
PV	= Portal vein
RRA	= Right renal artery
SMA	= Superior mesenteric artery
St	= Stomach

Fig. 7.175

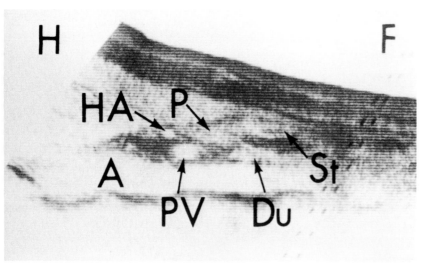

Fig. 7.176

Lymphadenopathy

Ultrasound examination of the retroperitoneum can detect lymphadenopathy, although computed tomography is the diagnostic procedure of choice, for a great deal of the retroperitoneum can be obscured by bowel air when performing an ultrasonic examination. Figures 7.177–7.180 are examples of lymphadenopathy in the high retroperitoneum and porta hepatis region. Figure 7.177 is a transverse scan of the high retroperitoneum in which we see a large mass anterior to the aorta and inferior vena cava. The stomach is displaced anteriorly. This lymphadenopathy, secondary to lymphoma, yielded a solid mass which was somewhat more lucent than the liver. Figure 7.178 is an example of lymphadenopathy in the region of the porta hepatis. The aorta is in a normal location anterior to the spine. In this instance, however, the inferior vena cava is anteriorly displaced. Most of the lymphadenopathy is situated within the porta hepatis. Numerous relatively sonolucent masses surrounding the structures of the porta hepatis are seen. The portal vein, hepatic artery, and common hepatic duct are displaced anteriorly by the enlarged lymph nodes.

Figure 7.179, a longitudinal scan of the abdomen, illustrates tumor involving the caudate lobe and the high retroperitoneum. The important finding in this case is elevation of the superior mesenteric artery above the aorta by a mantle of nodes. Figure 7.180 is another longitudinal scan with multiple nodes beneath the liver. Many of the nodes are relatively lucent. This is a fairly characteristic appearance of lymphadenopathy. Although the nodes are lucent, they do not demonstrate through transmission as would be seen in a fluid-filled structure.

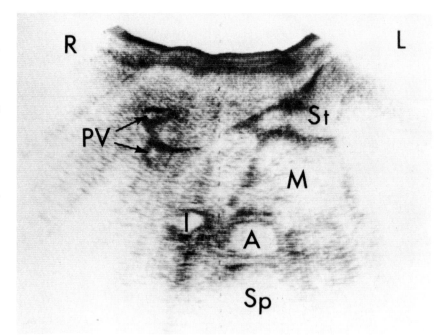

Fig. 7.177

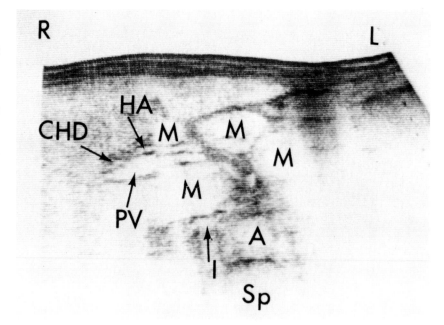

Fig. 7.178

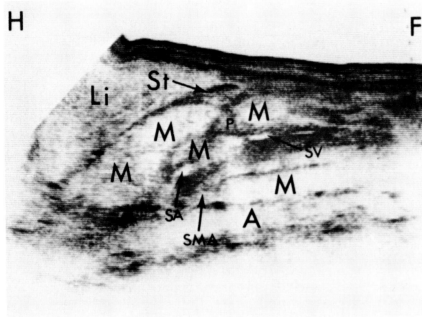

A	=	Aorta
CA	=	Celiac axis
CHD	=	Common hepatic duct
Cr	=	Crus of the diaphragm
Du	=	Duodenum
F	=	Foot
H	=	Head
HA	=	Hepatic artery
I	=	Inferior vena cava
L	=	Left
Li	=	Liver
M	=	Lymphadenopathy
P	=	Pancreas
PV	=	Portal vein
R	=	Right
SA	=	Splenic artery
SMA	=	Superior mesenteric artery
Sp	=	Spine
St	=	Stomach
SV	=	Splenic vein

Fig. 7.179

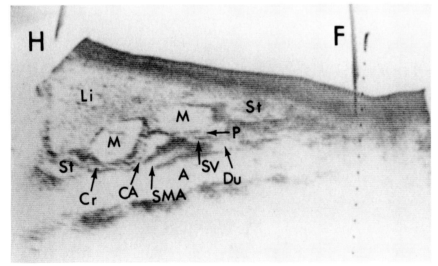

Fig. 7.180

Retroperitoneal Lymphadenopathy

Figures 7.181–7.184 are examples of lymphadenopathy and its relationship to the inferior vena cava. Figure 7.181 is a longitudinal scan of the inferior vena cava which demonstrates a large lymph node on its posterior aspect. This lymph node is actually situated posterior to the right renal artery. It is displacing this vessel and the inferior vena cava anteriorly.

Figure 7.182 is a longitudinal scan demonstrating lymphadenopathy both anterior and posterior to the inferior vena cava. The inferior vena cava is narrowed as it is pinched between the enlarged lymph nodes. Again, the right renal artery is situated anterior to the lymphadenopathy.

An interesting case of testicular carcinoma is found in figure 7.183. Numerous enlarged lymph nodes surround the inferior vena cava. Near the caudal portion of the inferior vena cava, the lymph nodes markedly compress its lumen. Within the lumen of the inferior vena cava is an echogenic mass secondary to thrombus from the tumor.

A transverse scan of the same case (fig. 7.184) demonstrates dramatic lymphadenopathy anterior to the spine. In this instance the lymphadenopathy is elevating the aorta and the inferior vena cava from the spine. The right renal artery is seen to be elevated off the spine, along with the abdominal aorta.

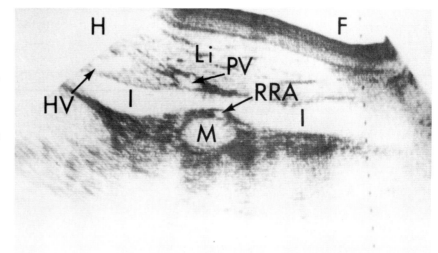

Fig. 7.181

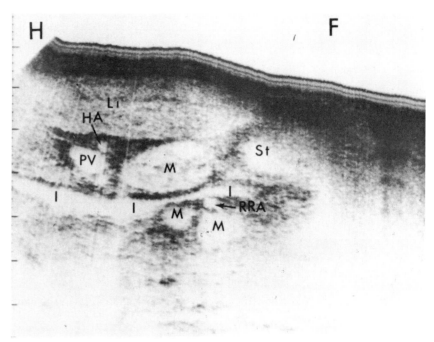

Fig. 7.182

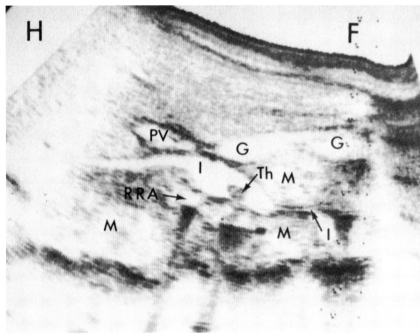

Fig. 7.183

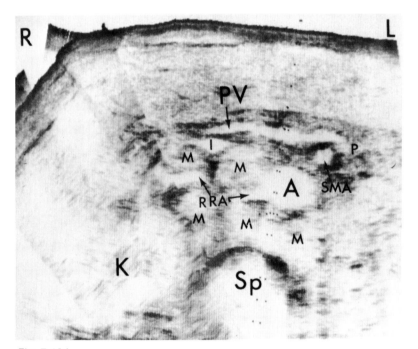

Fig. 7.184

A	=	Aorta
F	=	Foot
G	=	Gallbladder
H	=	Head
HA	=	Hepatic artery
HV	=	Hepatic vein
I	=	Inferior vena cava
K	=	Right kidney
L	=	Left
Li	=	Liver
M	=	Lymphadenopathy
P	=	Pancreas
PV	=	Portal vein
R	=	Right
RRA	=	Right renal artery
SMA	=	Superior mesenteric artery
Sp	=	Spine
St	=	Stomach
Th	=	Metastatic thrombus from testicular tumor

Retroperitoneal Lymphadenopathy

These four figures are examples of retroperitoneal lymphadenopathy involving the left side of the abdomen. Figure 7.185 is a transverse scan of the upper abdomen and retroperitoneum in which we see a large echogenic mass situated posterior to the inferior vena cava. The larger component of the mass, however, is situated to the left of the aorta and posterior to the superior mesenteric artery. The mass is relatively sonolucent and consistent with retroperitoneal lymphadenopathy.

Figure 7.186 illustrates a similar case with a mass situated between the aorta and left kidney. In this instance we can visualize elevation of the left renal vein as it drapes over the retroperitoneal lymphadenopathy. A coronal scan (fig. 7.187) of the same patient is an attempt to visualize the retroperitoneal mass in another plane. The left kidney is situated lateral to this large mass. The mass is seen between the kidney and aorta on this coronal scan.

Figure 7.188 is an example of massive retroperitoneal adenopathy anterior to the aorta, over the left retroperitoneum, and in the region of the porta hepatis. These large sonolucent masses are consistent with lymph node enlargement. In this instance, it is difficult to visualize the lumen of the aorta. This has been previously reported as the ultrasonic silhouette sign in which acoustic interfaces are lost by surrounding tumor tissue. The portal vein is surrounded both anteriorly and posteriorly by lymphadenopathy. The left kidney is displaced posteriorly by the large left-sided retroperitoneal mass.

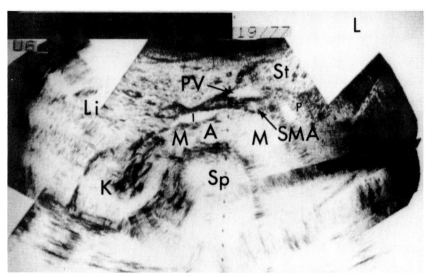

Fig. 7.185

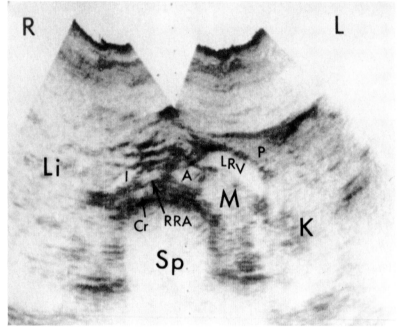

Fig. 7.186

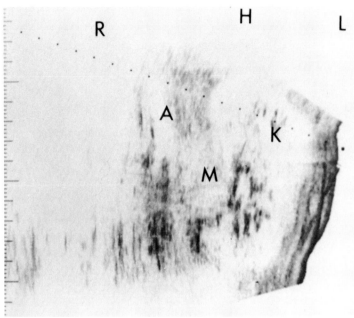

Fig. 7.187

A	= Aorta
Bo	= Bowel
Cr	= Crus of the diaphragm
H	= Head
I	= Inferior vena cava
K	= Kidney
L	= Left
Li	= Liver
LRV	= Left renal vein
M	= Massive lymphadenopathy
P	= Pancreas
PV	= Portal vein
R	= Right
RRA	= Right renal artery
S	= Spleen
SMA	= Superior mesenteric artery
Sp	= Spine
St	= Stomach

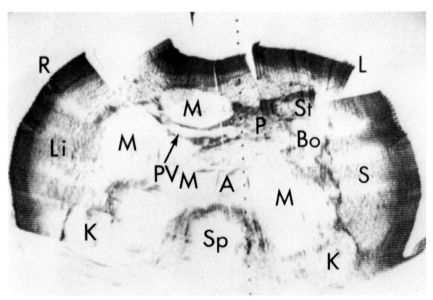

Fig. 7.188

Retroperitoneal Lymphadenopathy

A transverse scan (fig. 7.189) demonstrates a large retroperitoneal mass displacing the aorta to the right side. The left kidney is markedly displaced to the left side of the abdomen and in the position that we usually find the spleen. The spine is not situated in the middle of the abdomen. This patient demonstrated marked asymmetry of the abdomen when scanned by ultrasound. The left side of the abdomen was markedly enlarged, secondary to massive lymphadenopathy.

Figure 7.190 is a coronal scan of a patient with the left kidney displaced laterally by a large mass. Also present within the left kidney is evidence of hydronephrosis. The hydronephrosis was secondary to obstruction of the ureter by this large mass. A transverse scan of the lower abdomen (fig. 7.191) demonstrates a large mass secondary to lymph node enlargement displacing the aorta anteriorly off of the spine. Figure 7.192 is a longitudinal view of the same patient. It dramatically illustrates the abdominal aorta displaced anteriorly off the spine by the retroperitoneal lymphadenopathy.

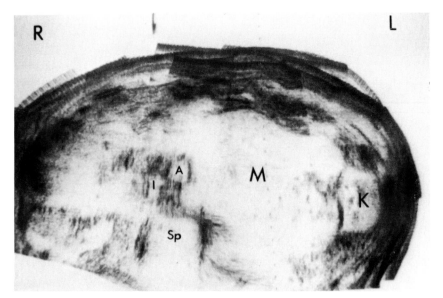

Fig. 7.189

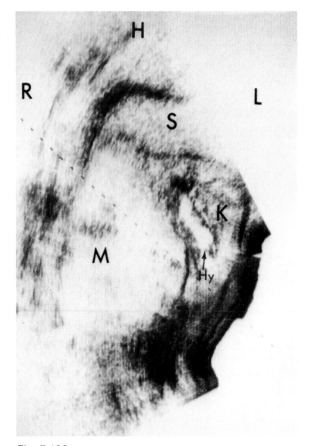

Fig. 7.190

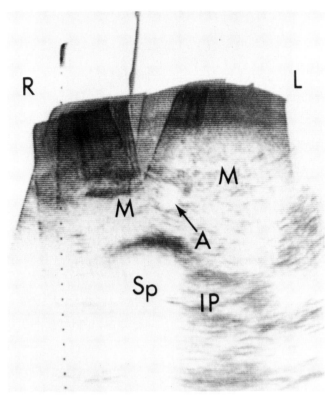

A = Aorta
F = Foot
H = Head
Hy = Hydronephrosis
I = Inferior vena cava
IP = Iliopsoas muscle
K = Kidney
L = Left
M = Lymphadenopathy
R = Right
S = Spleen
Sp = Spine

Fig. 7.191

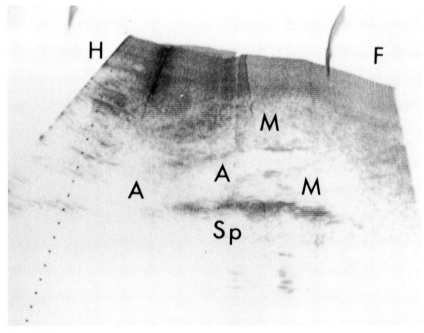

Fig. 7.192

Lymphadenopathy

A transverse scan of the mid abdomen (fig. 7.193) demonstrates multiple sonolucent masses on the left side. These are secondary to mesenteric adenopathy. The aorta is in its normal position, directly anterior to the spine. The lymphadenopathy was within the mesentery. Figure 7.194 is a transverse scan of the retroperitoneum near the bifurcation of the aorta. In this instance, the inferior vena cava is visualized. The massive lymphadenopathy, however, has obscured visualization of the aorta. As mentioned earlier, this is consistent with the ultrasonic silhouette sign.

One anatomical area that can be quite difficult to delineate on ultrasound examination is near the bifurcation of the aorta and inferior vena cava. Since these two vessels bifurcate, numerous circular sonolucencies are visualized at this site. This is also a confusing area on CAT examination. In a transverse scan (fig. 7.195) obtained near the bifurcation of the aorta, the inferior vena cava is visualized in its normal position and before it bifurcates. However, the two circular structures situated anterior and to the left of the inferior vena cava are secondary to the right common iliac artery and the left common iliac artery. An extra mass is present in this region. This represents lymphadenopathy. It is obvious how difficult this area can be to visualize adequately when these vessels begin to bifurcate.

Figure 7.196 is a transverse scan of the right lower quadrant with lymphadenopathy situated anterior to the right iliopsoas muscle. We very often are asked to examine this area to rule out an appendiceal abscess. In this instance, we did find a mass in this patient, secondary to lymphadenopathy.

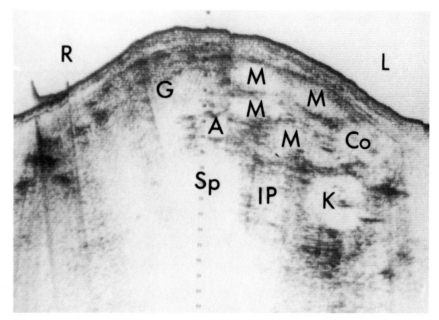

Fig. 7.193

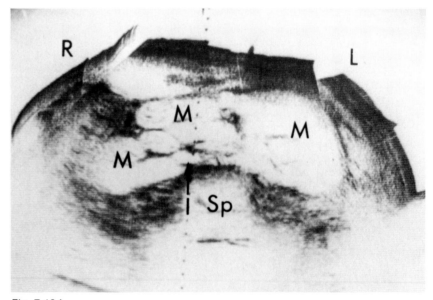

Fig. 7.194

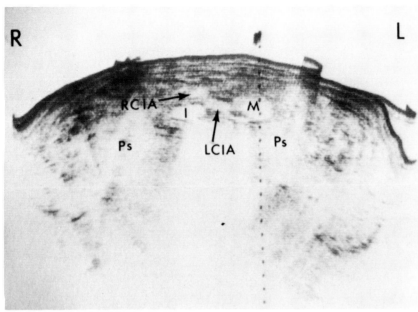

A	=	Aorta
Co	=	Colon
G	=	Bowel gas
I	=	Inferior vena cava
IP	=	Iliopsoas muscle
K	=	Kidney
L	=	Left
LCIA	=	Left-common iliac artery
M	=	Lymphadenopathy
Ps	=	Psoas muscle
R	=	Right
RCIA	=	Right-common iliac artery
Sp	=	Spine

Fig. 7.195

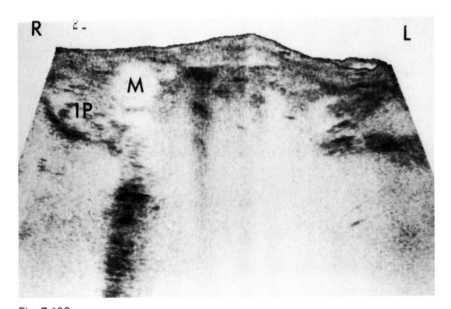

Fig. 7.196

Retroperitoneal Tumors

Although masses arising from lymphadenopathy are the most common cause
for retroperitoneal solid masses on ultrasound, there are other sites of origin
for solid tumors. Figure 7.197 is a transverse scan of a 30-year-old woman who
was known to have extensive retroperitoneal neuroblastoma. In this transverse
scan, we see a large echogenic mass
situated anterior to the aorta and the
inferior vena cava. Two tubular structures are present within the mass, and
those represent the hepatic and splenic
arteries, which are displaced anteriorly
by the retroperitoneal mass. The mass
is solid in nature, with numerous echoes
noted throughout and extensively involving the upper abdomen. The portal
vein is displaced anteriorly by the mass,
along with the right lobe of the liver.

Figure 7.198 is a transverse scan of a
60-year-old woman with a retroperitoneal liposarcoma. In this instance, the
mass is situated posterior to the portal
vein. It is highly echogenic, indicating its
solid nature. The portal vein is displaced
anteriorly as it drapes over the large
retroperitoneal mass.

Figure 7.199 is a transverse scan of a
55-year-old woman with a synovial sarcoma of the lower extremity resected
previously. Follow-up examinations
demonstrated the development of a
large mass in the left upper quadrant.
This eventually was diagnosed as
metastatic synovial sarcoma. A transverse scan of the upper abdomen (fig.
7.199) demonstrates a large mass in the
left upper quadrant. The extent of the
mass is indicated by the asymmetry of
the abdominal wall. It differs from the
previous two in that numerous sonolucent areas are present within it. These
sonolucent areas are secondary to
necrosis and liquifaction of the solid
tumor. It is common for extremely large
masses to have sonolucent areas secondary to necrosis and hemorrhage.

Figure 7.200 is a longitudinal scan of
a 55-year-old man who had a partial
gastrectomy for a leiomyosarcoma. He
was later found to have recurrent leiomyosarcoma. An ultrasound examination was done of the left lateral abdomen. The longitudinal scan shows a

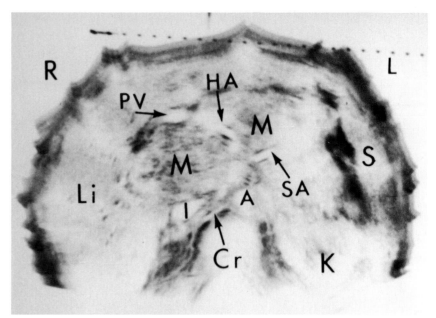

Fig. 7.197

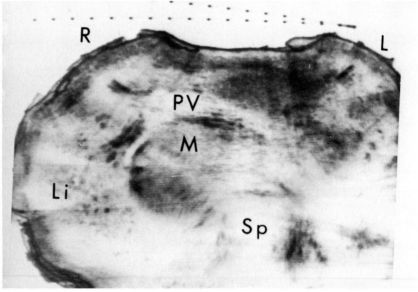

Fig. 7.198

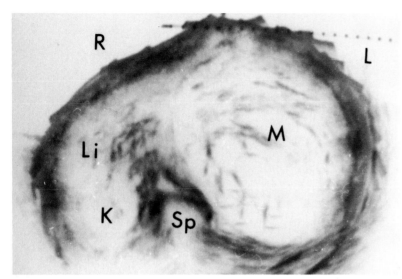

Fig. 7.199

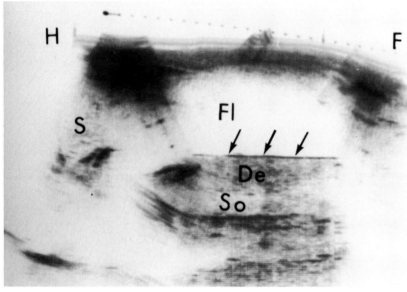

Fig. 7.200

large mass caudal to the spleen. This mass has three components to it. The anterior portion is sonolucent, secondary to fluid. Deep to the fluid area is a highly echogenic region, secondary to debris. A fluid level (arrows) is seen between the fluid and debris. Finally, the deep portion of the mass was solid in nature. This large recurrent leiomyosarcoma shows the various physical ultrasonic appearance of large necrotic tumors.

SOURCE: The cases for figures 7.197–7.200 are provided through the courtesy of Dr. B. Green, M. D. Anderson Hospital, Houston, Texas.

A	=	Aorta
Arrows	=	Fluid level (fig. 7.200)
Cr	=	Crus of the diaphragm
De	=	Debris
F	=	Foot
Fl	=	Fluid
H	=	Head
I	=	Inferior vena cava
K	=	Kidney
Li	=	Liver
M	=	Solid retroperitoneal tumor
PV	=	Portal vein
R	=	Right
S	=	Spleen
SA	=	Splenic artery
So	=	Solid component to the tumor
Sp	=	Spine

Psoas Abscess

When evaluating the retroperitoneum, large fluid-filled masses may be detected by ultrasound. The following cases are examples of psoas abscesses.

Figure 7.201 is a transverse scan with a large fluid-filled mass representing a psoas abscess anterior to the iliopsoas muscle. Ultrasound techniques could not distinguish this from a hematoma, urinoma, lymphocele, or other fluid-filled collection. Figure 7.202 is a longitudinal scan with a large psoas abscess situated inferior to the lower pole of the right kidney. Again, this sonolucent mass could be consistent with other fluid-filled structures. The findings of some internal echoes on the back wall are highly suggestive of either an abscess or a hematoma.

Figures 7.203 and 7.204 are scans of a different patient that demonstrate an extremely unusual ultrasonic finding. In figure 7.203 a psoas abscess situated on the left side, lateral to the spine, is seen. Normal iliopsoas muscle is seen on the right side, at the level of the transverse colon. Scanning more caudally, the abscess took on a bilobed appearance (fig. 7.204). This most likely indicates the continuation of the psoas abscess into the psoas and iliacus muscles.

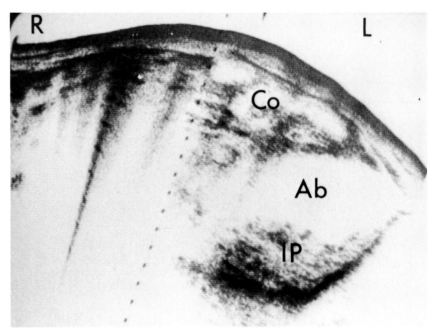

Fig. 7.201

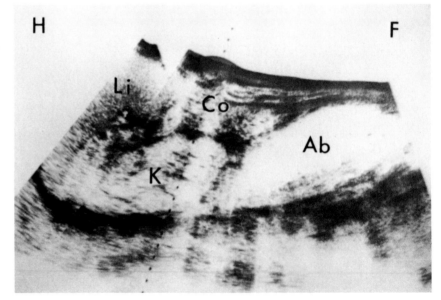

Fig. 7.202

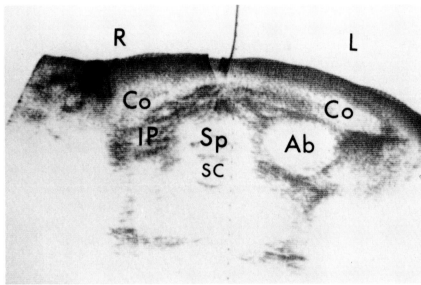

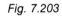
Fig. 7.203

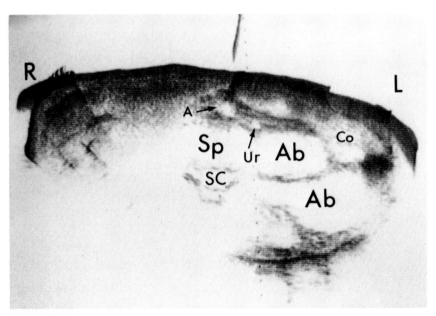

Fig. 7.204

A	=	Aorta
Ab	=	Abscess
Co	=	Colon
F	=	Foot
H	=	Head
IP	=	Iliopsoas muscle
K	=	Kidney
L	=	Left
Li	=	Liver
R	=	Right
SC	=	Spinal canal
Sp	=	Spine
Ur	=	Ureter

Perinephric Abscess and Hematoma

Ultrasound is an excellent means for evaluating the perinephric region for any fluid collection. Figures 7.205 and 7.206 are scans obtained from an extremely unusual case with rather dramatic ultrasound findings. The patient was in an automobile acident approximately 2 weeks prior to admission. She noted the gradual increase in the size of her abdomen on the right side over a 2-week period. Figure 7.205 is a transverse scan of the right abdomen at the time of admission. We see a large relatively sonolucent mass in the right abdomen. Marked asymmetry of the abdominal wall is indicated by the surface echoes. The spine is situated somewhat to the left of midline. This mass has through transmission present. Within it are some echoes indicating that it is not completely fluid. The findings would be consistent with a hematoma or an abscess.

At surgery, an infected hematoma was found. The dramatic finding was noted in figure 7.206, a longitudinal scan over the midline. The aorta is well seen along with the splenic vein, pancreas, and superior mesenteric artery. Situated anterior to the pancreas is the right kidney displaced over the midline by the large infected hematoma. Although the kidney and pancreas are retroperitoneal organs, it is amazing how far they can be displaced in the retroperitoneum.

Figure 7.207 is a transverse scan of a patient with a large left perinephric abscess. The right kidney is in normal position, adjacent to the spine. The left kidney is displaced anteriorly and laterally by a large perinephric collection. Figure 7.208 is a transverse scan of another patient with a large sonolucent collection representing a retroperitoneal hematoma. In this instance the left kidney is displaced medially and anteriorly. The borders of the kidney are difficult to see, since the hematoma involved a portion of the posterior aspect of the kidney.

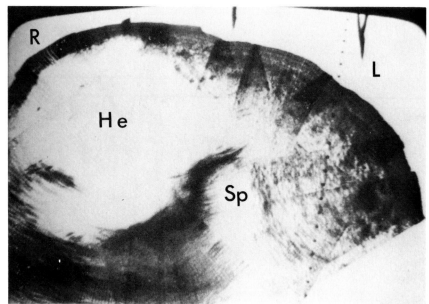

Fig. 7.205

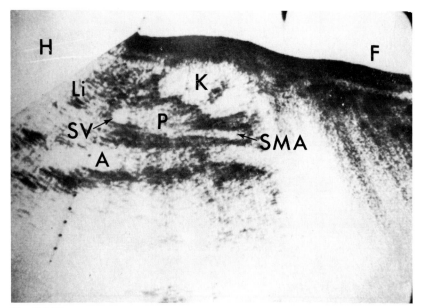

Fig. 7.206

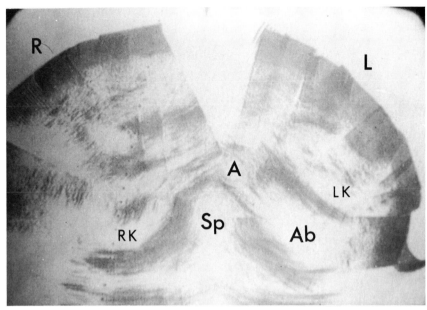

Fig. 7.207

A	= Aorta
Ab	= Abscess
Du	= Duodenum
F	= Foot
GB	= Gallbladder
H	= Head
He	= Right retroperitoneal hematoma
I	= Inferior vena cava
K	= Kidney
L	= Left
Li	= Liver
LK	= Left kidney
P	= Pancreas
R	= Right
RK	= Right kidney
SMA	= Superior mesenteric artery
SMV	= Superior mesenteric vein
Sp	= Spine
St	= Stomach
SV	= Splenic vein

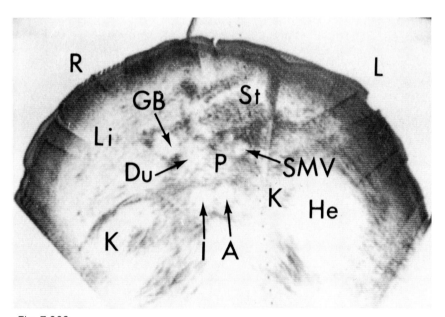

Fig. 7.208

Retroperitoneal Lymphoceles

Lymphoceles usually present as fluid collections within the abdomen. Usually, they are basically echo-free. They may, however, demonstrate echoes secondary to debris and fibrosis. Figures 7.209 and 7.210 are examples of large lymphoceles following retroperitoneal lymph node resection. In figure 7.209, a large fluid collection is noted just beneath the umbilical level. A second fluid collection is present just above the urinary bladder. This lower fluid collection, however, has some echoes within it when compared to the more cephalad collection. Figure 7.210 is a transverse scan of the lymphocele in the umbilical region. The fluid is completely echo-free, draping over the abdominal aorta.

Figure 7.212 is a lymphocele with multiple echoes within it. This would be difficult to distinguish from an abscess or hematoma. It did represent a lymphocele with debris. The lymphocele was causing hydronephrosis of the right kidney (fig. 7.211).

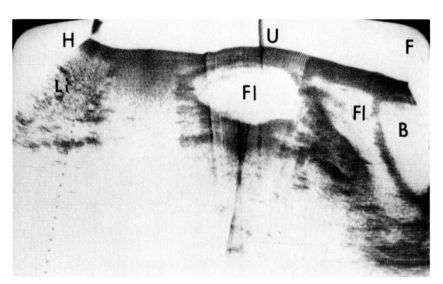

Fig. 7.209

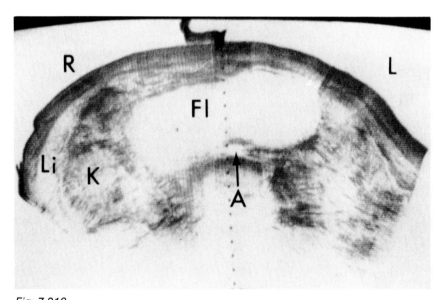

Fig. 7.210

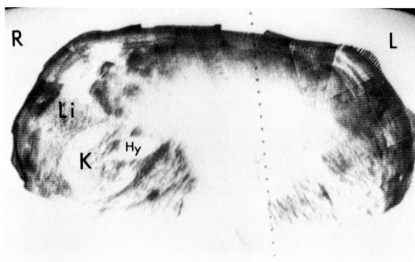

Fig. 7.211

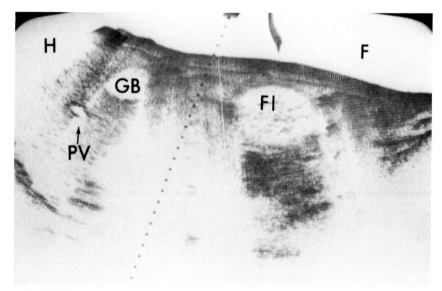

Fig. 7.212

A = Aorta
B = Urinary bladder
F = Foot
FI = Fluid in the lymphocele
GB = Gallbladder
H = Head
Hy = Hydronephrosis
K = Kidney
L = Left
Li = Liver
PV = Portal vein
R = Right
U = Umbilical level

The Normal Scrotum

Examination of the normal scrotum easily can be performed with conventional contact scanners. The scrotum is supported on a rolled towel and is gently scanned in the transverse planes without stabilization (figs. 7.213 and 7.214). The median raphe represents a highly attenuative area, on either side of which the finely granular echogenicity of the glandular elements of the testes can be seen. The ductus deferens is visualized along the posterior medial aspect of each testis as a relatively circular echofree area. The epididymis is not usually resolved normally, but it passes on the posterolateral aspect of the testes. Five-MHz transducers usually are used with a short internal focus. The slightly increased level of echogenicity at the focal plane can frequently be appreciated on the scans (fig. 7.214).

Longitudinal scans of the testes are usually best performed with a contact scanner after the palpable epididymis has been aligned directly posterior to the glandular elements of the testes. The scrotum is stabilized in this position, and the longitudinal scan is performed (fig. 7.215). More recently, high resolution real-time systems with a built-in water delay have become available. The field of view is considerably smaller (3 x 4 cm), but the degree of detail is rather remarkable (fig. 7.216). The superficial scrotal areas can be appreciated, and the potential space created by the tunica vaginalis can often be seen as an echogenic line. The fine homogeneous texture of the glandular elements of the testes is even more evident.

In an evaluation of the scrotum, symmetry is the key as in any paired organ. Most of the time, the testes are symmetrical unless there has been atrophy related to a previous insult such as a mumps orchitis or trauma.

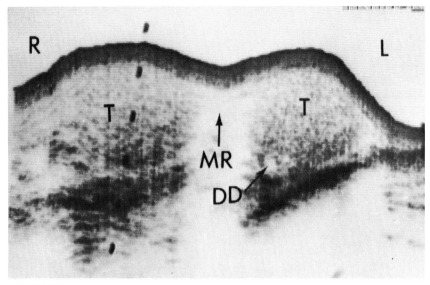

Fig. 7.213

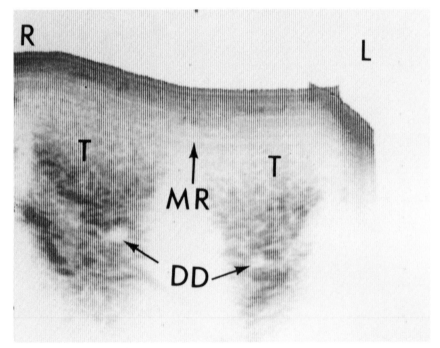

Fig. 7.214

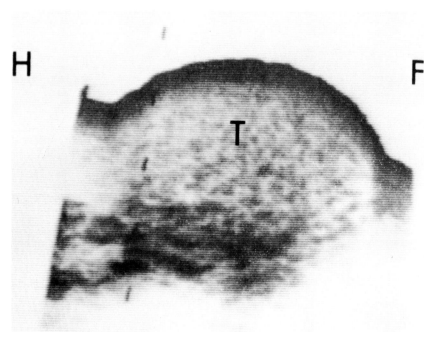

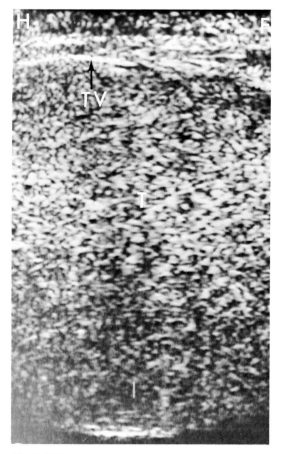

DD = Ductus deferens
F = Foot
H = Head
L = Left
MR = Median raphe
R = Right
T = Testis
TV = Tunica vaginalis

Fig. 7.215

Fig. 7.216

Epididymitis

In uncomplicated acute epididymitis, the ductus deferens and epididymis are enlarged as a result of the inflammatory process. In addition, the epididymal area loses echogenicity, and on sonograms the epididymis appears as a nonechogenic cord running along the underside of the glandular elements of the testes (figs. 7.217 and 7.218). Careful scanning is required to ensure a tissue plane between the epididymis and the testis.

In some patients, a focal area of orchitis may develop adjacent to the epididymis, particularly in the rete testis region (fig. 7.219). This pattern is indistinguishable from an occult neoplasm which may be the underlying etiology to the epididymitis. These two entities can be distinguished only after serial examination following antibiotic therapy. In the case of acute epididymitis associated with focal orchitis, the echogenicity of the epididymal area will return, and the glandular elements of the testes will return to a normal homogenous texture (fig. 7.220).

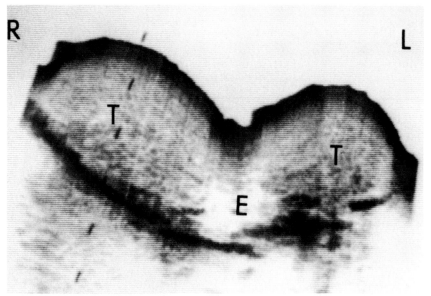

Fig. 7.217

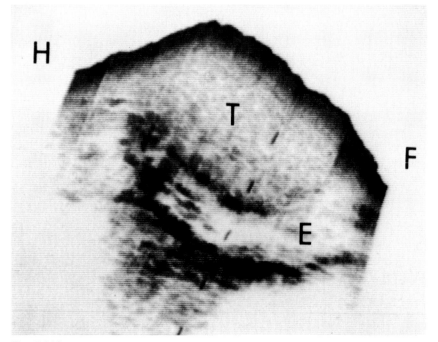

Fig. 7.218

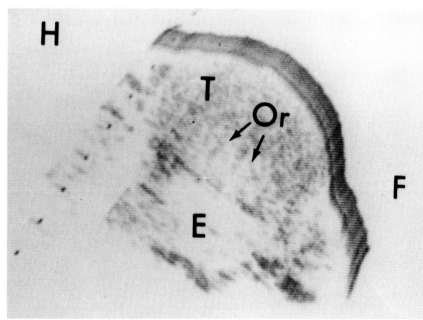

Fig. 7.219

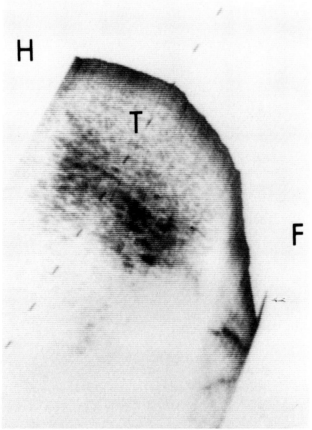

Fig. 7.220

E = Epididymis
F = Foot
H = Head
L = Left
Or = Orchitis
R = Right
T = Glandular elements of testes

Acute Epididymitis in Association with an Occult Neoplasm

Neoplasms of the testis may present initially as acute epididymitis. On ultrasonogram, the thickened epididymis with the decreased echogenicity characteristic of epididymitis will be observed (figs. 7.221 and 7.222). Usually, multiple tomographic scans of the testes will demonstrate an indistinct junction between the epididymis and testis (fig. 7.222) or a focal abnormality in the texture of the glandular elements of the testis. As indicated in the previous case, such a finding can also be due to associated orchitis. In the case of an underlying tumor, however, serial examination after antibiotic therapy will demonstrate no resolution of the junctional zone between the testis and epididymis and frequently will show further evidence of focal texture abnormalities within the testis (figs. 7.223 and 7.224).

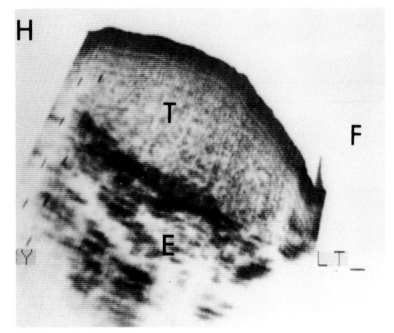

Fig. 7.221

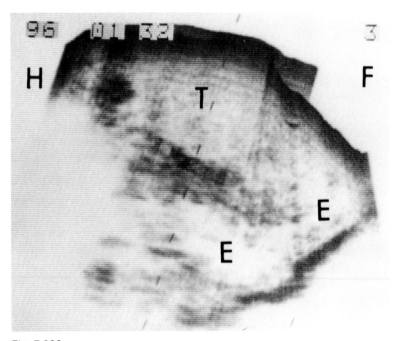

Fig. 7.222

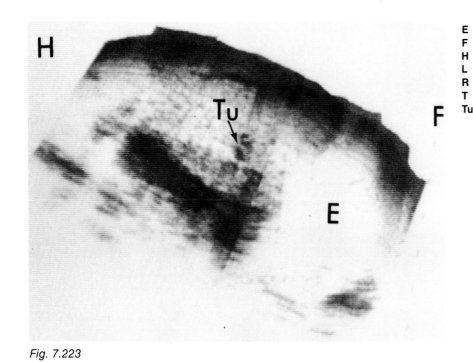

E = Epididymis
F = Foot
H = Head
L = Left
R = Right
T = Glandular elements of testis
Tu = Tumor

Fig. 7.223

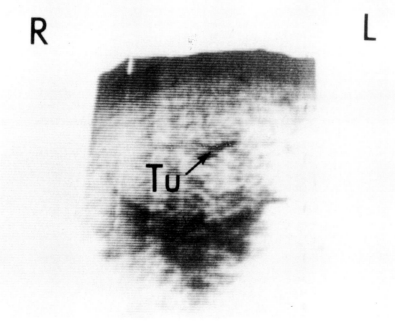

Fig. 7.224

Epididymitis and Reactive Hydrocele

During an acute episode of epididymitis, a reactive hydrocele may form. In most cases, this is identified as a simple fluid area with fairly smooth margins and no internal echogenicity (figs. 7.225 and 7.226). The abnormally thickened epididymis also is identified.

During a more severe form of epididymitis, the reactive hydrocele may take on an irregular configuration with multiple septations and adhesions (figs. 7.227 and 7.228). Although the acoustic texture of the glandular elements of the testes remains normal, this type of fluid collection is indistinguishable from a periepididymal abscess. The complex types of reactive hydroceles usually require either aspiration or surgical exploration for differentially diagnostic purposes.

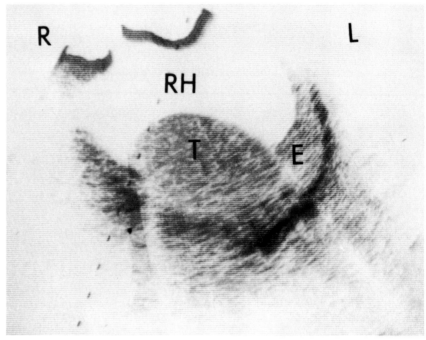

Fig. 7.225

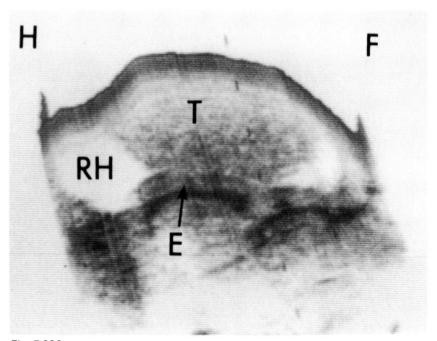

Fig. 7.226

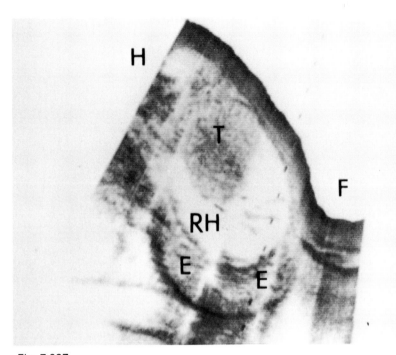

E = Epididymis
F = Foot
H = Head
L = Left
R = Right
RH = Reactive hydrocele
T = Glandular elements of testis

Fig. 7.227

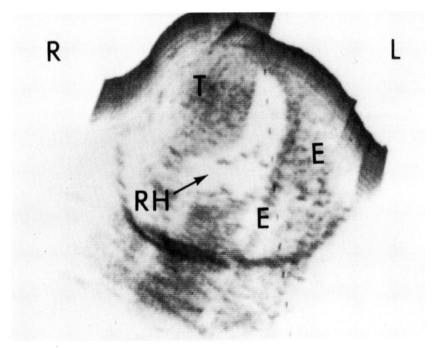

Fig. 7.228

Epididymitis with Reactive Hydrocele and Abscess

The difficulty in distinguishing an un-complicated reactive hydrocele from a peritesticular abscess in association with acute epididymitis is illustrated by the following two cases. Figures 7.229 and 7.230 represent a noninfected re-active hydrocele, whereas figure 7.231 represents a peritesticular abscess. The normal opposite scrotum is provided for comparison (fig. 7.232). In both cases, the glandular elements of the testis are normal. The surrounding fluid collec-tions contain some irregularities of the wall, scattered debris, and internal sep-tations. In cases of an associated testic-ular abscess, the acoustic texture of the glandular elements of the testis become abnormal. In all of these patterns, surgi-cal exploration is usually required for a final differential diagnosis and treat-ment.

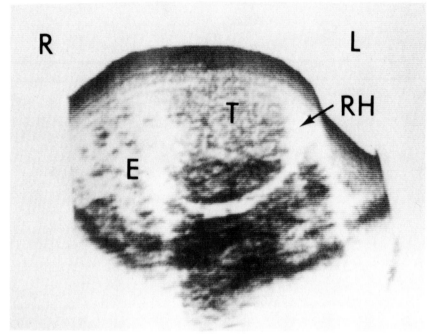

Fig. 7.229

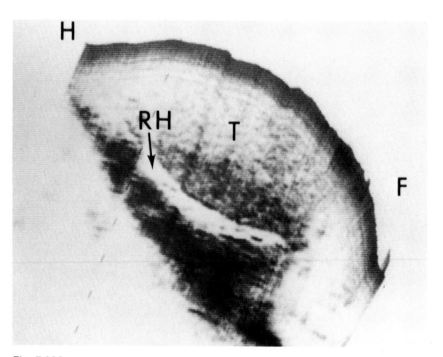

Fig. 7.230

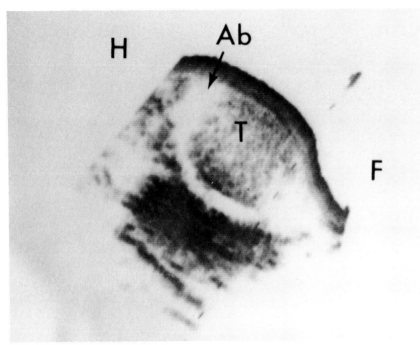

Fig. 7.231

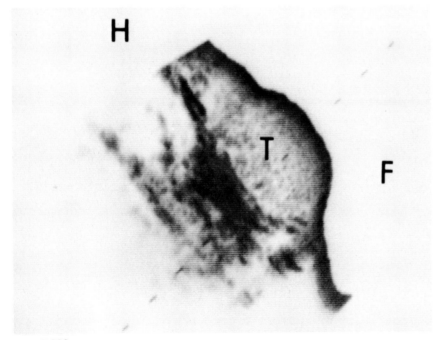

Fig. 7.232

Ab = Abscess
E = Epididymis
F = Foot
H = Head
L = Left
R = Right
RH = Reactive hydrocele
T = Glandular elements of testis

Acute Scrotal Torsion and Trauma

Two frequently encountered pathologies in the differential diagnosis of the acutely enlarged scrotum are acute torsion and acute scrotal trauma. Acute torsion of the testes may demonstrate a number of ultrasonic patterns. In some cases, the entire scrotal contents are abnormal in organization and texture (fig. 7.233). All layers of the scrotum seem involved, and a reactive hydrocele may be present. In addition, the acoustic texture of the glandular elements of the testes is usually abnormal. This picture may mimic that of a testicular abscess.

In other cases of acute torsion the actual twisted vascular pedicle can be resolved (fig. 7.234). The consistent abnormality in torsion of the testes is a lack of attachment of the epididymis to the scrotal tissues. This provides a pedicle upon which torsion can occur. The typical features of involvement of the entire scrotum, a reactive hydrocele, and an abnormal acoustic texture to the glandular elements of the testes again are seen.

In the evaluation of acute trauma to the scrotum, the viability of the testes must be established. Careful comparative scanning of the scrotum in a case with a viable testis with a hemorrhagic hydrocele demonstrates the complex mass surrounding the glandular elements of the testis, this represents the hemorrhagic hydrocele. In addition, the two testes appear equal in size and acoustic texture (figs. 7.235 and 7.236). If any abnormality in testicular texture is noted, the probability of damage to the glandular elements of the testes is increased.

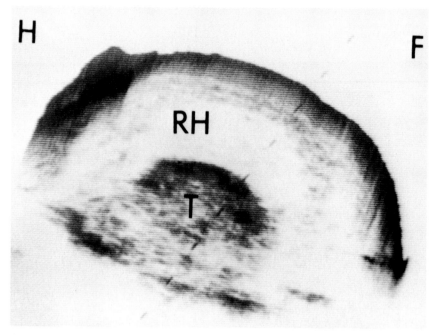

Fig. 7.233

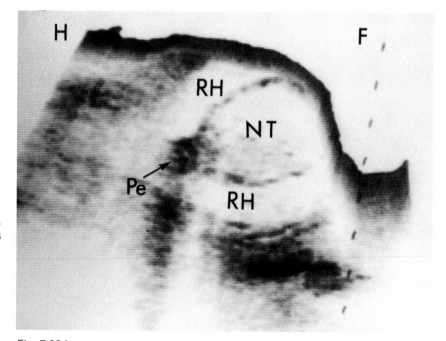

Fig. 7.234

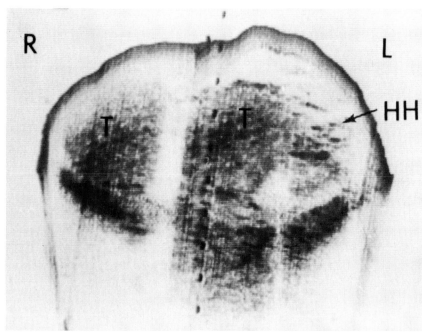

F = Foot
H = Head
HH = Hemorrhagic hydrocele
L = Left
NT = Necrotic testis
Pe = Vascular pedicle
R = Right
RH = Reactive hydrocele
T = Glandular elements of testis

Fig. . .235

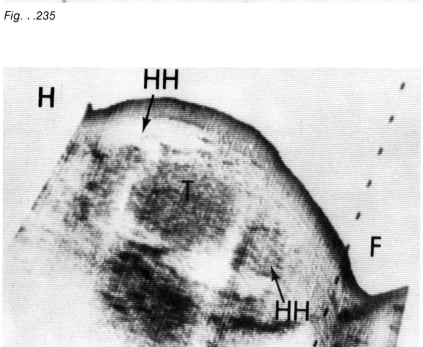

Fig. 7.236

Chronic Scrotal Epididymitis; Spermatocele

Chronic epididymitis and spermatocele frequently present as chronic enlargements of the scrotum. The extratesticular nature of the process, although frequently difficult to ascertain clinically, can be determined in 80% of cases on ultrasonogram. In chronic epididymitis, a focal or generalized thickening of the epididymis is noted. The cleavage plane between the epididymis and glandular elements of the testes should be preserved. If this finding is not demonstrated on the sonogram, the possibility of an underlying occult neoplasm cannot be ruled out. Uncomplicated chronic epididymitis usually presents as a solid type of epididymal thickening (figs. 7.237 and 7.238).

Another common scrotal mass is the spermatocele (figs. 7.239 and 7.240). It appears as a cystic accumulation of sperm, usually in a ductule leading from the epididymis to the testes, near the head of the epididymis. These accumulations may arise as a result of trauma or as a sequela to chronic epididymitis (fig. 7.240). In the case of the latter, findings of chronic epididymitis will frequently be present. Spermatoceles are usually round and do not deform the glandular elements of the testis.

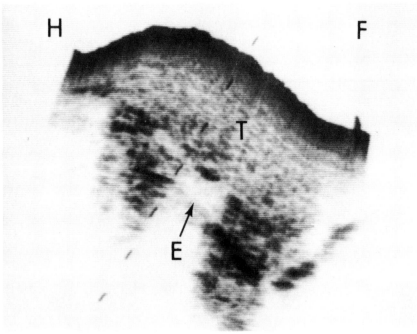

Fig. 7.237

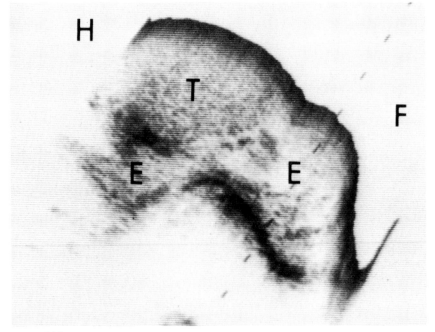

Fig. 7.238

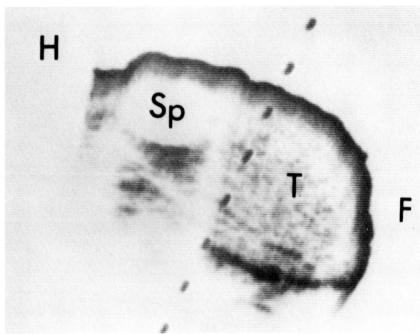

Fig. 7.239

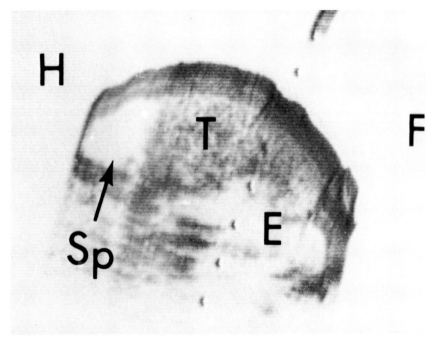

Fig. 7.240

E   = Epididymis
F   = Foot
H   = Head
Sp = Spermatocele
T   = Glandular elements of testis

Chronic Scrotal Epididymal Cyst; Varicocele

Another common sequela to epididymitis is the development of small cysts along the course of the epididymis (figs. 7.241 and 7.242). The fluid collections are usually well circumscribed and reside along the course of the epididymis. They may contain some wall thickness or internal debris. Because of their close proximity to the rete testis area, they may deform the testis to the extent that the extratesticular nature of the process is difficult to ascertain. Other sequelae of epididymitis, such as a spermatocele, also may be visualized (fig. 7.242).

A similar feeling mass clinically may be observed in the case of varicocele. In this instance, one or more veins within the ductus deferens and spermatic cord may be dilated and appear as serpiginous fluid areas along the posterior aspect of the scrotum (figs. 7.243 and 7.244). Although the ultrasonic picture may simulate that of chronic epididymitis or an epididymal cyst, there is usually little deformity of the glandular elements of the testis.

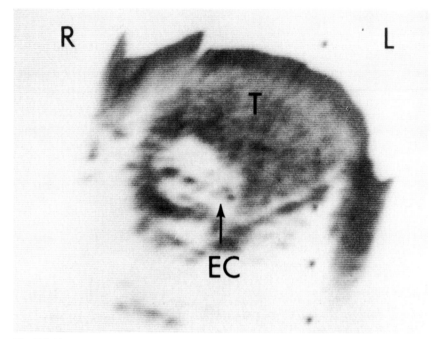

Fig. 7.241

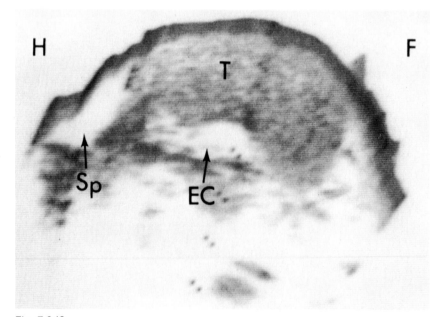

Fig. 7.242

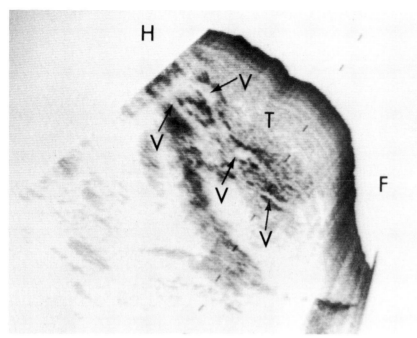

Fig. 7.243

EC = Epididymal cyst
F = Foot
H = Head
L = Left
R = Right
Sp = Spermatocele
T = Glandular elements of testis
V = Varix

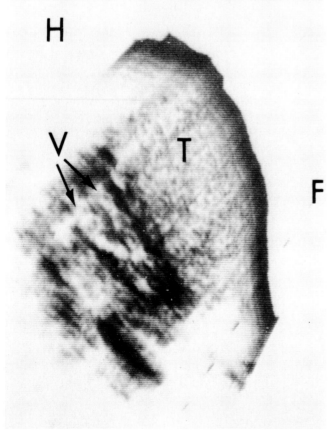

Fig. 7.244

Chronic Scrotal Hydrocele

Hydroceles are probably the most commonly encountered scrotal masses. Frequently, the simple fluid nature of the mass can be ascertained by transillumination. A surprising number of hydroceles, however, do not transilluminate, making the clinical distinction from a malignant process difficult. Furthermore, the tense nature of the hydrocele may give the scrotum a rock-hard feeling. The hallmark of a simple hydrocele on ultrasonogram is the presence of a simple fluid collection surrounding the testes, with the exception of the area of attachment to the scrotum in the region of the epididymis (figs. 7.245 and 7.246). Since hydroceles may be congenital or associated with prior trauma, infection, or occult neoplasms, careful analysis of the acoustic texture of the glandular elements of the testes is important. In this regard, it should be recalled that the relative echogenicity of the testes beyond the fluid area may appear different from the opposite testis, just on the basis of the inappropriate time-gain compensation through the fluid. Therefore, the time-gain compensation must frequently be changed to assess more accurately the true texture. Another technique is to manually compress the fluid in front of the testis and rescan the patient.

In the presence of a hydrocele, considerably more detail may be seen around the head of the epididymis (figs. 7.247 and 7.248). Either the entire head may be visualized, or the vestigial appendages of the appendix epididymis and appendix testis may be resolved. A rather dramatic amount of detail may be appreciated with the newer high-resolution, small-field view scanners (fig. 7.248).

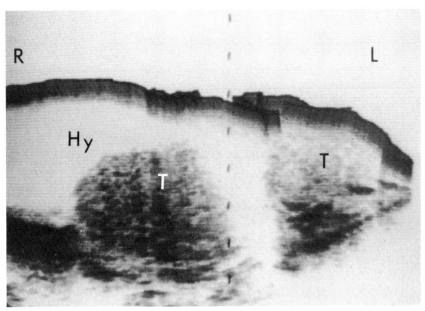

Fig. 7.245

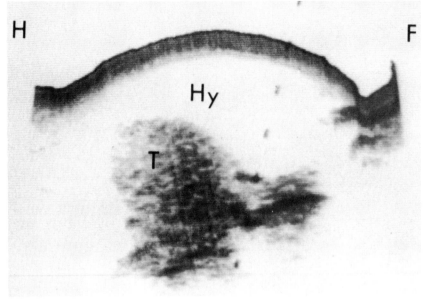

Fig. 7.246

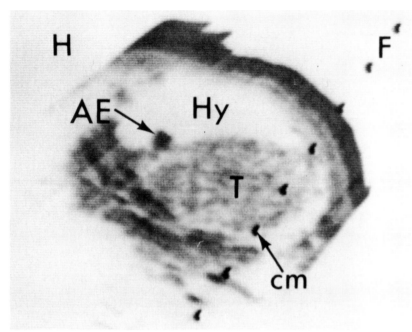

Fig. 7.247

AE = Appendix epididymis
AT = Appendix testis
cm = Centimeter marker
E = Epididymis
F = Foot
H = Head
Hy = Hydrocele
L = Left
R = Right
T = Glandular elements of testis

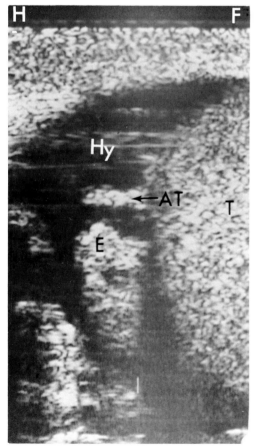

Fig. 7.248

Chronic Primary Testicular Tumors

Testicular tumors present as masses generally confined to the glandular elements of the testes. Usually, there is focal or generalized enlargement of the testis within the scrotum without significant alteration of the surrounding layers and epididymis, unless associated epididymitis is present. The key ultrasonic feature is the inhomogeneity of the acoustic texture of the testis with areas of decreased and increased reflectivity (figs. 7.249 and 7.250). Occasionally, minimal enlargement of the testis is evident, but with a diffusely abnormal, generally decreased echogenicity, as compared to the opposite side (fig. 7.251). On rare occasions, a primary testicular tumor will present as a predominantly cystic mass with some septations and internal solid elements (fig. 7.252). This pattern has made the differential diagnosis of testicular neoplasm extremely difficult.

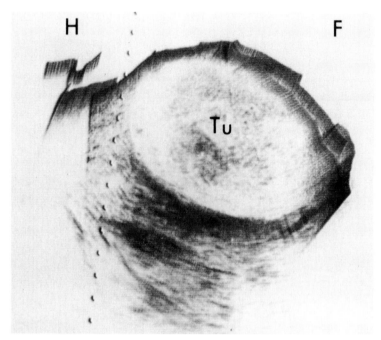

Fig. 7.249

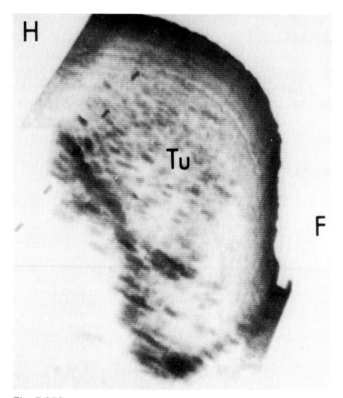

Fig. 7.250

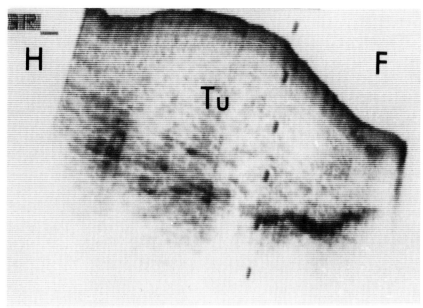

F = Foot
H = Head
T = Glandular elements of testis
Tu = Tumor

Fig. 7.251

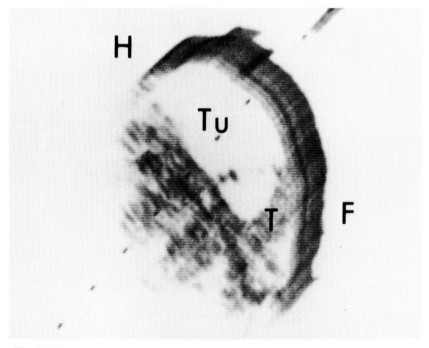

Fig. 7.252

Mimicing Testicular Tumors

A number of benign chronic scrotal processes, because of their combined testicular and extratesticular appearance, mimic primary neoplasms of the testis. Hydroceles, particularly when they are posttraumatic or sequelae of epididymitis, may be so large or so deforming that they can mimic the cystic type of primary testicular neoplasm (figs. 7.253 and 7.254). A history of trauma cannot often be elicited, and surgical exploration is necessary for a final diagnosis.

Similarly, the various stages of subacute and chronic torsion can present as mixed or solid scrotal masses which appear in part to involve the testis (figs. 7.255 and 7.256). The ultrasonic patterns may be bizarre, presenting with mixed cystic and solid components or as solid components markedly deforming the residual testicular elements. Again, in a surprising number of cases, the acute episode is never noted historically, and surgical exploration is necessary for differential diagnosis.

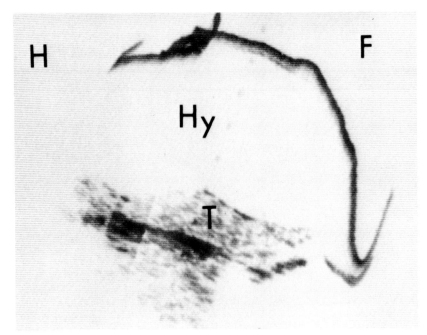

Fig. 7.253

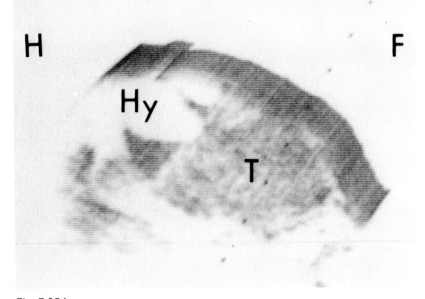

Fig. 7.254

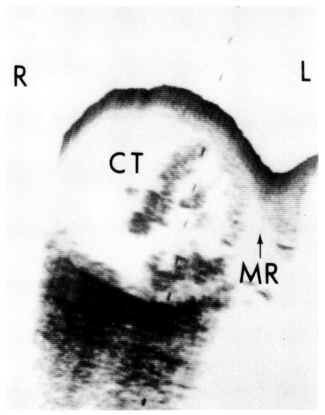

CT = Chronic torsion
F   = Foot
H   = Head
Hy = Hydrocele
L   = Left
MR = Median raphe
R   = Right
T   = Glandular elements of testis

Fig. 7.255

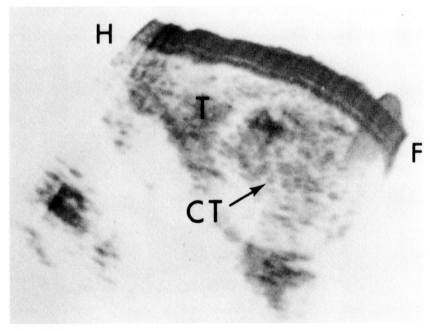

Fig. 7.256

Chronic Scrotal Masses That Mimic Primary Testicular Neoplasms

Granulomatous epididymitis is another entity that may mimic primary testicular neoplasm. It frequently occurs with associated orchitis, leading to permanent scarring and sometimes calcification within the testis. The onset is often insidious; therefore, the process presents as a chronic scrotal mass. On ultrasonograms, a thickened epididymis is frequently observed. However, associated textural changes within the glandular elements of the testes raise the suspicion of an occult, associated neoplasm (figs. 7.257 and 7.258). If this diagnosis is entertained, evidence for tuberculosis or other granulomatous disease can be sought elsewhere and appropriate therapy instituted. In many cases, however, surgical exploration is necessary for the final diagnosis.

Another entity which can present as a complex interscrotal mass involving both the extratesticular and testicular elements is a hernia (fig. 7.259). When the hernia contains fat which may lead to high reflectivity, attenuation, and scattering of the sound, resulting in a distorted picture to the testis, differentiation from neoplasm can be particularly difficult.

Finally, the glandular elements of the testis may be a site for metastatic disease. This is particularly true in cases of leukemia in children (fig. 7.260). Unless the primary diagnosis is already established, the ultrasonic picture can closely mimic primary neoplasm.

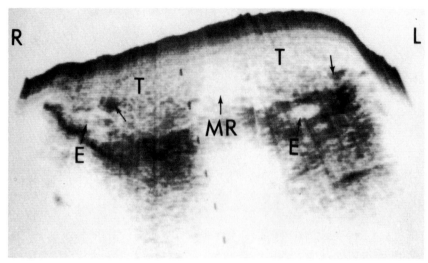

Fig. 7.257

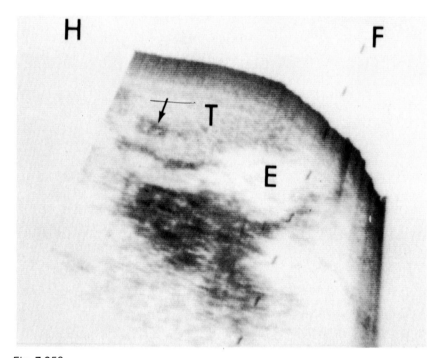

Fig. 7.258

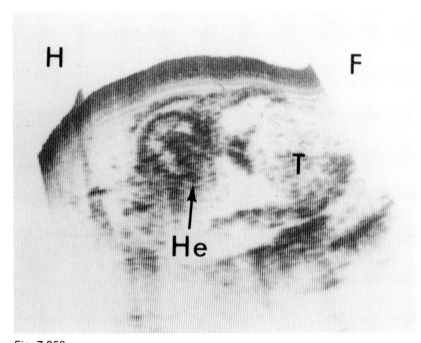

Fig. 7.259

Arrows = Textural abnormalities within
glandular elements of testis
E = Epididymis
F = Foot
H = Head
He = Hernia
L = Left
MR = Median raphe
R = Right
T = Glandular elements of testis

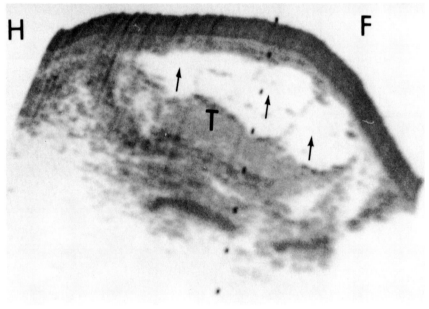

Fig. 7.260

Occult Neoplasms

One of the most important indications for ultrasonic scanning of the scrotum is to detect occult neoplasms in patients who present with retroperitoneal and mediastinal adenopathy. The scrotum will frequently be clinically negative, and it is uncertain whether there is an underlying small primary neoplasm. In this clinical setting, tumors have been readily detected on ultrasound as small focal abnormalities in the testicular texture (figs. 7.261 to 7.263). They generally demonstrate a decreased echogenicity and often a striking attenuation of the sound beam. Two of these tumors are demonstrated in the present series of cases, and a normal opposite testicle is shown for comparison (fig. 7.261). Occasionally, although the scrotum is clinically negative and the involved testis is normal in size, a diffusely abnormal texture is evident when compared to the opposite testicle (fig. 7.264). Again in these situations, the acoustic texture is generally decreased in echogenicity. In the pathological examination of these testes it often is necessary to take multiple sections to demonstrate tumor cells. On the sonograms, the major portion of the mass may represent a desmoplastic reaction.

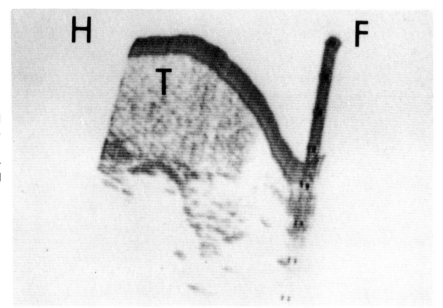

Fig. 7.261

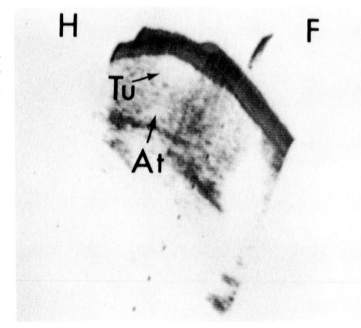

Fig. 7.262

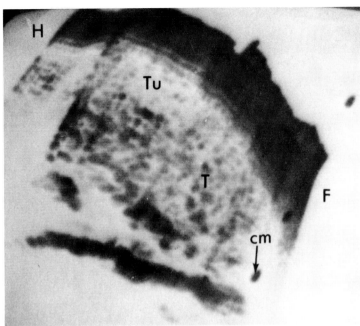

Fig. 7.263

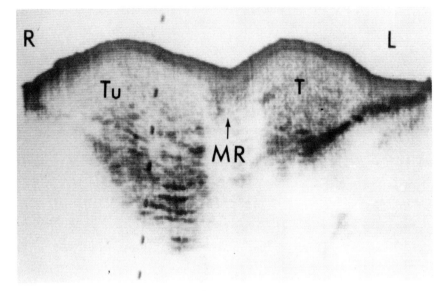

Fig. 7.264

At	= Attenuation
cm	= Centimeter marker
F	= Foot
H	= Head
L	= Left
MR	= Median raphe
R	= Right
T	= Glandular elements of testis
Tu	= Tumor

8.
Ultrasonography of the General Abdomen: Peritoneal Cavity, Bowel and Mesentery, and Abdominal Wall

Anthony A. Mancuso, M.D.

Introduction

Sonography has become widely accepted as the initial imaging examination of choice for evaluating abdominal masses and suspected fluid collections. The sonographer's major job is to define the origin and extent of pathology and thereby to direct the course of the remaining diagnostic evaluation (Bearman, Snaders, and Oh 1973; Kangarloo et al. 1977; Leopold and Asher 1972; Maklad, Doust, and Baum 1974; Meyers 1970; Taylor et al. 1978; Wicks, Silver, and Bree 1978). Accurate differential diagnosis is possible with ultrasound, but it often depends more on clinical observations than on specific sonographic findings. A final diagnosis usually requires biopsy, paracentesis, or other confirmatory studies.

This chapter considers several areas of interest in abdominal ultrasonography: (1) the abdominal wall; (2) the peritoneal cavity and spaces; (3) the bowel and mesentery; and (4) the diaphragm. These areas are often lumped into a general discussion of the abdominal viscera, leading to only a passing consideration of their participation in intraabdominal sonographic abnormalities. Moreover, the gastrointestinal tract creates a large proportion of the artifacts, justifying its separate consideration.

Technique

General Working Principles

The diagnostic imager's most important working principle is that a study is most useful when used to answer a specific, well-formulated question from the referring physician. When studies are done as surveys or to "rule out pathology" they tend to be much less informative.

A flexible attitude toward the technique of examination is also important. We should never hesitate to change the patient's position in whatever manner necessary to produce an adequate study. For example, decubitus views are extremely useful to determine whether a fluid collection is free, contained in bowel, or loculated. Furthermore, to keep errors related to artifacts at a minimum, potential pathological findings should always be confirmed in two views at right angles to one another.

While reading the following sections and reflecting on the sonographic appearance of this normal anatomy and the pathological changes it undergoes, several basic questions will serve as a useful framework for examination and interpretation (see tables 8.1 and 8.2).

1. What is the sonographic nature of the lesion: free fluid—simple or complex or localized abnormalities—simple cystic, mixed solid-cystic, solid?
2. Does the finding represent a significant abnormality, or is it a normal structure mimicking pathology?
3. What is the origin and extent of the abnormality, using vector analysis (Whalen, Evans, and Shanser 1971)?
4. Are there any associated or specific findings that might help in the differential diagnosis?
5. How can I vary the technique of examination better to answer these questions?

The principles inherent in these questions are important to keep in mind while performing or interpreting any ultrasound examination. The following sections will emphasize an overall approach while considering the limitations and pitfalls of the examination in individual areas.

Patient Preparation

The preparation of the patient depends on the goals of the examination. If the patient is acutely ill, and a specific question is raised—such as "Does the patient have a subdiaphragmatic abscess?"—then there need not be any preparation, and the examination can be limited to the area designated. More often circumstances are not so acute, and some degree of preparation is possible and desirable. Routinely, the patients are kept without oral intake overnight, or at least are asked not to eat any fat-containing foods for approximately 12–18 hours prior to the study. This usually insures visualization of the normal, distended gallbladder and may reduce gastrointestinal air content. If barium studies precede sonography within two days, bowel preparation is necessary. The barium-filled bowel may impair sound transmission or mimic an abnormal mass (Sarti and Lazere 1978).

Since gas represents a barrier to the transmission of sound, some attempt to reduce the volume of gas in the gastrointestinal tract is a good idea. Investigators have met with some limited success in improving sound transmission following preparation with oral Simethi-

cone (Sommer and Filly 1977; Sommer, Filly, and Laing 1977). Water has been instilled in the stomach in order to reduce its gas content while producing a sonographic window for looking at the left upper quadrant. The water does not produce the desired sonographic window, because accompanying microbubbles of gas usually cause the sound to be dispersed (Yeh and Wolf 1977a). Such a maneuver may, however, allow the differentiation of the stomach from an abnormal left upper quadrant mass. Obviously a distended urinary bladder greatly facilitates examination of the lower abdomen because it displaces gas-filled bowel.

Anatomy of the General Abdomen

Abdominal Wall

The abdominal wall can be studied in detail with a 3.5- or 5-MHz short internal-focus transducer, with single-pass scanning technique, and with the time-gain compensation curve set as we might for a thyroid study. The skin-transducer interface produces the initial "bang." Deep to this dark, linear echo is the relatively sonolucent subcutaneous plane, a fat and fibrous tissue zone producing variable amounts of low-level echoes. The exact appearance and thickness of this subcutaneous plane varies with its fat content.

The fascia surrounding the musculature of the abdominal wall produces strongly reflective surfaces, so that the musculofascial plane consists of a relatively thick, sonolucent muscular zone bracketed by two thin, very echogenic fascial interfaces (Spangen 1976). The parietal peritoneum echoes blend with those of the deep fascia of the abdominal wall. Consequently, normal peritoneum is not seen as a distinct structure (Hollinshead 1967; Spangen 1976).

Abdominal Cavity and Lesser Sac

The abdominal and pelvic cavities should always be considered a continuum; the pelvis represents the most dependent portion of this large space. For the purposes of discussion, however, we will consider the abdominal cavity to end inferiorly at the pelvic brim. Superiorly, it is bound by the diaphragm where the parietal peritoneum is firmly adherent to the diaphragmatic fascia (Hollinshead 1967). Anteriorly and posteriorly, the parietal peritoneum is separated from the abdominal wall and retroperitoneum, respectively, by varying amounts of fat and connective tissue (Hollinshead 1967).

Separation of the peritoneal cavity into several compartments produces a useful framework for understanding how the movement of fluid or spread of tumor and infection is channeled along the natural pathways the normal anatomy creates (Hollinshead 1967; Meyers 1970; Proto, Lane, and Marangola 1976). The transverse mesocolon divides the abdominal cavity into supra- and inframesocolic spaces. The root of the small bowel mesentery runs obliquely from slightly to the left of midline at the ligament of Trietz to the cecum, thereby separating the inframesocolic compartment into two infracolic spaces. The right infracolic space is much smaller and does not communicate as readily as the left with the pelvis (Meyers 1970; Proto, Lane, and Marangola 1976).

The infracolic spaces are bound externally by paracolic gutters which may serve as communications between the pelvis and supramesocolic compartments; the degree of communication varies from side to side. On the right, the paracolic gutter is deeper and leads to the subhepatic space and its posterosuperior extension, the hepatorenal fossa (Morrison's pouch) (Hollinshead 1967; Meyers 1970; Proto, Lane, and Marangola 1976). The hepatorenal fossa is a paravertebral space and, therefore, the most fluid-dependent of the upper abdominal cavity spaces when the patient is supine (Meyers 1970; Proto, Lane, and Marangola 1976). These basically subhepatic spaces freely communicate with the right subphrenic space (Hollinshead 1967; Meyers 1970; Proto, Lane, and Marangola 1976).

The lesser peritoneal sac also communicates with the subhepatic spaces (Hollinshead 1967; Meyers 1970). Anteriorly, it is bound by the lesser omentum. The right free edge of the lesser omentum forms the hepatoduodenal ligament and the anterior wall of the epiploic foramen (foramen of Winslow). The remainder of the lesser omentum spreads to join with the mesentery of the stomach, contributing to several ligaments between the stomach, liver, spleen, and diaphragm; this forms the anterior wall, the closed superior recesses, and the left lateral borders of the lesser sac (Hollinshead 1967). The inferior border of the lesser sac is the transverse mesocolon. The very important relationship of the posteroinferior wall of the lesser sac to the pancreas must always be kept in mind.

The falciform ligament separates the right and left subphrenic spaces, though they may communicate anteriorly (Proto, Lane, and Marangola 1976). The left subphrenic and subhepatic spaces are in gross continuity and may be thought of as either entirely subphrenic or perihepatic. The phrenicocolic ligament attaches the colon to the left hemidiaphragm and forms an effective barrier between the relatively shallow left paracolic gutter and the perihepatic and perisplenic spaces (Meyers 1970; Proto, Lane, and Marangola 1976).

Normal Bowel and Mesentery

The intestinal tract, from the stomach to the rectum, is usually distended with varying amounts of air. These highly reflective air-soft tissue interfaces are responsible for most of the artifacts encountered in abdominal scanning and are easily identified. Occasionally, the intestinal tract is distended with fluid, in which case it may look like complex or simple fluid collections.

Various parts of the gastrointestinal tract are often collapsed; the exact identification of the visualized, nondistended gastrointestinal tract depends on the related anatomic landmarks. A good example is the collapsed gastric antrum lying anterior to the pancreas (Sample and Sarti 1978; Sample 1977). The pattern typical of collapsed portions of the gastrointestinal tract consists of a central, highly reflective, usually linear echo representing mucous and admixed air. If the bowel is fluid-filled, it will have a central sonolucency (fluid contents) surrounded by the high-level mucosal echoes. A peripheral sonolucency of varying thickness represents the bowel wall which surrounds the collapsed or fluid-filled lumen. This is in turn surrounded by a highly reflective interface representing the serosal surface of the bowel and closely related mesenteric attachments (Sample and Sarti 1978; Sample 1977).

Stomach

The appearance of the collapsed "hollow viscus," typically seen in longitudinal scans, is secondary to the gastroesophageal junction which lies just anterior to the aorta and is surrounded by the crura of the diaphragm (Sample 1977; Sample and Sarti 1978). The stomach's appearance is otherwise variable. It usually contains enough air to obscure the left upper quadrant. At times, it contains fluid, food, and small amounts of air and, therefore, may mimic a complex mass lesion or lesser sac fluid collection. Often, the gastric antrum is collapsed and can be seen lying immediately anterior to the pancreas; the more inferior part of the lesser sac then represents only a potential space. The central linear echo of the collapsed antrum and surrounding sonolucent stomach wall should not be mistaken for the pancreas and the pancreatic duct (Sample 1977; Sample and Sarti 1978).

Small Bowel

The duodenum, taken with the gallbladder and proper vascular landmarks forms a triad which helps to localize the pancreatic head (Sample 1977; Sample and Sarti 1978). While the duodenum is a useful landmark, it is also a source of serious artifacts. When it contains gas, reverberation artifacts can mimic pancreatic mass lesions. Reproduction of findings by scanning in oblique and perpendicular planes becomes mandatory when a gas-filled duodenum is suspected of such treachery (Sample 1977; Sample and Sarti 1978). At times, the highly reflective gas-filled duodenum mimics a gallbladder filled with calculi, but these often can be differentiated by observing a "clean" shadowing pattern (without reverberation artifacts) in the case of calculi as opposed to the "dirty" shadowing (with reverberation artifacts) caused by a gas-filled duodenal bulb or sweep. Fluid-filled second and third portions of the duodenum create pseudomasses in the pancreatic or retroperitoneal areas. At the ligament of Treitz, fluid in the duodenum might mimic an adrenal mass or retroperitoneal lymphadenopathy (Sample 1977; Sample and Sarti 1978).

The small bowel also has a variable appearance. When the bowel is distended with fluid, valvulae and bowel contents are sometimes visible. More often, even with its relatively small air content, the small bowel obscures areas of interest within the abdomen. Collapsed small bowel without much air produces an amorphous echogenic pattern filling the mid to lower abdomen. Sometimes this collapsed bowel takes on a faint, serpiginous, or stacked appearance indicative of its origins.

Large Intestine

The collapsed transverse colon will often be seen, especially on longitudinal sections, somewhat inferior to the plane of the pancreas and stomach. The gas-containing hepatic flexure may produce artifacts simulating gallbladder disease much the same as those produced by the duodenum. Observing "dirty" versus "clean" shadowing patterns again may aid in differentiation.

The omentum and the mesenteries are usually not distinctly visible unless they are either diseased, or a large amount of peritoneal fluid is present. These structures are, therefore, discussed in greater detail in the sections dealing with pathology and, more specifically, with ascites.

The important working principle here is that the appearance of the bowel varies with its contents and degree of distension. Moreover, its appearance is often characteristic. As a source of artifacts the bowel may be responsible for abnormal findings such as localized fluid collections. As a useful anatomic landmark, its recognition may result in a more accurate diagnosis.

Pathology of the Abdominal Wall

Masses and fluid collections may arise in or involve the subcutaneous plane, musculofascial plane, peritoneal surface, or intraabdominal compartment (see table 8.1). Following localization, the basic internal consistency of the abdominal area is considered, and it helps to rank differential possibilities (see table 8.3); the clinical circumstances usually determine which is most likely. The differential diagnosis of predominantly cystic areas limited to the abdominal wall usually includes seroma, abscess, and hematoma. Rarely, a cystic or necrotic tumor may be present. Ventral hernias with air- or fluid-filled bowel are also included in the differential diagnosis when the clinical setting is appropriate. Abdominal wall defects without herniated bowel may also be seen (Spangen 1976). A solid mass with homogenous internal architecture may appear sonolucent and mimic the internal consistency of a fluid collection; through transmission, however, will be absent. The differential diagnosis of predominantly solid processes includes tumor, clotted blood, and induration.

Artifacts generated by the abdominal wall are mainly related to rib attenuation and loss of the acoustic coupling at the skin-transducer interface. Scars often cause a break in the skin-transducer couple; moreover, because of their dense fibrous tissue content, they attenuate sound and produce significant artifacts, even when the skin-transducer contact is maintained.

Fluid Collections in the Peritoneal Cavity

Free Fluid—Simple or Complex?

Fluid accumulations in the peritoneal cavity as seen at sonography may be free, loculated, or contained in bowel (see table 8.2). Changing the patient's position and observing the movement of the fluid area will usually determine the nature of the accumulation. If not, it may be useful to wait several minutes or, if possible, have the patient walk around before rescanning the area. Real-time scanning is also valuable in this setting because the movement of fluid in bowel due to peristasis can be documented (Yeh and Wolf 1977b).

Free fluid may be either simple or complex in appearance (see tables 8.2 and 8.3). Simple fluid collections have no internal echo pattern and form very smooth, well-defined interfaces with the surrounding tissues. Such fluid collections may be loculated. Complex fluid collections either have some sort of internal echo pattern, such as septae or floating debris, or form thickened and/or irregular interfaces with the surrounding anatomical structures.

Simple ascites is most often a transudate resulting from a metabolic disturbance; it may, however, just as well originate from an inflammatory or neoplastic focus. Complex ascites is more likely to be the result of an inflammatory or neoplastic process. These generalizations should not be carried too far. Any time free fluid is present, associated findings, such as localized masses or evidence of metastatic disease, should be sought to help clarify the etiology (see table 8.2). In trauma cases the fluid may represent blood, and a source of the bleeding can be sought; such an investigation might include looking for subcapsular splenic or hepatic hematomas and/or fractures of the liver, spleen, or retroperitoneal viscera. Occasionally, thickening of the peritoneal surfaces will indicate diffuse or localized tumor involvement.

Fluid Movement

The following factors influence the movement of fluid in the peritoneal cavity and its localization in various compartments.

1. The position of the patient
2. The amount of fluid (Goldberg et al. 1973; Proto, Lane, and Marangola 1976; Yeh and Wolf 1977b)
3. The peritoneal organs, reflections, and ligaments (see anatomy section) (Meyers 1970; Proto, Lane, and Marangola 1976; Yeh and Wolf 1977b)
4. The presence of adhesions
5. Where the fluid originates (Proto, Lane, and Marangola 1976; Yeh and Wolf 1977b)
6. What process is responsible for the fluid being present (Meyers 1970)
7. Intraperitoneal pressure (movement secondary to changes in respiration and related changes in hydrostatic pressure) (Meyers 1970; Proto, Lane, and Marangola 1976; Yeh and Wolf 1977b)
8. Density of the fluid (Proto, Lane, and Marangola 1976)

Logical patterns of flow can be predicted by considering the patient's position in light of the previous anatomical discussion. These predicted flow patterns agree with those observed during cadaver studies on fluid movement within the peritoneal cavity and agree basically with the actual clinical experience (Meyers 1970; Proto, Lane, and Marangola 1976; Yeh and Wolf 1977b). Experimentally, fluid amounts as small as 100–200 cm^2 can be detected sonographically (Goldberg et al. 1973; Proto, Lane, and Marangola 1976). Clinically, small collections are typically seen in the right paracolic gutter; lateral, and at times, anterior to the liver; and in the subhepatic spaces (Proto, Lane, and Marangola 1976; Yeh and Wolf 1977b). The sonolucency of preperitoneal fat anterior to the liver must not be interpreted as a fluid collection.

When right-sided fluid collections are larger, they tend to fill out the subhepatic space and hepatorenal fossa, extending from there to the right subphrenic space. Subhepatic space fluid may also enter the lesser sac. Flow across the midline may be restricted by the falciform ligament (Meyers 1970; Proto, Lane, and Marangola 1976; Yeh and Wolf 1977b). Flow between the left supramesocolic space and paracolic gutter is limited on the left by the phrenicocolic ligament so that if fluid is present in the left subphrenic region, it most likely originated in the supramesocolic compartment (Meyers 1970). There is free communication among the right, upper, and lower abdominal compartments via the deeper, unobstructed right paracolic gutter (Meyers 1970).

Ascites and Its Associated Effects on Bowel, Mesentery, and Liver

Large ascitic collections present no problem in detection but do produce some interesting sonographic phenomena. Fluid in tense ascites will surround, compress, and displace the liver, causing it to have a more richly echogenic appearance than usual (Yeh and Wolf 1977b). When the liver is surrounded by fluid, other peritoneal attachments such as the falciform ligament and the lesser omentum become visible (Yeh and Wolf 1977b). Furthermore, the usual anatomical landmarks in the high retroperitoneum are obscured by the posteriorly and medially displaced bowel and mesentery.

As the ascites increases in volume, the normal mesentery tends to collect around the lines of its posterior peritoneal attachment producing a highly reflective group of echoes in the mid and upper abdomen. With a very fatty mesentery, the echo pattern tends to spread out more, because the mesentery is more buoyant and assumes a more vertical orientation. With a less fatty and, therefore, less buoyant mesentery, the echoes tend to clump and collapse posteriorly (Yeh and Wolf 1977b).

Normal bowel floats or sinks in ascitic fluid, depending on its relative air and fluid content. The bowel usually appears as echogenic clumps arranged in an arcuate fashion around the vertically oriented mesentery (Yeh and Wolf 1977b). Occasionally, the bowel may be seen in cross section as a rounded prominence at the end of a fingerlike mesenteric projection. Adhesions may be seen extending from the bowel to the abdominal wall (Yeh and Wolf 1977b).

Localized Peritoneal Abnormalities

After studying the origin and extent (see tables 8.1 and 8.2) of a peritoneal abnormality and determining that it is most likely localized disease, the sonographic features of the localized mass or fluid collection can be scrutinized. Consideration of the internal consistency, borders, and associated findings aids greatly in weighing the differential diagnosis and directing further diagnostic evaluation (Doust and Thompson 1978; Fleischer et al. 1978; Kressel and Filly 1978; Wicks, Silver, and Bree 1978; Yeh and Wolf 1977c). Any classification of this type leads to obvious overlapping of differential possibilities so that this categorization is intended only as a

Table 8.1.

Characteristics of Localized Abnormal Masses of the Abdomen

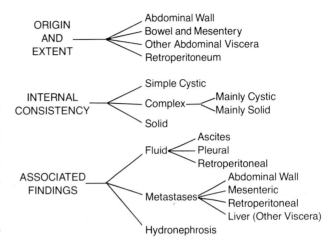

Table 8.2.

Characteristics of Abnormal Fluid Collections of the Abdomen

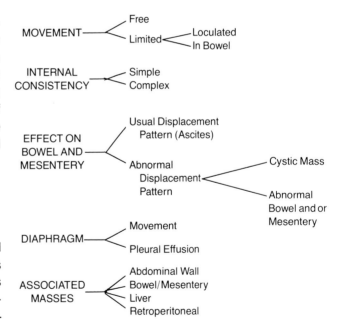

Table 8.3.

Sonographic Characteristics as an Aid to Differential Diagnosis

FREE FLUID COLLECTIONS*	Internal Echoes	Borders	Increased Through Transmission	Usual Differential Diagnosis	Less Common Diagnosis
Simple	No	Smooth, Distinct	Yes	Ascites— Transudate or Exudate	Hematoma, Abscess, Fluid in Bowel
Complex	Septated, Debris	Irregular, Thickened, Indistinct (Fuzzy)	Yes	Malignant Ascites, Inflammatory Exudate with Adhesions Simple Ascites with Preexisting Adhesions	Bowel plus contents See Complex, Mainly Cystic, Localized Abnormalities
LOCALIZED ABNORMALITIES					
Simple Cystic	No	Smooth, Regular, Distinct	Yes	Loculated Ascites, Cysts	Abscess, Hematoma, Fluid in Bowel, Pseudocyst, Duplication or Mesenteric Cyst
Complex, Mainly Cystic	Septa, Debris, Fluid Levels	Smooth, Regular to Irregular, Thickened, Indistinct	Yes, Prominently	Abscess, Hematoma, Pseudocyst, Bowel, Loculated Ascites, Ovarian Neoplasm	Lymphocele, Duplication, Mesenteric Cyst, Abnormal Bowel, (Infarcted, Obstructed)
Complex, Mainly Solid	High-level Calcium, Air (Microbubbles) Septa, Debris, Solid Elements, Cystic Foci	Regular and Smooth to Irregular, Thickened, Indistinct	Yes, Often Subtle	Pelvoabdominal Neoplasm (Lymphoma Sarcomas, Benign Mesenhymal Tumors) with Necrosis	Abnormal Bowel (Infarcted), Abscess, Hematoma
Solid	High-level Calcium, Homogeneous and Almost Sonolucent, Homogeneous and Obvious Internal Architecture, Variable Gray Tones	Regular, Smooth to Irregular and Indistinct	No	Neoplasm, Lymphoma, Sarcoma, Benign Mesenchymal Tumor	Barium in Bowel Gastrointestinal-tract Masses Tumor, or Intussusception Hematoma Abscess (None)

*Loculated fluid; see localized abnormalities

general aid to differential diagnosis. Again, our more important job is either to guide the clinician to appropriate further studies or to outline the extent of disease for accurate planning of therapy.

The gain settings must be scrupulously set when examining for localized or small fluid collections. A fluid area with some internal debris may "fill in" and be missed if gain settings are too high (Doust and Thompson 1978). Homogeneous solid abnormalities may be mistaken for fluid areas if gains are too low (Doust and Thompson 1978; Yeh and Wolf 1977c). Sometimes, examination at two different gain settings is required to avoid these pitfalls (Doust and Thompson 1978).

Loculated Ascites

Nonpyogenic inflammatory conditions (e.g., pancreatitis) produce fluid collections which spread as expected along existing anatomic pathways. Their inflammatory nature may, however, allow them to dissect along the large and small bowel mesenteries which provide a direct path to literally any quadrant (Meyers 1970). More often, the mesentery and the parietal and visceral peritoneum wall off these processes near their site of origin. Thus, whenever fluid becomes loculated, the differential diagnosis is shifted toward an inflammatory etiology, even when no internal echoes are present (see table 8.3). Evaluation of the margins of the fluid area then becomes extremely important. At times, a fuzzy, irregular border may be the only differentiating characteristic between inflammatory or neoplastic exudate and simple ascites that has become loculated due to preexisting adhesions. In this setting, a fluid-filled loop of bowel must always be considered a possible source of the findings and excluded by changing the patient's position or by real-time examination.

Abscess

Abscesses present most often as complex, predominantly cystic masses (Doust and Thompson 1978; Fleischer et al. 1978; Taylor et al. 1978) (see table 8.3). Their classic appearance is of elliptical sonolucent masses with thick and irregular margins (Doust and Thompson 1978). They tend to be under tension and displace surrounding structures (Doust and Thompson 1978; Gerzof, Robbins, and Birkett 1978). A septated

appearance may result from previous or developing adhesions. Necrotic debris may produce internal echoes; at times such debris may be seen "floating" within the abscess. Occasionally, fluid levels are seen (Fleischer et al. 1978), probably because of the settling of debris which alters the acoustic properties of the fluid in the more dependent parts of the abscess cavity. Gas-containing abscesses present varying echo patterns; the general appearance is that of a densely echogenic mass with or without acoustic shadowing and otherwise increased through transmission. Mixed, solid, and cystic calcium-containing mass lesions such as a teratoma may mimic the sonographic pattern of a gas-containing abscess, but the clinical history and plain film evaluation usually will exclude them from the diagnosis (Kressel and Filly 1978).

Peritonitis and resultant abscess formation may be a generalized or localized process. Once such pathology has been discovered, its extent should be determined. Multiloculated abscesses or multiple collections should be documented and their size determined as accurately as possible to aid in planning drainage and for improved accuracy in follow-up studies (Kim et al. 1977; Maklad, Doust, and Baum 1974). Lesser-sac abscesses deserve some separate attention. The slitlike epiploic foramen usually seals off the lesser sac from inflammatory processes extrinsic to it (Meyers 1970). If the inflammatory process begins within the lesser sac, such as with a pancreatic abscess, the sac may be involved in addition to other secondarily affected peritoneal spaces. Differential consideration of simple and complex lesser-sac fluid collections should always include pseudocyst, pancreatic abscess, and gastric outlet obstruction. A normally fluid-filled stomach should always be excluded.

Subphrenic abscesses also present some unique diagnostic problems. The left upper quadrant is particularly difficult to examine. Placing the patient into the right lateral decubitus position and scanning along the coronal plane of the body as well as prone scanning using the spleen as a sonographic window will insure a more complete examination of the left upper quadrant. Pleural effusion should not be mistaken for subdiaphragmatic fluid collections. If clarification is necessary, the patient may be scanned upright, so that the pleural fluid, diaphragm, and subphrenic region relationships can be shown (Haber, Asher, and Freimanis 1975; Landay and Harless 1977). The diaphragm must always be identified and its excursion quantiated when looking for subphrenic abnormalities (Haber, Asher, and Freimanis

1975; Landay and Harless 1977). Subcapsular collections of fluid within the liver may mimic loculated subphrenic fluid. The intraabdominal fluid may be differentiated by its smooth border and its tendency to conform to the contour of the liver while it displaces the liver medially, rather than to indent the border locally as subcapsular fluid might. Sometimes the differentiation of subphrenic abscess from localized simple ascites may be difficult. Often the margins of the fluid collection are the only clue to its inflammatory nature. Preperitoneal fat anterior to the liver may also mimic a localized fluid collection.

Computed Tomography versus Ultrasound Techniques

Some investigators have suggested that the CAT scan is better than ultrasound for the detection and delineation of the extent of intraabdominal abscesses (Daffner et al. 1978). Others point out that computed tomography is a useful adjunct to percutaneous drainage of intraabdominal fluid collections (Gerzof, Robbins, and Birkett 1978). To date, however, no well-controlled, comparative study of computed tomography and ultrasound techniques and their relative usefulness and reliability has been performed. Clearly, when ultrasound does not produce a diagnostic examination or does not sufficiently show the extent of the abnormalities, computed tomography is indicated. Available data indicate that ultrasound by itself is both a sensitive and reliable way to look for intraabdominal fluid collections; it should, therefore, be used as a primary screening test in this regard (Maklad, Doust, and Baum 1974; Meyers et al. 1972).

Hematoma

Hematomas run the gamut of possible sonographic appearances (see table 8.3). The appearance of a hematoma at any given time depends on where the clot is in its natural history of organization from lysis to resorption stages. The sonographic correlates of this process are roughly homogenous solid to complex cystic to cystic. As a hematoma ages, it tends to appear as a complex fluid area containing echogenic clumps (Doust and Thompson 1978). Hematomas may become infected and any stage may be sonographically indistinguishable from abscess. Hematomas in the hepatic or splenic

subcapsular areas may mimic subphrenic fluid; differential criteria for this problem were discussed previously. The clinical setting usually decides the issue, though in the more acute stages the density data available from CAT scans can also be more definitive.

Lymphoceles

These fluid collections generally look like loculated, simple fluid collections, though they may have a more complex, usually septated morphology (see table 8.3). Differentiation from loculated ascites is usually possible because the mass effect of a lymphocele which is under tension will displace the surrounding organs (Doust and Thompson 1978; Fleischer et al. 1978). Differentiation from other fluid collections is mainly made on clinical grounds.

Other Mainly Cystic Complex Masses

Other possible etiologies for predominantly cystic complex masses must be considered in localized abdominal abnormalities (see table 8.3). Multiple adherent loops of fluid-filled normal or "matted" abnormal bowel may look exactly like a complex predominantly cystic mass. Furthermore, ascites combined with adhesions and bowel gives a similar appearance. Such abnormalities can be differentiated from masses arising from other pelvic and abdominal viscera or the retroperitoneum by determining the vector of the mass effect on the surrounding anatomy (Haller et al. 1978; Kim et al. 1977; Whalen, Evans, and Shanser 1971; Wicks, Silver, and Bree 1978; Yeh and Wolf 1977b). For example, large pelvoabdominal masses related to cystic ovarian tumors are notoriously difficult to differentiate from complex ascites with abnormal bowel unless the bowel is actually displaced posteriorly and superiorly by a mass. With massive complex pathology and a possibly associated ascites, a definitive evaluation as to origin and extent may not be possible with ultrasound. In these circumstances, computed tomography may be used for a more definite evaluation.

Other Localized Peritoneal Abnormalities

Predominantly solid and homogenously solid masses may arise from the bowel and mesentery or, rarely, from the peritoneal surfaces (see tables 8.1 and 8.3). These masses are discussed in detail under their respective anatomical categories. Abscess and hematoma are included in the morphologic group of complex, predominantly solid masses; however, this morphology is more often the result of primary neoplasms complicated by either necrosis or hemorrhage (see table 8.3).

Peritoneum

The peritoneal lining is not seen as a distinct structure during sonography unless it is thickened. Thickening is usually secondary to metastatic implants or to direct extension of tumor from the viscera or mesentery. Primary mesotheliomas occur rarely. In our experience, such processes are almost universally associated with malignant ascites when patients present for sonography. Thickening of the peritoneal lining may also be related to inflammation. In this case, the margin will become ill-defined and thickened. The peritoneum also may form adhesions that help to limit the spread of inflammatory processes.

Bowel and Mesentery Pathology

sonographically, bowel masquerades as amorphous, solid masses; mixed, solid, and cystic masses; complex fluid collections; and loculated fluid collections. It also produces many artifacts. For these reasons, abnormal and normal bowel enter the differential diagnosis of mass lesions and fluid collections in the abdomen and pelvis more often than expected. Changing the patient's position often helps determine whether such findings are related to bowel. Examination with real-time capabilities is a very useful adjunct, for it allows us direct observation of fluid movement in response to peristalsis. Consequently, although bowel enters the differential diagnosis more often than expected, it usually can be excluded.

Mass Lesions

Solid masses found on ultrasound examination to arise from various parts of the gastrointestinal tract have been described by several authors (Kremer, Lohmoeller, and Zollner 1977; Peterson and Cooperberg 1978;

Walls 1976; Weissberg, Scheible, and Leopold 1977). The pattern common to all descriptions is a solid, basically sonolucent mass with a central, usually linear, echo. This pattern results from infiltration and resultant thickening of the bowel wall surrounding the lumen with its highly reflective mucus and gas content. This appearance is only an exaggeration of the pattern described for normal, collapsed bowel (Sample 1977; Sample and Sarti 1978). The expression "target-like" abdominal mass has been coined to describe these lesions. The "target-like" or "double-ring" configuration is also seen in cases of intussusception (Weissberg, Scheible, and Leopold 1977). Whenever a mass with this configuration is seen at ultrasound, bowel, in some form, should be considered as its origin.

Fresh barium in the bowel will prevent through transmission of sound (Sarti and Lazere 1978). Furthermore, and perhaps more importantly, as the barium settles, its acoustic properties change and allow better through transmission of the sound. At the same time, however, the settled barium may then be mistaken for a pathological echogenic, intraluminal mass lesion (Sarti and Lazere 1978). An abdominal X-ray can help settle the issue.

It is only rarely that primarily cystic or mixed solid and cystic masses that arise from the bowel and mesentery can be seen at ultrasound (Haller et al. 1978; Goldberg, Capitanio, and Kirkpatrick 1972; Kim et al. 1977; Wicks, Silver, and Bree 1978). Duplications of the gastrointestinal tract and biliary system should always be considered in a primarily cystic lesion when it is adjacent to bowel or the biliary tree respectively (Wicks, Silver, and Bree 1978). Benign mesenchymal tumors and teratomas are also uncommon sources of primary mesenteric or bowel abnormalities seen at sonography. Ultrasound is nonspecific in the differential diagnosis of such an abnormality; vector analysis, however, will usually indicate the origin of the mass lesion and define its relationships to the surrounding anatomy (Haller et al. 1978; Kim et al. 1977; Whalen, Evans, and Shanser 1971). In all of these possibly malignant abdominal masses, evidence of metastatic disease to the retroperitoneum or liver should always be sought (see table 8.1).

The appearance of bowel in the presence of ascites has been outlined and should be reviewed at this point if necessary. In cases where massive, complex ascites is present, it is often difficult to tell whether a mass plus the ascites is responsible for the image or whether the findings are due to fluid and related abnormal bowel and mesentery. If the bowel was displaced, a mass is more likely. If the bowel and mesentery are pathologically involved their response to the pressure of intraabdominal fluid will be altered. For example, when the mesentery is diffusely involved with metastatic disease, instead of floating or collapsing medially and posteriorly, it usually appears as a large echogenic mass surrounded by bowel.

Obstruction

Obstruction of the gastrointestinal tract may produce sonographic patterns which appear quite bizzare until dilated. Abnormal bowel is considered as an etiology. The level of obstruction can, at times, be accurately predicted; the distended stomach is a prime example (Boychuk, Lyons, and Goodhan 1978; Teele and Smith 1977; Zimmerman 1978). When gastric outlet obstruction is suspected, other diagnostic possibilities including lesser sac abscess, pseudocyst, and a recent meal should be excluded.

Numerous, serpiginous, fluid-filled loops of bowel may be clumped together or appear to be stacked upon one another when a relatively distal obstruction is present. A closed-loop obstruction may present as a complex mass, indistinguishable from an abscess (Doust and Thompson 1978). Duodenal obstruction may produce a striking tubular sonolucency in the expected location; we have seen such a case secondary to duodenal hematoma. In the fetus, if a portion of the gastrointestinal tract is persistently distended, the possibility of bowel obstruction should be relayed to the pediatrician (Zimmerman 1978).

Infarcted bowel produces an extremely amorphous, mixed, solid, and cystic sonographic pattern. At times, the infarcted bowel may take on the somewhat serpiginous character described for obstructed bowel. The appearance is, of course, nonspecific but should raise the index of suspicion for bowel infarction in the appropriate clinical setting.

In general, abnormal and normal bowel enter the differential diagnosis of abdominal masses and fluid collections with great frequency. When abnormalities in the abdomen are encountered, bowel always should be considered as a possible origin. Usually, it can be excluded as a source of the abnormal findings. Other studies will sometimes be necessary to settle the issue.

References

Altemeier, W. A.; Culbertson, W. R.; Fullen, W. D.; and Shook, C. D. Intra-abdominal abscesses. *Am. J. of Surg.* 125:70–79, 1973.

Bartrum, R. J. Practical considerations in abdominal ultrasonic scanning. *N. Engl. J. Med.* 291:1068–1070, November 1974.

Bearman, S.; Snaders, R. C.; and Oh, K. S. B-scan ultrasound in the evaluation of pediatric abdominal masses. *Radiology* 108:111–117, July 1973.

Boychuk, R. B.; Lyons, E. A.; and Goodhan, T. K. Duodenal atresia diagnosed by ultrasound. *Radiology* 127:500, May 1978.

Conrad, M. R.; Landay, M. J.; and Khoury, M. Pancreatic pseudocysts: unusual ultrasound features. *Am. J. Roentgenol.* 130:265–268, February 1978.

Daffner, R.; Halber, M.; Morgan, C.; Trought, W.; Thompson, W.; and Rice, R. CT in the diagnosis of intraabdominal abscess. Presented at International Symposium and Course on Computed Tomography, Miami Beach: March 1978.

Doust, B. D., and Thompson, R. Ultrasonography of abdominal fluid collections. *Gastrointest. Radiol.* 3:273–279, 1978.

Fleischer, A. C.; James, A. E.; Millis, J. B.; and Julian, C. Differential diagnosis of pelvic masses by gray scale sonography. *Am. J. Roentgenol.* 131:469–476, September 1978.

Haller, J. O.; Schneider, M.; Kassner, E. G.; Slovis, T. L.; and Perl, L. J. Sonographic evaluation of mesenteric and omental masses in children. *Am. J. Roentgenol.* 130:269–274, February 1978.

Gerzof, S. G.; Robbins, A. H.; and Birkett, D. H. Computed tomography in the diagnosis and management of abdominal abscesses. *Gastrointest. Radiol.* 3:287–294, 1978.

Goldberg, B. B.; Capitanio, M. A.; and Kirpatrick, J. A. Ultrasonic evaluation of masses in pediatric patients. *Am. J. Roentgenol.* 116:677–684, November 1972.

Goldberg, B. B.; Clearfield, H. R.; Goodman, G. A.; and Morales, J. O. Ultrasonic determination of ascites. *Arch. Intern. Med.* 131:217–220, February 1973.

Haber, K.; Asher, W. M.; and Freimanis, A. K. Echographic evaluation of diaphragmatic motion in intraabdominal diseases. *Radiology* 114:141–144, January 1975.

Hollinshead, H. W. *Textbook of anatomy*, second edition. New York: Harper and Row Publishers, 1967.

Holt, S., and Samuel, E. Multiple concentric ring sign in the ultrasonographic diagnosis of intussusception. *Gastrointest. Radiol.* 3:307–309, 1978.

Kangarloo, H.; Sukov, R.; Sample, W. F.; Lipson, M.; and Smith, L. Ultrasonographic evaluation of juxta-diaphragmatic masses in children. *Radiology* 125:785–787, December 1977.

Kim, E.; Goldman, S. M.; Minkin, S. D.; and Salik, J. O. Contralateral displacement of abdominal viscera by a retroperitoneal liposarcoma: ultrasonic demonstration. *J. Clin. Ultrasound* 5:117–120, April 1977.

Kremer, H.; Lohmoeller, G.; and Zollner, N. Primary ultrasonic detection of a double carcinoma of the colon. *Radiology* 124:481–482, August 1977.

Kressel, H. Y., and Filly, R. A. Ultrasonographic appearance of gas-containing abscesses in the abdomen. *Am. J. Roentgenol.* 130:71–73, January 1978.

Landay, M., and Harless, W. Ultrasonic differentiation of right pleural effusion from subphrenic fluid on longitudinal scans of the right upper quadrant: importance of recognizing the diaphragm. *Radiology* 123:155–158, April 1977.

Leopold, G. R., and Asher, W. M. Diagnosis of extra-organ retroperitoneal space lesions by B-scan ultrasonography. *Radiology* 103:133–138, July 1972.

Lutz, H. T., and Petzoldt, R. Ultrasonic patterns of space occupying lesions of the stomach and the intestine. *Ultrasound Med. Biol.* 2:129–132, 1976.

Maklad, N. F.; Doust, B. D.; and Baum, J. K. Ultrasonic diagnosis of postoperative intra-abdominal abscess. *Radiology* 113:417–422, November 1974.

Meyers, M. A. The spread and localization of acute intraperitoneal effusions. *Radiology* 95:547–554, June 1970.

Meyers, M. A.; Whalen, J. P.; Peele, K.; and Berne, A. S. Radiologic features of extraperitoneal effusions. *Radiology* 104:249–257, August 1972.

Peterson, L. R., and Cooperberg, P. L. Ultrasound demonstration of lesions of the gastrointestinal tract. *Gastrointest. Radiol.* 3:303–306, 1978.

Proto, A. V.; Lane, E. J.; and Marangola, J. P. A new concept of ascitic fluid distribution. *Am. J. Roentgenol.* 126:974–980, 1976.

Sample, W. F. Techniques for improved delineation of normal anatomy of the upper abdomen and high retroperitoneum with gray-scale ultrasound. *Radiology* 124:197–202, July 1977.

Sample, W. F., and Sarti, D. A. Computed body tomography and gray scale ultrasonography: anatomic correlations and pitfalls in the upper abdomen. *Gastrointest. Radiol.* 3:243–249, 1978.

Sarti, D. A., and Lazere, A. Reexamination of the deleterious effects of gastrointestinal contrast material on abdominal echography. *Radiology* 126:231–232, January 1978.

Sommer, G., and Filly, R. A. Patient preparations to decrease bowel gas: evaluation by an ultrasonographic measurement. *J. Clin. Ultrasound* 5:87–88, April 1977.

Sommer, G.; Filly, R. A.; and Laing, F. C. Use of simethicone as a patient preparation for abdominal sonography. *Radiology* 125:219–222, October 1977.

Spangen, L. Ultrasound as a diagnostic aid in ventral abdominal hernia. *J. Clin. Ultrasound* 3:211–213, 1976.

Taylor, K. J. W.; Sullivan, D. C.; Wasson, J. F. M.; and Rosenfield, A. R. T. Ultrasound and gallium for the diagnosis of abdominal and pelvic abscesses. *Gastrointest. Radiol.* 3:281–286, 1978.

Teele, R. L., and Smith, E. H. Ultrasound in the diagnosis of idiopathic hypertrophic pyloric stenosis. *N. Engl. J. Med.* 296:1149–1150, May 1977.

Walls, W. J. The evaluation of malignant gastric neoplasms by ultrasonic B-scanning. *Radiology* 118:159–163, January 1976.

Weissberg, D. L.; Scheible, W.; and Leopold, G. R. Ultrasonographic appearance of adult intussusception. *Radiology* 124:791–792, September 1977.

Whalen, J. P.; Evans, J. A.; and Shanser, J. Vector principle in the differential diagnosis of abdominal masses: the left upper quadrant. *Am. J. Roentgenol.* 113:104–118, September 1971.

Wicks, J. D.; Silver, T. M.; and Bree, R. L. Giant cystic abdominal masses in children and adolescents: ultrasonic differential diagnosis. *Am. J. Roentgenol.* 130:853–857, May 1978.

Yeh, H. C., and Wolf, B. S. Ultrasonic contrast study to identify stomach tap water microbubbles. *J. Clin. Ultrasound* 5:170–174, June 1977a.

Yeh, H. C., and Wolf, B. S. Ultrasonography in ascites. *Radiology* 124:783–790, September 1977b.

Yeh, H. C., and Wolf, B. S. Ultrasonography and computed tomography in the diagnosis of homogeneous masses. *Radiology* 123:425–428, May 1977c.

Zimmerman, H. B. Prenatal demonstration of gastric and duodenal obstruction by ultrasound. *J. Can. Assoc. Radiol.* 29:138–141, June 1978.

CASES
Dennis A. Sarti, M.D.
W. Frederick Sample, M.D.

Normal Anatomy

Ultrasound examination of the abdomen outside of the various organs has received relatively little attention. A thorough understanding of the anatomy is extremely helpful in doing a general search of the abdomen. Figure 8.1 is a schematic drawing which shows the relationship among the various peritoneal spaces. The mesenteric attachments of the large bowel form the major boundaries of the peritoneal cavity. Above the transverse mesocolon is the supramesocolic space. Inferior to the transverse mesocolon is the inferior mesocolic space. The root of the small bowel mesentery separates the inframesocolic spaces into right and left compartments. The right and left paracolic gutters are lateral to the ascending and descending colon, respectively. The phrenococolic ligament (arrows) limits communication among the left subphrenic, the perihepatic, and the perisplenic spaces and the paracolic gutter. Freer communication is present on the right side among the subhepatic space, the subphrenic space, and the lesser sac. Communication with the subhepatic space and the lesser sac occurs through the foramen of Winslow. The dotted lines in figure 8.1 outline the pancreatic region situated posterior to the lesser sac.

Figure 8.2 is a sagittal section intended to depict the mesenteric relationships of bowel, retroperitoneum, and the peritoneal spaces. The lesser sac, a potential space, is bounded anteriorly by the stomach and its mesentery, inferiorly by the mesentery (arrow) of the transverse colon, and posteriorly by the retroperitoneal structures. The pancreas and the third portion of the duodenum are situated in the retroperitoneum deep to the lesser sac. The small bowel and its mesenteric attachment (arrow) are inferior to the lesser sac. The potential space of the lesser sac can enlarge and separate the distance between the stomach and the pancreas. When an ultrasound examination is performed on

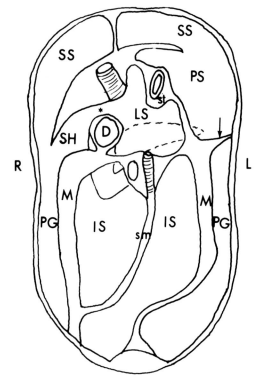

Fig. 8.1

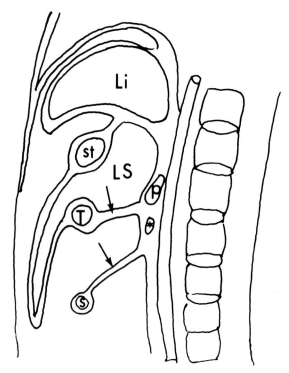

Fig. 8.2

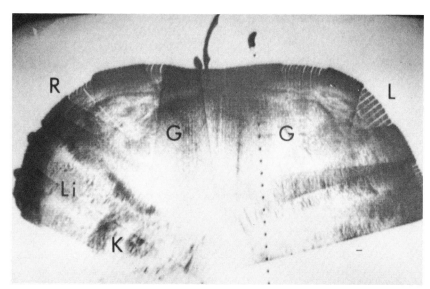

Fig. 8.3

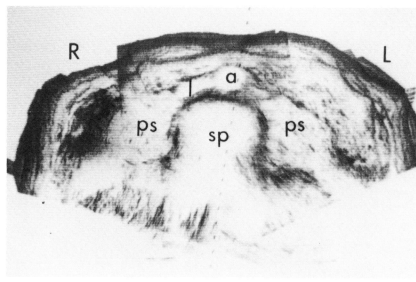

Fig. 8.4

a normal individual, the stomach rests directly on top of the pancreas in most instances.

Ultrasound examination of the abdomen is often obscured by bowel air. Figure 8.3 is a typical example of an air-filled study. Bowel gas yields a high amplitude echo with no through transmission. The abdominal cavity and retroperitoneal region cannot be evaluated when bowel gas is present. If large amounts of fluid were present in the potential spaces of the peritoneum, however, they would displace the bowel gas, and the ultrasound would yield important information. Figure 8.4 is a transverse scan of an airless abdomen. In this instance, we can see the aorta, inferior vena cava, psoas muscles, and spine. All of the structures anterior to the aorta represent collapsed and airless bowel.

*	=	Foramen of Winslow
A	=	Aorta
D	=	Duodenum
G	=	Bowel gas
I	=	Inferior vena cava
IS	=	Inframesocolic space
K	=	Kidney
L	=	Left
Li	=	Liver
LS	=	Lesser sac
M	=	Mesenteric attachments of the large bowel
p	=	Pancreas
PG	=	Pericolic gutter
PS	=	Perisplenic space
ps	=	Psoas muscle
R	=	Right
S	=	Small bowel
SH	=	Subhepatic space
sm	=	Small bowel mesentery
Sp	=	Spine
SS	=	Subphrenic space
St	=	Stomach
T	=	Transverse colon

Normal Anatomy of the Abdomen

Figure 8.5 is a schematic drawing of the abdominal wall with the skin as the superficial structure. Deep to the skin is the fibrofatty subcutaneous tissue which is extremely variable in thickness and causes great havoc to the passage of sound waves. Individuals with large amounts of subcutaneous fat scatter sound quite dramatically and yield extremely poor images. Deep to the subcutaneous fat is the musculofascial plane for which ultrasound can give a strong inner face. The peritoneum is then seen inferior to the muscle plane.

Figure 8.6 is an ultrasound examination demonstrating superficial structures. The skin surface coincides with the strong initial echo arising from the transducer-skin interface. Deep to the skin surface is the subcutaneous fat. This has a coarse echo appearance to it with areas of lucency separated by strong linear echoes. Deep to the subcutaneous fat is the rectus muscle and the peritoneal fat. The relationship of these structures can be seen quite well in figure 8.6. The stomach gives a characteristic "bull's-eye" appearance of the bowel and structures deep to it can be visualized.

A longitudinal scan of the abdomen from the xiphoid to the symphysis pubis (fig. 8.7) yields a fairly characteristic appearance to the upper abdomen. Deep to the liver and the collapsed stomach, we can see the hepatic artery, superior mesenteric vein, and pancreas. Visualization of these structures is possible because of the collapsed stomach. The pelvic structures can also be visualized well secondary to a distended urinary bladder. The uterus is seen deep to the urinary bladder. The anatomy between the urinary bladder and the stomach, however, is completely obscured due to the overlying bowel air.

The diaphragm and subhepatic space are also important areas for examination by ultrasound. The scan in figure 8.8 was performed with the purpose of demonstrating diaphragmatic motion. This is relatively easy to do. Two scans are obtained on the same image. A first scan is performed in deep inspiration; a

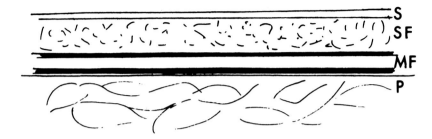

Fig. 8.5

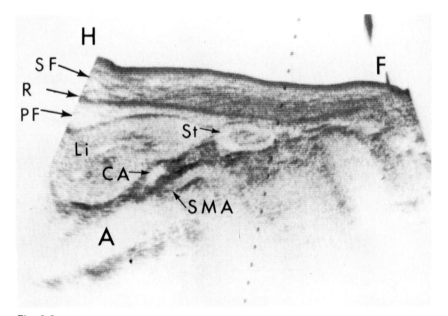

Fig. 8.6

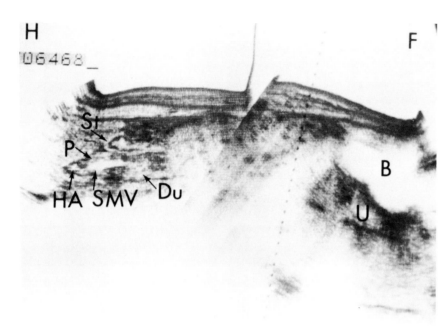

Fig. 8.7

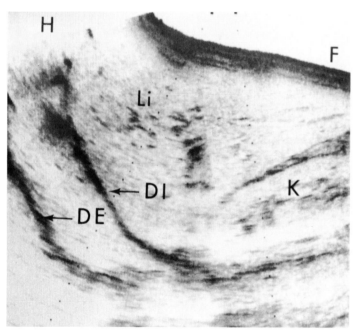

Fig. 8.8

second, in deep expiration. The amount of diaphragmatic motion can then be documented. This procedure is extremely helpful in a patient with a pleural effusion on the right side. Fluoroscopy is not useful in this situation because of silhouetting of the diaphragm by pleural fluid.

We are, however, dealing with acoustic waves in ultrasound, and the diaphragm is readily visualized above the liver, whether or not a pleural effusion is present.

A	=	Aorta
B	=	Urinary bladder
CA	=	Celiac axis
DE	=	Diaphragm during expiration
DI	=	Diaphragm during inspiration
Du	=	Duodenum
F	=	Foot
H	=	Head
HA	=	Hepatic artery
K	=	Kidney
Li	=	Liver
MF	=	Musculofascial plane
P (fig. 8.5)	=	Peritoneal cavity
P	=	Pancreas
PF	=	Peritoneal fat
R	=	Rectus muscle
S	=	Skin
SF	=	Subcutaneous fat
SMA	=	Superior mesenteric artery
SMV	=	Superior mesenteric vein
St	=	Stomach
U	=	Uterus

Rectus Hematoma; Peritoneal Abscess

Ultrasound is an excellent diagnostic tool for the evaluation of masses within or adjacent to the abdominal wall. The subcutaneous fat appears most often as a relatively lucent area just beneath the skin surface. The rectus muscle on thin individuals will be a strong echogenic line. On more well developed individuals, both of its walls can be seen, with soft echoes of the muscle itself present within. Figures 8.9 and 8.10 are of a patient with a palpable mass in the left lateral anterior abdomen following a traumatic episode. Ultrasound examination demonstrated a sonolucency within the rectus muscle. Figure 8.9 is a longitudinal scan through the mid portion of the mass. The rectus muscle is seen above and below the mass. It is outlined by two strong linear echoes. The width of the rectus muscle is within normal limits both superior and inferior to the mass. In its mid portion, however, is a sonolucent mass which turned out to be a rectus hematoma. It is definitely within the rectus muscle, increasing its thickness. A transverse section of the same patient (fig. 8.10) demonstrates the hematoma within the rectus muscle on the left side of the abdomen.

Occasionally, sonolucent masses are seen adjacent to the muscle wall. Often, it will be difficult to determine whether or not they are within the subcutaneous tissue, rectus muscle, or adjacent peritoneal cavity. Figures 8.11 and 8.12 are scans of a patient who had undergone previous surgery. Intraperitoneal abscess was suspected. Ultrasound examination demonstrated a sonolucent mass in the left upper abdomen. A transverse section (fig. 8.11) demonstrates the rectus muscle anterior to the abscess. In this situation, the rectus muscle is displaced anteriorly. The mass, therefore, is within the peritoneal cavity, pushing the rectus muscle anteriorly. It is not situated within the rectus muscle and does not spread apart both of its borders. Figure 8.12 is a longitudinal scan through the abscess. The rectus muscle again is seen displaced anteriorly. At surgery, a loculated abscess

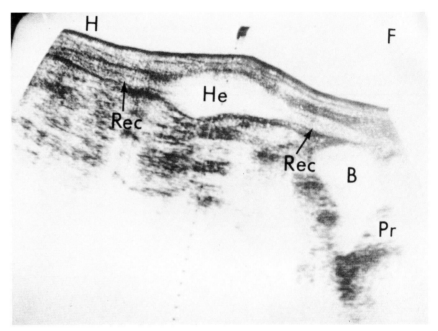

Fig. 8.9

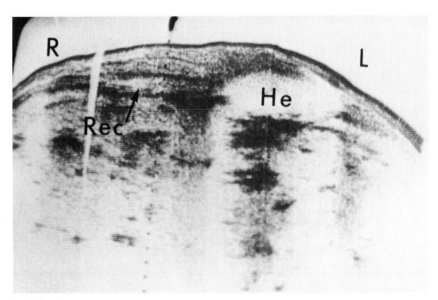

Fig. 8.10

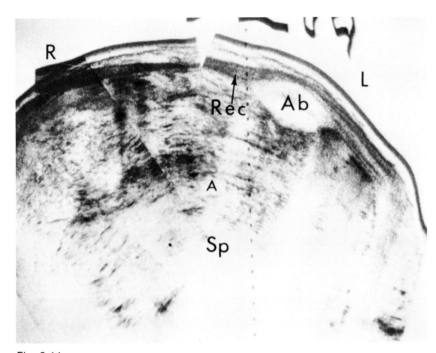

Fig. 8.11

with adherent edematous omentum was found.

A = Aorta
Ab = Abscess
B = Bladder
F = Foot
H = Head
He = Hematoma
L = Left
Pr = Prostate
R = Right
Rec = Rectus muscle
Sp = Spine

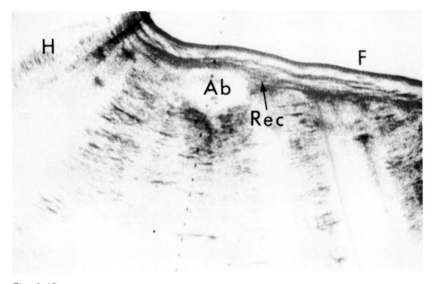

Fig. 8.12

Abdominal Fluid Collections

Numerous clinical entities within the abdomen can yield a fluid-filled mass on ultrasound. Figures 8.13 and 8.14 are of a patient with vague abdominal pain. An ultrasound survey scan was performed. During the course of the examination, a small loculated fluid collection was noted in the right lower abdomen beneath the rectus muscle. Because of the vague abdominal pain, aspiration under ultrasonic guidance was performed. The fluid that was collected was found to be serous. Cultures were negative. This sterile serous collection would have been almost impossible to detect and diagnose without the aid of ultrasound. The interesting point in this case is that we can see the serous collection just beneath the rectus muscle. We could not distinguish this from an abscess or loculated hematoma.

Often, we see numerous masses within the abdomen that represent fluid-filled or food-filled bowel. The stomach, duodenum, small bowel, and colon can be distended with something other than gas. These can be confused for pseudocysts, abscesses, or tumors. Therefore, it is important to recognize the potential masslike appearance of normal bowel.

Figure 8.15 is an example of normal structures yielding a masslike appearance. The gallbladder is easily seen on the right side of the abdomen and is not usually confused for a mass. The duodenum, however, (fig. 8.15) may be confused for a mass near the head of the pancreas. It can appear as air-filled, fluid-filled, or food-filled. In this instance, it is fairly well collapsed and yields a circular or "bull's-eye" appearance very suggestive of normal bowel. Figure 8.15 also demonstrates a mass over the anterior left abdomen which represents the stomach. Posterior to the stomach is the superior mesenteric artery and superior mesenteric vein. The stomach could be easily confused for an abscess or possible pseudocyst. Therefore, if there is any question it is important to perform the examination again 24 hours later after keeping the patient without oral

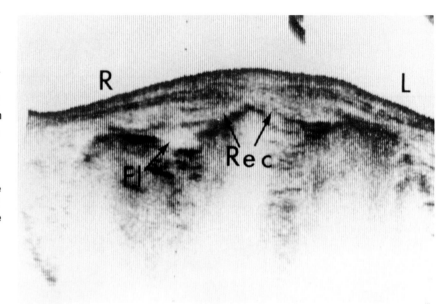

Fig. 8.13

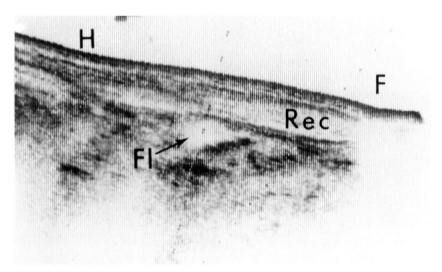

Fig. 8.14

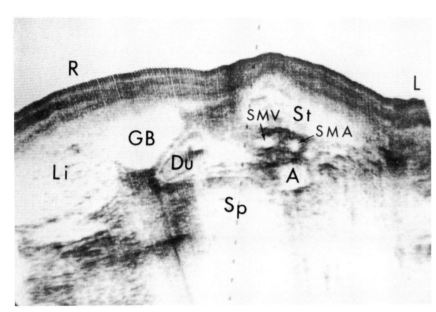

Fig. 8.15

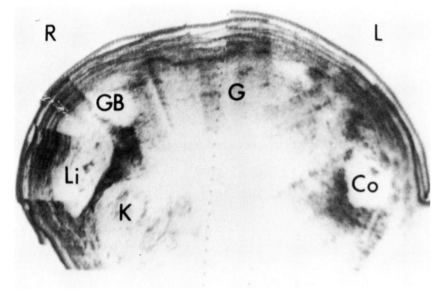

Fig. 8.16

intake overnight or use real-time ultrasound.

Infrequently, the large bowel will present difficulty on ultrasound exam. Figure 8.16 is an example of the presence of fluid and some feces in the descending colon. This could be easily misinterpreted as an abscess in the area. The patient had a history of diarrhea. Again, follow-up examination 24 hours later usually will remove any doubt as to whether or not a loop of bowel is masking as a pathological entity.

A = Aorta
Co = Descending colon
Du = Duodenum
F = Foot
Fl = Sterile serous fluid collection
G = Bowel gas
GB = Gallbladder
H = Head
K = Kidney
L = Left
Li = Liver
R = Right
Rec = Rectus muscle
SMA = Superior mesenteric artery
SMV = Superior mesenteric vein
Sp = Spine
St = Stomach

Ascites

Abdominal fluid frequently can be easily detected with ultrasound. In fact, ultrasound examination is more sensitive to a minimal amount of fluid than is physical examination. Numerous types of fluid may be found in the abdominal cavity. These may include hematoma and abscess. The most common cause of diffuse fluid in the peritoneal cavity, however, is ascites. Although ascites may loculate in unusual locations, there are certain anatomical areas in which it can be detected easily by ultrasonic examination. Figure 8.17 is a transverse section of the right upper quadrant. It demonstrates a characteristic finding in ascites in which the liver capsule (arrows) is displaced away from the right lateral abdominal wall by ascitic fluid. We do not normally see the liver capsule since it is in direct contact with the abdominal wall. With the sonolucent ascitic fluid adjacent to the abdominal wall, however, the strong echo arising from the liver capsule gives a sharp easily recognizable border.

Figure 8.18 is a transverse section in the upper abdomen with ascites in the hepatorenal angle. This is a very common early site for ascitic fluid detection. Since this is a dependent portion of the upper abdomen, ascitic fluid often will be noted in this region. Again we see the strong sharp echo of the liver capsule (arrows), displaced away from the retroperitoneum adjacent to the right kidney.

Figure 8.19 is a transverse scan in the upper abdomen. Again, ascitic fluid is seen displacing the liver capsule (arrows) away from the right lateral abdomen. A similar appearance is also present in the left upper quadrant in the location of the spleen. The splenic capsule also yields a highly reflective interface, since it is being displaced away from the left lateral abdomen. Ascitic fluid is interposed between the left lateral abdominal wall and the splenic capsule in a manner similar to the liver.

In a longitudinal scan of the right lower quadrant (fig. 8.20), we see ascites. Numerous bowel loops are noted to be floating within the ascitic fluid. The ascites is following the contour of the iliopsoas muscle as it fills the entire right

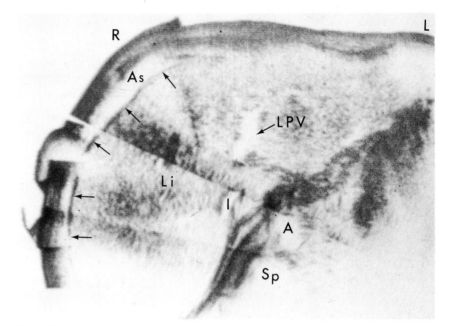

Fig. 8.17

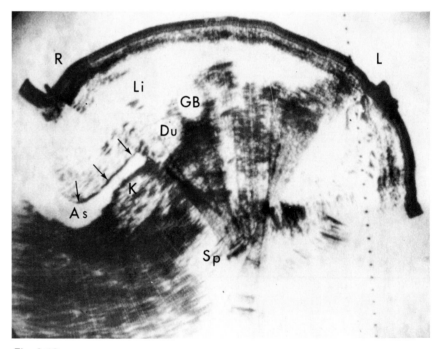

Fig. 8.18

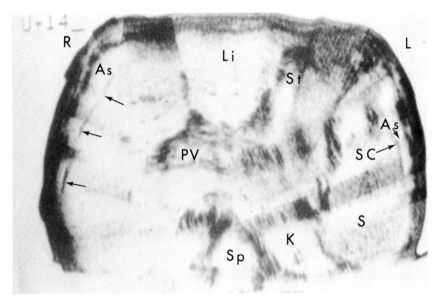

Fig. 8.19

lower quadrant. This is a frequent site of collection for ascitic fluid.

A	=	Aorta
Arrows	=	Liver capsule displaced away from the right abdominal wall by ascitic fluid
As	=	Ascites
Bo	=	Loops of bowel floating in ascitic fluid
Du	=	Duodenum
GB	=	Gallbladder
H	=	Head
I	=	Inferior vena cava
IP	=	Iliopsoas muscle
K	=	Kidney
L	=	Left
Li	=	Liver
LPV	=	Left portal vein
PV	=	Portal vein
R	=	Right
S	=	Spleen
SC	=	Splenic capsule displaced away from the abdominal wall
Sp	=	Spine
St	=	Stomach
U	=	Umbilical level

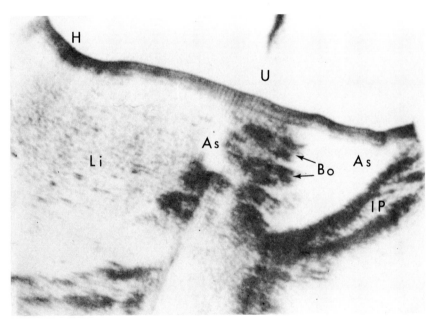

Fig. 8.20

Ascites

Very small collections of ascitic fluid can be present in the lesser sac. Figure 8.21 is an excellent example of ascitic fluid noted posterior to the liver and anterior to the pancreas. This small linear lucency normally is not present. Whenever a small sonolucency is seen just posterior to the liver, loculated ascites, abscess, or hematoma should be considered. A very smooth plane, separating the liver from the pancreas and stomach is demonstrated. These findings are highly consistent with a small loculated ascitic fluid collection in the lesser sac.

Occasionally, ascitic fluid collection can be quite massive. Figure 8.22 is of a patient with chronic ethanol abuse who entered the hospital with a massively distended abdomen. Ultrasound examination demonstrated the abdomen to be mainly fluid-filled, consistent with severe ascites. The liver is markedly compressed and displaced away from the lateral right abdominal wall. The liver capsule represents a sharp border on ultrasound, indicating the intraabdominal collection. The gallbladder is well seen with fluid both within and outside the gallbladder wall. Occasionally, we can see the falciform ligament in a patient with this severe ascites. Another characteristic of severe ascites are bowel loops displaced centrally by the large amount of fluid.

Figures 8.23 and 8.24 are examples of fairly massive ascites visible in the lower abdomen and pelvis. A longitudinal scan of the right lower quadrant (fig. 8.23) demonstrates ascites. Bowel loops are seen floating within the ascitic fluid along with their mesenteric attachment. Figure 8.24 gives a characteristic picture of ascitic fluid situated in the pelvis. The urinary bladder is nearly completely collapsed, with only a small amount of urine present. Fluid is seen in the pelvis, with bowel loops floating within the ascites. This should not be confused with a distended urinary bladder, since the bowel loops give a characteristic circular indentation in the ascitic fluid.

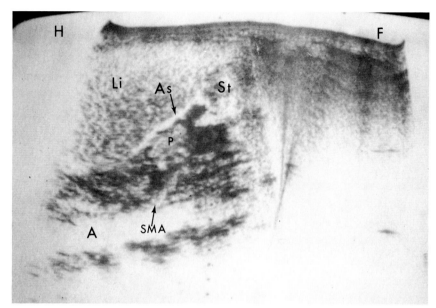

Fig. 8.21

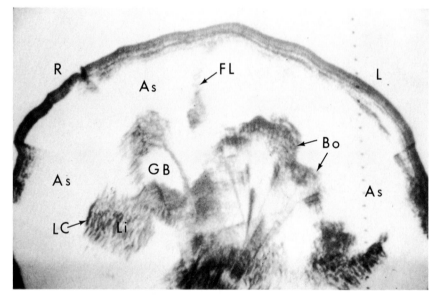

Fig. 8.22

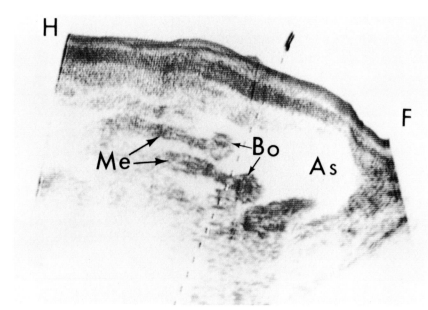

A   = Aorta
As   = Ascites
B   = Urinary bladder
Bo   = Bowel loops
F   = Foot
FL   = Falciform ligament
GB   = Gallbladder
H   = Head
L   = Left
LC   = Liver capsule
Li   = Liver
Me   = Mesenteric attachment of the
         bowel loops
P   = Pancreas
Pu   = Symphysis pubis
R   = Right
SMA = Superior mesenteric artery
St   = Stomach
U   = Umbilical level

Fig. 8.23

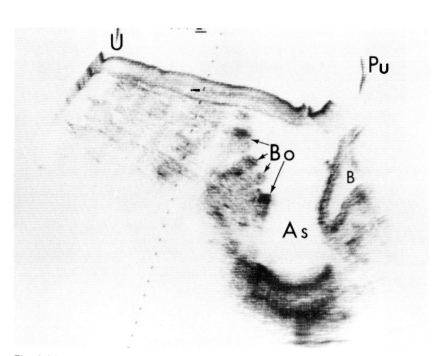

Fig. 8.24

Malignant Ascites; Hemorrhagic Leiomyoma

Very often fluid is noted in the peritoneal cavity and assumed to be secondary to ascites. Often, however, clues indicate that this is not the typical ascites seen most commonly in chronic ethanol abuse. Figure 8.25 shows ascitic fluid in the lower abdomen and pelvis. It does not have the typical appearance of free-floating bowel loops. Here we see evidence of a soft tissue mass adjacent to the abdominal wall, and just superior to the urinary bladder. Findings of irregular soft tissue masses in this region indicate malignancy. This, along with fluid in the pelvis, gives the suggestion of malignant ascites. This patient happened to have metastatic melanoma of the pelvis and anterior abdominal wall. The bowel loops are situated more centrally and are not floating as freely in the ascitic fluid as is usually seen in simple ascites.

Figure 8.26 is of a patient with a metastatic lesion noted in the peritoneal cavity. The only reason we were able to identify this on ultrasound was that the metastatic lesion was made easily visible because of the surrounding ascitic fluid. The ascitic fluid displaces the liver away from the lateral abdominal wall giving a visual window to the area of the metastatic implant.

It is not unusual to see an abdomen nearly completely fluid-filled without the characteristic bowel loops floating within it. Often this will be misdiagnosed as ascites. Numerous pelvic entities, however, may yield large fluid-filled masses which fill nearly the entire abdominal cavity. A very common entity that will cause this is an ovarian tumor with a large amount of fluid. The case in figures 8.27 and 8.28 was an unusual instance of a large hemorrhagic uterine leiomyoma which filled nearly the entire abdomen. This degenerating fibroid was nearly completely fluid-filled. The transverse scan (fig. 8.27) over the mid abdomen shows that nearly the entire abdomen is fluid-filled. We do not, however, see the characteristic floating bowel loops present within the fluid. Therefore, the diagnosis of ascites is eliminated. There are some linear echoes (arrows) in the left lateral abdomen, but they do

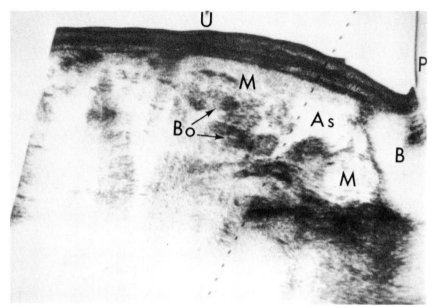

Fig. 8.25

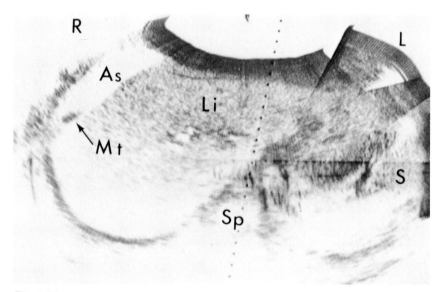

Fig. 8.26

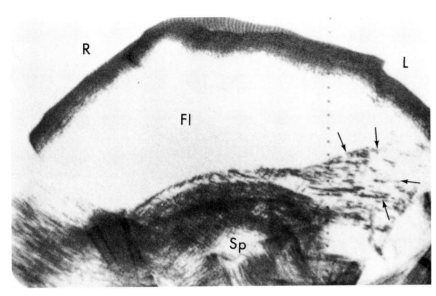

Fig. 8.27

not have the characteristic appearance of bowel loops with attached mesentery. Figure 8.28 is a longitudinal scan of the upper abdomen of this patient. The liver is displaced quite cephalad by this fluid-filled mass. Again, the characteristic bowel and mesentery are not seen floating within the abdominal fluid; this means we are not dealing with ascites.

Arrows	=	Solid component to the hemorrhagic leiomyoma
As	=	Ascites
B	=	Urinary bladder
Bo	=	Bowel loops
D	=	Diaphragm
F	=	Foot
Fl	=	Fluid in a hemorrhagic leiomyoma
H	=	Head
L	=	Left
Li	=	Liver
M	=	Malignant melanoma
Mt	=	Peritoneal metastasis
P	=	Symphysis pubis
R	=	Right
S	=	Spleen
Sp	=	Spine
U	=	Umbilical level

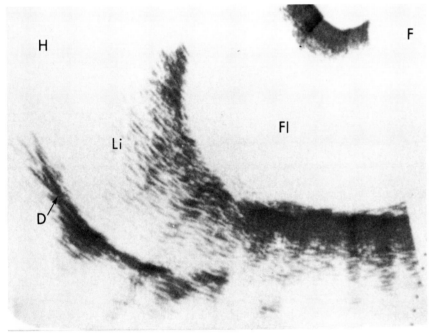

Fig. 8.28

Peritonitis;
Left-Upper-Quadrant
Abscess

When ascites is present in the abdomen
the fluid visualized with ultrasound is
usually relatively echo-free, unless
there has been previous surgery. Other
types of fluid may be present in the peritoneal cavity. When pus or blood is present, there often will be internal echoes
noted within the fluid because of debris
and fibrosis or clot formation. This is one
general way of distinguishing ascites
from other forms of fluid collection.

Figures 8.29 and 8.30 are scans of a
patient with diffuse peritonitis secondary
to bowel perforation. A longitudinal scan
over the right abdomen (fig. 8.29) demonstrates a fluid collection anterior to
the right lobe of the liver. Within the fluid
collection are numerous curvilinear echoes (arrows) which help to distinguish it
from simple ascites. A longitudinal scan
(fig. 8.30) was obtained of the right lower
quadrant. Again we see numerous curvilinear echoes present within the fluid.
The patient has diffuse peritonitis. It is
clear that the fluid collection is somewhat different than in the previous cases
of ascites. There is much more evidence of debris within the fluid, and this
is highly consistent with either pus or
hematoma.

Figures 8.31 and 8.32 are of a patient
with a large left-upper-quadrant abscess following surgery for colonic carcinoma. Figure 8.31 demonstrates
bowel loops floating within the fluid. The
abscess shows evidence of linear echoes (arrows) within the fluid collection.
A longitudinal scan of the left lateral abdomen (fig. 8.32) also shows numerous
linear echoes within the abscess. Again,
ascites tends to be relatively echo-free
as it displaces organs and bowel loops.
Abscesses and hematomas within the
abdomen tend to give more internal
echoes.

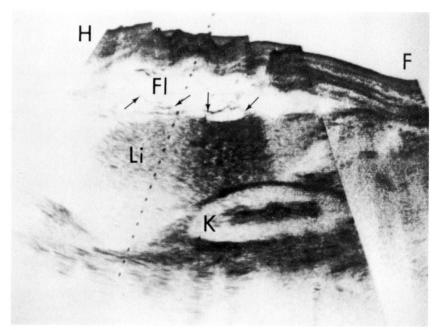

Fig. 8.29

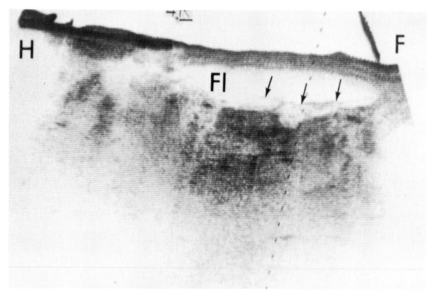

Fig. 8.30

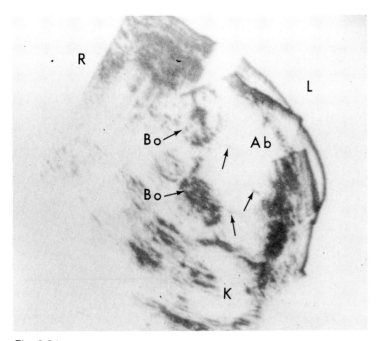

Fig. 8.31

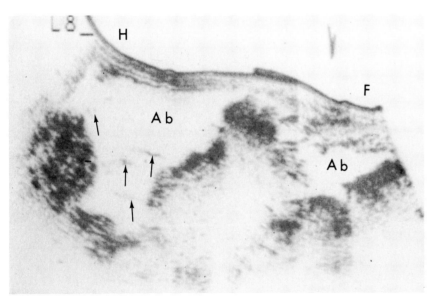

Fig. 8.32

Ab	= Left upper quadrant abscess
Arrows	= Internal echoes within the fluid, indicating debris
Bo	= Bowel loops
F	= Foot
Fl	= Fluid secondary to peritonitis
H	= Head
K	= Kidney
L	= Left
Li	= Liver
R	= Right

Intraabdominal Abscesses

Often a patient will be sent to the ultrasound laboratory with the provisional diagnosis of an intraabdominal abscess. Ultrasound is an excellent means for visualizing intraabdominal abscesses if there is no intervening bowel air between the transducer and the mass. Abscesses can present in a variety of appearances. If the abscess is recent and suppurative, it will appear as a fluid-filled mass. If, however, the abscess is of a chronic nature, with a large amount of debris, it can present as a solid mass and be mistaken for a tumor. Figure 8.33 is of a patient who was examined to rule out a right upper quadrant abscess. The longitudinal scan over the right upper abdomen demonstrates a subdiaphragmatic abscess anterior to the liver and just inferior to the right hemidiaphragm. It could also represent ascites, hematoma, or a bile leak. It is extremely difficult to distinguish among these entities by ultrasound. However, the clinical history often contributes to the ultrasonic findings and leads to a correct diagnosis.

In an unusual case (fig. 8.34), a patient was examined for vague rightupper-quadrant pain. Initially, the study was done to rule out cholelithiasis. During the course of the examination, a sonolucent mass in the lateral abdomen was noted. This decubitus transverse scan shows a sonolucent mass lateral to the liver. Because of this finding, associated with the vague right-upperquadrant pain, the patient was taken to surgery. Chronic appendicitis with a walled-off chronic abscess lateral to the liver at the location noted on ultrasound was found.

An abscess frequently will present with a large amount of debris and give the appearance of a solid mass on ultrasound. Figures 8.35 and 8.36 are of a patient found to have a subhepatic abscess at operation. The ultrasonic findings demonstrated a solid mass noted in the epigastric region beneath the left lobe of the liver. The numerous echoes within the abscess lead to the confusing picture of a solid lesion within the upper abdomen. This, however, was secondary to a chronic abscess filled with a

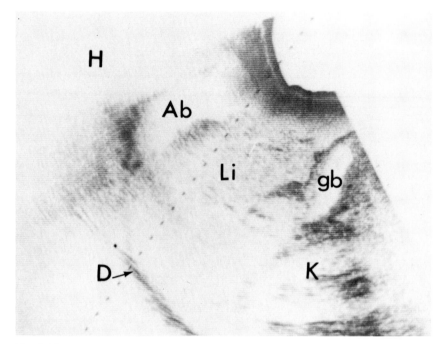

Fig. 8.33

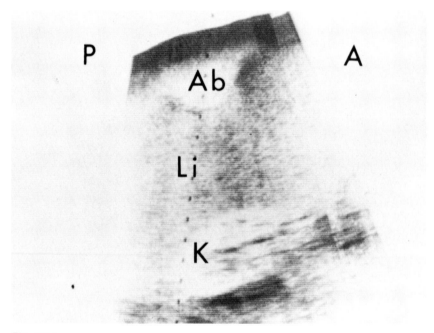

Fig. 8.34

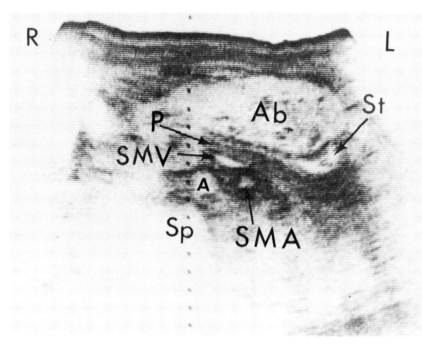

Fig. 8.35

large amount of debris. It could also be misinterpreted for a stomach filled with food. The transverse scan (fig. 8.35), however, demonstrates a small amount of fluid within the stomach. The pancreas is seen posterior to the abscess and stomach. The longitudinal scan (fig. 8.36) shows the abscess to be in the subhepatic region.

A	=	Aorta
A	=	Anterior (fig. 8.34)
Ab	=	Abscess
D	=	Diaphragm
F	=	Foot
GB	=	Gallbladder
H	=	Head
K	=	Kidney
L	=	Left
Li	=	Liver
P	=	Pancreas
P	=	Posterior (fig. 8.34)
R	=	Right
SA	=	Splenic artery
SMA	=	Superior mesenteric artery
SMV	=	Superior mesenteric vein
Sp	=	Spine
St	=	Stomach

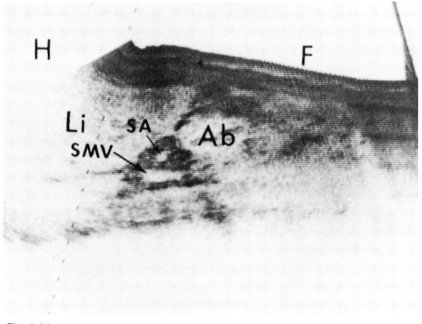

Fig. 8.36

Edematous Omentum; Duodenal Hematoma

Figures 8.37 and 8.38 are of a patient with an ultrasonic picture highly consistent with a left upper quadrant abscess. At surgery, however, no abscess was found. The patient, a 62-year-old man, was admitted with the diagnosis of colonic cancer. He was operated on, and a colostomy was performed. Three weeks after the operation there was a fever spike, and an ultrasound examination was performed. Figures 8.37 and 8.38 demonstrate a relatively sonolucent mass with some linear echoes present within it. It was situated superior, lateral, and anterior to the spleen. The finding was highly consistent with a left-upper-quadrant abscess. The patient underwent surgery, and the left upper quadrant was explored. No abscess or hematoma was noted. The left upper quadrant, however, had a large amount of markedly edematous omentum which most likely had been viewed as this relatively lucent mass. We have seen one other case in which markedly edematous omentum was present without evidence of frank pus. If a mass in the abdomen is highly suggestive for an abscess, the possibility of adherent edematous omentum also should be considered.

Figures 8.39 and 8.40 are of a young boy who had been involved in an auto accident. The upper-gastrointestinal series demonstrated a duodenal outlet obstruction. Ultrasound examination shows evidence of fluid in the duodenum and stomach. A mass is near the fourth portion of the duodenum. It was found to be secondary to a retroperitoneal hematoma of the fourth portion of the duodenum. Figure 8.40 is an excellent example of a fluid-filled antrum and pyloric region of the stomach. The hematoma has a mixed echo pattern with echogenic and sonolucent regions. Abscesses and hematomas can yield similar appearances on ultrasound. They can be nearly sonolucent, indicating their fluid-filled nature. Areas of hematomas with clotted blood or chronic abscesses can, however, present as echogenic masses which are difficult to distinguish from soft tissue tumors.

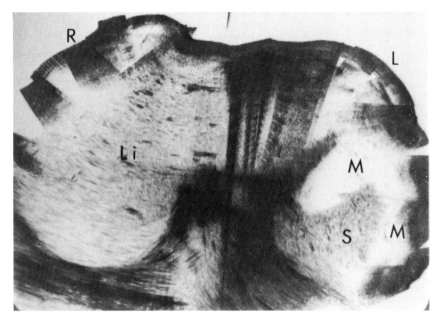

Fig. 8.37

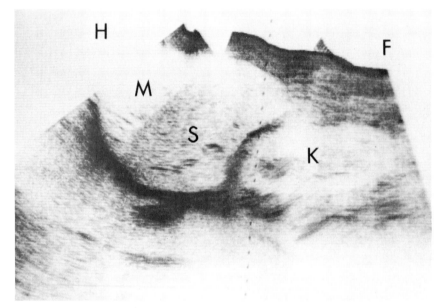

Fig. 8.38

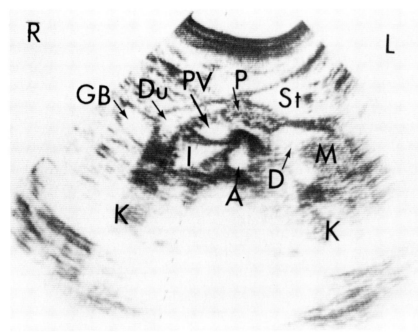

Fig. 8.39

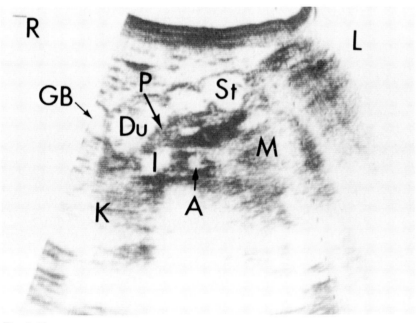

Fig. 8.40

A = Aorta
D = Fourth portion of the duodenum
Du = Duodenum
F = Foot
GB = Gallbladder
H = Head
I = Inferior vena cava
K = Kidney
L = Left
Li = Liver
M = Edematous omentum (figs. 8.37 and 8.38)
M = Duodenal and retroperitoneal hematoma (figs. 8.39 and 8.40)
P = Pancreas
PV = Portal vein
R = Right
S = Spleen
St = Stomach

Pleural Effusions Presenting as Abdominal Masses

Figure 8.41 is a transverse scan obtained of a patient with carcinoma of the left lung. Initially, there appears to be a large fluid-filled mass in the left upper quadrant. The diagnostic possibilities include a pancreatic pseudocyst, ascites, abscess, or possibly a fluid-filled stomach with gastric outlet obstruction. The longitudinal scan, however, (fig. 8.42) demonstrates a large pleural effusion. This scan was obtained in the right lateral decubitus position following the left axillary line. A completely filled left hydrothorax is seen. The diaphragm has been inverted by the large hydrothorax on the left side.

Pleural fluid frequently is confused for ascites. Figures 8.43 and 8.44 are of a 38-year-old man with a long history of alcohol abuse. He had a previous history of ascites and pleural effusion. The pleural effusion was negative for cytology and bacterial culture. A transverse scan of the right upper abdomen (fig. 8.43) demonstrates ascitic fluid lateral to the liver. Posterior to the liver we see the pleural effusion in the posterior sulcus. The diaphragm can be visualized between the ascitic fluid and the pleural effusion. A longitudinal scan of the right upper quadrant (fig. 8.44) shows the pleural effusion superior to the diaphragm, while ascitic fluid is noted inferior to the diaphragm. Since pleural fluid is present in the right pleural space, we are able to see the posterior aspect of the thorax (arrows). Normally, this cannot be seen when air is present in the lungs. When visualizing the echoes of the thorax, fluid or a solid material has to be present superior to the diaphragm in order to demonstrate the posterior thorax this far cephalad.

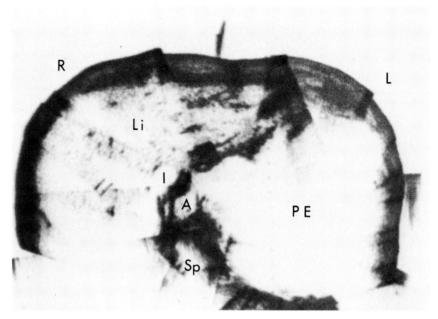

Fig. 8.41

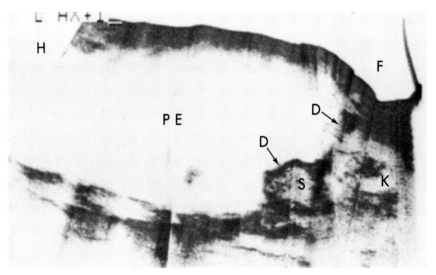

Fig. 8.42

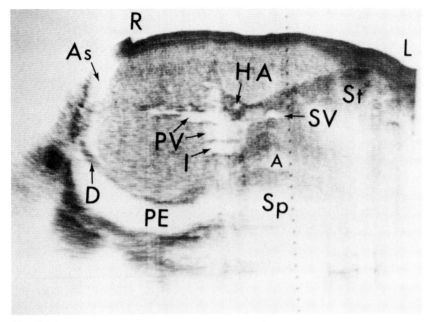

Fig. 8.43

A	= Aorta
Arrows	= Posterior right thoracic wall
As	= Ascites
D	= Inverted diaphragm
F	= Foot
H	= Head
HA	= Hepatic artery
I	= Inferior vena cava
K	= Kidney
L	= Left
Li	= Liver
PE	= Pleural effusion
PV	= Portal vein
R	= Right
S	= Spleen
Sp	= Spine
St	= Stomach
SV	= Splenic vein

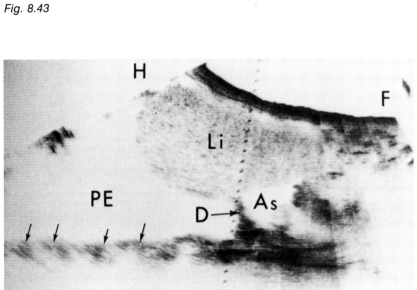

Fig. 8.44

Intra-Abdominal Metastasis; Small Bowel Obstruction

Figures 8.45 and 8.46 are of a 62-year-old man who entered the hospital with an enlarging abdominal mass. Ultrasound examination demonstrated a strongly echogenic soft tissue mass adherent to the anterior abdominal wall. It was approximately 4–5 cm in thickness and had an irregular inner surface. Ascitic fluid was noted posterior to the mass. Bowel loops were seen floating within the ascitic fluid. A percutaneous biopsy of the mass revealed diffuse adenocarcinoma. A barium enema demonstrated an "apple-core" lesion of the transverse colon, indicating a primary colonic carcinoma. The patient had metastatic adenocarcinoma to the peritoneum and abdominal wall, as documented by ultrasound. This was an unusual case of soft-tissue tumor adherent to the abdominal wall accompanied by malignant ascites, and ultrasound was an excellent means for evaluating its extent.

Occasionally, numerous fluid-filled circular and tubular structures are seen within the abdomen. The possibility of obstructed loops of bowel should always be considered. Figures 8.47 and 8.48 are of a patient with small bowel obstruction. We see the bowel loops in both transverse and longitudinal scans. The transverse scans in figure 8.47 show the bowel loops to be circular and oval in shape. There may be some confusion with an ovarian neoplasm. The longitudinal scans in figure 8.48, however, demonstrate a more tubular appearance to the bowel loops. These findings are highly consistent with obstructed fluid-filled bowel loops which can be confirmed by demonstrating peristaltic activity with real-time examination.

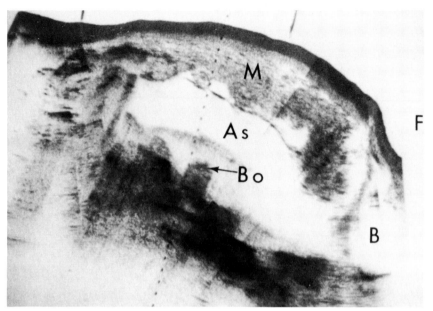

Fig. 8.45

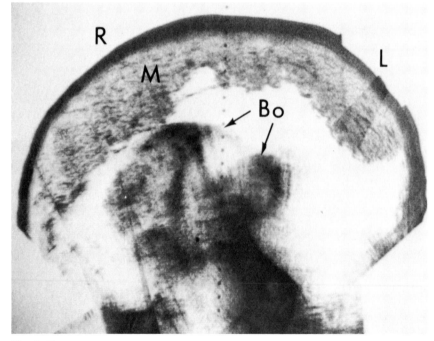

Fig. 8.46

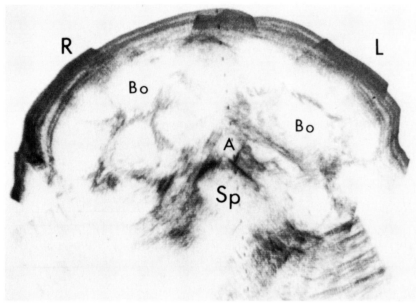

A	= Aorta
As	= Malignant ascites
B	= Urinary bladder
Bo (figs. 8.45 and 8.46)	= Bowel loops
Bo (figs. 8.47 and 8.48)	= Fluid-filled bowel loops
F	= Foot
H	= Head
K	= Kidney
L	= Left
M	= Metastatic adenocarcinoma
R	= Right
Sp	= Spine

Fig. 8.47

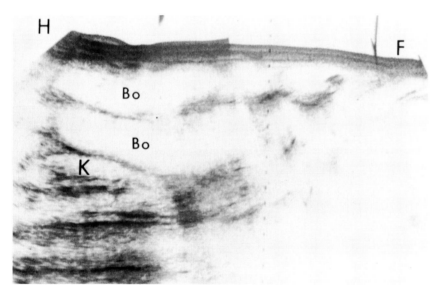

Fig. 8.48

Obstructed Bowel; Intussusception

Fluid-filled bowel loops give a fairly characteristic echo appearance on ultrasound. Numerous tubular and circular sonolucencies are present throughout the abdomen. Figures 8.49 and 8.50 are scans from two different patients with bowel obstruction. A longitudinal scan (fig. 8.49) demonstrates numerous tubular, fluid-filled bowel loops. These are due to a small bowel obstruction. The valvulae conniventes (arrows) can actually be seen within one of the loops of bowel giving a linear echo across the bowel lumen. Figure 8.50 is a transverse scan of a different patient with bowel obstruction. Multiple tubular and circular fluid-filled structures are seen. Bowel obstruction gives an ultrasonic picture very different from ascites or abscesses. Ascites will tend to have the fluid collect laterally, with the echogenic bowel loops noted centrally. Abscesses resolve as loculated or localized areas of fluid masses. However, with bowel obstruction the abdomen is filled with tubular or sausagelike sonolucent masses which lead to the correct diagnosis. Also, real-time examination often can detect peristaltic activity.

Figures 8.51 and 8.52 are scans of a patient who had a previous small bowel bypass for obesity. Because of intermittent abdominal pain, an ultrasound study was performed. A transverse scan of the mid abdomen (fig. 8.51) demonstrates a large mass draped over the spine. This mass has a lucent periphery with a strong echogenic central portion. A longitudinal scan (fig. 8.52) gives a similar appearance. At surgery, the patient was found to have intussusception of the blind loop segment. This large target or "bull's-eye" appearance has been reported in intussusception and gastrointestinal tumors.

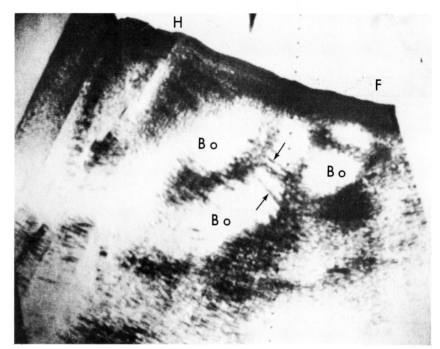

Fig. 8.49

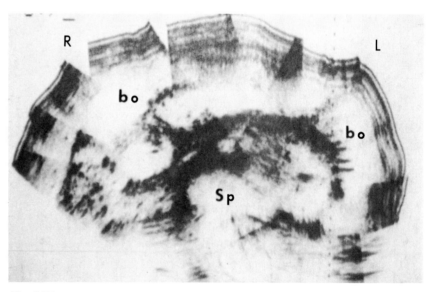

Fig. 8.50

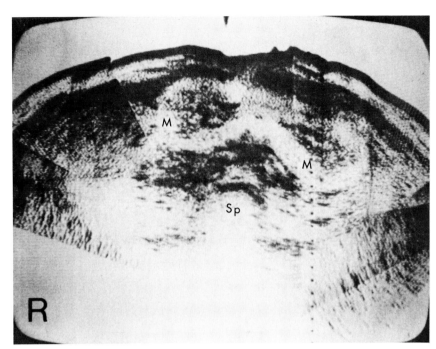

Arrows = Valvulae conniventes
B   = Bowel loops
Bo   = Small bowel fluid-filled loops
H   = Head
F   = Foot
L   = Left
Li   = Liver
M   = Intussusception
R   = Right
Sp   = Spine

Fig. 8.51

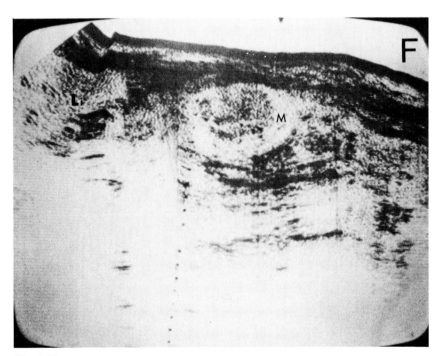

Fig. 8.52

Infarcted Bowel;
Duodenal Duplication Cyst

Fluid-filled obstructed bowel loops usually give a fairly characteristic ultrasonic appearance without a confusing etiological picture. Figures 8.53 and 8.54, however, show a patient sent for a pelvic ultrasound examination because of lower abdominal pain. The study demonstrated numerous sonolucent masses with very thick walls. These turned out to be infarcted bowel loops. At the time of examination, the possibility of an ovarian mass was considered quite likely. Figures 8.53 and 8.54 demonstrate numerous circular sonolucencies with fluid centrally. The bowel walls were thickened and edematous, which gives us a picture different from normal bowel obstruction in which the walls are quite thin. At surgery, numerous bowel loops were present in the pelvis and not only were obstructed but also markedly thickened and edematous from infarction.

Figures 8.55 and 8.56 are ultrasound examinations of a 17-year-old young man admitted with a 6-day history of abdominal pain. The ultrasound examinations demonstrated a large mass in the right upper quadrant. The mass had numerous echoes within it; through transmission, however, was noted posteriorly. This is best evident in the longitudinal scan (fig. 8.56). At surgery, the mass was found to be a duplication cyst of the duodenum. The ultrasonic appearance would be consistent with an abscess, hematoma, or pancreatic pseudocyst with debris. There was nothing specific to suggest a duplication cyst. We have seen other duplication cysts of the duodenum which have been completely sonolucent, indicating that only fluid is present.

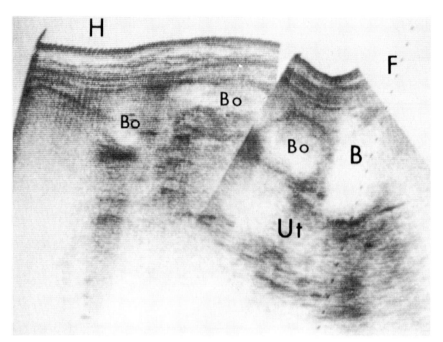

Fig. 8.53

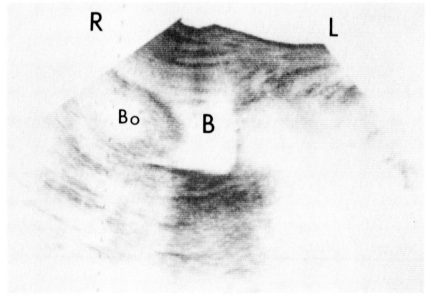

Fig. 8.54

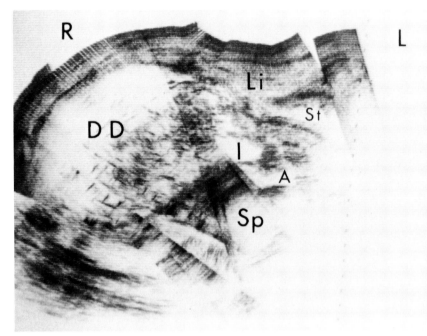

Fig. 8.55

A = Aorta
B = Urinary bladder
Bo = Infarcted bowel loops
DD = Duplication cyst of the duodenum
F = Foot
H = Head
I = Inferior vena cava
L = Left
Li = Liver
R = Right
Sp = Spleen
St = Stomach
Ut = Uterus

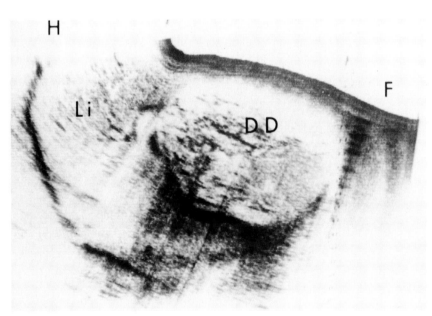

Fig. 8.56

9.
Ultrasonography of Thyroid and Neck Masses

Catherine Cole-Beuglet, M.D.

Introduction

The clinical application of thyroid sonography was not established until 1967 (Fujimoto et al. 1967). This late development is surprising, considering the superficial location of the gland which lies approximately 2 cm below the skin of the anterior neck. But contrary to expectations, it was its superficial location and its size that made early attempts at sonic imaging of the thyroid so difficult. Before water-bath scanning, the standard 2.25 MHz transducers were large-diameter crystals, which when pulsed with an electric current, produced a strong opening bang and a reverberation echo up to 2 cm thick. As a consequence, the thyroid gland was lost within it. Water-bath scanning eliminated this problem, and the tissues immediately below the skin surface could be imaged. Furthermore, the awkwardness resulting from contact scanning of the angular neck contour was eliminated because water-bath scanning allowed easier manipulation of the transducer in the water (Skolnick and Royal 1975).

With the advent of gray scale imaging techniques thyroid sonography became an established clinical examination. Gray scale recording of low-level amplitude information from the internal structure of the gland facilitated the differentiation of normal from pathological conditions (Jellins et al. 1975). Contact scanning became technically easier when transducers with smaller diameters were developed. Resolution improved with the use of higher-frequency crystals. The best thyroid images are obtained using gray scale water-bath B-scanning (Jellins et al. 1975; Sackler et al. 1977; Wagai, Ishihara, and Kobayashi et al. 1976). Recently, real-time imaging with enclosed water-bath, high-frequency transducers has proved valuable for the examination of the internal tissue texture and pulsations of thyroid and neck masses (Hassani and Bard 1977).

Imaging of the parathyroid glands has become a reality with the use of high-frequency transducers. The location of both the normal and enlarged glands is recordable and very important to surgeons attempting parathyroid removal (Crocker, Bautovich, and Jellins 1978; Sample, Mitchell, and Bledsoe 1978).

When examining patients with thyroid abnormalities, inspection and palpation of the gland is performed to determine the type of enlargement, either diffuse or nodular. Radionuclide studies using thyroid-tissue-specific tagged iodine are performed to identify the gland. Both the iodine uptake and imaging contribute to the evaluation of the gland's function and morphology. The size, location, and relative function of the gland or nodules within the gland are recorded. Glandular tissue in ectopic sites will also concentrate the radioactive iodine. If an area of the gland does not take up the radioactive isotope, it is designated as a cold nodule. A review of the literature shows these areas represent malignant change in approximately 20% of cases subjected to pathological studies (Blei, Gooding, and Rector 1977; Rosen, Walfish, and Miskin 1974). Cold nodules can also represent simple cysts, cystic degeneration, or hemorrhage within solid tissue, such as adenomas, hyperplasia, or thyroiditis (inflammation) (Perlmutter, Goldberg, and Charkes 1975; Sanders and Sanders 1977). Isotope studies do not differentiate the different types of cold nodules. Ultrasound B-scans give the internal composition of these nodules and of the thyroid gland (Shaub and Wilson 1975b; Walfish et al. 1977). The anteroposterior dimensions of the gland and nodules are measured. It should be noted that this information is unavailable on two-dimensional isotope images. The volume of the gland may be calculated using the three dimensions measurable on the sonic study (Rasmussen and Hjorth 1974). This is useful information when calculating the dose of radioisotopes for therapy. Serial B-scans may be performed to assess the response to therapy or the progression of disease.

Anatomy of the Thyroid Gland

The thyroid, an endocrine gland, develops as a bud from the ventral surface of the primitive pharynx. A mass forms at the base of the tongue and with fetal growth migrates inferiorly in the midline to its final position at the base of the neck opposite the fifth to the seventh cervical vertebrae. Aberrant tissue is found along the course of this duct, from the foramen caecum at the back of the tongue, to the midline anterior to the trachea and thyroid cartilage. If it migrates further, thyroid tissue can be found in the superior mediastinum in a retrosternal position. The duct normally obliterates during fetal life. If it fails to do so, cysts form along the tract. The subhyoid area is the commonest site, and a mass in this location may disappear beneath the hyoid bone when the patient swallows.

The thyroid gland has two lobes which straddle the trachea in an H or U shape. A thin section in the inferior portion, the isthmus, crosses in front of the trachea and covers the second, third, or fourth rings. It is variable in size, or it may be absent. Occasionally, an extra lobe, the pyramidal lobe, extends upward from the isthmus in the midline.

The apex of each lobe extends between the sternothyroid and inferior constrictor muscles of the pharynx. The lateral surface is covered by the infrahyoid muscles, the sternothyroid, sternohyoid, and omohyoid muscles. The medial surface rests on the trachea, the inferior constrictor muscle of the pharynx, and the esophagus. The recurrent laryngeal nerve runs between these tubular passages. The posterior surface is in contact with the paired parathyroid glands, the prevertebral muscle, the longus colli, the sympathetic trunk, and the carotid sheath. This sheath contains the common carotid artery medially, the internal jugular vein laterally, and the vagus nerve between them posteriorly. The gland is covered by a thin fibrous capsule that is adherent to it and a sheath from the pretracheal layer of deep cervical fascia. The parathyroids usually lie outside the thyroid capsule but may rest within it and be adjacent to the posterior thyroid tissue. The thyroid lobes move upward when a person swallows.

Technique

Ultrasound examination of the thyroid is usually preceded by an isotope examination. It is of the utmost importance that the masses in the neck designated as nonfunctioning on the isotope study be marked on the patient's skin surface with a felt pen. The patient is placed in a supine position with a folded pillow or bolus under the shoulder to hyperextend the neck. Contact solution, either mineral oil or a water-soluble gel, is applied to the skin.

For gray scale contact B-scanning a 5-MHz narrow-diameter short internal-focus transducer will resolve lesions less than 1 cm in size. The detail of 1-mm tissue architecture is resolved with a 7 or 10-MHz transducer. Larger masses, called goiters, may require a 3.5-MHz transducer. The time gain compensation curve is set at a gentle slope starting immediately at the skin surface. Cross-sectional tomograms of the neck starting just above the suprasternal notch are made at 1-cm intervals to the superior limits of the gland. Longitudinal scans from the midline to the lateral margin of the gland on each side are done at 0.5-cm intervals. The scanner arm is angled 10–15° medially for the longitudinal tomograms. Because of the difficulty in moving the transducer over the angular neck surface, it is advisable to steady it by placing the two outside fingertips of the hand holding the transducer on the skin surface. Simple sector scans over the palpable nodule at different sensitivity settings aid in the determination of the internal tissue texture of the nodule as compared with the adjacent thyroid tissue. The margins of the palpable nodule are marked on the image with the centimeter scale or graticule before the image is recorded.

Water-bath scanning is performed by placing a polyethylene drape, supported by a stand, over the neck of the patient. Contact solution is applied to the skin between the neck and the drape. Warm water, preferably 37° C, is poured into the supported drape to a depth equal to the depth of the tissue to be examined. Air bubbles trapped between the skin and the drape are smoothed away with one finger. The transducer is lowered into the water and guided in transverse or longitudinal sections over the gland (Sackler et al. 1977). It is difficult to maintain a constant distance between the transducer and the skin surface. Consequently, armatures have been developed to hold the transducer and allow mechanical transverse scanning at preset increments (Jellins et al. 1975; Wagai, Ishihara, and Kobayashi 1976).

Another approach to water-bath scanning involves the use of water-filled polyethylene bags or gloves which are draped over the neck. Contact solution is applied to both surfaces of the bags. The patient can assist in holding the closed water bag in position. The transducer is moved along the top surface to obtain a water-bath scan. The time compensation gain curve is set at a rising slope starting at the skin line.

With hand-held sector, linear, or phased array scanners, the scanner head is placed directly over the thyroid nodule and images at different gain settings are observed and recorded with the transducer in the same position. These may also be used in a water bath. Real-time imaging allows identification of the pulsations of the common carotid artery and intrathyroid arteries as well as changes in caliber of the internal jugular veins. These reference landmarks aid in the distinction between intrinsic mass pulsations and transmitted pulsations from adjacent vessels (Hassani and Bard 1977).

Landmarks for identification on every thyroid scan are the anterior wall of the trachea in the midline, the carotid sheath laterally, and the strap muscles of the neck. The air in the trachea reflects the sound beam, and this results in a midline shadow under the strong anterior tracheal-wall interface. Reverberation echoes often occur within this acoustic shadow. The carotid sheath along the posterior lateral margin of the thyroid contains the common carotid artery. Its walls image as strong echo-reflective surfaces. On a transverse single-sweep scan they may appear as two parallel echoes, whereas on a compound scan, a circle is imaged when the lateral walls reflect the sound beam. On longitudinal scans, the demonstration of two parallel strong echo-reflective surfaces at the posterior lateral margin of the gland indicates the lateral boundary of the lobe. The fluid-filled artery lumen acts as an echo-free reference standard to be compared with echo-free spaces within the thyroid gland. The walls of the external jugular vein give weaker echo reflections. The echo-free vein varies in size with respiration, attaining maximum diameter with a Valsalva maneuver. The strap muscles of the neck appear anterior and lateral to the gland and are relatively echo-free compared to the gland. Imaging of the prevertebral muscles posteriorly marks adequate penetration for visualization of the entire thyroid gland area.

The normal thyroid gland images on a gray scale B-scan as a fine homogeneous reflective pattern. The parenchyma images through diffuse reflections, and is thus independent of the angle of inclination of the sonic beam (Jellins et al. 1975). The fibrous tissue capsule is not imaged unless thickened. The gland measures 1–2 cm in anteroposterior dimension and 4–6 cm in length.

Pathology of the Thyroid Gland and Neck

Fluid-Filled Areas

On a gray scale B-scan, a circumscribed echo-free area with a well-defined posterior border represents a simple cyst. The accentuation of echoes usually seen behind liquid-filled areas may be absent in the neck without sufficient thyroid tissue behind the cyst to demonstrate this enhancement phenomenon. A review of a reported series of thyroid nodules designated as cold on isotope studies and examined with ultrasound shows an incidence of simple cyst in 11–22% of pathologically verified cases (Miller, Zafar, and Karo 1974; Shaub and Wilson 1975b; Solgaard, Grytter, and Rasmussen 1975). Cysts may be aspirated by percutaneous puncture with a fine needle and the fluid sent for cytological evaluation (Jensen and Rasmussen 1976; Miller, Zafar, and Karo 1974; Walfish et al. 1977).

Developmental thyroglossal duct cysts are present as midline neck masses. They may extend from the base of the tongue to the isthmus of the gland in front of the trachea. On an ultrasound B-scan, these are echo-free, well-outlined masses. Debris within the cyst may give rise to mobile low-amplitude echoes. One-third of these midline masses will contain functioning thyroid tissue which can be imaged on radioisotope iodine or fluorescent studies (Blei, Gooding, and Rector 1977; Blum and Goldman 1975). On an ultrasound scan, solid tissue will be imaged along margins of the echo-free space, or solid tissue may project into the echo-free space. The tissue has the fine, diffuse, echo-reflective pattern similar to normal thyroid parenchyma. Infected cysts or abscesses presenting as tender midline swellings give a similar appearance on an ultrasound examination. Fistulas may connect to the skin surface of the anterior neck when these infected cysts spontaneously drain.

Solid Areas

Often, palpable small nodules display an internal texture on a B-scan that is uniform and cannot be separated from the normal adjacent thyroid tissue. The boundary may not be imaged, and the position of the nodule can be outlined only when the margins of the nodule are marked on the image. These nodules generally represent benign adenomas. With higher-frequency real-time water-bath scanners, less than 1-mm thick capsules of these adenomas have been outlined as a relatively echo-poor boundary surrounding the nodule (Hassani and Bard 1977). Microscopic evaluation of the capsule of adenomas is required to differentiate benign nodules from pure carcinomas. As adenomas enlarge, they tend to displace adjacent structures, and the trachea may be deviated from the midline. The ipsilateral carotid sheath may be displaced laterally, posteriorly, or anteriorly. Benign tumors over 4 cm in diameter often show cystic degeneration, imaged sonically as crescent or irregular echo-free areas within solid tissue. Scattered low-level echo reflections may be present within the echo-free spaces.

Large thyroid glands weighing over 50 g are called goiters. The gland may be diffusely enlarged or composed of multiple nodular regions (USAF Institute of Pathology 1968). Rapid enlargement of one area may represent hemorrhage into a nodule. This is imaged as an irregular echo-free space with solid tissue projections within it (Perlmutter, Goldberg, and Charkes 1975; Walfish et al. 1976). Colloid, a jelly like mucoprotein, forms in these nodular areas and appears as echo-free spaces which do not have well-defined margins. These complex, mixed, solid, and cystic areas require further investigation either by fine needle aspiration or pathological examination (Blum 1977; Walfish et al. 1977).

The majority of malignant lesions of the thyroid gland image as complex, mixed, solid, and echo-free spaces on ultrasound examination. Strong echo attenuation of malignant tissue has been reported in thyroid malignancy (Crocker et al. 1974). If the mass lesion is irregular in shape or has displaced or become adherent to the surrounding structures, infiltration may be suggested.

Thyroid masses containing calcification image as strong echo-reflective surfaces with shadowing posteriorly. The presence of punctate calcifications can be visualized on a radiography of the neck. Characteristic psammoma-type calcifications are associated with papillary carcinoma. Coarse calcifications generally occur in benign masses, nodular goiters, or cysts (USAF Institute of Pathology 1968; Gooding 1978).

Diffuse enlargement of the gland occurs in thyroiditis. On a B-scan a low-amplitude, uniform echo-reflective pattern may involve the entire gland or one lobe. The alteration in the echo pattern is believed to represent inflammation and edema of the glandular tissue (Blum et al. 1977). Diffuse lymphomatous infiltration of the thyroid may give a similar appearance. With chronic fibrous thyroiditis (Riedel's struma) there is replacement of the thyroid tissue by dense scar tissue and fibrous tissue (USAF Institute of Pathology 1968). To image these glands requires higher-sensitivity settings than those required for a normal gland. Strong echo-reflective surfaces are recorded, and the glandular tissue has an inhomogenous pattern.

Thyroid Exophthalmus

Individuals with exophthalmus exhibit anterior protrusion of the globe in the orbit. This unilateral or bilateral condition may be due to an endocrine etiology, usually hyperthyroidism, a diffuse enlargement of the thyroid gland seen in Graves' disease. The soft tissues behind the globe increase in bulk as a result of both edema fluid and cellular infiltration in this enclosed space (Coleman 1972). Gray scale ultrasound B-scans of the orbit demonstrate these retrobulbar soft-tissue alterations. The adipose-tissue echo reflections are increased and appear spread apart with scalloped margins. The rectus muscles hypertrophy, and this increase in size is measurable. Muscle shadows over 2 mm in diameter are considered enlarged. With endocrine exophthalmus, the inferior rectus muscle often demonstrates the first measurable change. Orbital symptoms may precede the presentation of clinical thyroid disease. Advanced eye changes are due to edema of the optic nerve, which images sonically as enlargement of the optic nerve diameter and also contains low-level echo-reflective surfaces (Coleman et al. 1972; Werner, Coleman, and Franzen 1974).

Orbital echography is the most specific noninvasive examination for the diagnosis of endocrine exophthalmus. The demonstration of these features on a B-scan eliminates the possibility of a space-occupying tumor in the retrobulbar compartment causing the exophthalmus. Surgical exploration of the orbit is not required for this diagnosis (Werner, Coleman, and Franzen 1974). Computed tomography of the orbit does not demonstrate the inferior rectus muscle, which is often the first enlarged in this condition. Hypertrophy of the other rectus muscles is only demonstrated in more advanced stages with this radiographic technique. Consequently, gray scale ultrasound B-scans are the simplest, most precise method for making this diagnosis.

Other Neck Masses

When imaged, the paired parathyroid glands lie along the posterior medial surface of the thyroid lobes. Both superior and inferior glands may be in aberrant locations. With contact gray scale scanning, a sector sweep of the angle between the trachea and the esophagus on each side helps outline the glands. Solid masses, 5 mm in size, must be differentiated from the recurrent laryngeal nerve and inferior thyroid artery in this groove (Sample, Mitchell, and Bledsoe 1978). Masses larger than 5 mm usually represent enlarged glands, either hyperplasia or tumor (Sample, Mitchell, and Bledsoe 1978). The parathyroid tissue gives a fine echo-reflective pat-

tern of slightly decreased amplitude when compared to that of thyroid tissue.

Masses in the lateral neck, that fail to take up radioactive iodine, are suitable for ultrasound studies to evaluate their internal composition. Well-defined echo-free structures in the area of the angle of the jaw usually represent branchial cleft cysts. These embryonic remnants can contain lymphoid tissue in their walls. Newborns or infants with lateral neck masses may demonstrate a fluid-filled cavity representing cystic hygroma. These are congenital in origin and consist of lymphoid tissue in the walls of fluid-filled spaces (Hunig 1976).

Salivary gland masses are generally imaged as solid areas. Diffuse enlargement of the gland or localized nodules represent tumors, often the benign mixed type. They are solitary, round, or oval, 2–5-cm masses, and are well outlined and encapsulated (Baker and Ossoinig 1977; Southwick 1976; Wagai, Ishihara, and Kobayashi 1976). Traumatic pseudocysts may form after damage to the duct structure of a salivary gland. Lymphomas that infiltrate the gland give an appearance of an enlarged gland with diffuse low-level echo reflections.

Cervical adenopathy presenting as masses in the lateral neck image as nodular solid masses with low-level echo-reflective surfaces. No posterior shadowing is present unless the nodes contain calcification.

Carotid body tumors are solid masses found at the upper end of the common carotid artery near the birfurcation. They are encapsulated and exhibit transmitted pulsations from the artery. Gray scale sonography of these tumors shows low-level echo reflections that appear homogeneous (Southwick 1976).

Gray scale ultrasonography has defined the internal tissue texture of thyroid and neck masses in a manner never before possible. Consequently, it has altered their clinical management. It has allowed refined indications for fine-needle aspiration biopsy and altered indications for surgical intervention (Blum 1977; Jensen and Rasmussen 1976; Rosen, Walfish, and Miskin 1974; Walfish et al. 1977). Continued development of gray scale and real-time equipment as well as research into the evaluation of additional ultrasound features including impedance, echo scattering, cross section, and velocity measurements is aimed at the possibility of precise pathological tissue characterization (Jellins et al. 1975; Wagai, Ishihara, and Kobayashi 1976). This would add valuable clinical information and further alter the management of these conditions, eliminating the need for needle or surgical biopsy.

References

Baker, S., and Ossoinig, K. C. Ultrasonic evaluation of salivary glands. Pp. 1109–1118 in *Ultrasound in medicine*, eds. D. White and R. E. Brown. New York: Plenum Press, 1977.

Blei, C. L.; Gooding, G. R.; and Rector, W. Ultrasonic and fluorescent scanning: a combined non-invasive diagnostic approach to extra-thyroidal neck lesions. *Am. J. Surg.* 134(3):369–74, September 1977.

Blum, M. Managing the solitary thyroid nodule: role of needle biopsy (Editorial). *Ann. Intern. Med.* 87(3):375–77, September 1977.

Blum, M., and Goldman, A. B. Improved diagnosis of "non-delineated" thyroid nodules by oblique scintillation scanning and echography. *J. Nucl. Biol. Med.* 16(8):713–15, August 1975.

Blum, M.; Passalaqua, A. M.; Sackler, J. P.; and Pudlowski, R. Thyroid echography of subacute thyroiditis. *Radiology* 125:795–98, December 1977.

Coleman, D. J. Reliability of ocular and orbital diagnosis with B-scan ultrasound. 2. Orbital diagnosis. *Am. J. Ophthalmol.* 74(4):704–18, October 1972.

Coleman, D. J.; Jack, R. L.; Franzen, L. A.; and Werner, S. C. High resolution B-scan ultrasonography of the orbit. V. Eye changes of Graves' disease. *Arch. Ophthalmol.* 88(5):465–71, November 1972.

Crocker, E. F.; Bautovich, G. J.; and Jellins, J. Gray-scale echographic visualization of a parathyroid adenoma. *Radiology* 126:233–34, January 1978.

Crocker, E. F.; McLaughlin, A. F.; Kossoff, G.; and Jellins, J. The gray-scale echographic appearance of thyroid malignancy. *J. Clin. Ultrasound* 2(4):305–6, December 1974.

Damascelli, B.; Cascinelli, N.; Livraghi, T.; and Veronesi, U. Pre-operative approach to thryoid tumors by a two-dimensional pulsed echo technique. *Ultrasonics* 6(4):242–3, October 1968.

Freimanis, A. K. Ultrasonic imaging of neoplasms. *Cancer* 37(1 Suppl.):496–502, January 1976.

Fujimoto, Y.; Oka, A.; Omoto, R.; and Hirose, M. Ultrasonic scanning of the thyroid gland as a new diagnostic approach. *Ultrasonics* 5:177–80, July 1967.

Gooding, G. A. W. Ultrasonic appearance of a thyroid nodule invested in eggshell calcification. *J. Clin. Ultrasound* 6:1–72, 1978.

Hassani, N., and Bard, R. Evaluation of solid thyroid neoplasms by gray-scale and real-time ultrasonography. Pp. 1153–1154 in *Ultrasound in medicine*,

eds. D. White and R. E. Brown. New York: Plenum Press, 1977.

Hunig, R. Ultrasonic diagnosis in pediatrics. The state of the art of ultrasonic diagnosis in pediatrics today, Part 1. *Pediatr. Radiol.* 4(2):108–16, February 13, 1976.

Jellins, J.; Kossoff, G.; Wiseman, J.; Reeve, T.; and Hales, I. Ultrasonic gray-scale visualization of the thyroid gland. *Ultrasound Med. Biol.* 1(4):405–10, March 1975.

Jensen, F., and Rasmussen, S. N. The treatment of thyroid cysts by ultrasonically guided fine needle aspiration. *Acta Chir. Scand.* 142(3):209–11, 1976.

Miller, J. M.; Zafar, S. U.; and Karo, J. J. The cystic thyroid nodule. Recognition and management. *Radiology* 110(2):257–61, February 1974.

Perlmutter, G. S.; Goldberg, B. B.; and Charkes, N. D. Ultrasound evaluation of the thyroid. *Semin. Nucl. Med.* 5(4):299–305, October 1975.

Rasmussen, S. N., and Hjorth, L. Determination of thyroid volume by ultrasonic scanning. *J. Clin. Ultrasound* 2(2):143–47, June 1974.

Rosen, I. B.; Walfish, P. G.; and Miskin, M. The use of B-mode ultrasonography in changing indications for thyroid operations. *Surg. Gynecol. Obstet.* 139(2):193–97, August 1974.

Sackler, J. P.; Passalaqua, A. M.; Blum, M.; and Amorocho, L. A spectrum of diseases of the thyroid gland as imaged by gray-scale water bath sonography. *Radiology* 125(2):467–72, November 1977.

Sample, W. F.; Mitchell, S. P.; and Bledsoe, R. C. Parathyroid ultrasonography. *Radiology* 127:485–490, May 1978.

Sanders, A. D., and Sanders, R. C. The complementary use of B-scan ultrasound and radionuclide imaging techniques. *J. Nucl. Med.* 18(3):205–20, March 1977.

Shaub, M. S., and Wilson, R. L. The single non-functioning thyroid nodule: a new approach to diagnosis and treatment. *West. J. Med.* 122(4):321–22, April 1975a.

Shaub, M. S., and Wilson, R. L. The ultrasonic evaluation of nonfunctioning thyroid nodules. *West. J. Med.* 123(4):265–68, October 1975b.

Skolnick, M. L., and Royal, D. R. A simple and inexpensive water bath adapting a contact scanner for thyroid and testicular imaging. *J. Clin. Ultrasound* 3(3):225–27, September 1975.

Solgaard, S.; Grytter, C.; and Rasmussen, S. N. Detection of thyroid cysts by ultrasonic examination. *Acta Chir. Scand.* 141(6):495–98, 1975.

Southwick, H. W. Advances in detection and diagnosis of head and neck tumors. *Cancer* 37(1 Suppl):604–11, January 1976.

Taylor, K. J.; Carpenter, D. A.; and Barrett, J. J. Gray-scale ultrasonography in the diagnosis of thyroid swellings. *J. Clin. Ultrasound* 2(4):327–30, December 1974.

Thijs, L. G., and Wiener, J. D. Ultrasonic examination of the thyroid gland. Possibilities and limitations. *Am. J. Med.* 60(1):96–105, January 1976.

United States Armed Forces Institute of Pathology. *Atlas of tumor pathology, fasicle on tumors of the thyroid*. Washington, D.C., 1968.

Wagai, T.; Ishihara, A.; and Kobayashi, S. Diagnostic ultrasound in thyroid and salivary gland diseases. Pp. 176–88 in *Present and future in diagnostic ultra-sound*, eds. I. Donald and L. Salvator. Rotterdam: Kooyker Scientific Publications, 1976.

Walfish, P. G.; Hazani, E.; Strawbridge, H. T.; Miskin, M.; and Rosen, I. B. Combined ultrasonic and needle aspiration cytology in the assessment and management of hypofunctioning thyroid nodule. *Ann. Intern. Med.* 87(3):270–74, September 1977.

Walfish, P. G.; Miskin, M.; Rosen, I. B.; and Strawbridge, H. T. Application of special diagnostic techniques in the management of nodular goiter. *Can. Med. Assoc. J.* 115(1):35–40, July 3, 1976.

Werner, S. C.; Coleman, D. J.; and Franzen, L. A. Ultra-sonographic evidence of a consistent orbital involvement in Graves' disease. *N. Engl. J. Med.* 290(26):1447–1450, June 27, 1974.

CASES
Dennis A. Sarti, M.D.
W. Frederick Sample, M.D.

Normal Thyroid

Figure 9.1 is an anatomical drawing of the neck of the region of the thyroid gland. The lobes of the thyroid are situated on each side of the trachea. A small isthmus of the thyroid is seen anterior to the trachea. On ultrasound examination, the trachea will appear as a strong echo posterior to the isthmus. Deep to the trachea will be a shadow secondary to air in the trachea. The lobes of the thyroid are situated on each side of the trachea and are usually fairly symmetrical. Posterior to the trachea is the esophagus. We usually do not see the esophagus on an ultrasound examination, since it is situated posterior to the air-filled trachea. Lateral to the lobes of the thyroid are the common carotid artery and the deep jugular vein. This major neurovascular bundle also includes the vagus nerve. The carotid artery and the jugular vein can be visualized on ultrasound. Posterior to the lobes of the thyroid is situated the inferior thyroid artery and the recurrent laryngeal nerve. This is the minor neurovascular bundle which will be referred to in subsequent cases in this chapter. It is

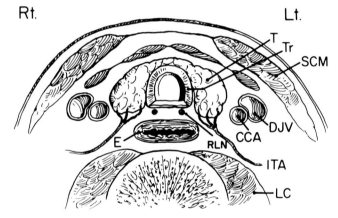

Fig. 9.1

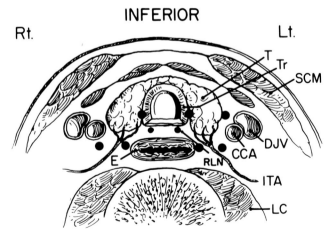

Fig. 9.2

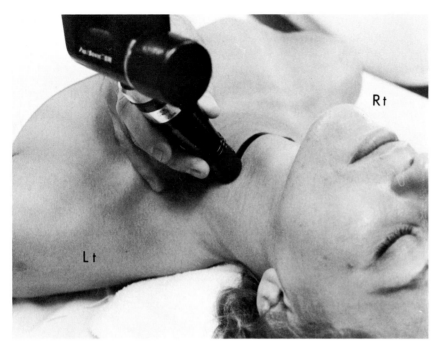

Fig. 9.3

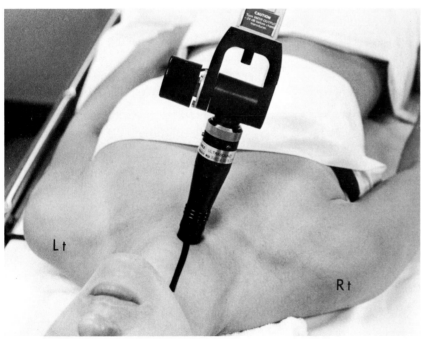

Fig. 9.4

parathyroid glands are usually present. The upper-pole parathyroid glands are fairly consistent in location, situated just deep to the thyroid lobes. Figure 9.2 is an anatomical drawing of the location of the parathyroid glands posterior to the inferior poles of the thyroid. There is more variation in the inferior parathyroid glands which are demonstrated as the dark circles in figure 9.2. We can see that the parathyroid glands are in close proximity to the minor neurovascular bundle, which is composed of the inferior thyroid artery and the recurrent laryngeal nerve. The parathyroid glands can be confused for the minor neurovascular bundle on an ultrasound examination.

Figure 9.3 is an example of a transverse scan of the thyroid. This is a direct contact scan as opposed to a water-bath scan. The gel is applied directly to the patient's neck. In figure 9.3, the transverse scan is examining the left lobe of the thyroid. The transducer is placed at approximately a 45° angle over the neck, and this gives good skin contact and excellent visualization of the thyroid and parathyroid region. Figure 9.4 is an example of a longitudinal scan of the right lobe of the thyroid. The angulation of the transducer maintains excellent skin contact and also lines up the thyroid gland anterior to the longus colli muscle. This is important in an evaluation of the thyroid, but it is especially important in examining the parathyroid gland, for this angulation will place the parathyroid region between the longus colli muscle and the thyroid lobe.

Black circles =	Common locations of the inferior parathyroid glands (fig. 9.2)
CCA =	Common carotid artery
DJV =	Jugular vein
E =	Esophagus
ITA =	Inferior thyroid artery
LC =	Longus colli muscle
Lt =	Left
RLN =	Recurrent laryngeal nerve
Rt =	Right
SCM =	Sternocleidomastoid artery
T =	Thyroid
Tr =	Trachea

extremely important in attempting to evaluate parathyroid adenomas. Posterior to the esophagus and trachea are the muscles situated anterior to the cervical vertebrae. The longus colli muscles are also important anatomical landmarks in the evaluation of the thyroid and parathyroid.

The parathyroid glands are situated posterior to the lobes of the thyroid. Four

Normal Thyroid

Figure 9.5 is a transverse scan of a thyroid gland with fairly symmetric lobes bilaterally. The thyroid has an even homogeneous echo pattern throughout. Situated between the thyroid lobes is the strong echo and shadow of the trachea. There is no sound passing through the trachea because it is air-filled. Deep to the lobes of the thyroid are the longus colli muscles. These are extremely important landmarks when evaluating the parathyroid region. The parathyroid area is situated between the thyroid and the longus colli muscles. Lateral to the lobes of the thyroid are circular sonolucencies representing the carotid artery. In this scan, the jugular veins are not visible. The size of the jugular veins varies greatly from patient to patient.

In figure 9.6, the lobes of the thyroid are slightly less echogenic than those in figure 9.5. They are, however, fairly even in echogenicity and amplitude when the right and left lobes are compared. Again, the trachea is present between the lobes of the thyroid. The strong curvilinear echo of the trachea is seen deep to the isthmus of the thyroid. The common carotid arteries are the circular sonolucencies lateral to the lobes of the thyroid. The jugular veins are seen lateral to the common carotid arteries. The longus colli muscles are situated anterior to the vertebral bodies of the cervical region. Between the longus colli muscles and the lobes of the thyroid is the minor neurovascular bundle. This is comprised of the inferior thyroid artery and recurrent laryngeal nerve. It is extremely important to identify the minor neurovascular bundle and not misdiagnose it as a parathyroid lesion.

The normal parathyroid is approximately 5 mm in thickness or less. We cannot distinguish the normal parathyroid from the minor neurovascular bundle. Therefore, anything 5 mm in thickness or smaller is considered within normal limits. If a mass is situated between the lobe of the thyroid and the longus colli muscle, which is larger than 5 mm, then the diagnosis of a parathyroid adenoma is made.

Figure 9.7, another transverse scan,

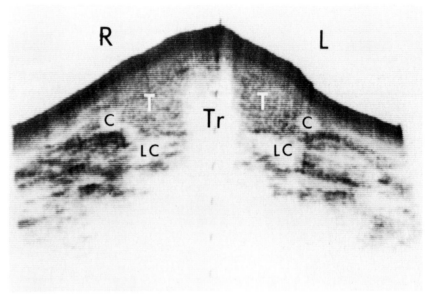

Fig. 9.5

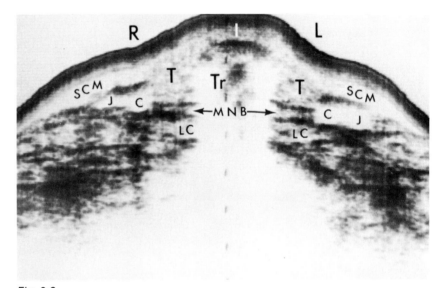

Fig. 9.6

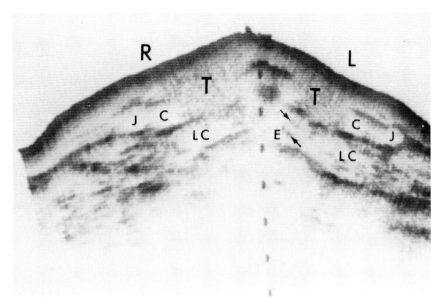

Fig. 9.7

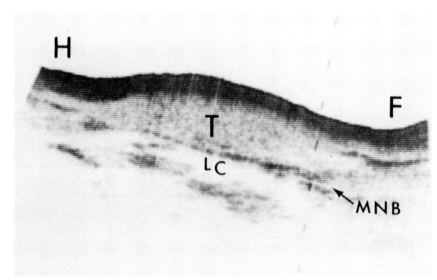

Fig. 9.8

demonstrates thyroid lobes that are slightly asymmetric, with the right side larger than the left. The carotid arteries and the jugular veins are lateral to the lobes of the thyroid. The longus colli muscles are seen deep to the lobes of the thyroid. In this scan, a mass is situated posterior to the left lobe of the thyroid. This would be extremely worrisome for a parathyroid adenoma, but it represents the esophagus. The esophagus is situated slightly more to the left side in the neck, and it can be visualized posterior to the left lobe of the thyroid in many instances. The best way to identify the esophagus is to visualize the highly echogenic central mucosa (arrows). With high-resolution real-time examination, the patient can be given water, and air and water can actually be seen bubbling through the esophagus.

Figure 9.8 is a longitudinal scan of the thyroid performed with a medial angulation of the transducer which provides good skin contact and lines up the thyroid and longus colli muscle. This gives excellent visualization of the lobe of the thyroid and parathyroid anatomy. A small tubular lucency, located between the longus colli muscle and lobe of the thyroid, is secondary to the minor neurovascular bundle.

Arrows = Esophageal mucosa (fig. 9.7)
C   = Carotid artery
E   = Esophagus
F   = Foot
H   = Head
I   = Isthmus of the thyroid
J   = Jugular vein
L   = Left
LC = Longus colli muscle
MNB = Minor neurovascular bundle comprising the inferior thyroid artery and the recurrent laryngeal nerve
R   = Right
SCM = Sternocleidomastoid muscle
T   = Thyroid
Tr = Trachea

Normal Thyroid

Figures 9.9–9.12 are examples of scans obtained from a high-resolution, real-time scanner which provides excellent visualization of the thyroid anatomy. A longitudinal scan (fig. 9.9) demonstrates the sternocleidomastoid muscle as a relatively sonolucent band anterior to the lobe of the thyroid. On the inferior portion of the thyroid are two tubular structures which represent the inferior thyroid veins. The dotted line in figure 9.9 is the scan plane which is obtained in figure 9.10. Figure 9.10, a transverse scan, shows the branching of the thyroid vein as two oval lucencies within the lobe of the thyroid. The trachea is the shadowed area near the medial aspect of the lobe of the thyroid.

Figure 9.11 is another example of a longitudinal scan of the lobe of the thyroid. The echogenic pattern is fairly even throughout the lobe. Deep to the thyroid is the longus colli muscle.

A transverse scan (fig. 9.12) shows the even echo pattern of the thyroid, deep to the sternocleidomastoid muscle. Lateral to the lobe of the thyroid is the carotid artery. Deep to the lobe of the thyroid and the carotid artery is the longus colli muscle. In this scan, we see a mass posterior to the lobe of the thyroid and secondary to the esophagus. In the central portion of the esophagus is a high amplitude echo which arises from the esophageal mucosa. With real-time capabilities, the patient can swallow either air or water and the air bubbling through the central portion of the esophagus can be visualized. This will confirm the diagnosis.

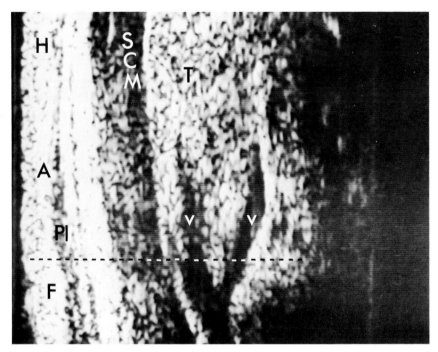

Fig. 9.9

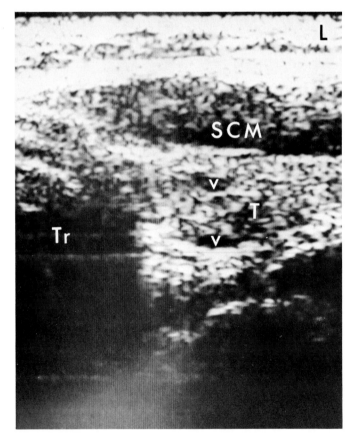

Fig. 9.10

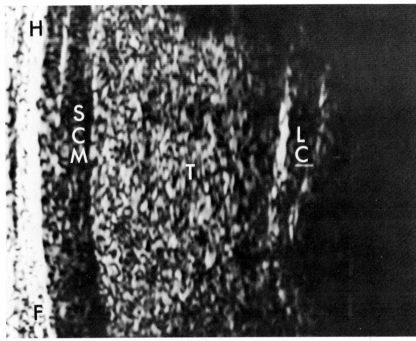

Fig. 9.11

A = Anterior
C = Carotid artery
Dotted line = Level of the transverse scan
of figure 9.10 (fig. 9.9)
E = Esophagus
F = Foot
H = Head
L = Left
LC = Longus colli muscle
Pl = Platysma muscle
Pos = Posterior
SCM = Sternocleidomastoid muscle
T = Thyroid
Tr = Trachea
v = Thyroid veins

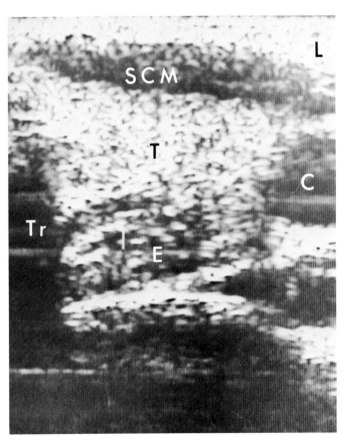

Fig. 9.12

Thyroid Cyst

The most common purpose for ultrasound examination of the thyroid is to examine a cold nodule found on isotope study. The function of the ultrasonographer is to determine whether or not a thyroid cyst is present. If a cyst is detected as the cause of the cold nodule, a follow-up study or a cyst puncture is the next step. If a solid lesion is detected, however, surgery must be considered.

Figure 9.13 is a transverse scan of a patient with a large cyst in the left lobe of the thyroid. The cyst is sonolucent with fairly sharp walls; it is situated medial to the carotid artery and jugular vein. The right lobe of the thyroid has a normal echogenic appearance. Figure 9.14 is a longitudinal scan of another patient with a cyst off the lower pole of the thyroid. The cyst is situated anterior to the longus colli muscle. As in other parts of the body, it has the characteristic of a fluid-filled structure; through transmission (arrows) is present. The mass is also completely sonolucent with fairly sharp borders.

Figure 9.15 is a transverse scan of another cyst with through transmission manifested by increased echogenicity to the left lobe of the thyroid compared with the right. If thyroid tissue is deep to a cyst, through transmission can be assessed. If the cyst is situated anterior to the vertebral bodies, however, through transmission cannot be assessed as in other parts of the body. Whenever a fluid-filled mass is situated anterior to a bone or air interface, the amount of through transmission cannot be assessed because of the high-amplitude echo arising from the bone or air interface.

Figure 9.16 is a longitudinal scan of another thyroid cyst situated in the lower pole of the thyroid. The cyst is anterior to the longus colli muscle. There is excellent visualization of through transmission (arrows) as the thyroid deep to the cyst has a higher amplitude along with the longus colli muscle.

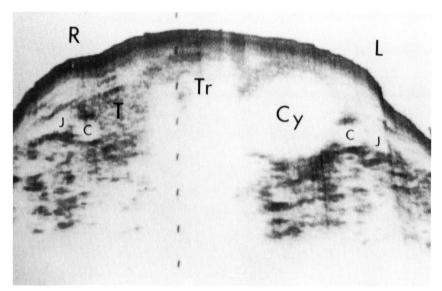

Fig. 9.13

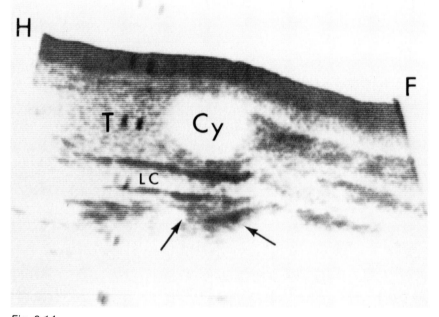

Fig. 9.14

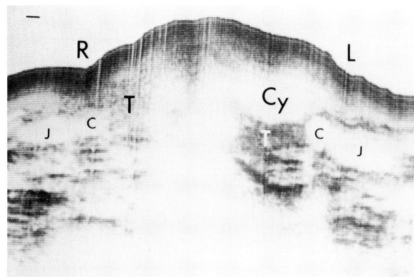

Arrows	=	Through transmission
C	=	Carotid artery
Cy	=	Thyroid cyst
F	=	Foot
H	=	Head
J	=	Jugular vein
L	=	Left
LC	=	Longus colli muscle
R	=	Right
T	=	Thyroid
Tr	=	Trachea

Fig. 9.15

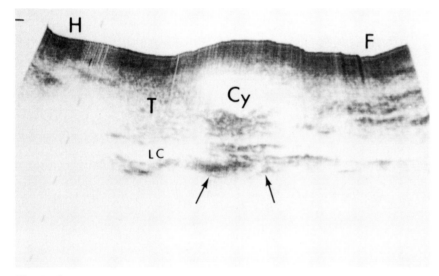

Fig. 9.16

Thyroglossal Cyst; Hemorrhagic Cyst

Figures 9.17 and 9.18 are scans obtained from a patient with a palpable mass which was felt to be slightly superior to the thyroid and situated in the midline. A longitudinal B-scan of the midline of the neck (fig. 9.17) demonstrates a sonolucency just beneath the skin surface. This turned out to be a thyroglossal cyst in the midline anterior to the trachea. On this scan the trachea presents as a strong echo with shadowing deep to it. Figure 9.18 is a high-resolution, real-time scan of a thyroglossal cyst. The cyst resolves as an echo-free area in the midline with prominent deep through transmission.

Occasionally, we will encounter a cystic mass that gives an extremely confusing ultrasonic picture. Figures 9.19 and 9.20 are examples of a thyroid cyst which was felt to be a solid mass on ultrasound examination. At surgery, it was found to be a cyst filled with clotted blood. The hemorrhagic cyst is seen in the right lobe of the thyroid (fig. 9.19). The carotid artery is on the right side, displaced posteriorly, and the right jugular vein is displaced laterally by the mass. A longitudinal scan (fig. 9.20) shows the hemorrhagic cyst in the lower pole of the thyroid. Numerous echoes are noted within the mass. These were the reason for the ultrasonic diagnosis of a solid lesion.

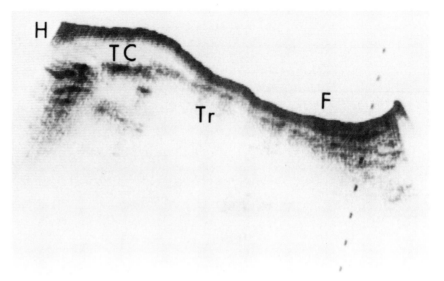

Fig. 9.17

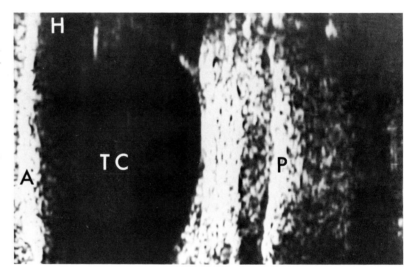

Fig. 9.18

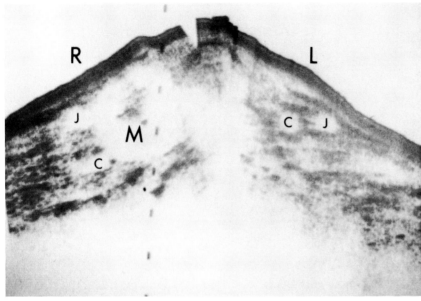

A	=	Anterior
C	=	Carotid artery
F	=	Foot
H	=	Head
J	=	Jugular vein
L	=	Left
M	=	Hemorrhagic cyst
P	=	Posterior
R	=	Right
T	=	Thyroid
TC	=	Thyroglossal cyst
Tr	=	Trachea

Fig. 9.19

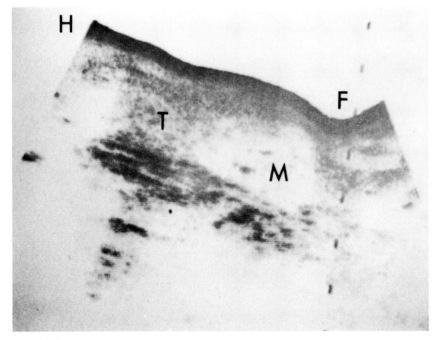

Fig. 9.20

Thyroid Adenoma

Thyroid adenomas present as solid lesions within the thyroid. They may have a lucent periphery on ultrasound. Figures 9.21 and 9.22 are scans obtained from a patient with a large thyroid adenoma found at surgery. The mass is seen on the left side of the thyroid. It is mainly echogenic in its central portion. A longitudinal scan (fig. 9.22) demonstrates a lucent periphery which is casting a shadow deep to it. The shadowing may be due to the velocity change and critical angle phenomenon discussed in the first chapter. The major portion of the mass, however, is echogenic. The effect of the mass on the skin can be seen (fig. 9.22) as the mass is protruding beneath the skin surface.

Figures 9.23 and 9.24 are examples of an extremely small thyroid adenoma diagnosed by ultrasound. In figure 9.24, a transverse scan using a high-resolution, real-time scanner, a small mass is visualized in the lateral aspect of the right lobe of the thyroid. It is just medial to the carotid artery and approximately 3–4 mm in diameter.

Initially, we failed to visualize the mass on B-scanning. After using the high-resolution real-time unit and finding the mass, we reexamined the patient with a B-scanner. Figure 9.23 is a longitudinal scan of the right lobe of the thyroid with an extremely subtle echogenic change over its lower pole. This subtle change (arrows) is the site of a small thyroid adenoma. It is approximately 4 mm in thickness.

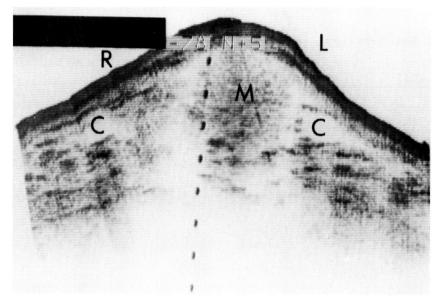

Fig. 9.21

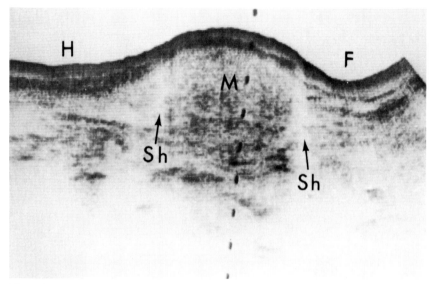

Fig. 9.22

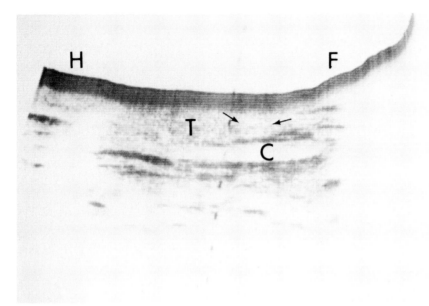

Fig. 9.23

Arrows = Small thyroid adenoma
C   = Carotid artery
F   = Foot
H   = Head
L   = Left
LC   = Longus colli muscle
M   = Thyroid adenoma
R   = Right
Sh   = Shadowing behind the lucent
          periphery of the adenoma
T   = Thyroid

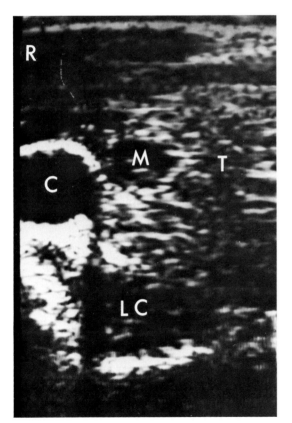

Fig. 9.24

Degenerating Thyroid Adenomas

The images on this page are scans from four different patients illustrating various presentations of thyroid adenomas. Figure 9.25 is a longitudinal scan of a patient with two thyroid adenomas of the left lobe found at surgery. A normal portion of the thyroid is seen in the superior region of the left lobe. Two thyroid adenomas (arrows) are seen in the mid and lower poles. A surrounding sonolucent rim is evident in both adenomas. Centrally, there is a highly echogenic region, which is characteristic of a thyroid adenoma.

The central echogenicity does not have any necrotic portion in figure 9.25. However, figure 9.26 is a longitudinal scan obtained from another patient with a large adenoma with a surrounding sonolucent rim (arrows). Within the sonolucent rim is a highly echogenic area. In the central portion of that echogenic region is a smaller sonolucency which may represent an area of early necrosis.

Figure 9.27 is a transverse scan of another patient with a thyroid adenoma of the right lobe. Again we visualize a surrounding sonolucent rim (arrows) with a more echogenic central portion. In this case, fluid is present within the central highly echogenic region, indicating necrosis and hemorrhage. In figure 9.28 a large amount of necrosis associated with a thyroid adenoma is visualized. The normal thyroid is situated in the upper left lobe. In the lower left lobe is an echogenic area surrounded by fluid and a second fluid component inferior to this. This is an example of severe degeneration in a thyroid adenoma.

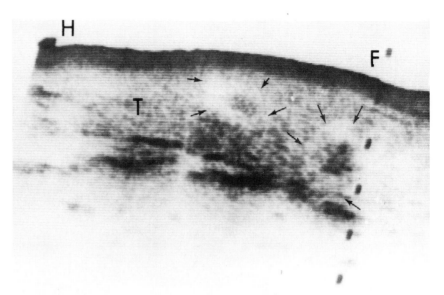

Fig. 9.25

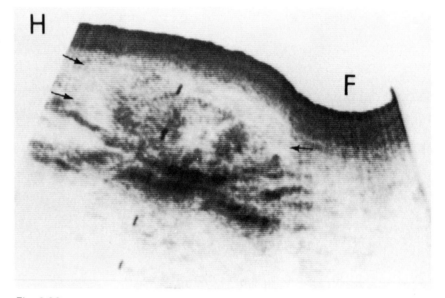

Fig. 9.26

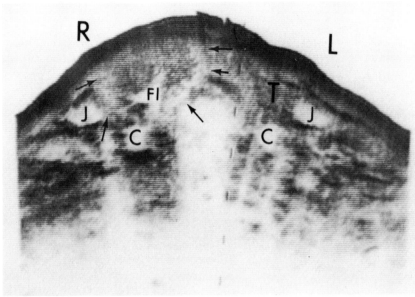

Fig. 9.27

Arrows = Thyroid adenoma
C = Carotid artery
F = Foot
Fl = Fluid indicating degeneration and necrosis
H = Head
J = Jugular vein
L = Left
M = Solid portion within a degenerating thyroid adenoma
R = Right
T = Thyroid

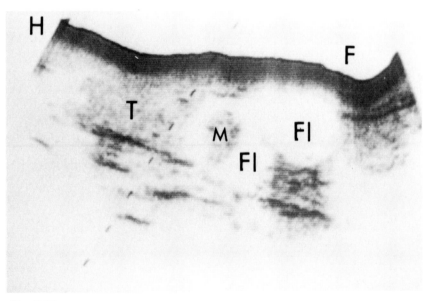

Fig. 9.28

Goiter

Diffuse enlargement of the thyroid consistent with a goiter gives an ultrasonic appearance of a solid echogenic mass throughout the thyroid. The echo pattern from a goiter is usually uneven and more coarse than seen in a normal thyroid examination. Figure 9.29 is a transverse scan obtained from a patient who had diffuse enlargement of the thyroid due to a goiter. Both lobes of the thyroid are enlarged along with the isthmus. The goiter has an uneven coarse echo pattern. A small fluid collection is noted in the mid portion of the massively enlarged isthmus.

Figure 9.30 is a scan of a patient with a goiter which involves predominantly the right lobe of the thyroid. This marked asymmetry would be difficult to distinguish from a large adenoma or carcinoma. A goiter presents as an echogenic mass which cannot be diagnosed as malignant or benign. Figures 9.31 and 9.32 are scans of a patient with a goiter undergoing necrosis and degeneration. The enlarged goiter presents as an uneven echogenic mass. Within the mass is a sonolucent fluid collection which indicates an area of necrosis.

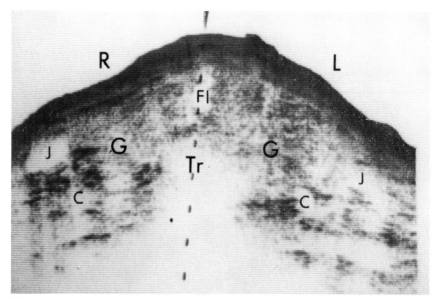

Fig. 9.29

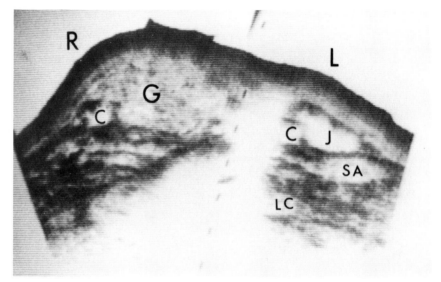

Fig. 9.30

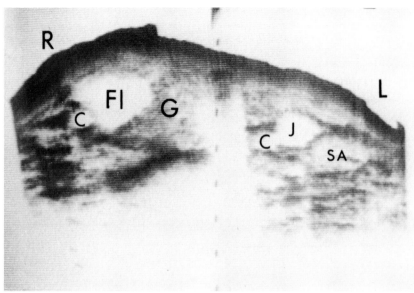

Fig. 9.31

C = Carotid artery
F = Foot
Fl = Fluid consistent with necrosis
     and degeneration
G = Goiter
H = Head
J = Jugular vein
L = Left
LC = Longus colli muscle
R = Right
SA = Scalenus anterior muscle
Tr = Trachea

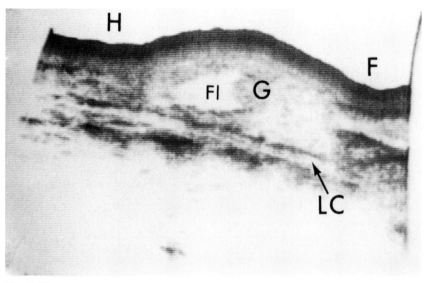

Fig. 9.32

Thyroid Carcinoma

Thyroid carcinomas usually present as solid masses on ultrasound examination. Their echo pattern is often uneven and irregular. Usually, it is relatively less echogenic than surrounding thyroid. Figure 9.33 is a transverse scan of the neck of a 24-year-old man who noted right neck swelling approximately 5 months prior to admission. This was disregarded until the patient noted some tenderness. He finally saw a physician and was admitted to the hospital. A large mass in the region of the right thyroid is seen in figure 9.33. It has an uneven echo pattern. Although it is relatively sonolucent, numerous echoes are noted within it. No enhanced through transmission is present. The findings are indicative of a large solid lesion on the right lobe of the thyroid. A relatively sonolucent, though solid, mass lateral to the carotid artery is also demonstrated. At surgery it was diagnosed as a metastatic lymph node. The larger mass was found to be a papillary carcinoma of the thyroid. Numerous metastatic lymph nodes were also present.

Thyroid carcinomas are usually irregular in their echo pattern and relatively less echogenic than the normal thyroid gland. In figure 9.34, however, we see a mass in the right lobe of the thyroid which is extremely echogenic. This mass was found at surgery to be a papillary adenocarcinoma. It is somewhat unusual in its high echogenicity.

Figures 9.35 and 9.36 are transverse scans of a 62-year-old man who had a previous goiter. The mass has an irregular echo pattern (fig. 9.35). In figure 9.36 a sonolucent fluid area is noted within the mass. Through transmission (arrows) is present deep to the mass. At surgery, this was found to be a mixed papillary follicular adenocarcinoma.

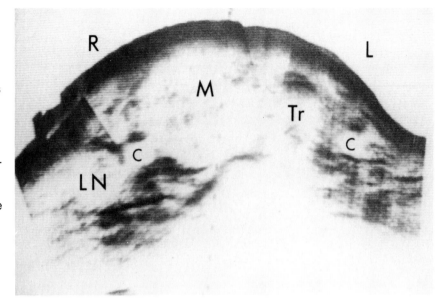

Fig. 9.33

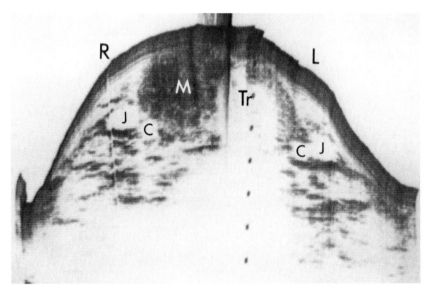

Fig. 9.34

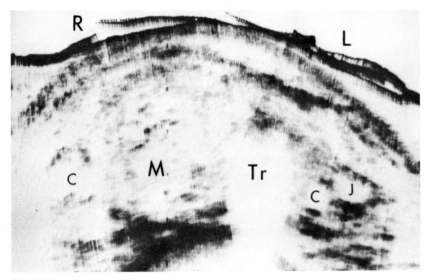

Fig. 9.35

SOURCE: The case for figures 9.35 and 9.36 are provided through the courtesy of Dr. Catherine Cole-Beuglet, Thomas Jefferson University Hospital, Philadelphia, Pennsylvania.

Arrows	=	Through transmission (fig. 9.36)
C	=	Carotid artery
Fl	=	Fluid
J	=	Jugular vein
L	=	Left
LN	=	Metastatic lymph node
M	=	Thyroid carcinoma
R	=	Right
Tr	=	Trachea

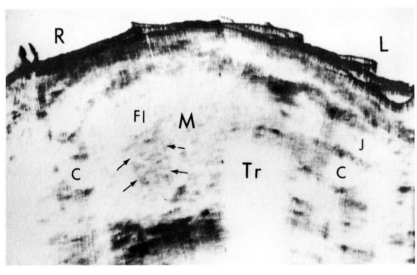

Fig. 9.36

Thyroiditis

Thyroiditis will present ultrasonic findings similar to those of other organs involved with diffuse inflammatory changes. Figures 9.37 and 9.38 are transverse and longitudinal scans of a patient with chronic thyroiditis. Diffusely enlarged thyroid lobes are visualized in figure 9.37. The lobes themselves have a decreased echogenic appearance. The diffuse sonolucent involvement of the thyroid is highly suggestive of inflammatory disease. Figure 9.38 is a longitudinal scan of the right lobe of the thyroid anterior to the longus colli muscle. Compared with the normal echogenic appearance of the thyroid seen in previous cases, the thyroid lobes in this case are much less echogenic than expected. The curvature of the skin (fig. 9.38) indicates thyroid enlargement.

Figures 9.39 and 9.40 are scans of a patient also diagnosed as having thyroiditis. In this instance, it was much more localized. The transverse scan (fig. 9.39) shows a large sonolucency on the right side. Within this sonolucent area is a fluid level (arrows). Aspiration of this cystic structure found cholesterol crystals which are consistent with the diagnosis of thyroiditis. The longitudinal scan of the right lobe of the thyroid demonstrates a 3-cm sonolucent mass. A fluid level (arrows) is also evident on the longitudinal scan.

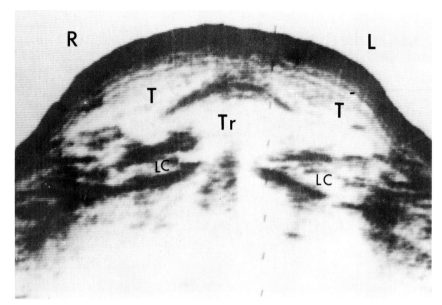

Fig. 9.37

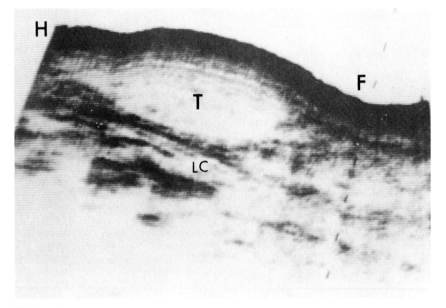

Fig. 9.38

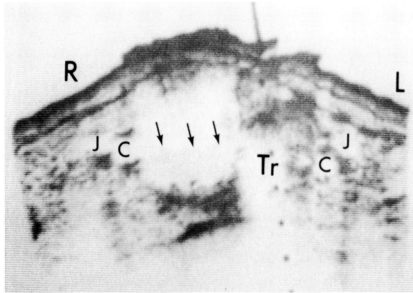

Arrows = Fluid level
C   = Carotid artery
F   = Foot
H   = Head
J   = Jugular vein
L   = Left
LC   = Longus colli muscle
R   = Right
T   = Thyroid
Tr   = Trachea

Fig. 9.39

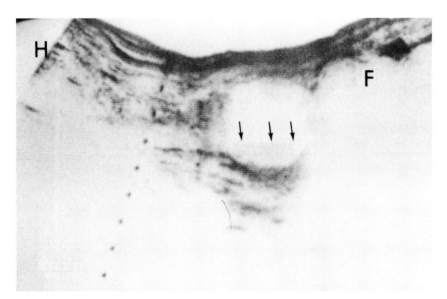

Fig. 9.40

Parathyroid Adenomas

Earlier in this chapter, in the section on normal anatomy, the relationship between the lobe of the thyroid, carotid artery, and the longus colli muscle was outlined (see figs. 9.1–9.12). This triangular relationship is extremely important in a parathyroid examination. There should be no mass between the lobe of the thyroid and the longus colli muscle which is greater than 5 mm in diameter. The minor neurovascular bundle, which is comprised of the recurrent laryngeal nerve and the inferior thyroid artery, is present in this location. If the size of such a mass is 5 mm or less, however, it is considered to be within normal limits. When a lesion is greater than 5 mm, we have ultrasonic criteria for the diagnosis of a parathyroid adenoma. Figures 9.41 and 9.42 are examples of a parathyroid adenoma deep to the superior pole of the thyroid. In figure 9.41, the relationship of the thyroid to the carotid artery and the longus colli muscle is seen. On the right side, there is a lucent area between the lobe of the thyroid and the longus colli muscle. At surgery, this lucent area proved to be a parathyroid adenoma of the superior right side. The adenoma measures approximately 7–8 mm which is above our criterion for normal. Figure 9.42 is a longitudinal scan of the same patient with the parathyroid adenoma deep and superior to the thyroid. In this plane, it is approximately 8–9 mm which is well above the 5-mm criterion.

Figures 9.43 and 9.44 are examples of a parathyroid adenoma deep to the inferior portion of the thyroid. In this instance, the adenoma is anterior to the longus colli muscle and medial to the carotid artery. It is in this position that one has difficulty distinguishing a parathyroid adenoma from the esophagus. Reference to the examples of normal thyroid gland at the beginning of this section will help to clarify what the esophagus looks like. It is usually seen on the left side between the lobe of the thyroid and the longus colli muscle. The strong central echo arising from esophageal mucosa, however, usually can be visualized. As mentioned earlier, high-resolution real-time studies with the pa-

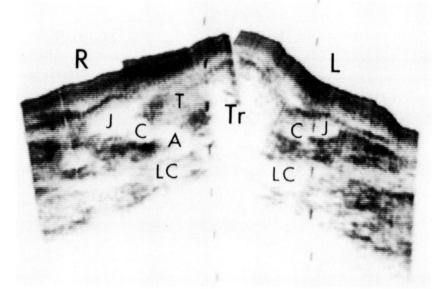

Fig. 9.41

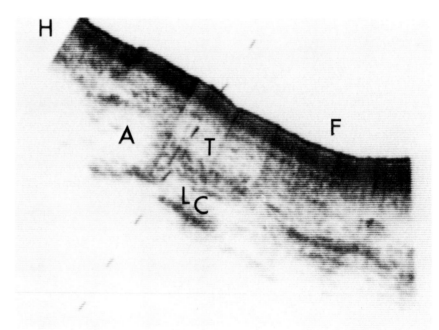

Fig. 9.42

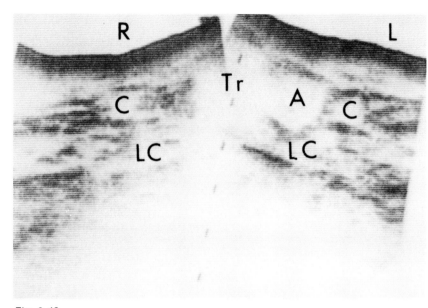

Fig. 9.43

tient swallowing give a better visualization of the esophageal mucosa. Figure 9.44 is a longitudinal scan of the same patient. The relatively sonolucent parathyroid adenoma anterior to the longus colli muscle and inferior to the left lobe of the thyroid is seen.

A = Parathyroid adenoma
C = Carotid artery
F = Foot
H = Head
J = Jugular vein
L = Left
LC = Longus colli muscle
R = Right
T = Thyroid
Tr = Trachea

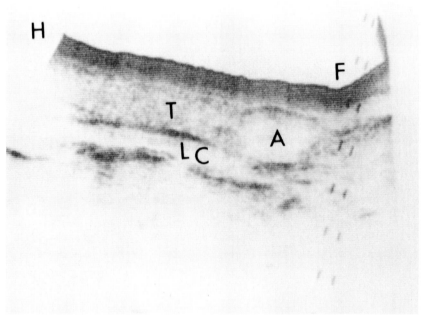

Fig. 9.44

Parathyroid Adenomas

When examining a patient with suspected parathyroid adenoma, it is important to visualize any lesion in both transverse and longitudinal planes. A correct identification of anatomical structures is more likely if two planes are used in the diagnosis. Figure 9.45 is a longitudinal scan of a patient with a rather large parathyroid adenoma which did not present any difficulties. In this instance, a relatively sonolucent parathyroid adenoma, measuring 12 × 20 mm, is seen deep to the inferior pole of the thyroid and anterior to the longus colli muscle. A transverse scan of the same patient (fig. 9.46) confirms this finding. Figure 9.46 demonstrates the lucent parathyroid adenoma on the left side of the neck, compared with the normal echogenicity of the right lobe of the thyroid. The parathyroid adenoma is situated anterior to the longus colli muscle. In this scan, the normal minor neurovascular bundles can be visualized bilaterally. The minor neurovascular bundles, composed of the recurrent laryngeal nerve and inferior thyroid artery, measure approximately 3 mm in thickness on these scans. It becomes clear, especially on the right side, how the minor neurovascular bundle presents a diagnostic problem when scanning a patient for a parathyroid adenoma. Presently, only the size criterion of greater than 5 mm gives the ultrasonic diagnosis of a parathyroid adenoma.

A sonolucent parathyroid adenoma which is slightly greater than our criterion of 5 mm is seen in figure 9.47. In this instance, the thickness of the parathyroid adenoma is approximately 6–7 mm. It is situated between the longus colli muscle and lobe of the thyroid. The minor neurovascular bundle is superior to the parathyroid adenoma and measures only 2 mm in thickness.

Figure 9.48 is an example of a false-negative ultrasonic diagnosis. In this instance, a small parathyroid adenoma is situated between the thyroid and longus colli muscle. It is slightly medial to the carotid artery. The thickness of the adenoma, however, is only 2–3 mm. This is below our criterion, therefore it was called normal on ultrasound examina-

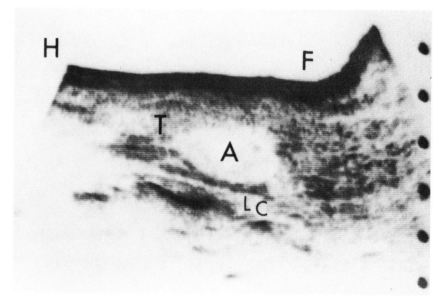

Fig. 9.45

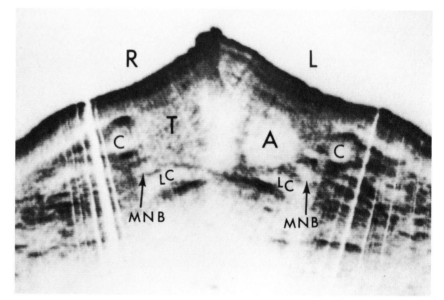

Fig. 9.46

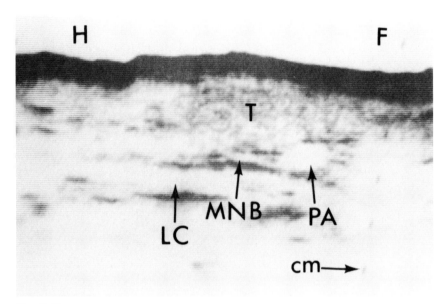

Fig. 9.47

tion. At surgery, however, a parathyroid adenoma was found in this location, approximately 3 mm in thickness but 1 cm in length. This misdiagnosis by ultrasound was caused by the size of the adenoma in its anteroposterior dimension.

A	=	Parathyroid adenoma
C	=	Carotid
cm	=	Centimeter markers
F	=	Foot
H	=	Head
L	=	Left
LC	=	Longus colli muscle
MNB	=	Minor neurovascular bundle
Pa	=	Parathyroid adenoma
R	=	Right
SCM	=	Sternocleidal mastoid muscle
T	=	Thyroid
Tr	=	Trachea

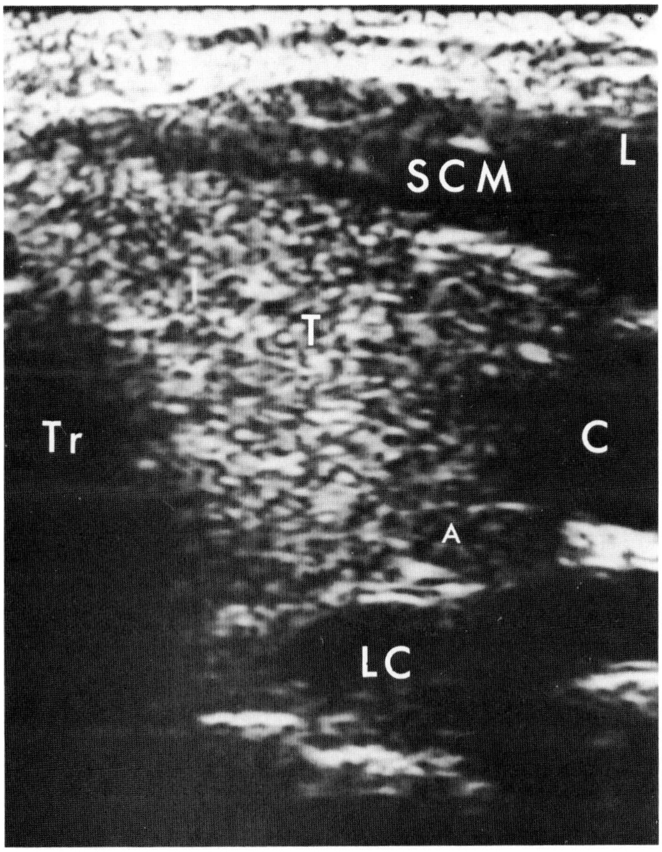

Fig. 9.48

Other Neck Masses

Ultrasound often may be requested to evaluate palpable neck masses which are unrelated to the thyroid. Figures 9.49 and 9.50 are scans of a patient who had recently had catheterization of her left jugular vein. The transverse scan (fig. 9.49) demonstrates a mass surrounding the jugular vein on the left side. The carotid and jugular vein on the right side are in the normal location and are normal in size. The jugular vein on the left is markedly enlarged. There is a circumferential mass (arrows) surrounding the lumen of the jugular vein. Figure 9.50 is a longitudinal scan of the left jugular vein. Again the lumen of the jugular vein surrounded by a large soft tissue mass (arrows) is seen. The mass was due to a jugular vein hematoma. This resolved completely with time.

Figure 9.51 is a transverse scan of a patient with a large palpable mass on the right side of the neck. This was found to be metastatic squamous cell carcinoma. Figure 9.52 is a transverse scan of another patient who had a palpable mass on the left side of the neck. This represented tumor recurrence from a thyroid carcinoma. Ultrasonography can evaluate mass lesions within the neck to determine whether they are fluid-filled or solid and, thereby, narrow the differential diagnosis.

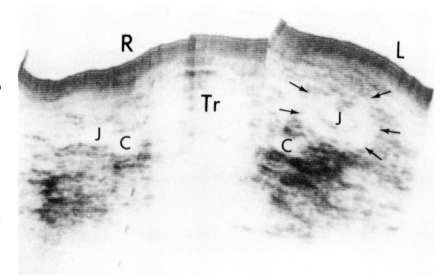

Fig. 9.49

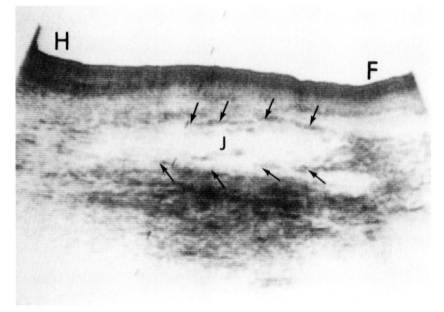

Fig. 9.50

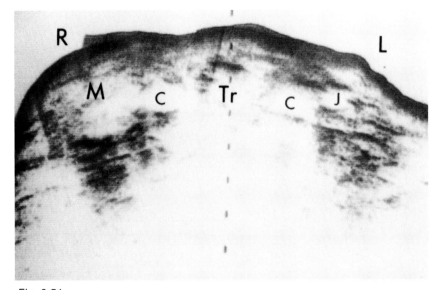

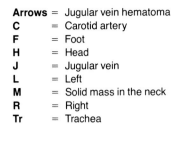

Arrows = Jugular vein hematoma
C = Carotid artery
F = Foot
H = Head
J = Jugular vein
L = Left
M = Solid mass in the neck
R = Right
Tr = Trachea

Fig. 9.51

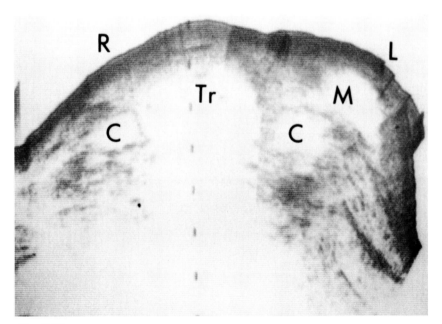

Fig. 9.52

Other Neck Masses

Figure 9.53 is a transverse scan of a patient with an extremely sonolucent mass in the region of the left thyroid. Although it is extremely sonolucent, the poor through transmission indicates the mass is solid. It can be compared to the normal right lobe of the thyroid. A CAT scan was performed (fig. 9.54). Here we visualize a soft-tissue density posterior to the left side of the trachea. There is an indentation on the tracheal lumen caused by this mass. The solid nature of the mass did not yield any specific diagnosis. At surgery, it was found to be a granular cell myoblastoma.

Figures 9.55 and 9.56 are scans of a patient with a supersternal notch mass diagnosed by ultrasound. The major portion of the mass is fluid-filled. Within the fluid-containing structure, however, is an echogenic region. The transverse scan (fig. 9.55) demonstrates tubular structures in the neck secondary to the subclavian vessels. The patient was taken to surgery, and a benign cystic teratoma was found in this region. The ultrasonic appearance is extremely suggestive of a benign cystic teratoma. Its location, however, is quite unusual.

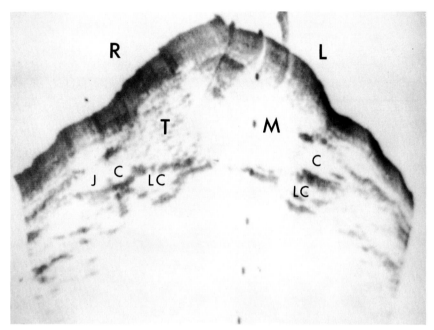

Fig. 9.53

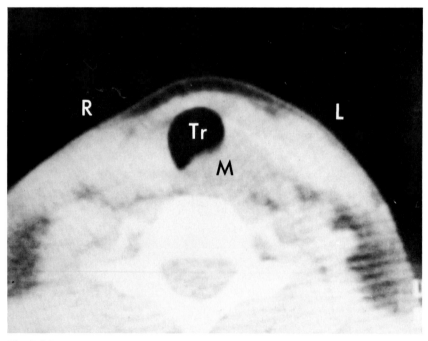

Fig. 9.54

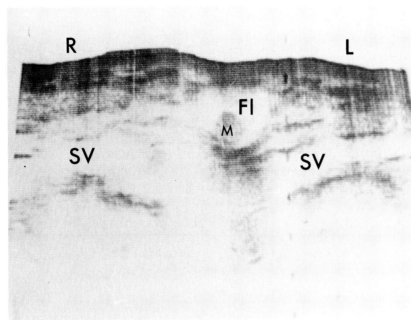

C   = Carotid artery
F   = Foot
Fl   = Fluid
H   = Head
J   = Jugular vein
L   = Left
LC   = Longus colli muscle
M   = Solid mass of the left neck
M   = Solid component (figs. 9.55 and
       9.56)
R   = Right
SV   = Subclavian vessels
T   = Thyroid
Tr   = Trachea

Fig. 9.55

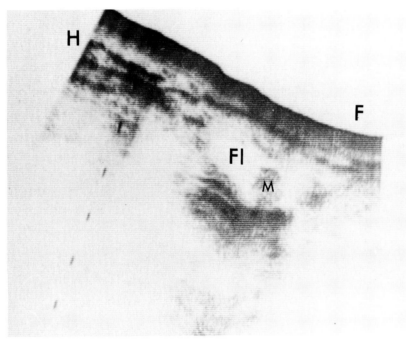

Fig. 9.56

10.
Ultrasonography of the Lower Extremity

Dennis A. Sarti, M.D.

Introduction

Diagnostic ultrasound has been used to study numerous organs within the abdomen. With ongoing technological innovations, however, other areas of the body are now scrutinized by the pulse of the piezoelectric crystal. Some of the more unusual areas now studied by ultrasound include the thyroid, parathyroid, carotid artery, chest wall, pleural space, and upper and lower extremities. Until recently, they had received little attention, although many are extremely amenable to ultrasonic examination. The lower extremity, for example, is well situated anatomically for such evaluation. Since the osseous structures are centrally located, they do not obstruct visualization of the soft tissues by ultrasound. The surrounding muscles and vessels can be examined quite easily by the application of oil to the skin. Furthermore, the lower extremity does not contain air and its centrally situated osseous structures can be avoided by circumferential or longitudinal scanning. Numerous pathological entities such as popliteal cysts, thrombophlebitis, cellulitis, popliteal artery aneurysm, hematoma, abscesses, and soft-tissue tumors can be identified by ultrasound.

Examination Technique and Normal Anatomy

A higher-frequency transducer such as a 5-MHz should be used in an examination of the lower extremity, since most of the areas of interest will be within the first 5–6 cm. Patients are scanned in the prone position with mineral oil applied to the popliteal region or any other region of interest to be examined. Longitudinal scans of the popliteal space are obtained by aligning the transducer plane parallel to the long axis of the leg. The popliteal region is then scanned at 1-cm intervals. A zero point of scanning is usually taken as the medial aspect of the knee (Moore, Sarti, and Louis 1975). This is done so that subsequent examinations cover a similar area. Only the mid portion of the popliteal space can be adequately scanned with the transducer arm perpendicular to the tabletop. As we move laterally or medially, skin contact is difficult to maintain because of the curvature of the posterior aspect of the leg. Therefore, the transducer arm is angled, so that skin contact is maintained, and scans proceed at 1-cm intervals along the medial and lateral aspect of the popliteal space.

Numerous normal structures may be visualized on

these longitudinal scans. A very strong echo is present deep to the muscle planes. Above the popliteal space, this strong echo is secondary to the femur. If more caudal, it is secondary to the tibia. Usually, the distal femur and proximal tibia are seen to flare out and enlarge in size at the knee joint. The muscle tissues of the thigh and calf present as echogenic regions and occupy nearly the entire scan posterior to the femur and tibia. Numerous strong curvilinear echoes can be seen within the soft-echo pattern of the muscle plane. These echoes are secondary to fascial planes separating the muscle bundles. On certain scans near the midline of the leg, a tubular structure secondary to the popliteal artery is visualized. This will be seen posterior to the femur, coursing in a soft curve over the posterior aspect of the knee, and then continuing slightly caudal over the tibia. It is important to recognize the normal course of the popliteal artery since masses may cause stretching or displacement of this vessel. Small sonolucent areas are occasionally present near the posterior aspect of the distal femur and the posterior aspect of the proximal tibia. These are secondary to fatty deposits. It is important to recognize these sonolucencies as normal variants so that a diagnosis of popliteal cyst will not be made.

Transverse scans of the popliteal space can be obtained of one or both legs on the same image. The initial scan is begun at the popliteal crease; this is given a zero reading. Scans are then obtained in a cephalad direction at 1-cm intervals and continued until the region of interest is covered. A second set of scans are begun caudal to the popliteal crease, also proceeding at 1-cm intervals. It is important to keep the transducer in contact with the skin surface as we scan over the curvature of the leg posteriorly in the transverse plane. If this is not done, poor acoustic coupling will lead to suboptimal scans. The muscle tissues and planes will present as echogenic regions posterior to the strong echoes of the femur and tibia. Occasionally, the popliteal artery will be seen as a small sonolucency within the muscle tissues. This most often occurs in the region of the distal femur. The popliteal artery, however, is more easily visualized on longitudinal rather than transverse scans.

If a palpable mass or an area of pain is situated in the lower extremity in a region other than the popliteal space, this area should be examined in at least two planes and covered in its entirety. (See p. 490 for additional comments on examination technique.)

Pathological Entities

Popliteal Cysts

Popliteal cysts usually arise secondary to some derangement or abnormality involving the knee joint. They are often a complication of rheumatoid arthritis, degenerative arthritis, trauma, and Reiter's syndrome (McDonald and Leopold, 1972). The etiology of a popliteal cyst is felt to be secondary to a valvular mechanism forcing the fluid in one direction out of the knee joint and into the cyst (Meire et al. 1974). Ultrasonic diagnosis of a popliteal cyst was first reported by McDonald and Leopold who demonstrated sonolucent masses in the popliteal space (1972). They were able to distinguish popliteal cysts from thrombophlebitis. Thrombophlebitis presented as diffuse enlargement of the tissue planes with no well-localized sonolucency, as is seen in cases of popliteal cysts. Later reports have documented excellent correlation between arthrography and ultrasound. Ultrasound can reliably detect cysts greater than 2 cm (Carpenter et al. 1976; Meire et al. 1974). Occasionally, cysts may be demonstrated by ultrasound which will not be seen on arthrography. This is due to the inability of contrast material to enter the cyst from the knee joint (Meire et al. 1974). It occasionally occurs when the cyst grows large enough to obstruct the communication.

Popliteal cysts most often are located in the popliteal space directly posterior to the knee joint and popliteal artery. They frequently are seen extending down into the soft tissue planes of the calf. Only rarely will they be noted to extend cephalad into the soft tissues of the thigh. If the cyst is filled with pannus or debris, it will present as an echo-filled mass (Meire et al. 1974). Through transmission, however, will be noted because of the fluid component in the cyst. Because of its noninvasive nature, ultrasound provides an ideal means for serially following the response of popliteal cysts to various forms of therapy such as a steroid injection into the cyst itself (Moore, Sarti, and Louis 1975).

As mentioned earlier, popliteal cysts are usually located posterior to the popliteal artery. We have seen an unusual case in which a traumatic cyst developed anterior to the popliteal artery and between it and the distal femur. This led to marked posterior displacement of the popliteal artery which had a tense, stretched appearance as it draped over the popliteal cyst. Popliteal cysts may be difficult to distinguish from well-loculated abscesses or hematomas. However, the clinical history in conjunction with the ultrasonic appearance usually leads to the correct diagnosis.

Leg Swelling

Leg swelling may be unilateral or bilateral, depending upon its etiology. The commonest causes are thrombophlebitis, cellulitis, and edema. Initially, ultrasonic evaluation of the popliteal space was performed to distinguish between popliteal cyst and thrombophlebitis (McDonald and Leopold 1972). Popliteal cysts occasionally may compress the popliteal vein (Swett, Jaffe, and McIff 1975). Since the clinical presentation of these two entities is similar, ultrasound provides an ideal means for distinguishing between them. Popliteal cysts present as a sonolucent mass in the popliteal space. Thrombophlebitis demonstrates diffuse enlargement of the leg with spreading of the tissue planes and slight increased sonolucency of the muscle echogenicity. Cellulitis and edema give a picture similar to that of thrombophlebitis. It is important to compare one leg to the other when attempting to make the diagnosis of thrombophlebitis and cellulitis. The normal side will provide a standard for size and echogenicity with which to compare the abnormal side (McDonald and Leopold 1972). In the case of bilateral edema, ultrasound is not as useful.

Popliteal Artery Aneurysms

Popliteal artery aneurysms are the commonest peripheral aneurysm (approximately 70%) (Scott, Scott, and Sanders 1977). They are very often bilateral and occur in elderly men with arteriosclerotic disease. The initial clinical complaint is usually pain or a palpable mass posterior to the knee. The ultrasonic findings of popliteal artery aneurysm include a sonolucency in the popliteal space (Sarti et al. 1976; Scott, Scott, and Sanders 1977; Silver et al. 1977). This is often situated more cephalad in the soft tissues of the thigh. This is an unusual location for a popliteal cyst. When a sonolucency is noted in this region, popliteal artery aneurysm should be considered most likely. Every effort should be made to identify the distal popliteal artery. Once this is identified, the transducer should be aligned, and an attempt should be made to demonstrate communication between the aneurysm and the popliteal artery. This is not always possible. If communication between the aneurysm and the distal popliteal artery is confirmed, however, the diagnosis of a popliteal artery aneurysm can be made. In many instances, demonstration of this communication is not possible due to the tortuosity of the popliteal artery, as seen in arteriosclerotic disease. Therefore, A-mode evaluation of the sonolucent mass is obtained. This will often demonstrate pulsatile characteristics, and the diagnosis of popliteal artery aneurysm can then be made (Moore, Sarti, and Louis 1975; Sarti et al. 1976; Silver et al. 1977). A popliteal cyst will not demonstrate A-mode pulsations. If the popliteal artery can be demonstrated in its entirety, and is shown to be separate from the sonolucent mass, a popliteal artery can be demonstrated in its entirety, and is shown to be separate from the sonolucent mass, a popliteal artery aneurysm can be ruled out. If a popliteal artery aneurysm is identified on the side in question, the opposite knee should also be examined because of the high incidence of bilateral aneurysms.

Abscess and Hematoma

The ultrasonic characteristics of abscesses and hematomas of the lower extremity are similar to those found elsewhere in the body. In examining for these entities, the area in question should be entirely covered. Swelling and pain will usually be present over the area in question. Abscesses and hematomas present mainly as sonolucent masses with somewhat irregular borders. If debris, fibrosis, or clot formation is present, internal echoes will be noted arising from the interfaces. Suppurative abscesses or hematomas containing unclotted blood will appear mainly sonolucent.

Soft-Tissue Tumors of the Lower Extremity

Those soft-tissue tumors of the lower extremity that have previously been reported include liposarcoma, neurofibroma, histiocytic lymphoma, undifferentiated sarcoma, and malignant fibrous histiocytoma (Birnholz 1973; Carpenter et al. 1976; Scott, Scott, and Sanders 1977). Soft-tissue tumors of the lower extremity will demonstrate disorganization of the normal muscle planes and present as echogenic masses. Occasionally, sonolucent portions of the mass will be noted if hemorrhage and necrosis of the tumor are present. Examination of the area should include longitudinal and transverse scans covering the entire extent of the lesion. We have noted a soft-tissue tumor of the upper thigh, extending into the iliopsoas muscle on the right side, and demonstrating disruption of the normal muscle planes.

Conclusion

The lower extremity lends itself extremely well to ultrasonic examinations, since no bone or air interfaces obscure visualization. The muscle planes are situated directly beneath the transducer. They can be visualized routinely with minimal difficulty. The only problem is poor acoustic coupling due to the curvature of the leg. Careful alignment of the transducer, however, will eliminate such problems. Among the numerous entities which may be diagnosed are popliteal cysts, popliteal artery aneurysm, thrombophlebitis, cellulitis, abscess, hematoma, and soft-tissue tumors. Ultrasonic evaluation of the lower extremity can prove extremely helpful in assisting the clinician in arriving at the correct diagnosis by yielding tissue information about the nature of various masses.

References

Birnholz, J. C. Ultrasound B-scanning. *Br. J. Radiol.* 46:317, 1973.

Carpenter, J. R.; Hattery, R. R.; Hunder, G. G.; Bryan, R. S.; and McLeod, R. A. Ultrasound evaluation of the popliteal space. Comparison with arthrography and physical examination. *Mayo Clin. Proc.* 51:498–503, 1976.

McDonald, D. G., and Leopold, G. R. Ultrasound B-scanning in the differentiation of Baker's cyst and thrombophlebitis. *Br. J. Radiol.* 45:729–732, 1972.

Meire, H. B.; Lindsay, D. J.; Swinson, D. R.; and Hamilton, E. D. D. Comparison of ultrasound and positive contrast anthrography in the diagnosis of popliteal and calf swellings. *Ann. Rheum. Dis.* 33:221–224, 1974.

Moore, C. P.; Sarti, D. A.; and Louis, J. S. Ultrasonographic demonstration of popliteal cysts in rheumatoid arthritis: a noninvasive technique. *Arthritis Rheum.* 18:577–580, 1975.

Sarti, D. A.; Louis, J. S.; Lindstrom, R. F.; Nies, K.; and London, J. Ultrasonic diagnosis of a popliteal artery aneurysm. *Radiology* 121:707–708, 1976.

Scott, W. W.; Scott, P. P.; and Sanders, R. C. B-scan ultrasound in the diagnosis of popliteal aneurysm. *Surgery* 81:436–441, 1977.

Silver, T. M.; Washburn, R. L.; Stanley, J. C.; and Gross, W. S. Gray scale ultrasound evaluation of popliteal artery aneurysms. *Am. J. Roentgenol.* 129:1003–1006, 1977.

Swett, H. A.; Jaffe, R. B.; and McIff, E. B. Popliteal cysts: presentation as thrombophlebitis. *Radiology* 115:613–615, 1975.

CASES
Dennis A. Sarti, M.D.
W. Frederick Sample, M.D.

Examination Technique for the Lower Extremity

Examination of the popliteal region is performed with the patient in the prone position. The scans are initially begun in the longitudinal plane (fig. 10.1). The transducer is aligned, paralleling the long axis of the leg, as is demonstrated on the right leg in figure 10.1. Scans are obtained at 1-cm intervals, coursing both medial and lateral to the midline of the leg. When scanning the lateral aspect of the leg, it is important to angle the transducer so that the transducer face is parallel to the skin. This will make skin contact much easier than if the transducer face is parallel to the table-top.

As scans are obtained near the mid axis of the leg, the popliteal artery will come into view as is demonstrated in figure 10.3. The popliteal artery is easily identified as a tubular structure coursing through the soft tissue echoes of the posterior aspect of the thigh and calf. It is seen posterior to the femur and tibia. It has a fairly smooth course as it drapes over the posterior aspect of the knee. Any masses in the popliteal region, such as a popliteal cyst, will present posterior to the popliteal artery in the soft-tissue echoes of the muscles of the back of the leg.

Transverse scans are obtained paralleling the popliteal crease (fig. 10.2). Scans are then obtained at 1-cm intervals cephalad and caudal to the popliteal crease until any unusual masses are covered in their entirety. It is important to maintain adequate skin contact while scanning the posterior aspects of the leg. Because of this, small sector scans over the posterior aspect of the leg are necessary. Figure 10.4 is a transverse scan of the leg with the sonolucent femoral condyles seen deep to the soft tissues of the muscles. The popliteal artery is present as a circular sonolucency nestled between the femoral condyles. This scan also demonstrates a curved

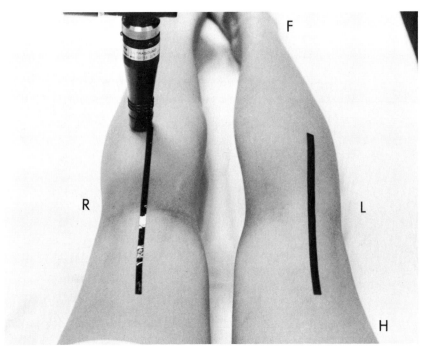

Fig. 10.1

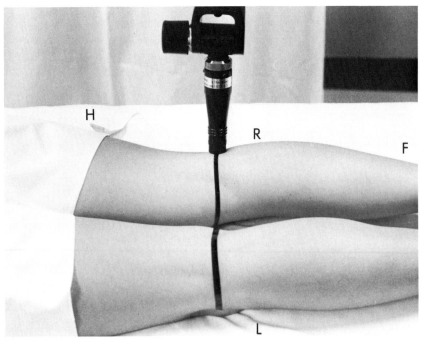

Fig. 10.2

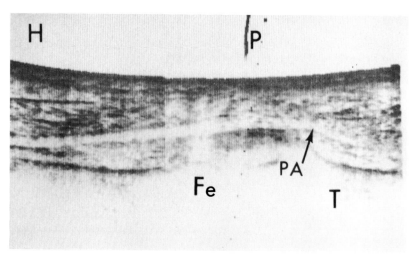

Fig. 10.3

sonolucent rim (arrows) caused by the articular cartilage over the femoral condyles. Any masses which would be present in the popliteal region would disrupt the coarse echo pattern of the soft tissues on the posterior aspect of the leg.

Arrows	=	Articular cartilage over the femur
Fe	=	Femur
F	=	Foot
H	=	Head
L	=	Left
La	=	Lateral aspect of the leg
Me	=	Medial aspect of the leg
P	=	Popliteal crease
PA	=	Popliteal artery
R	=	Right
T	=	Tibia

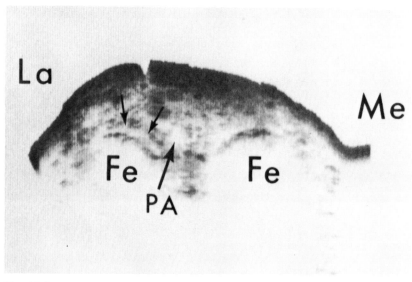

Fig. 10.4

Popliteal Cysts Associated with Rheumatoid Arthritis and Trauma

The soft tissues of the popliteal space normally fill in with a fairly even echo pattern on ultrasound examination. The strong echoes arising from the posterior aspect of the femur and tibia are easily seen. Whenever a cyst is present in the popliteal region, it usually appears as a sonolucent mass. Figures 10.5 and 10.6 are scans of the popliteal region of a patient with a long-standing history of rheumatoid arthritis. A longitudinal scan of the left leg (fig. 10.5) demonstrates the popliteal cyst as a sonolucent mass just posterior to the strong echo of the posterior aspect of the femur. Just caudal to the popliteal cyst is the strong echo of the tibia. The remainder of the muscles of the thigh and calf fill in with fairly even linear echoes. The popliteal crease is marked on the posterior aspect of the patient's leg for reference and future examinations. A transverse scan of both knees (fig. 10.6) illustrates the normal appearance of the popliteal region on the right side. There are diffuse echoes present within all of the soft tissues of the posterior leg. A cyst, however, will present as an easily identifiable sonolucency within the soft tissues. This is seen in a transverse scan on the left side. Cysts as small as 1–2 cm can be identified.

The case in figures 10.7 and 10.8 is an excellent example of a traumatic cyst. The patient is a young woman who had been running from 12 to 16 miles per day in preparation for an upcoming marathon. She noted the rather sudden onset of pain in the posterior left popliteal space. Ultrasound examination (fig. 10.7) demonstrated a sonolucent mass which is in an unusual location, anterior to the popliteal artery. Most cysts are situated in the soft-tissue space posterior to the artery. In figure 10.7 the popliteal artery is markedly elevated and lifted from the posterior aspect of the femur by the sonolucent mass which was felt to be a traumatic cyst.

The patient continued running for one week and noted a decrease in the amount of pain and in the palpable mass in the popliteal region. She returned for

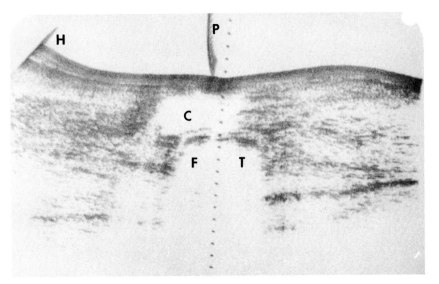

Fig. 10.5

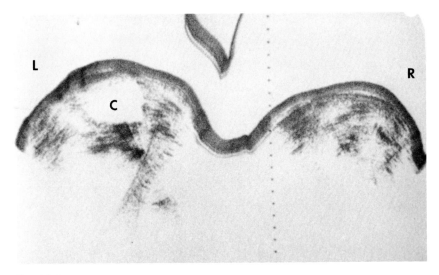

Fig. 10.6

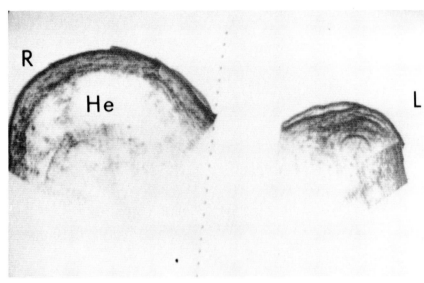

Arrows = Bulging left calf
F   = Foot
H   = Head
He = Hematoma
L   = Left
La = Lateral left calf
Me = Medial left calf
P   = Popliteal crease
R   = Right
T   = Tibia

Fig. 10.15

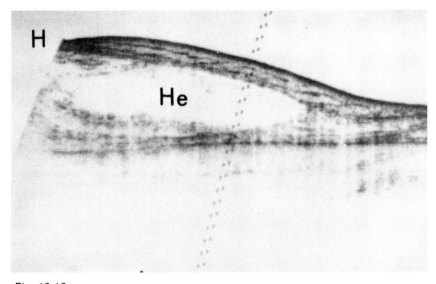

Fig. 10.16

Cellulitis; Echinococcal Cyst; and Soft-Tissue Tumor of the Thigh

Asymmetry of the legs often is found on transverse scans. There may not only be a difference in size, but occasionally also a difference in echogenicity. Figure 10.17 is a transverse scan of the right calf of a patient with an eventual diagnosis of cellulitis. The ultrasonic findings were confined mainly to the medial aspect of the calf. A relatively sonolucent appearance to the soft tissues of the medial aspect of the right calf is demonstrated. This was secondary to cellulitis in this region. Other pathology which could yield a diffuse sonolucent appearance includes thrombophlebitis, abscess, or hematoma.

An unusual case of echinococcal cyst of the proximal left thigh is shown in figures 10.18 and 10.19. The patient had undergone surgery two years earlier for a suspected soft-tissue tumor of the thigh, but the diagnosis at the time of surgery was echinococcal cyst. Two cysts were removed; a third was not resectable because of its proximity to vessels and nerves. The patient came to our ultrasonic laboratory after noting an increase in the size of the left thigh over the past six months. A longitudinal scan with through transmission of the anterior lateral aspect of the left thigh (fig. 10.18) demonstrates a large multiloculated mass which is mainly fluid-filled. Multiple septations, however, are evident. A transverse scan (fig. 10.19) over the anterior left thigh also demonstrates the multiloculated appearance to this echinococcal cyst.

Figure 10.20 is an example of a large soft-tissue tumor of the left thigh which has undergone necrosis. The patient was operated on and found to have a malignant fibrous histiocytoma. This mass was mainly solid. Areas of necrosis, however, as identified by a sonolucent component, were deep in the tumor adjacent to the femur. This soft-tissue mass demonstrates marked disruption of the normal muscle planes seen in the soft tissues of the thigh. The mixed solid/fluid echo pattern was highly suspicious for a necrotic tumor prior to surgery.

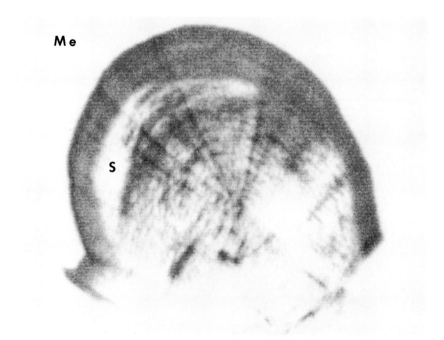

Fig. 10.17

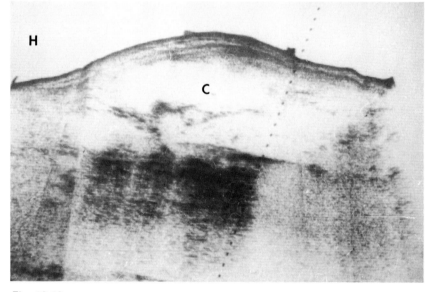

Fig. 10.18

C = Echinococcal cyst
F = Femur
fl = Fluid within the tumor
H = Head
M = Malignant fibrous histiocytoma
Me = Medial aspect of the right calf
P = Popliteal crease
S = Sonolucent soft tissue secondary
     to cellulitis

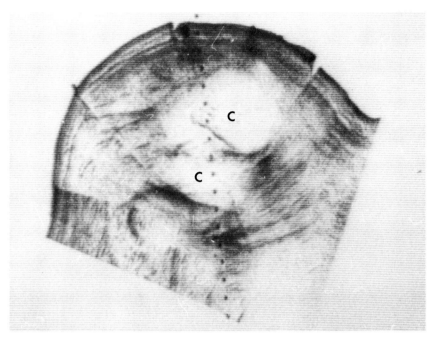

Fig. 10.19

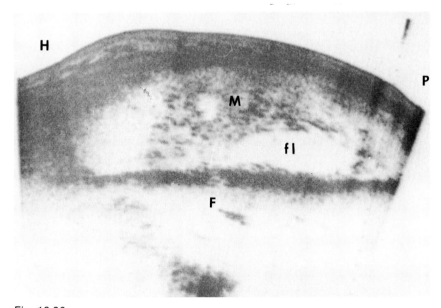

Fig. 10.20

Soft-Tissue Tumor of the Thigh and Upper Arm

Figures 10.21 and 10.22 are scans of the anterior right thigh and right ilio-psoas muscle of a woman who noted pain in the right leg after slipping while mopping the floor. She entered the hospital because of continuing pain that failed to resolve over 2–3 weeks. Figure 10.21 is the first portion of an ultrasound scan of the anterior right thigh. Disruption of the normal tissue planes is present in the muscles of the anterior thigh. A relatively sonolucent mass is noted in the anterior tissues of the thigh. This disruption was extremely worrisome. We do not see a marked amount of through transmission. The possibility of a tumor of the thigh was raised.

Examination was continued in a cephalad direction, and a pelvic study was finally performed. Figure 10.22 is a transverse scan of the pelvis with the urinary bladder filled. Indentation on the posterior right lateral aspect of the urinary bladder is caused by a large mass. This mass was situated in the right ilio-psoas muscle. We can see marked asymmetry of the iliopsoas muscles with the right side indenting the bladder wall. This patient was found to have undifferentiated metastatic carcinoma to the right iliopsoas muscle, which extended down the anterior muscle planes of the right thigh. The ultrasonic findings led to the diagnosis of a soft-tissue tumor in this unfortunate patient.

Figures 10.23 and 10.24 are ultrasound examinations of the right upper arm of a young man with a long-standing history of Hodgkin's disease. The bulging portion of the upper arm was found to be a soft-tissue tumor, later diagnosed as lymphomatous involvement of the upper arm. An interesting point of this study is the marked increased attenuation (arrows) present behind the soft-tissue mass. Therefore, it was not felt to be an abscess or a hematoma, both of which usually give posterior increased through transmission. This soft-tissue mass demonstrated increased attenuation that led to the suspicion of a soft-tissue tumor.

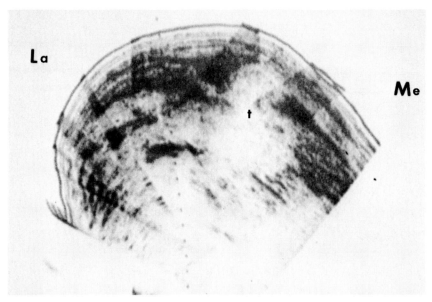

Fig. 10.21

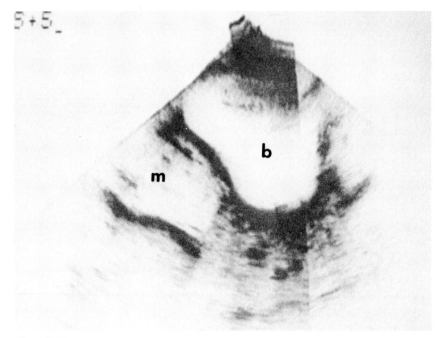

Fig. 10.22

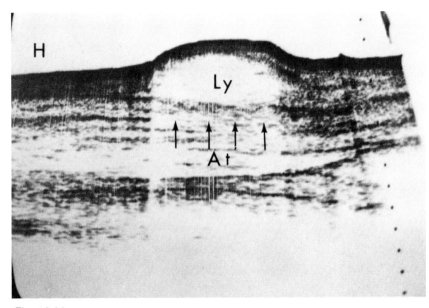

Fig. 10.23

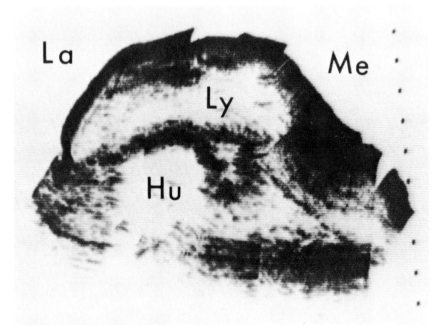

Fig. 10.24

At and arrows = Increased attenuation
through the tumor mass
b   = Urinary bladder
H   = Head
Hu   = Right humerus
La   = Lateral
Ly   = Lymphoma of the upper
arm
m   = Soft-tissue tumor of the
right iliopsoas muscle
Me   = Medial
t   = Soft-tissue tumor of the
right thigh

11.
Pelvic Ultrasonography

Barry Green, M.D.

Introduction

For a number of reasons, the ultrasound examination of the pelvis preceded the evaluation of higher abdominal structures by several years. The pelvic structures are few in number and are generally symmetrical in both men and women. Furthermore, a distended urinary bladder can serve to displace interfering bowel gas out of the pelvis, resulting in a window through which to evaluate the key pelvic structures. Gray scale technology has added a new dimension by improving resolution and allowing for observation of rather minor changes in the internal structures of these various organs. This chapter will discuss the gray scale anatomy of the pelvic bowl as well as the multiplicity of abnormalities that are encountered. Obstetrical aspects of the pelvis will be dealt with in chapter 12.

Examination Techniques

In the evaluation of the pelvis, it is mandatory that the patient's urinary bladder be moderately distended, usually just to the point of mild patient discomfort. This is usually achieved by having the patient drink several large glasses of water one-half hour prior to the examination. If the patient cannot drink liquids or if the bladder cannot be filled for other reasons, it can be filled via a Foley catheter. Bladder distention serves three major purposes: (1) displacement of bowel loops into the upper abdomen and out of the pelvis, (2) conduction of sound through which the deeper critical pelvic structures may be reached, and (3) an excellent reference "cyst" with which to compare other pelvic masses. On occasion it can be difficult to separate or distinguish masses from the bladder itself; in such instances, postvoiding views also are obtained.

The lack of attenuation through the urine enables us to use a 3.5-MHz, internal-focus transducer evaluation of the adult pelvis. When pelvic pathology extends higher into the abdomen, when adequate bladder distension is not achieved, or in obese patients, lower-frequency transducers (2.25 MHz) may be necessary.

The examination can be performed only with the patient in the supine position, since the sound impedance of the bony pelvis prevents prone scanning. Scans are performed in the sagittal and transverse planes at 1-cm intervals. Transverse scans are begun at the level of the umbilicus and are continued inferiorly to the level of the pubis. Longitudinal scans are obtained to both sides of the midventral line until the psoas muscles are encountered. These mark the lateral extent of the true pelvis. Oblique views will occasionally provide further information and will enable pockets of gas to be bypassed.

Generally, we employ compound scanning on the transverse views, although once a site of pathology is identified, sector scanning of the area of interest is performed. For additional information, see Bowie 1977; Leopold and Asher 1975; Sample 1977; and Sample, Lippe, and Gyepes 1977.

Normal Pelvic Anatomy

General Considerations

In the lower abdomen and upper pelvis, variable echoes with no particular pattern are obtained from normal bowel. Because of this gas and fluid, evaluation of this area with ultrasound is treacherous. As the scans continue deeper into the pelvis, the urinary bladder is encountered. Its shape depends upon the degree of distention. In general, the bladder tapers toward the anterior abdominal wall, with its apex pointed toward the umbilicus when viewed sagittally. In the transverse section, the bladder shape varies from almost round in the cephalad to nearly square in its caudal extent. Its internal contours are smooth. With gray scale techniques, artifactual reverberation echoes can be noted anteriorly. The left lateral wall of the bladder may be slightly flattened by the pelvic colon.

With newer gray scale techniques, the pelvic muscles that form the boundaries of the pelvic sidewalls are routinely visualized (Sample 1977; Sample, Lippe, and Gyepes 1977). In transverse scans, the obturator internus muscles are seen laterally, the piriform muscles posteriorly, and the iliopsoas muscle superolaterally. The iliopsoas muscle fans out laterally as one scans from the umbilicus inferiorly to the symphysis pubis. Various scanning angles can be used to show these muscle groups to better advantage. At higher levels, care must be taken not to confuse the iliopsoas muscles for the ovaries. The iliopsoas muscles have an echogenic central strip which is helpful in its identification. These various muscle bundles are quite symmetrical and should not be confused for masses. On longitudinal scans, 4–5 cm laterally, the psoas muscles are seen as solid bands coursing posteroanteriorly as they extend from the upper abdomen to the symphysis. If the transverse scans are extended around the outer aspect of the body, the iliac bones and proximal femurs, as well as the gluteal muscle masses, can be seen. For additional information, see Leopold and Asher 1975; Mittelstaedt, Gosink, and Leopold 1977; Morley and Barnett 1977; Sample 1977; and Sample, Lippe, and Gyepes 1977.

Female Pelvis

In the longitudinal scan, the uterine fundus, body, and cervix, and vagina are routinely demonstrated. The uterus is seen directly applied to the posterior aspect of the urinary bladder. Frequently, its entire length is visualized on one sagittal scan near the midline. As the scans proceed laterally, the fundus remains visible for several centimeters. The uterus is 6–8 cm in length by 3 cm in anteroposterior diameter by about 4 cm in width. The fundus can be difficult to visualize in the presence of severe retroversion. With the gray scale, the uterus has a fine, homogeneous echo pattern. The endocervical canal is seen as a linear echogenic central region in the lower cervical segment. On occasion, a linear echo representing the endometrial cavity also is seen in the center of the fundus on both transverse and longitudinal scans, particularly immediately preceding and during menstruation, as well as in the postpartum period and after dilatation and curettage. The vagina appears as three parallel lines at the lower portion of the uterus. Occasionally, the cervix is observed projecting into the vagina.

With careful scanning, the normal ovaries of premenopausal women can be seen with gray scale equipment in most cases (Sample 1977; Sample, Lippe, and Gyepes 1977; Zemlyn 1974). They are best seen as ellipsoid masses lying behind the bladder and lateral to the uterus on transverse scans. They generally measure $3 \times 2 \times 1$ cm, with the longest axis measuring up to 5 cm. They are usually not greater than 3 cm in any dimension and are usually about one-half the size of the uterus. In some cases, the proximal portions of the fallopian tubes and the suspensory ligaments can be seen separately from the uterus and ovary, particularly in the presence of ascites.

Male Pelvis

The normal prostate is not generally visualized, unless transverse scans with caudal angulation are obtained. On rare occasions, the normal seminal vesicles can be visualized in approximately the location of the normal female ovaries. For additional information, see Mittelstaedt, Gosink, and Leopold 1977.

Pathology of the Pelvis

Evaluation of the nonobstetrical pelvis deals essentially with the assessment of pelvic masses. These can be accurately localized, evaluated as to size and effect on surrounding organs and internal structures, and their internal character can be assessed (i.e., fluid-filled versus solid). Totally cystic lesions in women are almost always ovarian in origin. Multiple views and pictures should be obtained to demonstrate clearly that the mass is separate from the uterus. This can be difficult in the presence of large extrauterine masses which can obscure a small uterus. The site of origin of solid pelvic masses is less clear-cut. Useful information can be derived in a significant proportion of clinical disorders, although a specific histological diagnosis with ultrasound examination alone is not always possible. Serious diagnostic errors will be made unless all available clinical information is taken into consideration. A multiplicity of disorders, most of these mass-related, are encountered in the pelvis, and in women many involve or arise from the female organs. The ultrasonic appearances of many of these disorders will be discussed briefly.

Intrauterine Contraceptive Devices

Ultrasonography has been found useful for confirming the presence and identifying the type of contraceptive device within the endometrial cavity (Cochrane 1977; Cochrane 1975; Cochrane and Thomas 1972; Leopold and Asher 1975; Queenan, Kubarych, and Douglas 1975; Watt et al. 1977). Most of these devices are sufficiently different in acoustic impedence from the normal uterus, so as to be easily detected. The precise appearance depends upon the type of device used, the position of the device within the uterus, and the position of the device relative to the transducer. If the device cannot be identified within the uterine cavity with ultrasound, a radiograph is necessary to prove that it has not been spontaneously expelled. When the device has perforated the uterus it is seldom possible to visualize it ultrasonically, since it blends with the surrounding bowel echoes.

Uterine Neoplasms

Benign fibromyomata are the most common solid gynecological mass and are usually easily detected and identified with ultrasound (Cochrane 1975; Cochrane and Thomas 1974; Leopold and Asher 1975; von Micsky 1977). The usual ultrasonic appearance is that of an enlarged and irregularly shaped uterus. Most are directly related to the uterus, although parasitic and subserous nodules with long pedicles can present as masses separate from the uterus. Margination is moderate to poor. The bladder-mass interface tends to be irregular, thick, and of uneven width. Boundaries between other organs are poor. Gray scale sonograms of fibroids usually exhibit a finely speckled, homogeneous texture with fewer and coarser echoes than the normal uterus. More organized echo patterns or higher-level echoes within the homogeneous internal texture signify various types of degeneration. Transonicity may increase with hyaline or cystic degeneration. Calcifications may appear as highly echogenic areas, with or without acoustic shadowing.

Uterine leiomyosarcomas, carcinosarcomas, and mixed mesodermal tumors have an appearance virtually indistinguishable from a large degenerative uterus with fibroids, although they may exhibit large areas of hemorrhagic necrosis, bizarre patches of high intensity echoes, and malignant ascites (Cochrane 1975; von Micsky 1977).

Ultrasonography is presently of little help in the diagnosis of cervical and endometrial carcinoma. In advanced endometrial carcinoma, uterine enlargement with aggregates of high-intensity echoes within the endometrial cavity can be seen, but the appearance is in no way diagnostic of this condition and can be difficult to distinguish from a fibroid uterus. Pelvic sidewall extension of tumor mass from the uterus can be detected, although this is also usually obvious on clinical examination.

Ovary

The sonographic appearance of the multitude of ovarian masses has been described in some detail (Cochrane and Thomas 1974; Lawson and Albarelli 1977; Leopold and Asher 1975; Morley and Barnett 1977). Cystic masses are easily identifiable and have characteristic features. Their outline is clearly definable, and they are fully transonic, much like cysts elsewhere. In most cases, cysts of ovarian origin cannot be differentiated from other cystic pelvic masses. Endometriomas, hematomas, and inflammatory cystic masses may all appear as well-outlined, echo-free areas (Cochrane and Thomas 1974). Occasional echoes can be identified from within and generally arise from septae, blood, mucin, pus, malignant nodules, or dermoid elements. Several findings relative to cystic lesions can suggest malignancy (Morley and Barnett 1977; von Micsky 1977): (1) grossly thickened septae, (2) tumor nodules projecting into the cyst, (3) ascites, (4) grossly complex internal structure, (5) pelvic fixation, and (6) poor definition of the cyst wall.

Solid ovarian masses are echogenic. Benign solid masses are usually homogeneous and are acoustically attenuating, while malignant solid masses have an internal echo pattern that is inhomogeneous, and they tend to be less attenuating. The malignant lesions are poorly marginated with some pelvic fixation. Necrotic areas can be observed.

Some of the most frequently encountered ovarian masses will have the following diagnostically suggestive appearances.

1. Follicular Cyst. These vary in size from 3–10 cm in diameter, are thin-walled, unilocular, and tend to regress spontaneously.

2. Corpus Luteum Cyst. These are small, smooth-walled, unilocular, and can contain echoes and/or fluid level related to hemorrhage. They are common during early pregnancy with involution after the sixteenth week of gestation.

3. Parovarian Cyst. These cysts are very large, up to 15–18 cm in diameter, with thin walls. Most are unilocular, though they may contain a thin septum. Their ultrasonic features resemble follicular cysts and serous cystadenomas, and their anterior location can cause confusion for a filled urinary bladder (Haney and Trought 1978).

4. Theca Lutein Cyst. These sonolucent adnexal masses are usually multiple and bilateral and are associated with choriocarcinomas and hydatidiform moles. They are cystic in appearance with masses larger than 3 cm, appearing multilocular with septations (Fleischer et al. 1978).

5. Polycystic Ovaries. These may be unilateral or bilateral and present as enlarged ovaries with multiple, thin-walled cysts.

6. Endometriosis. Endometriomas are often bilateral and multiple, and are frequently located in the pouch of Douglas or behind the uterine fundus. They range in size from a few centimeters to 20 cm in width. They may be cystic, mixed, or solid. In the cystic type, the walls are shaggy and somewhat irregular, usually with some evidence of septation. These sonographically resemble hematomas or abscesses. The mixed type resemble pelvic inflammatory disease or other complex ovarian lesions. The solid lesions cannot be differentiated from solid ovarian masses (Sandler and Karo 1978).

7. Serous Cystadenoma. These are thin-walled, with occasional septa, and can vary in size from quite small to huge. Rarely are solid elements identified (Queenan, Kubarych, and Douglas 1975). They may rupture into the peritoneal cavity.

8. Mucinous Cystadenoma. These are usually unilateral, quite large, and multilocular. The septa are thin, although there may also be solid internal components despite benignity. They are more frequently septated than serous cystadenomas (Wicks, Silver, and Bree 1978).

9. Serous Cystadenocarcinoma. These lesions are complex cysts and contain solid areas with loss of capsular definition. Prominent septations can have an appearance like the spokes of a wheel. Malignant ascites is frequently observed. Regional nodal metastases are seen.

10. Mucinous Cystadenocarcinoma. The sonographic appearance resembles that of the serous counterpart, except that regional metastatic nodal enlargement is not observed.

11. Metastatic Ovarian Tumor (Krukenberg Tumor) (Birnholz 1976; Rochester and Levin 1977). They are relatively common, with approximately 50% originating in the gastrointestinal tract, 30% in the breast, 20% in the genital organs, and on rare occasion, from the bronchus. They vary in size, range from cystic to solid, are frequently bilateral, and are often accompanied by ascites. They cannot be differentiated from other ovarian neoplasms (Carnovale and Samuels 1976).

12. Benign Ovarian Teratoma (Dermoid). These are quite common and have a highly variable ultrasonic appearance (Cochrane 1975; Guttman 1977; Leopold and Asher 1975; Morley and Barnett 1977). Most are located anterior to the broad ligament, can be unilateral

or bilateral, and can be quite large. They can be entirely echo-free, may contain septa, may appear complex, and on occasion, will exhibit a fluid level due to the layering of sebacious material and hair. Acoustic shadowing from the hair ball may totally obscure the back wall of a large dermoid, a finding referred to as the "tip of the iceberg" sign (Guttman 1977). Recognition of this sign will prevent confusion with bowel gas. We have encountered several highly echogenic masses later proven to be hair-containing dermoids. Teeth or bone elements may also echo densely and exhibit acoustic shadowing. A common appearance is that of a complex mass with a focal solid area surrounded by a cystic zone and resembling an ectopic pregnancy.

13. Solid Ovarian Tumors (including both benign and malignant tumors such as fibromas, fibrosarcomas, granulosa cell tumors, Brenner tumors, dysgerminomas, malignant teratomas, leukemic infiltrates, etc.). There is no ultrasonographic feature diagnostic of any of these lesions. Most are difficult to differentiate from solid tumors of other origins within the pelvis. Their internal texture is variable although malignant tumors tend to show a greater tendency toward heterogenicity. Internal irregular cystic or semicystic areas indicate necrosis.

Pelvic Inflammatory Disease

In acute disease, through transmission is generally increased, and tissue planes are generally lost between adnexal structures, muscles, uterus, and bladder. The adnexae are edematous, and the uterus frequently is slightly enlarged with a loss of its normal echogenicity. The uterine changes last for only several days, while the adnexal thickening remains for weeks, although separation from the sidewall musculature eventually returns. Tubo-ovarian or pelvic abscesses present as thick-walled, irregular cystic masses in the adnexal and peri-uterine regions. They are frequently bilateral. These must be differentiated from normal muscles. Occasionally, they contain some solid debris.

In chronic pelvic inflammatory disease, one or both adnexae are thickened, and depending upon whether or not there is superimposed subacute disease, thickened adnexae may or may not be separable from the musculature. The uterus is of normal size and echogenicity. A pyosalpinx or tubo-ovarian abscess frequently is present, especially in gonococcal forms. A

hydrosalpinx may form. This is often funnel-shaped and can theoretically be separated from the ovary. These can have a complex appearance in complicated forms. For additional information, see Sample 1977; and Uhrick and Sanders 1976.

Pelvic Lymphadenopathy

Nodal enlargement in the pelvis is accurately evaluated with ultrasound (Freimanis 1975; Kobayashi, Takatani, and Kimura 1976; Leopold and Asher 1975; Mittelstaedt, Gosink, and Leopold 1977). Nodal masses are recognized as rounded, sausage-shaped, or lobular masses along the distribution of the iliac arteries, anterior to the iliopsoas muscles, and/or in a presacral location. They are often best appreciated on transverse scans where pelvic asymmetry can be a helpful clue to their presence. When large enough they impinge upon the posterior or lateral aspect of the bladder. Oblique scanning along the course of the iliac arteries may be helpful.

These masses tend to range from sonolucent in appearance to frankly echogenic. Lymphomatous masses tend to be more sonolucent, though with therapy, the nodal masses may shrink and develop an increased echo pattern (Freimanis 1975). In metastatic disease, the enlarged nodes tend to contain more echoes (Mittelstaedt, Gosink, and Leopold 1977). There is considerable overlap.

Assorted Nongynecological Solid Masses

Included in this group are masses related to colon carcinoma and lesions such as embryonal tumors, neural element tumors, soft tissue sarcomas, and other pelvic retroperitoneal malignancies. Most of these are located near the midline, a point which can help in differentiation from nodal malignancies, which tend to be more lateral in position. Most contain some echoes, and areas of both necrosis and calcification can be observed. As with solid tumors elsewhere, their ultrasonic appearance is rather nonspecific.

Abscess and Hematoma

In the pelvis, both abscesses and hematomas have

virtually identical appearances (Leopold 1973). They tend to be sonically complex but can be purely cystic in appearance. Both tend to localize in the posterior pelvis or anterior to the psoas muscle. They can simulate a true solid mass; for this reason, and in order to separate hematoma from abscess, pertinent history is essential. For additional information, see Cochrane 1975; Cochrane 1974; Doust, Quiroz, and Stewart 1977; Kaplan and Sanders 1973; Lawson and Albarelli 1977; and Mittelstaedt, Gosink, and Leopold 1977). CT evaluation of the bony pelvis, however, is the procedure of choice.

Tumors Arising from the Bony Pelvis

The value of ultrasound in assessment and follow-up of pelvic bony tumors is documented (de Santos and Goldstein 1977). Many of these tumors have a large soft-tissue component that is not readily appreciated clinically or by means of conventional radiographic examinations. Ultrasonography accurately demonstrates the true extent of extraosseous tumor and demonstrates its effects upon pelvic structures such as the urinary bladder.

Lymphocyst and Urinoma

These will present as either cystic or mixed elliptical masses within the cul-de-sac or anterior to the psoas muscles. They are usually echo-free, with sharp walls and potentiated through transmission, but septations can be observed when they are multilocular (Doust, Quiroz, and Stewart 1977). Both can mimic pelvic inflammatory disease and are difficult to distinguish from hematoma, abscess, or loculated ascites (Mittelstaedt, Gosink, and Leopold 1977). To diagnose lymphocyst it is helpful to have a recent history of renal transplant surgery (Phillips, Neiman, and Brown 1976) or deep nodal dissection. Urinoma usually is secondary to trauma.

Bladder and Prostate Gland

With conventional gray scale techniques, the urinary bladder can be reasonably assessed (Leopold and Asher 1975; Mittelstaedt, Gosink, and Leopold 1977). Bladder neoplasms, calculi, foreign bodies, and cathe-

ters can be observed. Tumors present as echogenic excrescences protruding into the bladder lumen. A lack of distensibility of the adjacent bladder wall can suggest invasion (Barnett and Morley 1971). Calculi usually are densely echogenic and demonstrate acoustic shadowing, much like gallstones.

An enlarged prostate gland will appear as a mass at the posterior bladder base (Leopold and Asher 1975; Mittelstaedt, Gosink, and Leopold 1977). Hypertrophy will appear smooth, with homogeneous distribution of internal echoes, while carcinoma will be more irregular with a coarse inhomogeneous internal echo pattern.

Recent advances using a transrectal transducer offer promise in the more accurate assessment of these two areas (Harada et al. 1977; Resnick, Willard, and Boyce 1977). Bladder and prostate malignancies can be more accurately detected, staged, and followed.

Pelvic Pseudomasses

Loculated ascites is easily confused for a true cystic pelvic mass (Conrad 1978; Yeh and Wolf 1977). Bowel loops tend to float on the ascites. The fluid has irregular margination, and real-time examination will show peristaltic movement of bowel loops within the ascitic fluid. True cystic masses push the bowel loops aside and are sharply marginated and/or encapsulated. Ascites collections will not indent the bladder (Doust, Quiroz, and Stewart 1977).

Fluid-filled and/or matted loops of bowel can simulate a true mass (Cochrane 1975; Kobayshi, Hellman, and Cromb 1972; Leopold and Asher 1975). These "pseudomasses" should not be constant or persistent. Changes in the patient's position will alter the appearance of the bowel loops, and real-time scanning will prove helpful. Repeat scan after a suitable interval of time should show a change.

A fecal-filled rectum has proved to be confusing on several occasions. This possibility should be excluded whenever a solid-appearing "mass" is seen posterior to the bladder in the midline. It is often better visualized on the transverse scans. Correlation with plain film of the pelvis and repeat examination after adequate cleansing enemas are recommended. A water enema with real-time examination during the enema has proved helpful in explaining the rectal echoes.

References

Barnett, E., and Morley, P. Ultrasound in the investigation of space occupying lesions of the urinary tract. *Br. J. Radiol.* 44:733–742, 1971.

Birnholz, J. C. Ultrasonography of ovarian masses (letter). *N. Engl. J. Med.* 294:906, 1976.

Bowie, J. D. Ultrasound of gynecologic pelvic masses: the indefinite uterus and other patterns associated with diagnostic error. *J. Clin. Ultrasound* 5:323–328, 1977.

Carnovale, R., and Samuels, B. I. Complex ovarian mass on ultrasonography: primary or metastatic tumor? (letter). *N. Engl. J. Med.* 294:446–447, 1976.

Cochrane, W. J. The value of ultrasound in the management of intrauterine devices. Pp. 387–440 in *Ultrasonography in obstetrics and gynecology*. Eds. R. C. Sanders and A. E. James, Jr. New York: Appleton-Century-Crofts, 1977.

Cochrane, W. J. Ultrasound in gynecology. *Radiol. Clin. North Am.* 13:457–466, 1975.

Cochrane, W. J., and Thomas, M. A. Ultrasound diagnosis of gynecologic pelvic masses. *Radiology* 110:649–654, 1974.

Cochrane, W., and Thomas, M. The use of ultrasound B-mode scanning in the localization of intrauterine contraceptive devices. *Radiology* 104:623–627, 1972.

Conrad, M. The use of ultrasound to diagnose a pseudomass effect secondary to abdominal ascites. *J. Clin. Ultrasound* 6:105–107, 1978.

de Santos, L.A., and Goldstein, H.M. Ultrasonography in tumors arising from the spine and bony pelvis. *Am. J. Roentgenol.* 129:1061–1064, 1977.

Doust, B. D.; Quiroz, F.; and Stewart, J. M. Ultrasonic distinction of abscesses from other intra-abdominal fluid collections. *Radiology* 125:213–218, 1977.

Fleischer, A. C.; James, A. E., Jr.; Krause, D. A.; and Millis, J. B. Sonographic patterns in trophoblastic disease. *Radiology* 126:215–220, 1978.

Freimanis, A. K. Echographic diagnosis of lesions of the abdominal aorta and lymph nodes. *Radiol. Clin. North Am.* 13:557–572, 1975.

Guttman, I. P., Jr. In search of the elusive benign cystic ovarian teratoma: application of the ultrasound "tip of the iceberg" sign. *J. Clin. Ultrasound* 6:403–406, 1977.

Haney, A. F., and Trought, W. S. Parovarian cysts resembling a filled urinary bladder. *J. Clin. Ultrasound* 6:53–54, 1978.

Harada, K.; Igari, D.; Tanahashi, Y.; Watanabe, H.; Saitoh, M.; and Mishina, T. Staging of bladder tumors by means of transrectal ultrasonography. *J. Clin. Ultrasound* 5:388–392, 1977.

Kaplan, G. N., and Sanders, R. C. B-Scan ultrasound in the management of patients with occult abdominal hematomas. *J. Clin. Ultrasound* 1:5–13, 1973.

Kobayashi, M.; Hellman, S.; and Cromb, E. *Atlas of ultrasonography in obstetrics and gynecology.* New York: Appleton-Century-Crofts, 1972.

Kobayashi, T.; Takatani, O.; and Kimura, K. Echographic patterns of malignant lymphoma. *J. Clin. Ultrasound* 4:181–186, 1976.

Lawson, T. L., and Albarelli, J. N. Diagnosis of gynecologic pelvic masses by gray scale ultrasonography: analysis of specificity and accuracy. *Am. J. Roentgenol.* 128:1003–1006, 1977.

Leopold, G. R. A review of retroperitoneal ultrasonography. *J. Clin. Ultrasound* 1:82–87, 1973.

Leopold, G. R., and Asher, W. M. Pp. 164–181 in *Fundamentals of abdominal and pelvic ultrasonography*, Philadelphia: W. Saunders Company, 1975.

Mittelstaedt, C. A.; Gosink, B. B.; and Leopold, G. R. Gray scale patterns of pelvic disease in the male. *Radiology* 123:727–732, 1977.

Morley, P., and Barnett, E. The ovarian mass. Pp. 333–356 in *Ultrasonography in obstetrics and gynecology*. Eds. R. C. Sanders and A. E. James, Jr. New York: Appleton-Century-Crofts, 1977.

Phillips, J. F.; Neiman, H. L.; and Brown, T. L. Ultrasound diagnosis of post-transplant renal lymphocele. *Am. J. Roentgenol.* 126:1194–1196, 1976.

Queenan, J. T.; Kubarych, S. F.; and Douglas, D. L. Evaluation of diagnostic ultrasound in gynecology. *Am. J. Obstet. Gynecol.* 123:453–465, 1975.

Resnick, M. I.; Willard, J. W.; and Boyce, W. H. Recent progress in ultrasonography of the bladder and prostate. *Trans. Am. Assoc. Genitourin. Surg.* 68:8–10, 1977.

Rochester, D.; Levin, B.; Bowie, J. D.; and Kunzmann, A. Ultrasonic appearance of the Krukenberg tumor. *Am. J. Roentgenol.* 129:919–920, 1977.

Sample, W. F. Pelvic inflammatory disease. Pp. 357–385 in *Ultrasonography in obstetrics and gynecology*. Eds. R. C. Sanders and A. E. James, Jr. New York: Appleton-Century-Crofts, 1977.

Sample, W. F.; Lippe, B. M.; and Gyepes, M. T. Gray-scale ultrasonography of the normal female pelvis. *Radiology* 125:477–483, 1977.

Sandler, M. A., and Karo, J. J. The spectrum of ultrasonic findings in endometriosis. *Radiology* 127:229–231, 1978.

Uhrich, P. C., and Sanders, R. C. Ultrasonic characteristics of pelvic inflammatory masses. *J. Clin. Ultrasound* 4:199–204, 1976.

von Micsky, L. I. Sonographic study of uterine fibromyomatoma in the non-pregnant state and during gestation. Pp. 297–331 in *Ultrasonography in obstetrics and gynecology.* Eds. R. C. Sanders and A. E. James, Jr. New York: Appleton-Century-Crofts, 1977.

Watt, I.; Watt, E.; Halliwell, M.; and Ross, F. G. M. Sonographic demonstration of intrauterine contraceptive devices. *J. Clin. Ultrasound* 5:378–382, 1977.

Wicks, J. D.; Silver, T. M.; and Bree, R. L. Giant cystic abdominal masses in children and adolescents: ultrasonic differential diagnosis. *Am. J. Roentgenol.* 130:853–857, 1978.

Yeh, H-C., and Wolf, B. S. Ultrasonography in ascites. *Radiology* 124:783–790, 1977.

Zemlyn, S. Comparison of pelvic ultrasonography and pneumography for ovarian size. *J. Clin. Ultrasound* 2:331–339, 1974.

CASES
Dennis A. Sarti, M.D.
W. Frederick Sample, M.D.

Technique for Pelvic Examination

When doing a pelvic ultrasound exam-ination, it is necessary to have the uri-nary bladder as distended as is comfort-able for the patient. This maneuver lifts the small bowel air out of the pelvis and provides an ultrasonic window through the urine-filled urinary bladder. In wom-en, it also elevates the pelvic organs to an area where they will be visible by the transducer beam.

The patient is examined in the supine position. Figure 11.1 is an example of a transverse scan obtained with the pa-tient in the supine position. There is slight cephalad angulation of the trans-ducer. When the urinary bladder is filled, the orientation of the uterus causes its fundus to lie somewhat anterior to the cervical area. This cephalad angulation of the transducer on transverse scans will place the sound beam more per-pendicular to the long axis of the uterus. Transverse scans can be obtained with the transducer perpendicular to the pa-tient's skin. Slight cephalad angulation, however, usually yields a better trans-verse examination of the uterus and adnexa.

Figure 11.2 is a longitudinal scan in the midline. Initially, it is useful to deter-mine the degree of bladder filling. The transducer has a caudal angulation ini-tially in figure 11.2. This gives excellent visualization of the vagina, and in men, of the prostate gland. As we reach the cervix and the uterus, the transducer continues in a more cephalad direction parallel to the long axis of the uterus.

On transverse scans, visualization of the posterior right pelvis is best obtained by scanning over the left side of the pa-tient, as is demonstrated in figure 11.3. Using the bladder as an ultrasonic win-dow, the transducer can be placed over the left side of the pelvis and angled toward the right. This will yield excellent visualization of the right pelvic wall and ovary. When examining the right ovary,

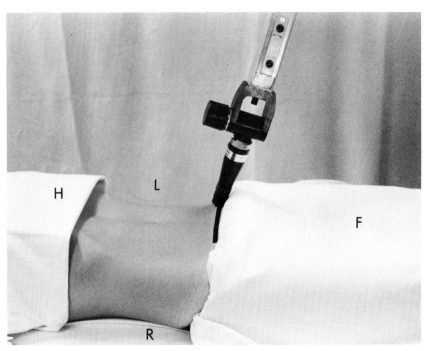

Fig. 11.1

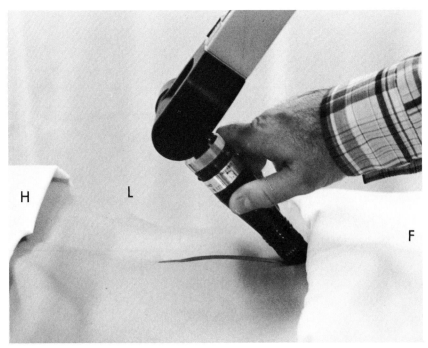

Fig. 11.2

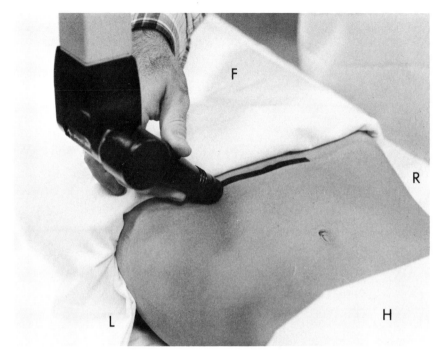

Fig. 11.3

a longitudinal scan should be obtained similar to that demonstrated in figure 11.4. Scanning the left side of the pelvis in a longitudinal plane with the transducer angled toward the right side will yield the best visualization of the right ovary in a longitudinal plane. The same is true for visualization of the left ovary. The right side of the patient is scanned with marked angulation toward the left side.

F = Foot
H = Head
L = Left
R = Right

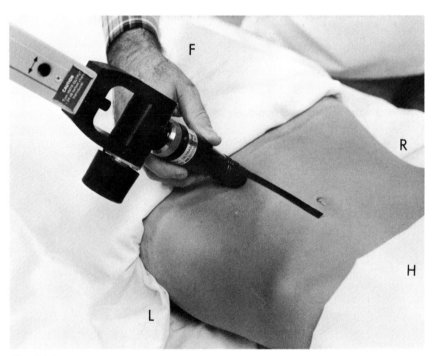

Fig. 11.4

Normal Longitudinal Scans

When the urinary bladder is well distended, the uterus is easily visualized posterior to it. With some caudal angulation, the vagina is well seen (fig. 11.5). When more cephalad, the cervix and the uterus come into view. Figure 11.5 is an example of the normal pear-shaped appearance of the uterus with fairly even echoes throughout the myometrium. We do not see any internal echoes within the uterus on this scan. The rectum and bowel loops are noted posterior to the uterus and vagina.

Figures 11.6–11.8 are longitudinal scans of the uterus with a linear echo seen within the myometrial echoes of the uterus. This linear echo is secondary to visualization of the endometrial cavity. This is normally seen during menstruation. The linear echo is not markedly thick and has a characteristically high-amplitude echo to it. In figure 11.8 sonolucency is seen secondary to fluid within the vagina. This is due to urine in the vagina which is not unusual to see with marked bladder filling.

Usually, indentation in the posterior bladder wall by the fundus of the uterus can be seen. In all of these scans we see the uterine indentation on the bladder wall in the longitudinal scans.

Figure 11.5 also demonstrates the suggestion of a large mass posterior to the uterus. However, this is secondary to a pseudomass which is very commonly seen in pelvic studies. It is due to a duplication artifact off the urinary bladder (see chapter 1).

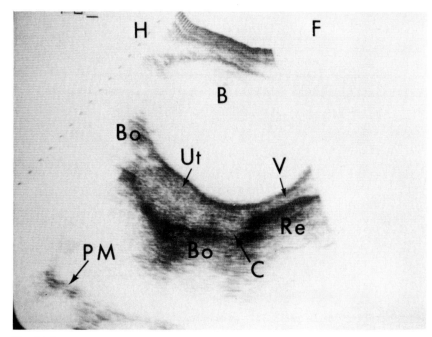

Fig. 11.5

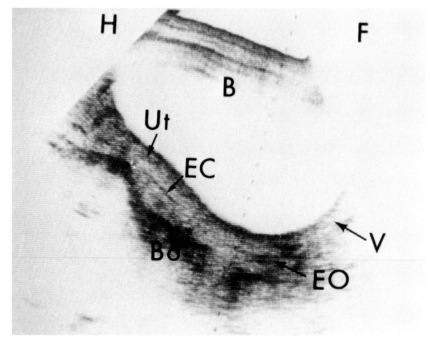

Fig. 11.6

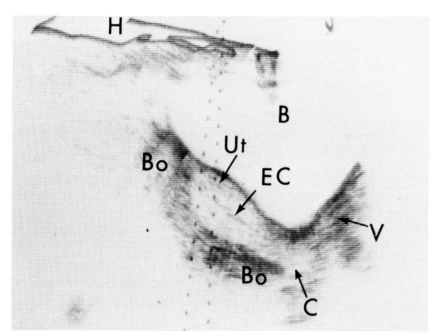

B   = Urinary bladder
Bo = Bowel
C   = Cervix
EC = Endometrial cavity
EO = External os
F   = Foot
FI = Fluid in the vagina
H   = Head
PM = Pseudomass
Re = Rectum
Ut = Uterus
V   = Vagina

Fig. 11.7

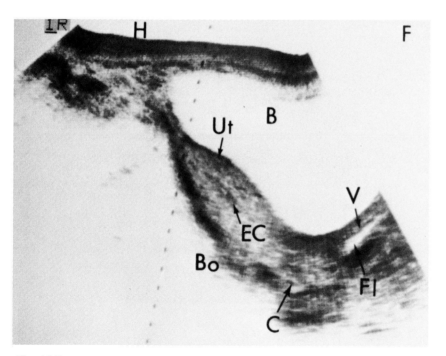

Fig. 11.8

Normal Longitudinal Scans

Figure 11.9, a longitudinal scan, demonstrates a linear echo within the uterus, secondary to visualization of the endometrial cavity. Around the endometrial cavity is a relatively sonolucent region (arrows). This usually can be visualized just prior to menstruation and may represent some edema of the uterine mucosa. A strong linear echo is also noted in the cervical region; this represents the external cervical os.

Occasionally, while scanning the uterus in the midline, an ovary in the cul-de-sac, posterior to the cervical region of the uterus, can be seen. Figure 11.10 is an example of an ovary in this location.

In figure 11.11 an ovary is seen in the midline. This time, however, it is situated superior to the fundus of the uterus. It has caused indentation (arrows) on the superior aspect of the urinary bladder. Indentation of the bladder by the uterus and ovaries is a normal occurrence. It is very important to become familiar with this indentation on the bladder wall, because it may be the only clue that a pelvic mass is present.

Figure 11.12 is an example of a questionable mass in the cul-de-sac region. However, it has a strong echogenic center and a relatively lucid periphery that is consistent with bowel.

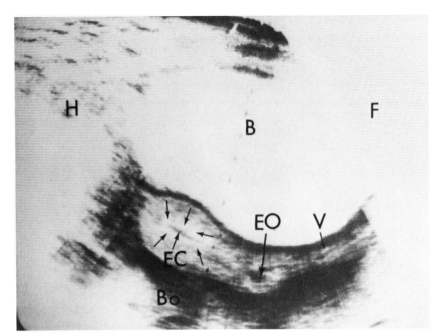

Fig. 11.9

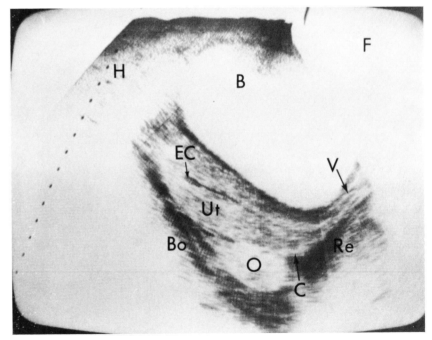

Fig. 11.10

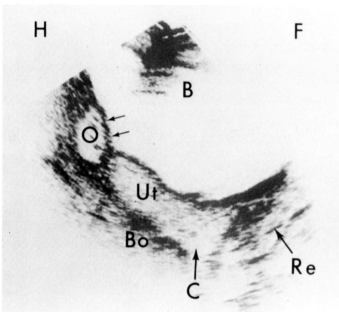

Fig. 11.11

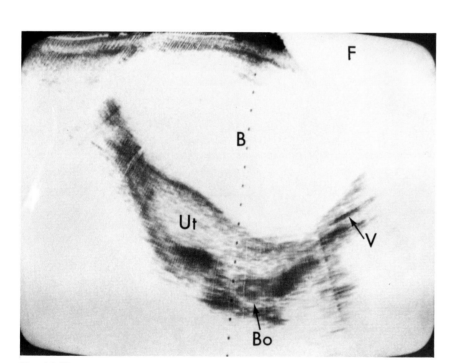

Fig. 11.12

Arrows = Lucencies surrounding the en-
dometrial cavity
B = Urinary bladder
Bo = Bowel
C = Cervix
EC = Endometrial cavity
EO = External os
F = Foot
H = Head
O = Ovary
Re = Rectum
Ut = Uterus
V = Vagina

Longitudinal Scans of the Normal Ovary

When examining the normal ovary, it is important to scan through the urinary bladder from the opposite side of the pelvis. For example, when scanning the right ovary, the transducer should be over the left lower abdomen and pelvis, angled toward the posterior right side of the bladder. This will yield the best visualization of the ovary on a longitudinal scan.

Figure 11.13 is a longitudinal scan of the right ovary. Here we see the soft echoes of the ovary situated posterior to the urinary bladder. It is important to note the indentation (arrows) of the ovary on the posterior bladder wall. This is a normal finding. As mentioned previously, indentation on the urinary bladder is important in detecting a pathological condition. Just deep to the ovary, we will see an echogenic region secondary to the piriform muscle.

In figures 11.14–11.16, several tubular structures are seen situated deep to the ovary. These tubular structures represent the internal iliac vessels. They are important landmarks and can be visualized fairly routinely. The ovary is situated anterior to them. In figure 11.16, we see another tubular structure situated deep to the ovary. This represents the ureter. The ovary has an oval appearance and gives a fairly homogeneous echo pattern which is often slightly less echogenic than that of the uterus.

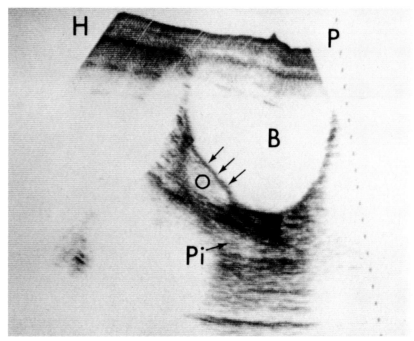

Fig. 11.13

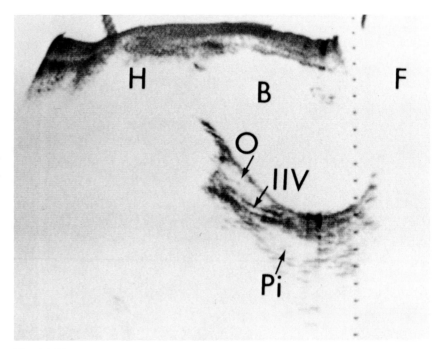

Fig. 11.14

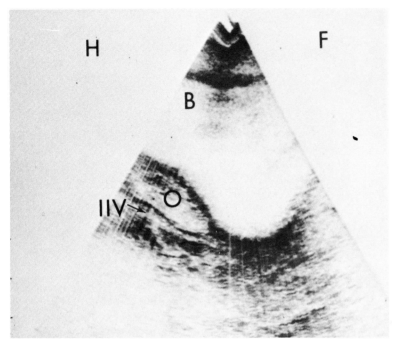

Fig. 11.15

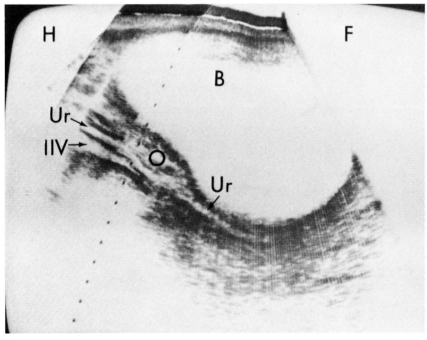

Fig. 11.16

Arrows = Indentation of the ovary on the urinary bladder wall
B = Urinary bladder
F = Foot
H = Head
IIV = Internal iliac vessels
O = Ovary
P = Level of the symphysis pubis
Pi = Piriform muscle
Ur = Ureter

Normal Transverse Scans

When attempting to visualize the vagina in a transverse plane, a caudal angulation of the transducer is often necessary. Figures 11.17 and 11.18 are examples of visualization of the vagina posterior and deep to the urinary bladder. The vagina appears as a strong linear central echo surrounded by a sonolucent rim. The strong echogenic area in the vagina is due to opposition of the vaginal mucosa. Deep to the vagina are echoes often seen arising from the rectum. Scanning more cephaladly, the uterus is visualized (figs. 11.19 and 11.20). Transverse scans through the uterus are made with the transducer arm angled more cephaladly. This places the transducer beam perpendicular to the body of the uterus.

Figure 11.19 demonstrates linear echos on the lateral pelvic wall, lateral to the urinary bladder. These echoes arise from the obturator internus muscle. They should not be confused with echoes arising from the ovary.

The ovary will come into view as a soft echogenic mass situated in the adnexa lateral to the uterus (fig. 11.20). On the left side of the uterus (fig. 11.20) is a highly echogenic region secondary to bowel loops, most likely the sigmoid colon. It is important to recognize the muscle planes in the pelvis so as not to confuse them with the ovary. The obturator internus muscles seen in figures 11.19 and 11.20 usually do not cause problems, because they are fairly thin and parallel the lateral urinary bladder wall.

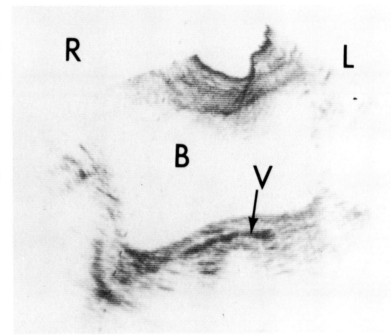

Fig. 11.17

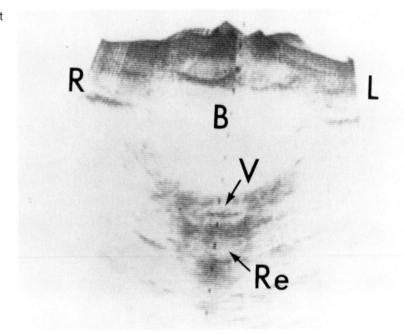

Fig. 11.18

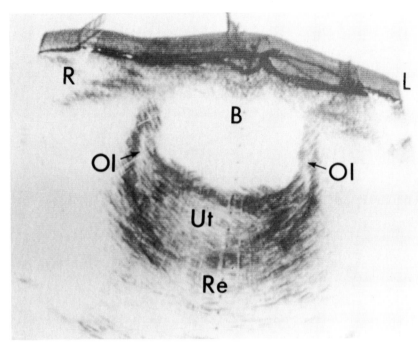

Fig. 11.19

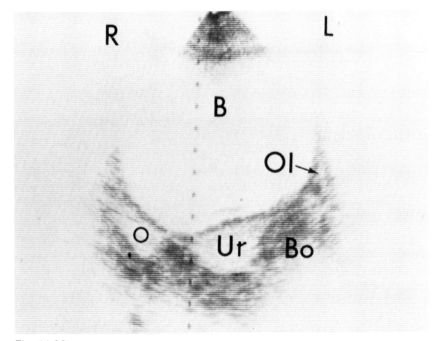

Fig. 11.20

B = Urinary bladder
Bo = Bowel
L = Left
O = Ovary
OI = Obturator internus muscle
R = Right
Re = Rectum
Ut = Uterus
V = Vagina

Normal Transverse Scans

As mentioned previously, it is important to recognize the various muscle bundles within the pelvis. Figure 11.21 demonstrates the right obturator internus muscle lateral to the urinary bladder. Just medial to this muscle, the right ovary can be seen to the right of the uterus. The ovary is situated just medial to the obturator internus muscle in this case.

Figure 11.22 shows two muscle groups which occasionally may be confused with the ovary or ovarian masses. The iliopsoas muscle is seen more anterior to the left ovary in figure 11.22. A characteristically strong central echo is present within the iliopsoas muscle, and this makes it fairly easy to recognize. A lucent region is also noted anterior to the iliopsoas muscle; this represents the external iliac vessels. In figure 11.22 we visualize the piriform muscle posterior to the left ovary. It is this muscle which usually is confused for the ovary.

Figure 11.23 demonstrates the right piriform muscle posterior to the fallopian tube and the uterus. The piriform muscle often will be confused with the ovary. Usually symmetry between the piriform muscles can be seen, but the rectum and sigmoid will occasionally obscure the left piriform muscle, yielding only visualization of the right side. This may be confused with the ovary. If there is any question, a longitudinal scan over the region will determine whether the ovary or the muscle is visualized.

Figure 11.24 demonstrates a mass posterior to the uterus and secondary to an ovary which has slipped into the region of the cul-de-sac. This is a common site for the ovary. We also see the fallopian tube draping along the lateral right aspect of the uterus. Again, the characteristic appearance of the iliopsoas muscle, with the strong central echogenic center, is seen.

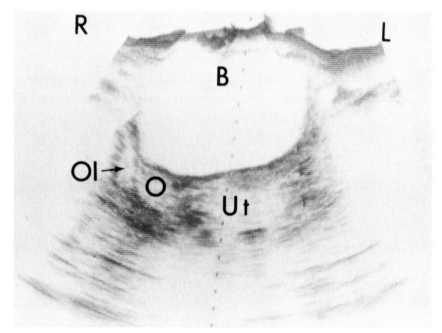

Fig. 11.21

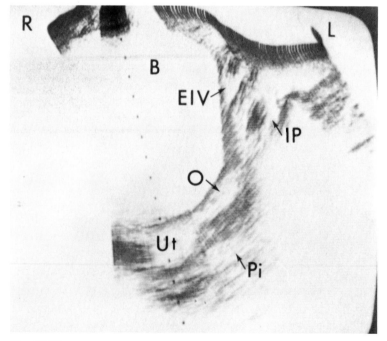

Fig. 11.22

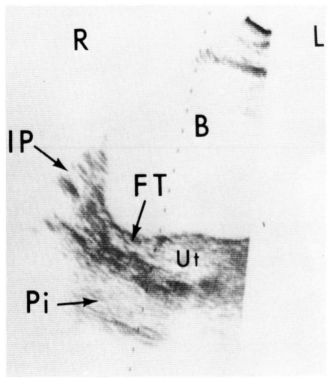

B   = Urinary bladder
EIV = External iliac vessels
FT = Fallopian tube
IP = Iliopsoas muscle
L   = Left
O   = Ovary
OI = Obturator internus muscle
Pi = Piriform muscles
R   = Right
Re = Rectum
Ut = Uterus

Fig. 11.23

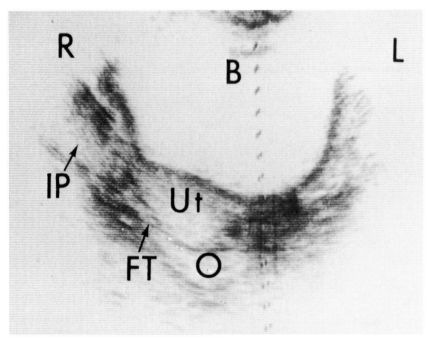

Fig. 11.24

Retroverted Uterus; Hysterectomy

Figure 11.25 is an example of a retroverted uterus. Usually the uterus is seen to parallel the superior border of the urinary bladder. However, occasionally a uterus is oriented posteriorly (fig. 11.25). The echo arising from the uterus are decreased in amplitude. This is not unusual in a retroverted uterus; the sound beam is passed through the long axis of the uterus which has marked attenuation. Occasionally a myoma is misdiagnosed. It is often very difficult to diagnosis a myomatous lesion on a retroverted uterus because of this finding.

A longitudinal scan of a patient with a previous hysterectomy (fig. 11.26) is fairly characteristic of a vagina continuing posteriorly and ending abruptly without any evidence of a uterus. Superior to the vagina we see only bowel air. Occasionally, a small cervical cuff may be present and may be mistaken for a small uterus.

Figures 11.27 and 11.28 are also examples of hysterectomy, since no uterus is identified. Only bowel air is noted superior to the urinary bladder, but fluid is present in the vagina in both instances. Fluid is often seen in the vagina when doing an ultrasound examination. Most likely, it represents urine. Since the urinary bladder has to be markedly distended, the patient may be unable to avoid urinating a small amount.

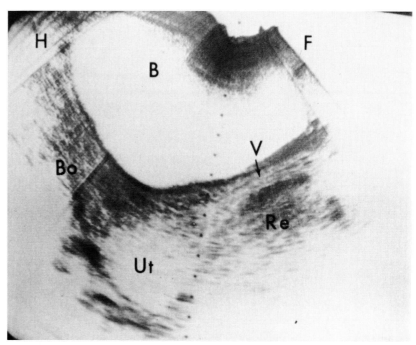

Fig. 11.25

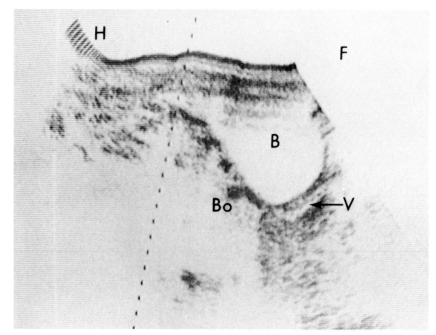

Fig. 11.26

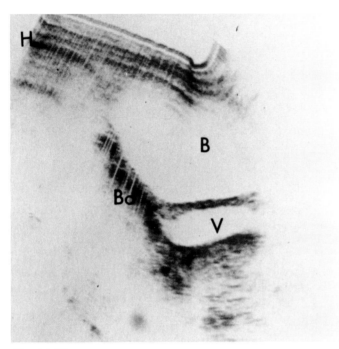

B   = Urinary bladder
Bo = Bowel air
F   = Foot
H   = Head
Re = Rectum
Ut = Retroverted uterus
V   = Vagina
v   = Vagina

Fig. 11.27

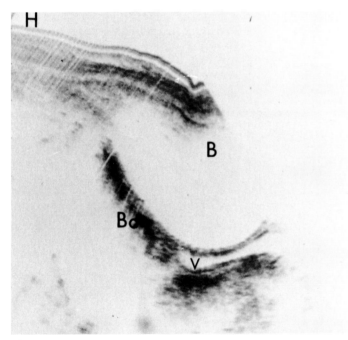

Fig. 11.28

Bicornuate Uterus

The patient in figures 11.29–11.32 is a 27-year-old woman who had had three pregnancies ending in a first or second trimester abortion. Because of this history, an ultrasound examination was performed, followed by a hysterosalpingogram. The diagnosis of a bicornuate uterus was made. The transverse scans (figs. 11.29 and 11.30) demonstrate myometrial echoes in the right and left pelvis consistent with a bicornuate uterus. Figure 11.30 is a slightly more cephalad transverse scan that shows further separation of the bicornuate uterus. The indentation on the bladder wall (arrows) by the uterus is noted. This is a normal finding in the pelvis. Posterior to the uterus are the piriform muscles which should not be mistaken for ovaries.

Figure 11.31 is a longitudinal scan through the long axis of the right uterus. Here we see some reverberations off the anterior wall of the urinary bladder, which is a normal finding in the pelvis. A longitudinal scan lining up the long axis of the left-sided uterus (fig. 11.32) demonstrates echoes within the endocervical cavity on this side. A hysterosalpingogram confirmed the diagnosis of the bicornuate uterus. This is a fairly characteristic appearance of this entity; it is best diagnosed on transverse scans through the cephalad portion of the uterus.

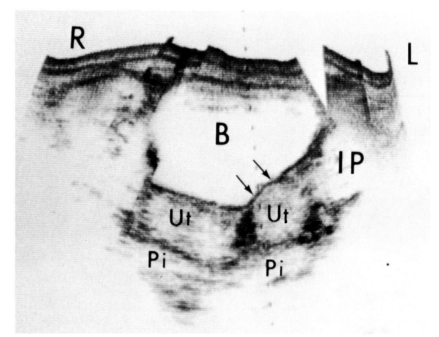

Fig. 11.29

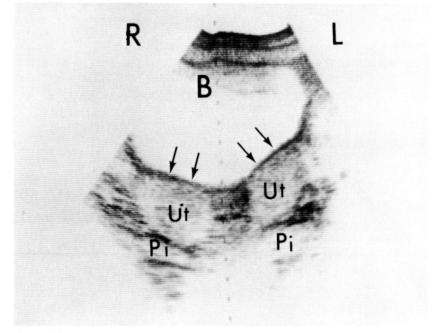

Fig. 11.30

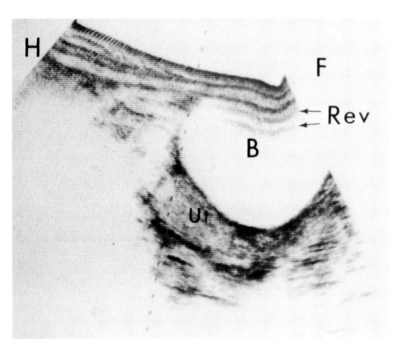

Fig. 11.31

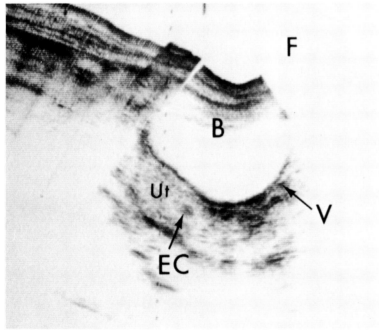

Fig. 11.32

Arrows = Indentation of the uterus on the urinary bladder wall
B   = Urinary bladder
EC = Endometrial cavity
F   = Foot
H   = Head
IP = Iliopsoas muscle
L   = Left
Pi = Piriform muscle
R   = Right
Rev = Reverberation artifacts in the urinary bladder
Ut = Uterus
V   = Vagina

Intrauterine Devices

The various intrauterine devices give fairly characteristic echo patterns within the endometrial cavity.

Figure 11.33 is a longitudinal scan through the uterus with a steplike appearance to the echoes arising within the endometrial cavity. This steplike appearance is characteristic of a Lippe's loop. Posterior to the central echoes is evidence of shadowing.

A longitudinal scan of the uterus (fig. 11.34) demonstrates a strong central echo arising from a Dalkon shield. This device presents an uninterrupted echogenic appearance without evidence of the steplike echoes noted in a Lippe's loop.

Figures 11.35 and 11.36 are longitudinal and transverse scans of a uterus containing a Copper 7 intrauterine device. Copper 7s and Copper Ts have a fairly characteristic appearance of a circular echo on transverse scans through the uterus. Longitudinal scans through the uterus show a fairly strong linear echo suggesting a small tubular structure approximately 2–3 mm in diameter.

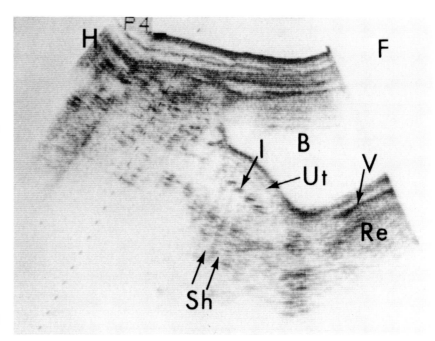

Fig. 11.33

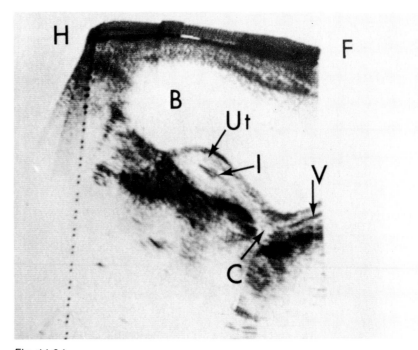

Fig. 11.34

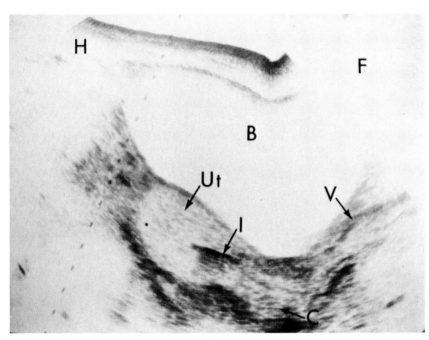

B = Urinary bladder
C = Cervix
F = Foot
H = Head
I = Intrauterine device
IP = Iliopsoas muscles
L = Left
O = Ovary
R = Right
Sh = Shadowing
Ut = Uterus
V = Vagina

Fig. 11.35

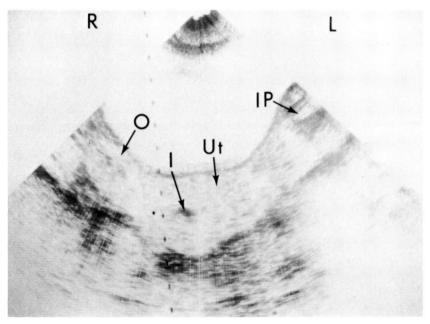

Fig. 11.36

Fibroid Uterus

Leiomyomas of the uterus are fairly common. Their appearance varies, depending mainly upon their size. Figures 11.37 and 11.38 are of a patient with a myoma in the posterior fundal region of the uterus. The difference in echogenicity between the myoma and the normal myometrium arising from the uterus and cervix is notable. The myoma is less echogenic than the normal myometrial echoes. A word of caution is in order when evaluating the fundal region of the uterus. Very often, the fundus of the uterus appears less echogenic than the mid and lower uterine segments. However, this is extremely dependent upon the degree of bladder filling. When the urinary bladder is not well filled, the fundal region of the uterus often will appear less echogenic, because a distended urinary bladder is not present anterior to it. We must remember that the through transmission from the urinary bladder increases the level of echoes arising from the uterus. Therefore, a misdiagnosis of a fundal myoma is very common when the urinary bladder is only partially filled.

Figures 11.39 and 11.40 are scans of a myoma that contains calcification. Calcifications are often present within a myoma. They give very strong echoes that are often accompanied by shadowing. The myoma in these scans yields a less echogenic appearance as compared to the normal myometrial echoes arising within the uterus. The transverse scan in figure 11.40 shows that the myoma is somewhat pedunculated and situated off the posterior left aspect of the uterus.

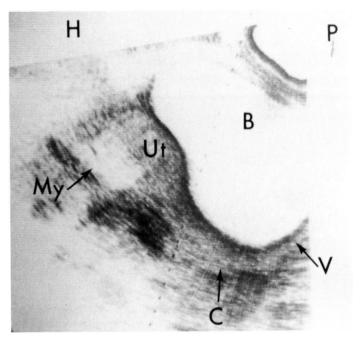

Fig. 11.37

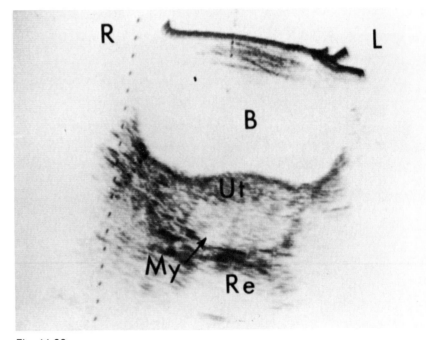

Fig. 11.38

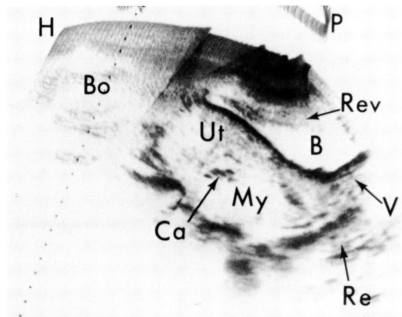

Fig. 11.39

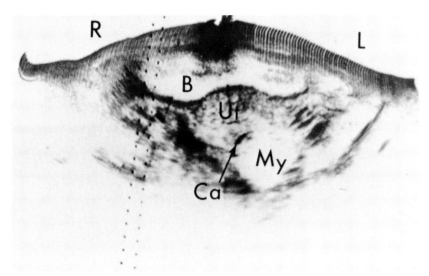

Fig. 11.40

B	= Urinary bladder
Bo	= Bowel
C	= Cervix
Ca	= Calcification
H	= Head
L	= Left
My	= Myoma
P	= Level of the symphysis pubis
R	= Right
Re	= Rectum
Rev	= Reverberation artifacts
Ut	= Uterus
V	= Vagina

Fibroid Uterus

Figure 11.41, a longitudinal scan, shows nearly the entire fundal region of the uterus containing a large myoma. The only normally appearing uterine echoes arise from the cervical region and the lower uterine segment. The myoma has a fairly homogeneous, relatively sonolucent appearance which is characteristic of a fibroid uterus.

Another longitudinal scan (fig. 11.42) demonstrates a uterus containing a large myoma. In this case, however, numerous echoes are present within the myoma. This is an instance of a fibroid uterus undergoing some degeneration. This can occur to such a severe degree that the uterus may occasionally be confused for a hydatidiform mole. The echoes are more irregular in a degenerating fibroid uterus than in a mole.

Figures 11.43 and 11.44 are of a patient with a large fibroid uterus, part of which was undergoing degeneration. The longitudinal scan (fig. 11.43) shows the myomatous uterus involving much of the entire abdomen. Again, the only normally appearing myometrial echoes are in the cervical region. There is relatively poor through transmission on the posterior aspect of the myoma, and this is another characteristic of fibroid lesions within the uterus. Figure 11.44 is a transverse scan of a myomatous mass with attenuation on the right side. The portion of the mass on the left side, however, does have some through transmission with a relatively sonolucent central area. This is due to fluid present within a degenerating fibroid uterus. When severe degeneration occurs, a myoma may appear relatively echo-free with through transmission secondary to fluid within its central portion.

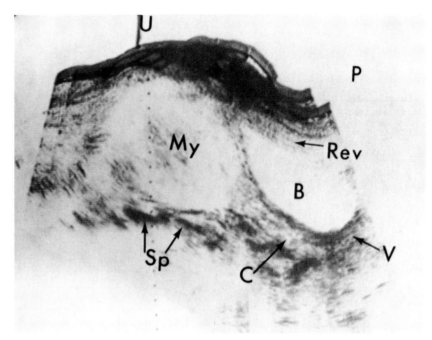

Fig. 11.41

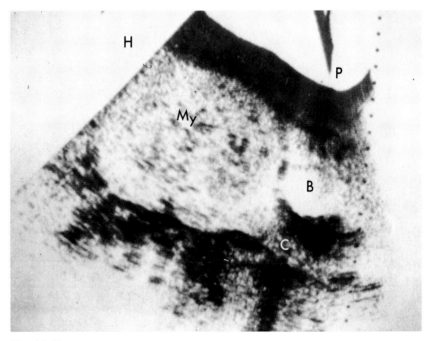

Fig. 11.42

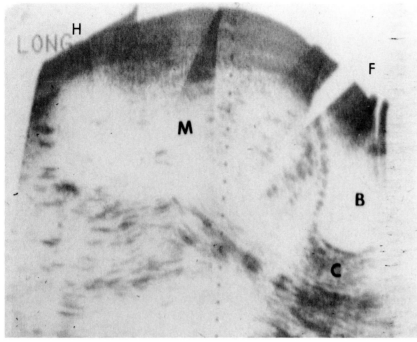
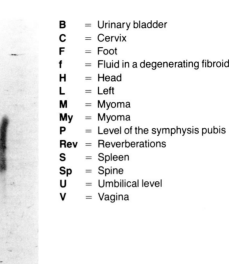

Fig. 11.43

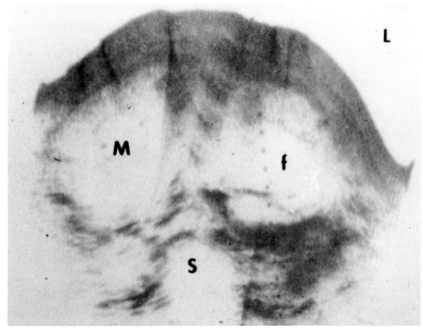

Fig. 11.44

Cervical Carcinoma; Mixed Mesodermal Sarcoma of the Uterus

Figures 11.45–11.47 are ultrasound scans of a patient with cervical carcinoma. Figure 11.45 is a longitudinal scan with a less echogenic cervical region which is also the site of the cervical carcinoma. The difference in echogenicity between the uterus and the cervix can be noted. The cervix is markedly enlarged with somewhat irregular borders, along with decreased echo amplitude. Figure 11.46 is a transverse section through the cervix in which we again see decreased echogenicity to the cervical carcinoma. Figure 11.47 is a transverse section, higher and through the normal portion of the uterus. We can note the normally appearing echo pattern of the myometrium in the uninvolved portion of the uterus. The decreased echogenicity in the cervical region is not specific for cervical carcinoma and could represent a cervical fibroid.

Figure 11.48 is a longitudinal scan of the pelvis and lower abdomen of a 58-year-old woman. Here we see enlargement of the uterus. The echogenicity of the uterus is somewhat irregular. Although this could represent involvement of the uterus with fibroids, a carcinoma of the uterus or other malignancy could not be ruled out. At surgery, a mixed mesodermal sarcoma of the uterus with numerous tumor implants throughout the pelvis was found.

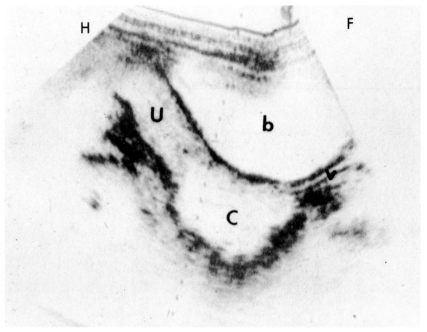

Fig. 11.45

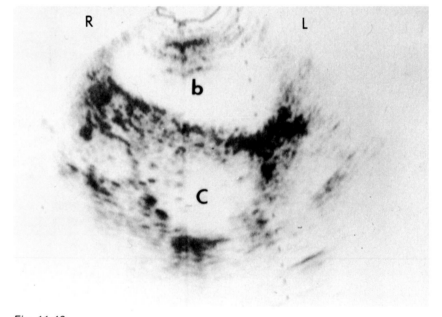

Fig. 11.46

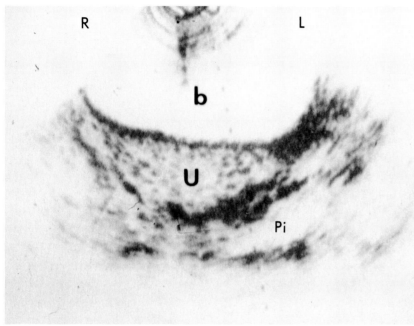

Fig. 11.47

SOURCE: The case in figure 11.48 is provided through the courtesy of Dr. B. Green, M. D. Anderson Hospital, Texas Medical Center, Houston, Texas.

b = Urinary bladder
C = Cervical carcinoma
F = Foot
H = Head
L = Left
Pi = Piriform muscle
R = Right
U = Uterus
Ut = Mixed mesodermal sarcoma of the uterus
V = Vagina

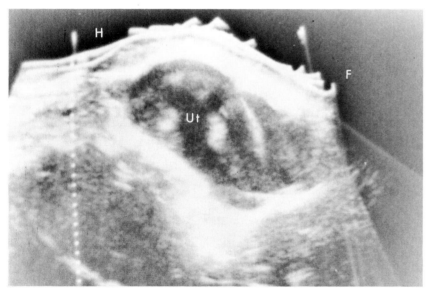

Fig. 11.48

Uterine Neoplasms

Figures 11.49 and 11.50 are scans of a 66-year-old woman with lower-abdominal pain and a palpable pelvic mass. Ultrasound examination demonstrated a large mass within the pelvis and lower abdomen. The echogenic portion of this mass was noted posterior to a sonolucent segment and was felt to be fluid. At surgery, adenocarcinoma of the endometrium was diagnosed. The ultrasound examination demonstrated evidence of necrosis of the tumor with fluid anteriorly and through transmission and echogenicity posteriorly. Uterine carcinoma is difficult to distinguish from a necrotic fibroid, but uterine carcinomas appear to undergo necrosis somewhat more frequently than fibroids.

Figures 11.51 and 11.52 are of an elderly woman admitted for severe pelvic pain and fever. The patient had a previous diagnosis of a large uterine mixed mesodermal sarcoma. The pelvic pain developed following radiation therapy. Ultrasound examination demonstrated an enlarged uterus. In the central and anterior portion of the uterus, a relatively sonolucent mass indicates the presence of fluid. At surgery, this turned out to be a necrotic abscess within a uterine mesodermal sarcoma. Again, uterine enlargement with fluid is present, indicating necrosis, hemorrhage, or abscess.

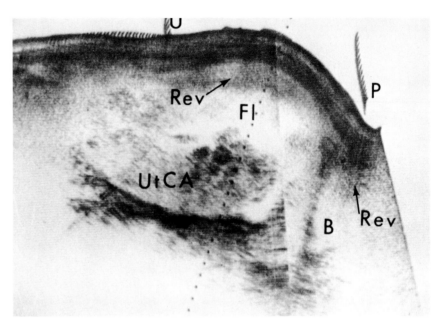

Fig. 11.49

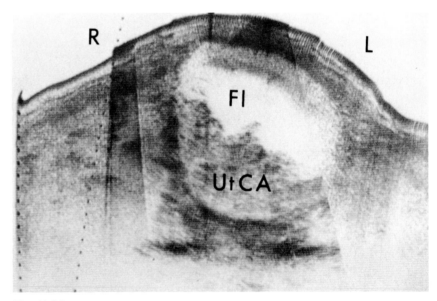

Fig. 11.50

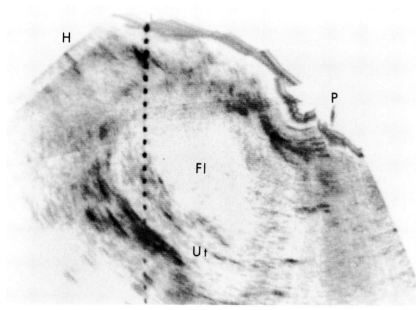

Fig. 11.51

SOURCE: The case for figures 11.51 and 11.52 is provided through the courtesy of Dr. B. Green, M. D. Anderson Hospital, University of Texas Medical Center, Houston, Texas.

Ab	=	Necrotic abscess within a mesodermal uterine sarcoma
B	=	Urinary bladder
Fl	=	Necrotic fluid within the adenocarcinoma
H	=	Head
L	=	Left
P	=	Level of the symphysis pubis
R	=	Right
Rev	=	Reverberations
U	=	Umbilical level
Ut	=	Uterus
UtCA	=	Adenocarcinoma of the uterus

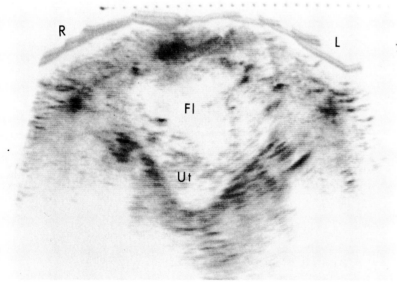

Fig. 11.52

Ovarian Cysts

Functional follicular cysts are encountered quite often during an ultrasound examination of the female pelvis. They can range in size from a few millimeters to large masses. The simple cysts have sonolucent centers with good through transmission and sharp borders. They usually do not cause any diagnostic problems or become confused with such things as abscesses, hematomas, or necrotic tumors. We look for the sharp borders and good through transmission to confirm the diagnosis of a simple ovarian cyst. A simple ovarian cyst seen on one examination will often disappear. We often see fluid in the cul-de-sac following spontaneous rupture of an ovarian cyst. This is a common finding.

Figure 11.53 is a transverse scan of a patient with a small 2-cm cyst of the right ovary. The left ovary is in the normal position. Just posterior to the left ovary and lateral to the uterus is a strong circular echogenic region which represents bowel. This often may be confused with an ovarian mass, especially with a dermoid. The echoes behind the ovarian cyst are of very high amplitude when compared to the echoes behind the left ovary. This is consistent with its fluid-filled nature.

A longitudinal scan of a different patient (fig. 11.54) demonstrates an ovarian cyst in the central portion of the ovary. Here we see the ovarian cyst is only 1 cm in size, but it stands out quite easily as a sonolucent mass within the soft echoes of the normal ovarian parenchyma. The strong border surrounding the ovarian cyst is fairly characteristic of a simple cyst.

Figures 11.55 and 11.56 are from a patient with a functional ovarian cyst of the left ovary. A transverse scan (fig. 11.55) demonstrates a sonolucent mass in the left adenexa, consistent with an ovarian cyst. Very strong echoes are seen posterior to the ovarian cyst, indicating through transmission. This may, however, be difficult to evaluate in many instances because of the strong echoes which arise from air-filled bowel. Numerous curvilinear strong echoes secondary to reverberations off a strong air-filled bowel interface are present on the left

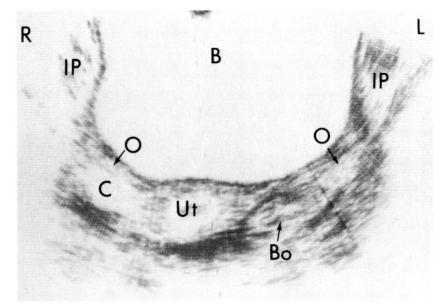

Fig. 11.53

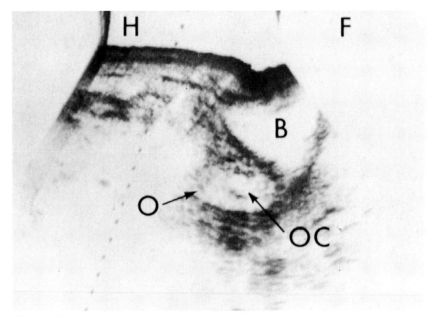

Fig. 11.54

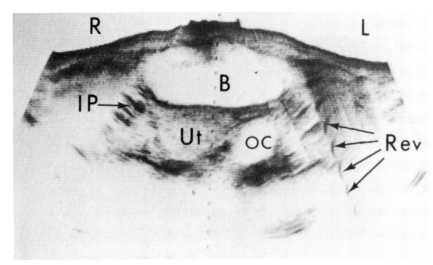

Fig. 11.55

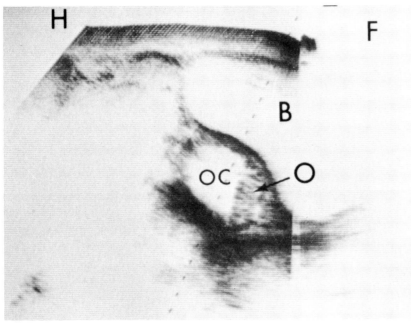

Fig. 11.56

side of the abdomen. This is a fairly common artifact in the pelvis. Figure 11.56 is a longitudinal scan of the same patient with the superior half of the ovary completely fluid-filled by the ovarian cyst. The caudal half of the ovary has a normal echogenic pattern to it consistent with a normal ovarian parenchyma. The indentation of the left ovary on the posterior aspect of the bladder wall is notable. This indentation becomes extremely important in evaluating pelvic masses, as will be shown in the following cases.

B   = Urinary bladder
Bo   = Bowel
C   = Ovarian cyst
F   = Foot
H   = Head
IP   = Iliopsoas muscles
L   = Left
O   = Ovaries
OC   = Ovarian cyst
R   = Right
Rev = Reverberation artifacts
Ut   = Uterus

Ovarian Cysts— Hemorrhagic and Theca-Lutein

Figure 11.57 is a longitudinal scan of a left ovary with a small 1-cm cyst in its superior portion. This is an excellent example of visualization of the ovary anterior to the internal iliac vessels. We often have difficulty locating the ovary on longitudinal scans unless the internal iliac vessels can be visualized. The normal parenchymogram of the ovary can be seen in the caudal portion with the sonolucent ovarian cyst present in the cephalad portion.

Figure 11.58 is a transverse scan of a patient with a large right adnexal mass which was not completely sono-lucent. It eventually was found to be a hemorrhagic ovarian cyst. The large right adnexal mass is sonolucent ante-riorly and represents a fluid-filled ovarian cyst. We see soft echoes on the posterior aspect of the mass as well as a fluid–fluid level secondary to hemor-rhage. An indentation on the posterior right bladder floor (arrows) is a con-sistent finding in large pelvic masses. Studying the bladder floor superior to the uterus a similar, although less dra-matic, indentation is seen. Whenever pelvic masses are easy to identify, the bladder floor finding is not critical. When echogenic masses blend into the strong echoes of the bowel-filled pelvis, how-ever, the indentation on the bladder floor can become extremely important.

Figures 11.59 and 11.60 are of a 24-year-old woman whose uterus had been evacuated for a hydatidiform mole 1 week prior to the ultrasound examina-tion. After evacuation of the uterus, she was still found to have a pelvic and abdominal mass. Scans performed at that time demonstrated multiple fluid-filled sonolucent masses in the pelvis and lower abdomen (figs. 11.59 and 11.60). A multiloculated appearance to the mass is demonstrated here, with numerous curvilinear echoes separat-ing the sonolucent fluid-filled areas. In figure 11.60, the uterus is seen posterior to the urinary bladder and separate from these fluid-filled masses. Theca-lutein cysts which are associated with hyda-tidiform moles were diagnosed. The

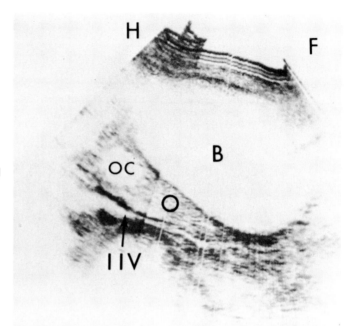

Fig. 11.57

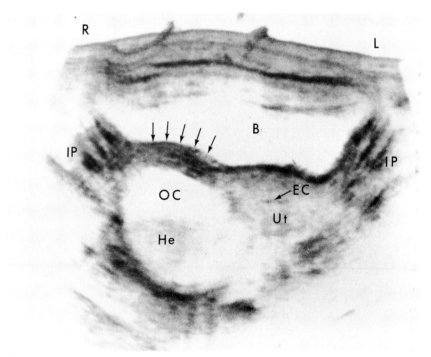

Fig. 11.58

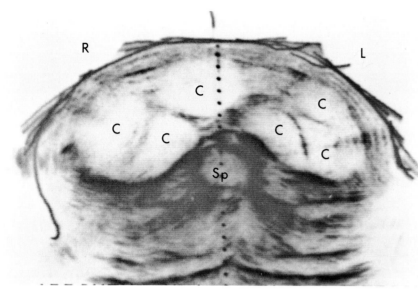

Fig. 11.59

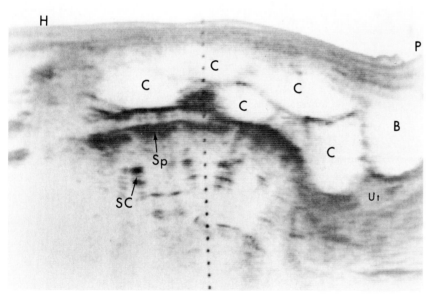

Fig. 11.60

multiloculated appearance cannot be distinguished from numerous such other entities as cystadenomas.

B	=	Urinary bladder
C	=	Theca-lutein cyst
EC	=	Endometrial cavity
F	=	Foot
H	=	Head
He	=	Hemorrhage in an ovarian cyst
IIV	=	Internal iliac vessels
IP	=	Iliopsoas muscles
L	=	Left
O	=	Ovary
OC	=	Ovarian cyst
P	=	Level of the symphysis pubis
R	=	Right
SC	=	Spinal canal
Sp	=	Spine
Ut	=	Uterus

SOURCE: The case for figure 11.158 is provided through the courtesy of Dr. R. Bree, Toledo Hospital, Toledo, Ohio. The case for figures 11.59 and 11.60 is provided through the courtesy of Dr. B. Green, M. D. Anderson Hospital, Texas Medical Center, Houston, Texas.

Polycystic Ovaries

Figures 11.61–11.64 are pelvic ultrasound scans of a 16-year-old girl referred for secondary amenorrhea. Examination was concentrated on the ovaries to determine their size and ethogenicity. A longitudinal scan in the midline (fig. 11.61) shows the uterus to be of normal size and stimulated. A stimulated uterus has a fundal region that is usually thicker and larger than the cervical region. The unstimulated uterus will have a small thin fundus with a smaller diameter than the cervical region (see figure 11.145).

A large sonolucent mass is also present posterior to the urinary bladder. This is a false mass (arrows) and secondary to an artifact. The duplication artifact of the urinary bladder can present as a false mass. This is a fairly common occurrence, and care must be taken not to misdiagnosis an extremely large sonolucent mass in the pelvis. The patient must return with varying bladder filling if any question of a false mass has been created by bladder duplication. In trying to find the ovaries, we can often follow the uterus until the fallopian tubes are visualized. A transverse scan (fig. 11.62) demonstrates the fallopian tubes quite well bilaterally. The piriform muscles could be confused for the ovaries on this patient. They are, however, situated somewhat posterior to the uterus and are fairly symmetrical in appearance. We see only the anterior and posterior borders of the piriform muscles, not the lateral borders.

Following the fallopian tubes, the ovaries can finally be identified bilaterally. A transverse scan (fig. 11.63), that is actually cephalad to the fundus of the uterus shows the uterus to be no longer in the central portion of the scan. Bowel gas is seen. If the fallopian tubes had not been followed, the piriform muscles in figure 11.62 might have been misinterpreted as the ovaries. In figure 11.63 we see the ovaries bilaterally. The right ovary is anterior to the internal iliac vessels. On this transverse scan, the ovaries have a much coarser appearance than those noted in previous examples. Numerous strong linear echoes are present within them.

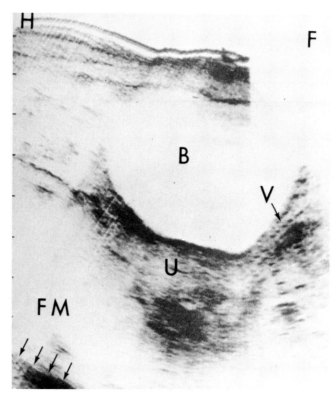

Fig. 11.61

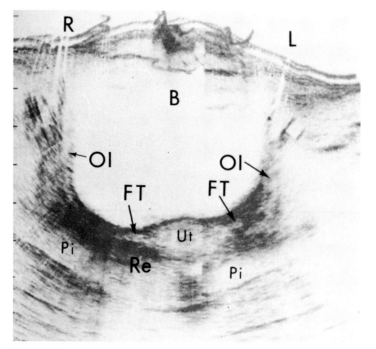

Fig. 11.62

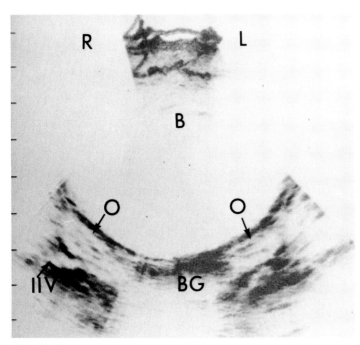

Fig. 11.63

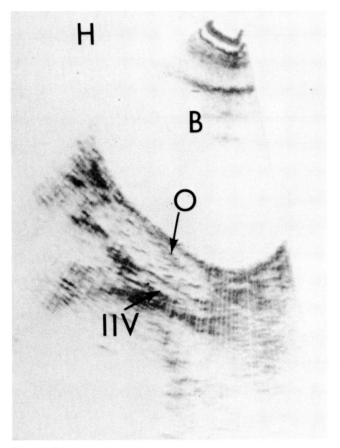

Fig. 11.64

Figure 11.64 is a longitudinal scan of the right ovary, which is seen anterior to the internal iliac vessels. Again, numerous curvilinear strong echoes within the ovary are noted. These are consistent with the walls of the numerous small cysts in these polycystic ovaries. The cysts are quite small in size. The lumen cannot actually be visualized but the sharp echogenic walls are demonstrated. This is fairly characteristic of polycystic ovaries. The patient also had hormonal levels which confirmed the diagnosis of polycystic disease.

B	=	Urinary bladder
BG	=	Bowel gas
F	=	Foot
FM and arrows	=	False mass due to bladder duplication artifact
FT	=	Fallopian tubes
H	=	Head
IIV	=	Internal iliac vessels
L	=	Left
O	=	Ovaries
OI	=	Obturator internus muscles
Pi	=	Piriform muscles
R	=	Right
Re	=	Rectum
U	=	Uterus
Ut	=	Uterus
V	=	Vagina

Mucinous Cystadenocarcinoma; Papillary Serous Cystadenocarcinoma

Figures 11.65 and 11.66 are scans of a 62-year-old woman with increasing abdominal distention. An intravenous pyelogram demonstrated no obstruction of the ureters; however, there was a soft-tissue density over the abdomen. Ultrasound examination demonstrated a multiloculated mass (figs. 11.65 and 11.66). It is a large mass with numerous fluid-filled areas separated by curvilinear echoes. This finding is fairly characteristic of a cystadenoma or cystadenocarcinoma of the ovaries. At surgery, a large 20-cm mass was found. Also present were numerous metastatic implants throughout the abdomen with nodules over the diaphragm, liver, gallbladder, right kidney, stomach, and omentum. The pathology report on this mass was mucinous cystadenocarcinoma. Mucinous and serous cystadenocarcinomas have a fairly similar appearance and cannot be distinguished with ultrasound. They present as a multiloculated fluid-filled mass with numerous curvilinear echoes within it.

Figures 11.67 and 11.68 are from another patient with an ultrasound examination demonstrating both a solid (arrows) and a fluid component to a rather large pelvic mass. This mixed-echo pattern is more suspicious for carcinoma because of the large solid component present within the mass. At surgery, it was found to be a papillary serous cystadenocarcinoma.

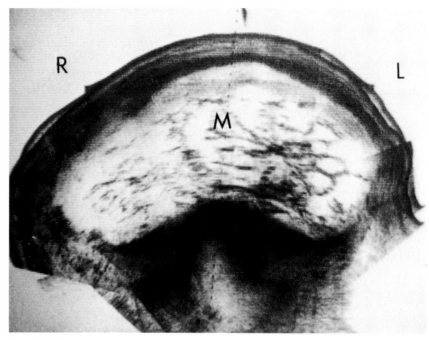

Fig. 11.65

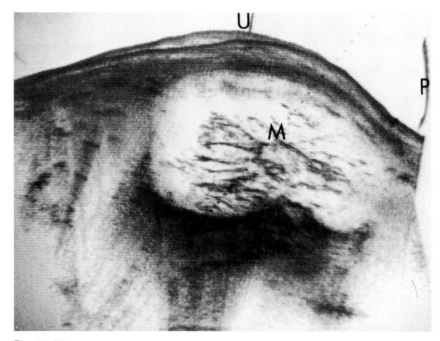

Fig. 11.66

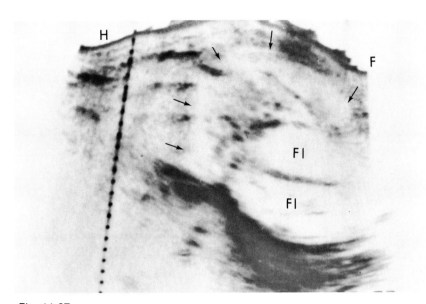

Fig. 11.67

SOURCE: The case for figures 11.65 and 11.66 was provided through the courtesy of Dr. B. Green, M. D. Anderson Hospital, University of Texas Medical Center, Houston, Texas.

Arrows = Solid component to a papillary serous cystadenocarcinoma
F = Foot
Fl = Fluid component to the mass
H = Head
L = Left
M = Mucinous cystadenocarcinoma
P = Level of the symphysis pubis
R = Right
U = Umbilical level

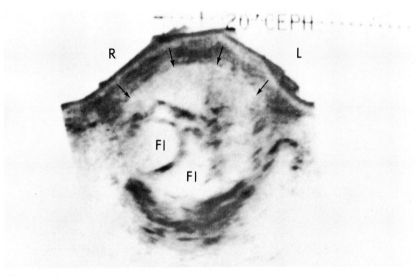

Fig. 11.68

Papillary Cystadenocarcinoma

Figures 11.69–11.72 are scans of a 14-year-old girl with increasing abdominal girth. An intravenous pyelogram was initially performed, and it indicated a suggestion of small bowel obstruction with areas of decreased density noted over the abdomen. Because of this, an ultrasound examination was done. This case is quite interesting in that it shows the various presentations of a cystadenocarcinoma. Figure 11.69 is a longitudinal scan of the abdomen and pelvis from the xyphoid to the symphysis pubis. Ascitic fluid is seen beneath the liver and in the pelvis. In figure 11.72 ascitic fluid is seen in the pelvis surrounding the uterus. Also noted in figures 11.69 and 11.72 is a large echogenic mass just above the ascitic fluid in the pelvis. It has a fairly homogeneous echogenic component to it, indicating the solid nature of this tumor.

A second component in this mass, however, is a more characteristic appearance of a cystadenocarcinoma. This is in the mid and upper abdomen. In figures 11.69, 11.70, and 11.71, numerous curvilinear echoes surrounding fluid-filled regions are noted. A transverse scan (fig. 11.71) of the midabdomen demonstrates the solid component of the mass along with the fluid and curvilinear echoes. In fact, the fluid-filled areas are highly suggestive of bowel loops, with which this entity could be confused. In papillary cystadenocarcinoma, however, the fluid-filled masses appear somewhat more irregular and disorganized than bowel loops. Examples of bowel obstruction are presented in the general abdomen chapter. Also noted in figures 11.70 and 11.71, is ascitic fluid in the right lateral gutter of the abdomen. At surgery, this mass was found to be a papillary cystadenocarcinoma. It had a large solid component in its inferior portion and a more characteristic fluid-filled component in the cephalad region.

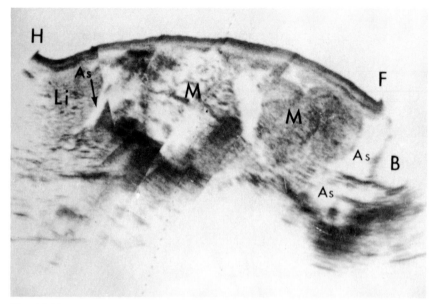

Fig. 11.69

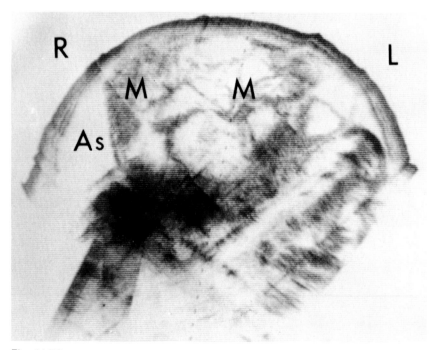

Fig. 11.70

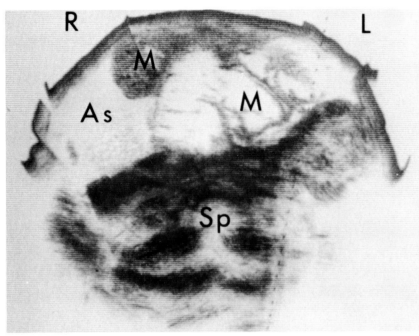

Fig. 11.71

As = Ascites
B = Urinary bladder
F = Foot
H = Head
L = Left
Li = Liver
M = Papillary cystadenocarcinoma
R = Right
Sp = Spine
Ut = Uterus

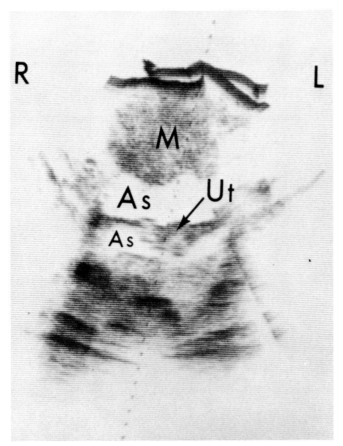

Fig. 11.72

Solid Ovarian Tumors

Solid ovarian tumors give an ultrasonic appearance of large echogenic masses within the pelvis. The ultrasonic appearance, however, is not very helpful in distinguishing one type of tumor from another. The major difficulty with a pelvic ultrasound examination of a solid ovarian tumor is the inability to distinguish it as separate from the uterus. If a complete separation of the uterus from the solid mass can be shown, an adnexal lesion can be diagnosed. If the lesion cannot be separated entirely from the uterus, however, the possibility of a uterine growth must be considered.

Figure 11.73 is a longitudinal scan that demonstrates a large mass superior to the uterus. The mass is markedly attenuating (arrows). The posterior wall of the mass is difficult to see because of this marked attenuation. The possibility of a pedunculated fibroid off the fundus of the uterus cannot definitely be ruled out. A fairly good interface is seen between the mass and the uterus. This case turned out to be a fibrosarcoma of the ovary. Fibrous tumors of the ovary can yield an ultrasonic appearance similar to that of fibroids of the uterus. The architecture of the tumor is usually fairly sonolucent with marked attenuation and poor through transmission, as is seen in a fibroid of the uterus.

Figure 11.74 is a longitudinal scan of a 10-year-old girl with a pelvic mass. Here we see a large sonolucent mass, separate from the uterus. Although the mass is extremely sonolucent, there is very poor through transmission deep to it. This may be confused for a cystic lesion. The lack of an extremely sharp posterior border and through transmission, however, indicates its solid nature by ultrasound. At exploration, a 10 x 5 x 3 cm, solid lobulated mass of the left ovary was found. It was diagnosed as a fibrosarcoma of the left ovary. Again, fibrous lesions of the ovary can be fairly sonolucent masses with poor through transmission similar to fibroid lesions of the uterus.

Figure 11.75 is a longitudinal scan of the pelvis of an 8-year-old girl with acute lymphocytic leukemia. A large, relatively lucent mass is seen posterior to the

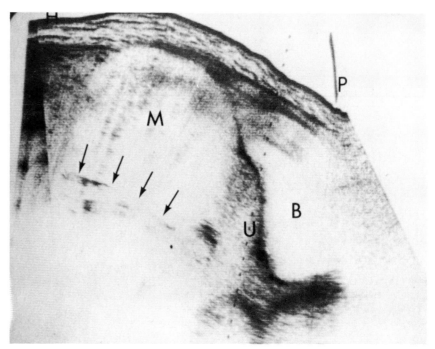

Fig. 11.73

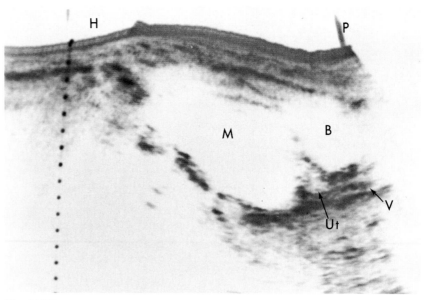

Fig. 11.74

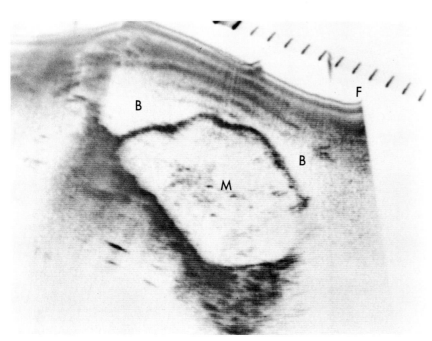

Fig. 11.75

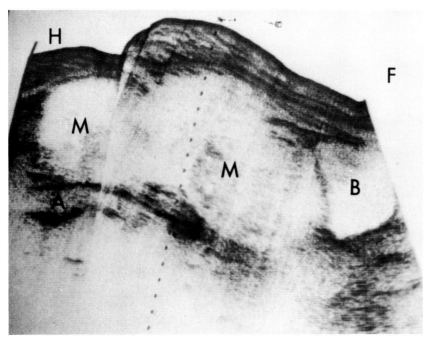

Fig. 11.76

urinary bladder. A marked irregular indentation on the posterior wall of the urinary bladder is also noted. Diffuse echoes are present within the mass, indicating the solid nature of this lesion. It turned out to be leukemic ovarian infiltrates.

Figure 11.76 is a longitudinal scan of the pelvis of a 27-year-old woman with increasing abdominal girth. Ultrasound demonstrated a large echogenic mass of the pelvis and abdomen. The distention of the abdominal wall by this mass can be seen. The solid nature was confirmed by numerous internal echoes and a poorly defined posterior wall with a lack of through transmission. This was found to be a dysgerminoma of the ovary. These rapidly growing tumors of the ovary cannot be distinguished by their ultrasonic appearance.

SOURCE: Figures 11.74 and 11.75 are provided through the courtesy of Dr. B. Green, M. D. Anderson Hospital, Texas Medical Center, Houston, Texas.

A	=	Aorta
Arrows	=	Lack of through transmission
B	=	Urinary bladder
F	=	Foot
H	=	Head
M	=	Solid ovarian mass
P	=	Level of the symphysis pubis
U	=	Uterus
Ut	=	Uterus
V	=	Vagina

Dysgerminoma

Figures 11.77 and 11.78 are ultrasound examinations of a 15-year-old girl with increased abdominal girth. Ultrasound examination demonstrated a large solid mass in the pelvis and abdomen. The anterior abdominal wall is distended secondary to the size of the mass. Within the mass are numerous strong echoes (arrows) which are of very high amplitude. An abdominal film demonstrated scattered calcifications throughout the abdomen, corresponding to these highly echogenic regions within the mass. Surgery demonstrated that this was a dysgerminoma. These tumors can grow extremely rapidly. They give an ultrasonic appearance of a solid lesion within the pelvis and abdomen.

Figures 11.79 and 11.80 are scans of a patient with dysgerminoma. This 13-year-old girl had had a large 20-cm dysgerminoma removed from the right ovary 1 year previously. Figure 11.79 is a transverse scan of the patient several months after surgery. The uterus is seen deviated slightly to the right. A mass in the left adnexal region represents the left ovary. The posterior left wall of the urinary bladder is seen to have a normal contour. The echogenicity of the ovary was somewhat worrisome at that time. It was decided to follow the patient serially with ultrasound examinations.

Figure 11.80 is a transverse scan of the same patient approximately 4 months after the exam in figure 11.79. We now see an enlargement of the left adnexal mass. An indentation present on the left posterior urinary blader wall (arrows) is also noted. Evaluation of the bladder wall is an excellent means for detecting pelvic masses or changes in any pelvic masses. Although this depends on the degree of bladder filling, it can provide important diagnostic information. The left ovary is now enlarged (fig. 11.80). An irregular echo pattern throughout it indicates a solid lesion. The patient was also found to have a dysgerminoma of the left ovary.

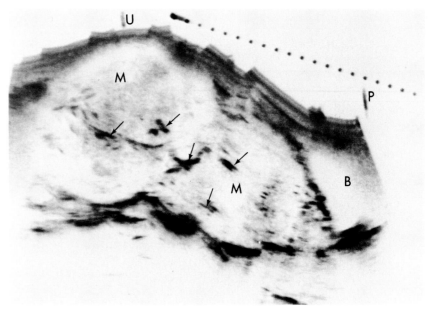

Fig. 11.77

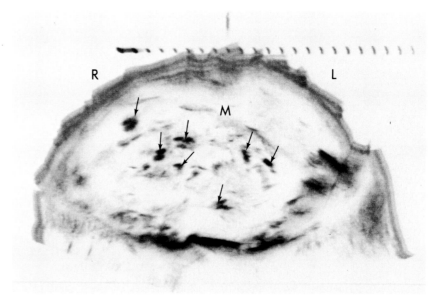

Fig. 11.78

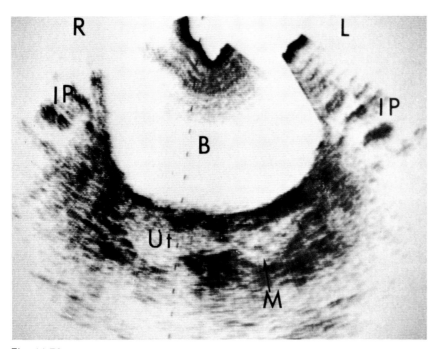

Fig. 11.79

SOURCE: The case for figures 11.77 and 11.78 is provided through the courtesy of Dr. B. Green, M. D. Anderson Hospital, Texas Medical Center, Houston, Texas.

Arrows = Areas of calcification in the dysgerminoma (figs. 11.77 and 11.78)

Arrows = Indentation on the bladder wall (fig. 11.80)

B = Urinary bladder
IP = Iliopsoas muscle
L = Left
M = Dysgerminoma
P = Level of the symphysis pubis
R = Right
U = Umbilical level
Ut = Uterus

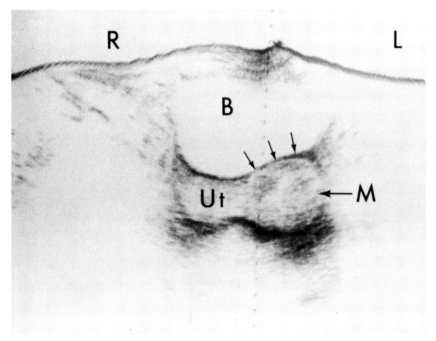

Fig. 11.80

Dermoids

Teratomas of the ovary can give various ultrasonic appearances. They can be entirely cystic, highly echogenic, or a mixture of the two.

Figure 11.81 is a longitudinal scan of a 14-year-old girl who underwent exploratory surgery for removal of a large pelvic mass. The ultrasonic findings were a large fluid-filled mass secondary to a cystic dermoid. This extended from the top of the urinary bladder to the xyphoid level. The cystic dermoid was found to contain 8000 cc of yellowish fluid. Cystic dermoids, which are mainly fluid-filled, present as a sonolucent mass within the pelvis or abdomen, similar to other ovarian cysts. This is an example of a dermoid filling the entire abdomen.

Figures 11.82–11.84 are ultrasound scans of a 48-year-old woman who noticed a slight increase in abdominal girth five years earlier. There was progressive increase in abdominal size through the years, with a suden rapid increase approximately 1 year before. Four months prior to admission, she noticed the onset of pain and a further increase in size of the abdomen. When she finally entered the hospital, an ultrasound examination revealed an extremely confusing picture. A longitudinal scan (fig. 11.82) demonstrates a solid component to the mass adherent to the anterior abdominal wall. The abdomen is filled with fluid with the uterus and bowel loops floating within it. Figure 11.83 is a transverse section through the mid abdomen with the solid mass seen anteriorly and the fluid in the dependent portions. Figure 11.84 is a transverse scan through the pelvis with fluid surrounding the uterus. We are easily able to identify the uterus in this case because of the linear echo arising from the endometrial cavity. It was originally felt to be a neoplastic tumor in the region of the solid mass with malignant ascites. At surgery, however, the patient was found to have a ruptured dermoid. Pathology revealed this to be a benign cystic teratoma with no evidence of malignancy. The ultrasound examination was extremely worrisome, for it suggested malignancy. The possibility

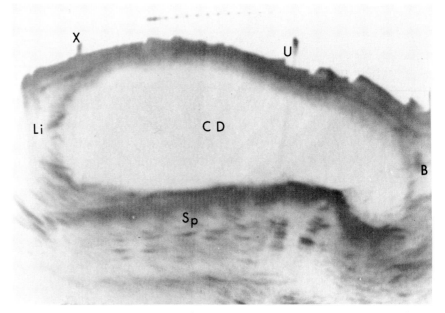

Fig. 11.81

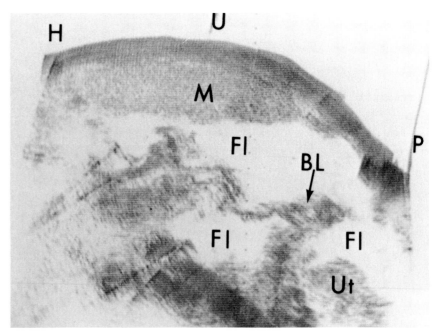

Fig. 11.82

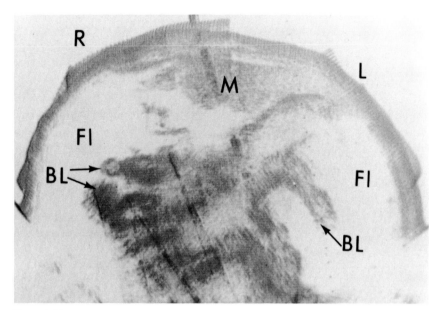

Fig. 11.83

of an ectopic pregnancy was also considered, since the anterior mass looked very much like placental tissue.

SOURCE: The case for Figure 11.81 is provided through the courtesy of Dr. B. Green, M. D. Anderson Hospital, University of Texas Medical Center, Houston, Texas.

B	=	Urinary bladder
Bl	=	Bowel loops
CD	=	Cystic teratoma
EC	=	Endometrial cavity
Fl	=	Fluid in the abdomen
H	=	Head
L	=	Left
Li	=	Liver
M	=	Solid component to the ruptured dermoid
P	=	Level of the symphysis pubis
R	=	Right
Sp	=	Spine
U	=	Umbilical level
Ut	=	Uterus
X	=	Xyphoid level

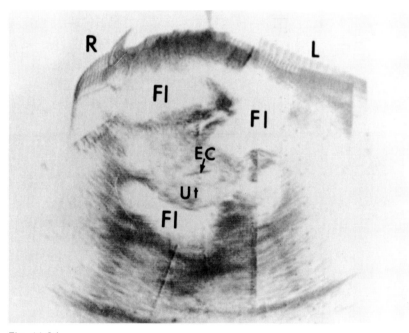

Fig. 11.84

Dermoids

Figures 11.85 and 11.86 are scans of a patient with ultrasound examination for a pelvic and abdominal mass. The uterus is displaced posteriorly on the longitudinal scan (fig. 11.85). A mass is impinging on the urinary bladder. It has a mixed pattern to it, with a large fluid component. Numerous echogenic areas, however, are noted and indicate a solid mass. In figure 11.86 we see numerous curvilinear echoes (arrows) suggesting septations running through this mass. This also turned out to be a dermoid. Dermoids have numerous elements within them which yield a mixed ultrasonic echo pattern. The possibility of a septated ovarian cyst, cystadenoma, or cystadenocarcinoma could not be ruled out by the ultrasonic findings.

The case in figures 11.87 and 11.88 was from a 23-year-old woman with a pelvic mass. In figure 11.87 we see the uterus displaced somewhat anteriorly by an extremely echogenic mass in the region of the cul-de-sac. The mass has somewhat ill-defined borders and is fairly difficult to see. It could be confused for bowel in the pelvis, except for the soft-echo appearance. Bowel usually is more echogenic. A pelvic X-ray (fig. 11.88) demonstrated a fat density in the pelvis. This indicated a dermoid. At surgery, a 13-cm, right ovarian mass was found which contained abundant sebum, hair, and a mixture of epidermis, dermal appendages, adipose tissue, and gastric mucosa. These echogenic dermoids usually contain a fair amount of hair and adipose tissue which yield high-level echoes on ultrasound.

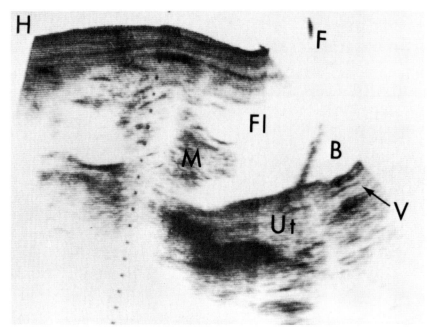

Fig. 11.85

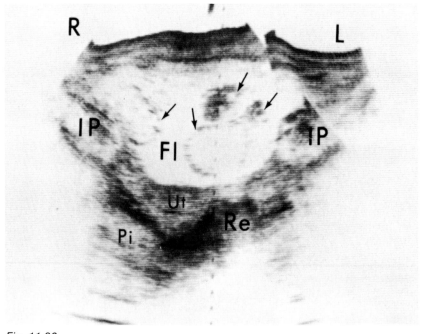

Fig. 11.86

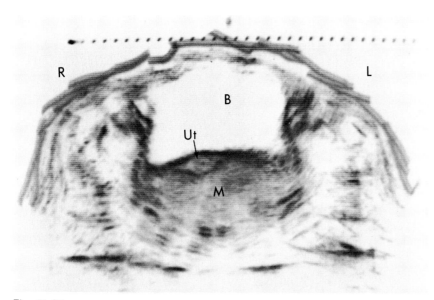

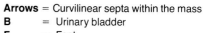

B　　= Urinary bladder
F　　= Foot
Fl　　= Fluid
H　　= Head
IP　　= Iliopsoas muscles
L　　= Left
M　　= Solid portion to the mass (fig. 11.85)
M　　= Mass posterior to the uterus (fig. 11.87)
Pi　　= Piriform muscle
R　　= Right
Re　　= Rectum
Ut　　= Uterus
V　　= Vagina

Fig. 11.87

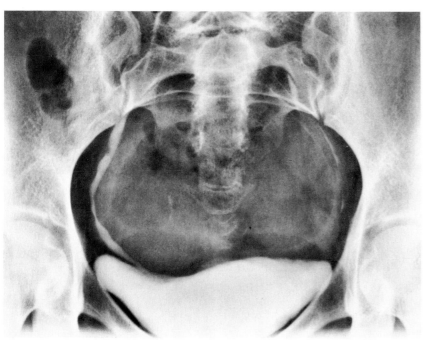

Fig. 11.88

Echogenic Dermoids

One of the most difficult lesions to detect with ultrasound is an extremely echogenic dermoid. Frequently, dermoids with high-amplitude echoes will be missed during a pelvic ultrasound examination. This is because the high-amplitude echoes arising from the dermoids blend in with the surrounding high-amplitude echoes of the bowel and rectum in the pelvis. Certain clues, however, help in detecting these lesions. If the referring gynecologist describes a large mass in the adnexa, and no lesion can be identified, it is extremely important to look for an echogenic dermoid.

Figures 11.89 and 11.90 are scans of a patient with left adnexal mass palpated by the referring physician. A transverse scan (fig. 11.89) demonstrates the extremely important sign of bladder wall indentation (arrows); this gives a clue as to the site and size of the mass. Here we see an extremely echogenic dermoid in the left adnexa displacing the uterus to the right side. The size of the mass can be measured from the bladder wall (arrows) to the piriform muscle on the left side. The mass could have been missed easily, except for the bladder wall indentation. Figure 11.90 is a longitudinal scan of the mass seen just inferior to a normal portion of the ovary. At surgery, a 7-cm dermoid was found, and this contained a large amount of sebaceous material along with hair and some adipose tissue. Usually, the dermoids containing a large amount of hair are the ones which will yield high-level echoes that can be lost in the pelvis.

Figures 11.91 and 11.92 are of another patient who presented with a pelvic mass on the right side, as noted by physical examination. Again we see the important sign of indentation on the bladder wall (arrows), this time on the right side. An echogenic mass is situated between the bladder wall and piriform muscle on the right side. The normal left ovary is seen between the uterus and the piriform muscle on the left side. A longitudinal scan of the right adnexa demonstrates the bladder wall indentation and the high-amplitude echo of the mass. It is obvious how easily this

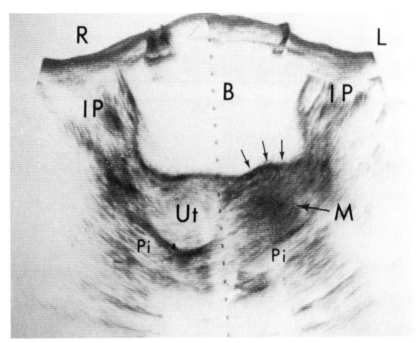

Fig. 11.89

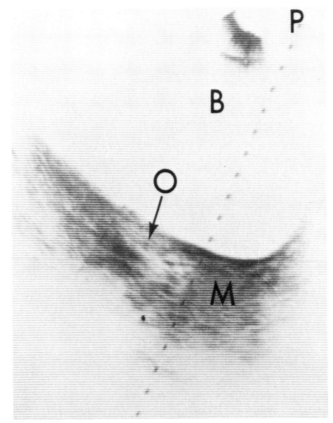

Fig. 11.90

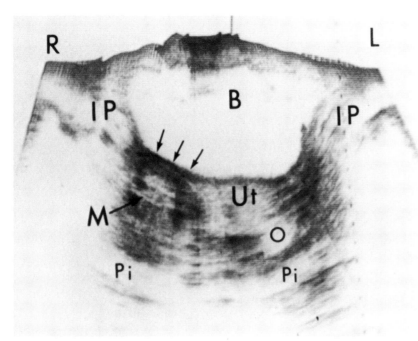

Fig. 11.91

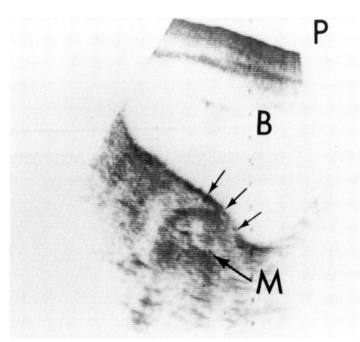

Fig. 11.92

mass might be lost in the high-amplitude echoes of the normal pelvis. If the referring physician states that there might be a large mass in the pelvis, we should be careful, for an echogenic dermoid could be missed on an ultrasound examination quite easily. It is extremely important to evaluate the contour of the bladder wall. This may provide the first clue that a mass is present. It is also extremely important to evaluate the high-amplitude echogenicity surrounding the uterus, ovaries, and normal pelvic musculature. If a region of echogenicity appears markedly different from the remainder of the pelvis, the possibility of an echogenic dermoid should be considered.

Arrows = Indentation on the bladder wall
B   = Urinary bladder
IP   = Iliopsoas muscle
L   = Left
M   = Echogenic dermoid
O   = Ovary
P   = Level of the symphysis pubis
Pi   = Piriform muscle
R   = Right
Ut   = Uterus

Pelvic Inflammatory Disease

Pelvic inflammatory disease presents an ultrasonic spectrum that depends upon the stage of infection. In an acute abscess, the masses within the pelvis will appear sonolucent and compatible with fluid. In a chronic abscess, however, the fibrosis and scarring will yield solid-appearing masses in the pelvis, which may be difficult to distinguish from neoplasms.

Figures 11.93 and 11.94 are of a 19-year-old young woman with a recent onset of pelvic pain. She was found clinically to have pelvic inflammatory disease and responded to antibiotics. Ultrasound examination demonstrated several fluid-filled areas in the right adnexal region compatible with tubal abscesses. The indentation on the urinary bladder wall indicating a right adnexal mass is notable. Fluid is seen in the tube as it loops over on itself in the right adenexa. The patient was found to have a positive gonococcal culture and responded well to antibiotic therapy.

Figures 11.95 and 11.96 are fairly characteristic pelvic scans of a patient with acute pelvic inflammatory disease. This 17-year-old girl had an onset of pelvic pain several weeks earlier. Pelvic ultrasound demonstrated fluid in the cul-de-sac. This sonolucent mass in the cul-de-sac does not appear to be as contained as we would see in an ovarian cyst or in an ovarian neoplasm. Rather, the fluid collection is noted in the cul-de-sac posterior to the uterus and filling the potential space of the lower peritoneal cavity. This was secondary to a collection of suppurative material in the cul-de-sac. The patient also responded well to antibiotics, leading to the diagnosis of pelvic inflammatory disease.

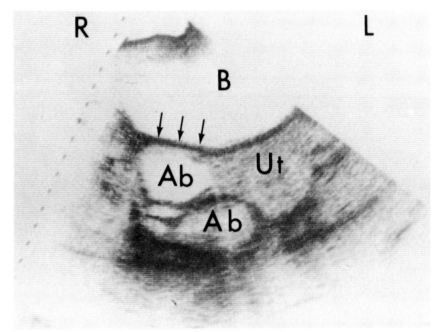

Fig. 11.93

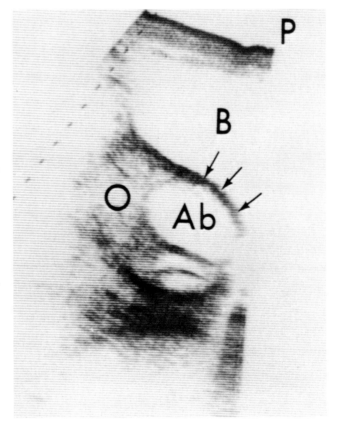

Fig. 11.94

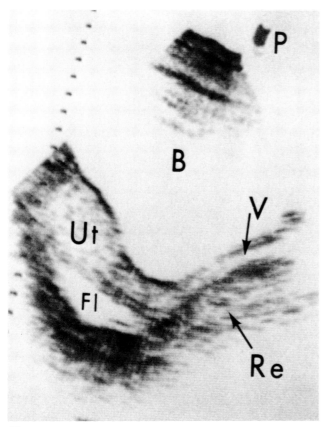

Fig. 11.95

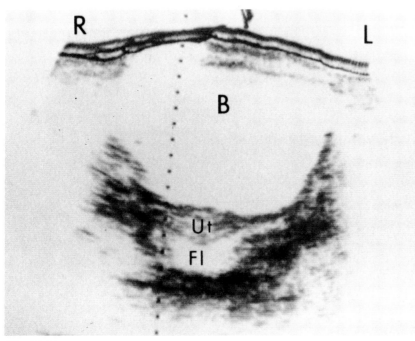

Fig. 11.96

Ab	=	Right adnexal abscess
Arrows	=	Indentation on the bladder wall
B	=	Urinary bladder
Fl	=	Fluid in the cul-de-sac
L	=	Left
O	=	Ovary
P	=	Level of the symphysis pubis
R	=	Right
Re	=	Rectum
Ut	=	Uterus
V	=	Vagina

Pelvic Inflammatory Disease

Pelvic inflammatory disease frequently is associated with an intrauterine device. Figure 11.97 is a longitudinal scan with a strong echo within the uterus, indicating an intrauterine device. This has a fairly characteristic appearance of a Copper 7 or a Copper T intrauterine device. Posterior to the uterus is a large sonolucent mass that is secondary to a cul-de-sac abscess. Here we see a somewhat irregular border to this sono-lucent mass, highly consistent with an abscess. The possibility of a hematoma could not be ruled out. Clinically, how-ever, the finding was consistent with pelvic inflammatory disease.

Often, long-standing pelvic inflam-matory disease leads to hydrosalpinx. This entity is actually a sterile collection that has been scarred and blocked with-in the fallopian tube. The sonolucent collection in the fallopian tube often gives a picture similar to an ovarian cyst.

Figure 11.98 is an example of a moderately sized hydrosalpinx in the right fallopian tube. Again we see inden-tation on the posterior bladder wall char-acteristic of a right adnexal lesion. The hydrosalpinx is extremely lucent, indi-cating its fluid-filled nature. The walls are fairly sharp, although not quite as sharp as we might see in a simple ovarian cyst.

Figures 11.99 and 11.100 represent a hydrosalpinx that is somewhat larger than the one in figure 11.98. The walls of this hydrosalpinx are slightly sharper than in the previous case. This one could be confused with an ovarian cyst, or possibly a cystadenoma.

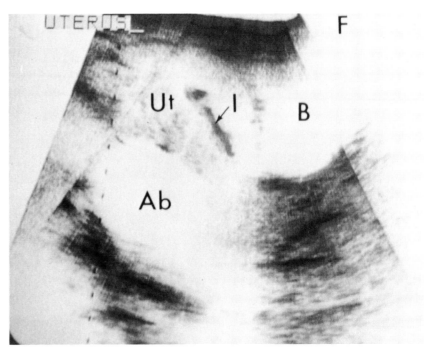

Fig. 11.97

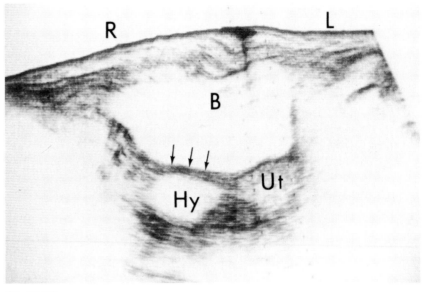

Fig. 11.98

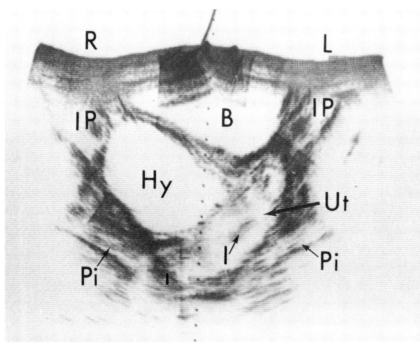

Ab   = Cul-de-sac abscess
Arrows = Indentation on the bladder wall
B   = Urinary bladder
F   = Foot
Hy = Hydrosalpinx
I   = Intrauterine device
IP   = Iliopsoas muscle
L   = Left
Pi   = Piriform muscle
R   = Right
U   = Umbilical level
Ut   = Uterus

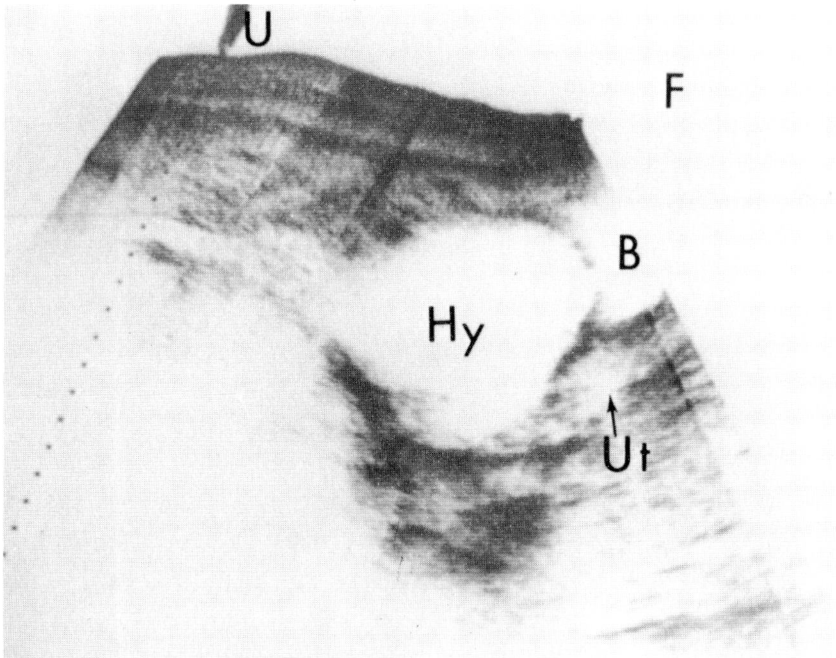

Fig. 11.99

Fig. 11.100

Pelvic Inflammatory Disease

Pelvic inflammatory disease also can appear to have a mixed echo pattern, rather than just a sonolucent echo pattern. Usually, when a mixed echo pattern of solid and cystic lesions is present, it is more characteristic of an abscess as is found elsewhere in the body. When a mixed echo pattern is present, the diagnosis of pelvic inflammatory disease with ultrasound is usually easier.

Figures 11.101 and 11.102 are of a patient with severe pelvic inflammatory disease associated with an abscess anterior to the uterus and thickening of the urinary bladder wall. There also is evidence of debris (arrows) within the urinary bladder itself. The relatively sonolucent collection between the uterus and bladder wall has an appearance more characteristic of an abscess. Irregular borders are demonstrated. The internal echoes arising from the abscess also have an appearance of debris rather than a solid nature. There is evidence of some through transmission through the abscess; again, this is somewhat characteristic.

Figures 11.103 and 11.104 are scans of a 21-year-old woman who had an intrauterine device removed 1 day previously because of pelvic pain. An ultrasound examination demonstrated two relatively lucent areas in the pelvis. It was difficult to visualize the uterus. Figure 11.103 is a transverse scan demonstrating the uterus in the mid pelvis. The borders of the uterus (arrows), however, are quite difficult to see because of the adherent adnexal masses. Bilateral abscesses are present. Because of the inflammatory reaction, the interface between the abscesses and the uterus may be quite difficult to see. The abscesses present with a mixed echo pattern in which a portion is relatively sonolucent, indicating suppurative material, and a portion is echogenic, indicating fibrosis and debris. Figure 11.104 is a longitudinal scan of the patient with the abscess collection posterior to the uterus.

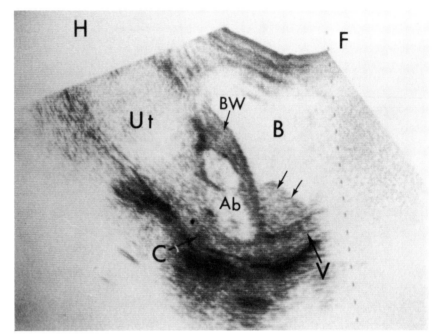

Fig. 11.101

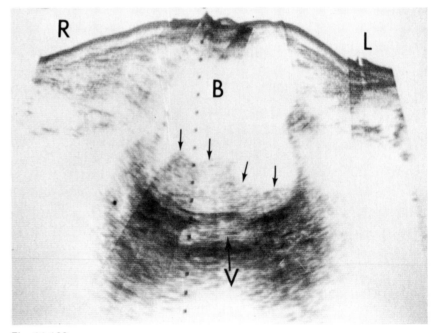

Fig. 11.102

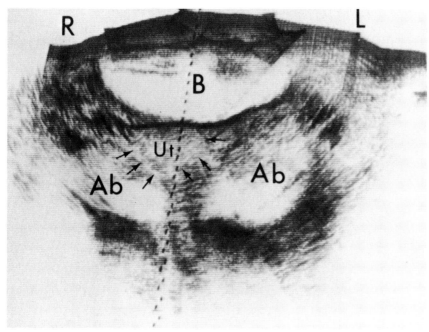

Fig. 11.103

Ab   = Pelvic abscess
Arrows   = Debris in the urinary blad-
               der wall
B   = Urinary bladder wall
BW   = Thickened   urinary   blad-
               der wall
C   = Cervix
F   = Foot
H   = Head
L   = Left
R   = Right
Ut   = Uterus
Ut and arrows = Uterus that is difficult to
               see secondary to sur-
               rounding abscess
V   = Vagina

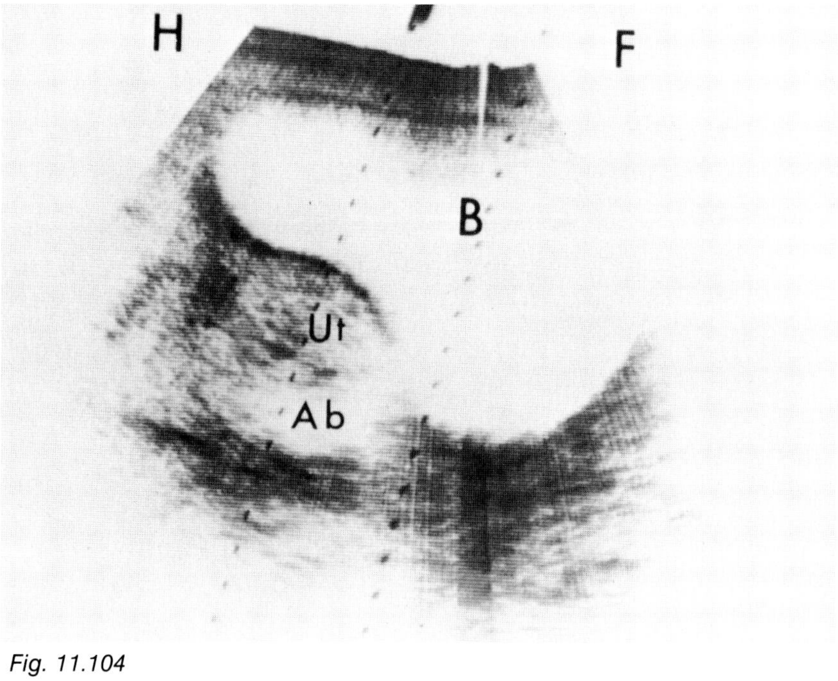

Fig. 11.104

Pelvic Inflammatory Disease

Occasionally, pelvic inflammatory disease can be so echogenic that a solid lesion of the pelvis may be diagnosed by ultrasound. Whenever a chronic abscess is present, the interfaces between the uterus and adnexa are difficult to distinguish with ultrasound due to the loss of an acoustic plane. Often a fibroid uterus or uterine tumor is considered when chronic pelvic inflammatory disease is present. The other possibility is an ovarian neoplasm.

Figure 11.105 is a transverse scan of a large pelvic mass. It is difficult to distinguish this from the uterus. A slight border, however, can be defined on the right side (small arrows). It is difficult to see because of the adherent abscess. Again we see indentation on the urinary bladder (large arrow) secondary to the right adnexal mass. This large abscess could be considered a solid ovarian tumor. Some through transmission is suggested, however, and this often can lead to the diagnosis of an abscess. It is important to have clinical information confirming the diagnosis of pelvic inflammatory disease.

In figure 11.106, a transverse scan, again it is difficult to see the uterus. There is the slight suggestion of a border to the uterus (arrows), but this is difficult to see because of the echogenic mass. This left mass was secondary to a chronic abscess in which the border to the uterus was lost because of inflammatory adhesions.

Figure 11.107 is an example of a right adnexal abscess that is more easily separated from the uterus. An interface between the uterus and the right adnexa actually can be seen, but the echogenicity and size of this abscess would be extremely worrisome for an ovarian neoplasm. Abscesses present a spectrum from fluid-filled to mixed to solid-appearing lesions in the pelvis. They can be confused for several other entities. Clinical correlation is extremely important in coming to the correct diagnosis.

Figure 11.108 shows an interesting case of pelvic inflammatory disease, which at first sight, could be confused

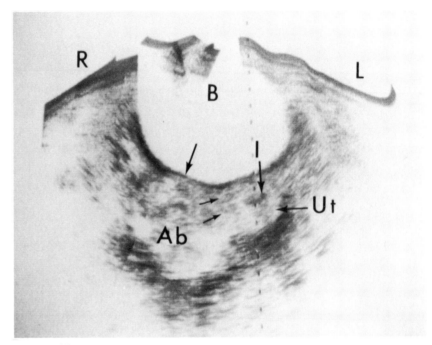

Fig. 11.105

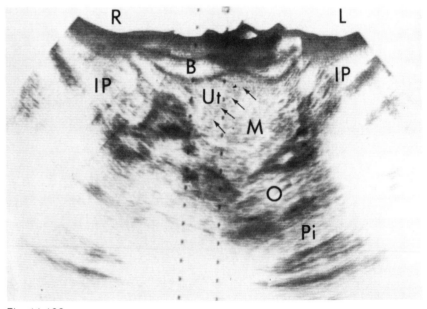

Fig. 11.106

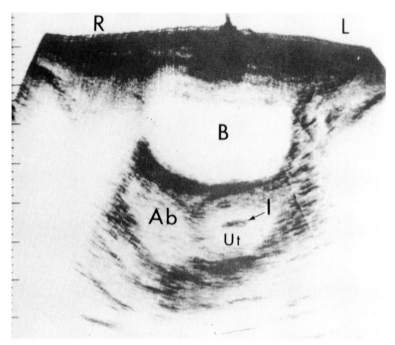

Fig. 11.107

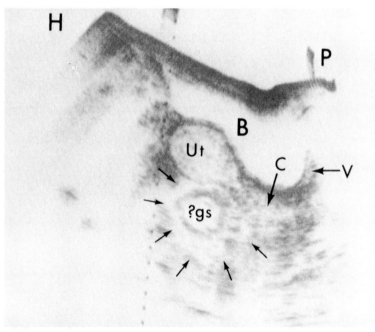

Fig. 11.108

for an ectopic pregnancy. Here we see a suggestion of a circular gestational sac. Surrounding this sac is a relatively sonolucent mass (arrows) which turned out to be a chronic abscess secondary to pelvic inflammatory disease.

SOURCE: The case in figure 11.108 is provided through the courtesy of Dr. F. Taber, Valley Presbyterian Hospital, Van Nuys, California.

Ab	=	Pelvic abscess
B	=	Urinary bladder
C	=	Cervix
?gs	=	Pelvic inflammatory disease suggesting an ectopic pregnancy
H	=	Head
I	=	Intrauterine device
IP	=	Iliopsoas muscle
Large arrow	=	Indentation on the urinary bladder
L	=	Left
M	=	Pelvic abscess
O	=	Ovary
P	=	Level of the symphysis pubis
Pi	=	Piriform muscle
R	=	Right
Small arrows	=	Uterine interface
Ut	=	Uterus
V	=	Vagina

Endometriosis

Endometriosis can be the great mimicker in pelvic ultrasound evaluation, similar to pelvic inflammatory disease. Just as in pelvic inflammatory disease, endometriosis can give a spectrum of ultrasonic appearances, ranging from a nearly completely sonolucent mass all the way to a highly echogenic solid. Figures 11.109–11.111 are of a patient with a large pelvic mass secondary to endometriosis. The large cephalic sonolucent portion of the mass is a fluid-filled endometrioma. A solid component to the endometriosis, however, is posterior to the uterus. The greater echogenicity of this region in the cul-de-sac is most likely due to clotted blood, debris, or fibrosis. A transverse scan of the same patient (fig. 11.111) demonstrates the endometrioma with soft echoes within it, just posterior and to the left of the uterus.

Figure 11.112 is of another patient with a large fluid-filled endometrioma in the left adnexa. The left adnexal mass is impinging on the posterior urinary bladder wall (arrows) as noted earlier. The endometrioma is displacing the left ovary away from the uterus. The ultrasonic findings of this endometrioma would not be specific for this entity. Other possibilities would include an abscess, an ovarian cyst, or possibly cystadenoma.

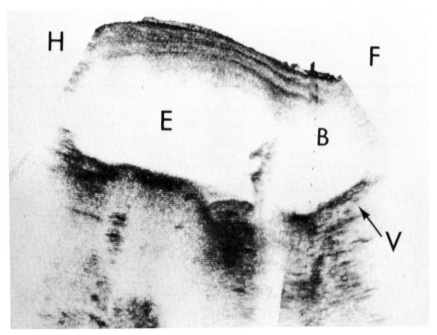

Fig. 11.109

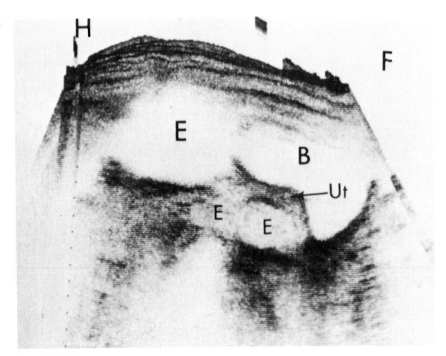

Fig. 11.110

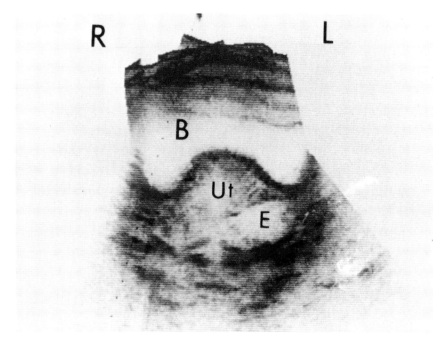

Fig. 11.111

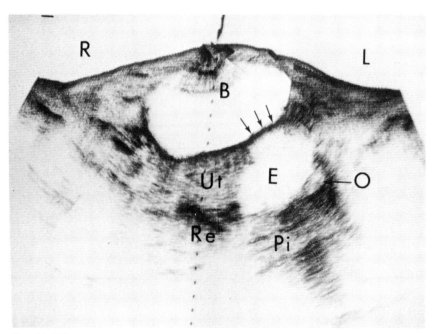

Fig. 11.112

Arrows = Indentation of the endometrioma
on the bladder wall
B = Urinary bladder
E = Endometriosis
F = Foot
H = Head
L = Left
O = Left Ovary
Pi = Piriform muscle
R = Right
Re = Rectum
Ut = Uterus
V = Vagina

Endometriosis

Figure 11.113 is a pelvic ultrasound scan of a 25-year-old woman with a large pelvic mass. The ultrasound demonstrated a large mixed mass superior to the uterus, which eventually was found to be an endometrioma. Within the sonolucent endometrioma are numerous echoes secondary to debris. Also present is a cul-de-sac endometrioma posterior to the uterus. This is an example of an endometrioma with a mixed echo pattern. It could not be distinguished from an abscess or an ovarian lesion.

Figures 11.114 and 11.115 are scans of a 34-year-old woman with carcinoma of the breast. She was noted to have pelvic masses on physical examination, and an ultrasound examination was performed. Here we see several large masses in the cul-de-sac and right adnexa. The mass in the cul-de-sac is solid in nature, and the interface between this mass and the uterus is quite difficult to see. The right adnexal mass has a sonolucent central fluid collection. With the patient's history, the possibility of ovarian neoplasm was considered quite likely. At surgery, however, she was found to have bilateral ovarian chocolate hemorrhagic cysts which indicated endometriosis rather than ovarian neoplasm. This case illustrates the marked difficulty in dealing with the ultrasonic findings of endometriosis. Because of its similarity to pelvic inflammatory disease, this entity can present as a spectrum of findings which can be confused with other pelvic pathology.

Figure 11.116 is another example of endometriosis with a very solid-appearing mass in the right adnexa, displacing the uterus to the left side. Again the possibility of a solid ovarian neoplasm could not be ruled out. This mass also could be consistent with a chronic abscess.

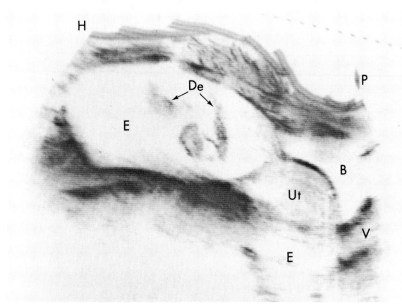

Fig. 11.113

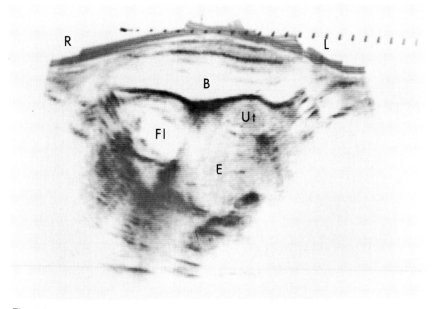

Fig. 11.114

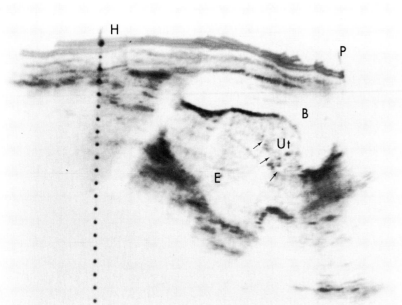

SOURCE: The cases in figures 11.113–11.115 are provided through the courtesy of Dr. B. Green, M. D. Anderson Hospital, University of Texas Medical Center, Houston, Texas.

Arrows	=	Separation between uterus and endometrioma
B	=	Urinary bladder
De	=	Debris
E	=	Endometrioma
Fl	=	Fluid in the endometrioma
H	=	Head
I	=	Intrauterine device
IP	=	Iliopsoas muscle
L	=	Left
P	=	Level of the pelvis
R	=	Right
Ut	=	Uterus
V	=	Vagina

Fig. 11.115

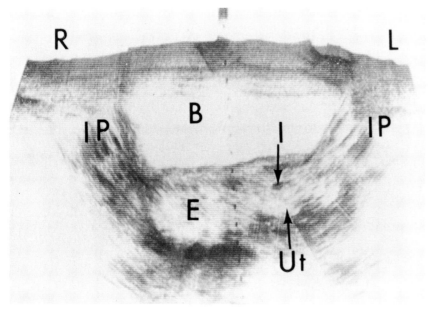

Fig. 11.116

Endometriosis

Figures 11.117 and 11.118 demonstrate a solid-appearing endometrioma in the right adnexa. The urinary bladder wall is indented, indicating a right adnexal mass. Although this endometrioma appears solid in nature, there is evidence of fluid in the cul-de-sac. The patient underwent surgery, and a large endometrioma involving the right ovary and posterior uterine wall was found.

Figures 11.119 and 11.120 are scans of a 26-year-old woman who entered the hospital complaining of lower-abdominal pain. Her abdominal pain started at age 18 and was associated with dysmenorrhea. The dysmenorrhea, however, disappeared when she was placed on oral contraceptives. In the preceding year the symptoms became worse, and she finally entered the hospital because of increasing abdominal pain associated with her menstruation. A pelvic ultrasound examination was performed (figs. 11.119 and 11.120). The transverse scan (fig. 11.119) demonstrates the uterus surrounded by a large echogenic mass. The interesting point in this case is that the mass penetrates the urinary bladder wall (arrows). The longitudinal scan demonstrates the uterus to be somewhat retroverted. The large endometrioma is difficult to separate from the fundus of the uterus. Again we see invasion of the urinary wall by this echogenic mass. At surgery, this patient was found to have an endometrioma involving the fundal portion of the uterus and posterosuperior aspect of the bladder wall. This portion of the urinary bladder had to be resected. Pathological examination demonstrated the urinary bladder wall to be involved with endometriosis. Ultrasound examination was extremely helpful in delineating the extent and nature of this disease.

It must be remembered that endometriosis can be situated any place in the abdomen. In this case, the finding of bladder wall thickening could not be distinguished from a bladder wall tumor. With the clinical history, however, the diagnosis of endometriosis was most likely.

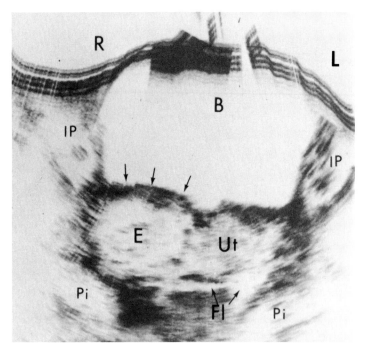

Fig. 11.117

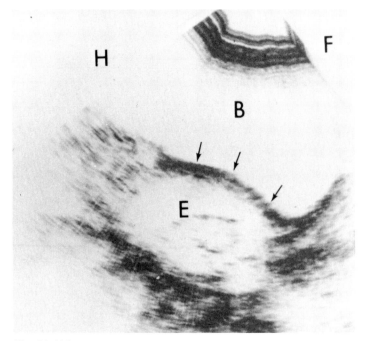

Fig. 11.118

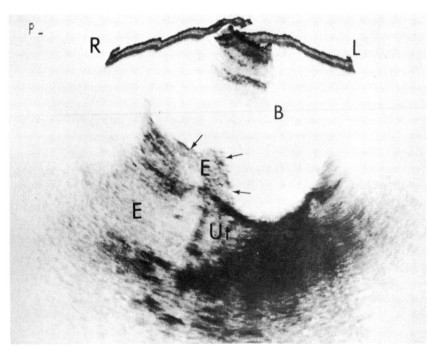

Fig. 11.119

Arrows = Indentation on urinary bladder wall (figs. 11.117 and 11.118)

Arrows = Urinary bladder wall invaded by endometriosis (figs. 11.119 and 11.120)

B = Urinary bladder
E = Endometrioma
F = Foot
Fl = Fluid
H = Head
IP = Iliopsoas muscle
L = Left
Pi = Piriform muscle
R = Right
Ut = Uterus

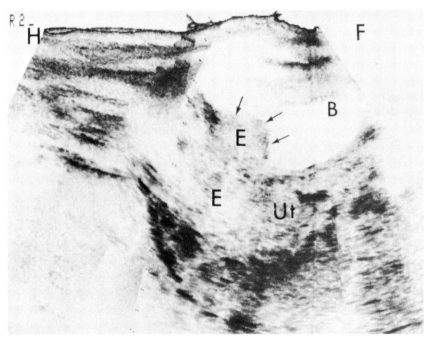

Fig. 11.120

Pelvic Lymphadenopathy; Burkitt's Lymphoma

Figures 11.121–11.123 are pelvic scans and a lymphangiogram obtained from a patient with stage III Hodgkin's disease. In the pelvis, as elsewhere in the body, lymphadenopathy presents as relatively sonolucent masses. The transverse scan (fig. 11.121) demonstrates the lymph nodes indenting the lateral superior aspect of the urinary bladder on the right side.

Figure 11.122 is a longitudinal scan of lymph node enlargement in the pelvis and lower abdomen. The characteristic feature of lymphadenopathy is usually a sonolucent mass with no marked enhanced through transmission. Such masses, however, are so sonolucent that they may be confused for cystic lesions.

Figure 11.123 is a lymphangiogram documenting the lymphadenopathy in the right pelvis and periaortic region.

Figure 11.124 is a transverse scan of a 5-year-old boy with abdominal pain and a large pelvic mass. The scan demonstrates a pelvic mass posterior to the urinary bladder and indentation on the posterior bladder wall. A barium enema demonstrated some narrowing of the rectum. The patient was found to have perirectal Burkitt's lymphoma.

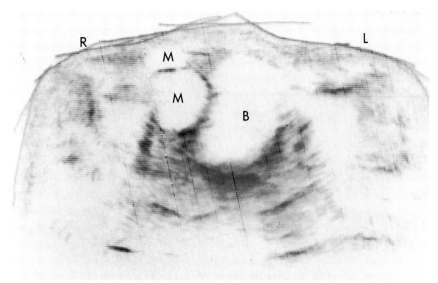

Fig. 11.121

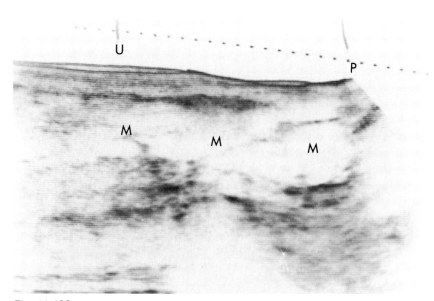

Fig. 11.122

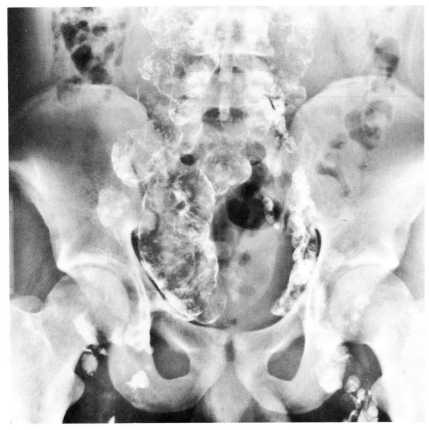

Fig. 11.123

SOURCE: The cases in figures 11.121–11.124 are provided through the courtesy of Dr. B. Green, M. D. Anderson Hospital, University of Texas Medical Center, Houston, Texas.

B = Urinary bladder
L = Left
M = Marked lymph node enlargement
P = Level of the symphysis pubis
R = Right
U = Level of the umbilicus

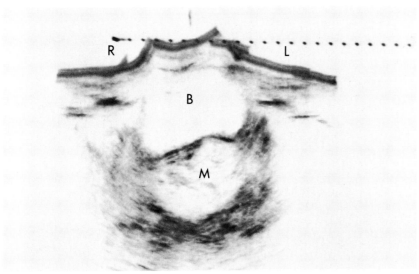

Fig. 11.124

Unusual Pelvic Tumors: Neuroblastoma; Adenocarcinoma of the Colon; and Liposarcoma

Numerous other pelvic masses may occur which do not have any distinguishing ultrasound characteristics. Figures 11.125 and 11.126 are examples of presacral neuroblastoma. This 16-year-old boy presented with a pelvic mass and urinary retention. The diagnosis of neuroblastoma was confirmed at open biopsy. A longitudinal scan of the pelvis (fig. 11.125) shows the urinary bladder displaced anteriorly by an echogenic mass. Posterior to the mass are strong curvilinear echoes representing calcification which is shadowing. Figure 11.126 is an intravenous pyelogram demonstrating hydronephrosis on the left side with some distention of the urinary bladder. In the pelvis a calcific density which corresponds to calcified neuroblastoma can be seen.

Figure 11.127 is a longitudinal scan of a woman with diffuse metastatic colonic carcinoma throughout the pelvis. A large mass is seen posterior to the urinary bladder. A portion of the mass is highly echogenic (arrows). Mucinous colonic carcinomas often give a high-amplitude echo. This patient had diffuse pelvic metastasis which impinged on the urinary bladder only slightly.

Figure 11.128 is a transverse scan of an elderly patient with recurrent pelvic liposarcoma. A large mass is seen posterior to the urinary bladder. There is no characteristic finding suggesting the etiology of this tumor. A Foley catheter is seen in place within the urinary bladder. This mass was found to be diffuse liposarcoma of the pelvis.

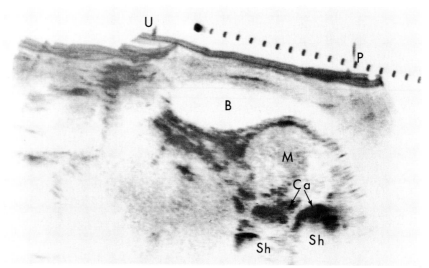

Fig. 11.125

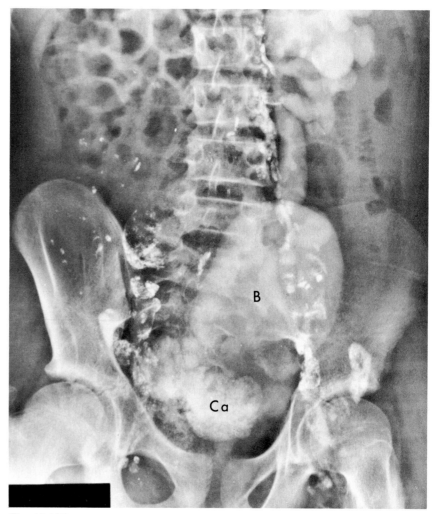

Fig. 11.126

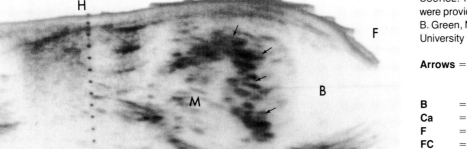
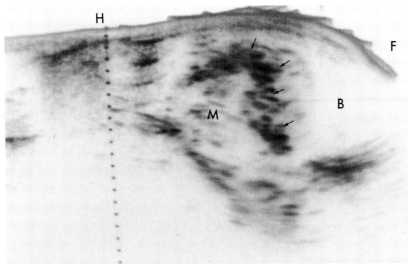

Fig. 11.127

SOURCE: The cases in figures 11.125–11.128 were provided through the courtesy of Dr. B. Green, M. D. Anderson Hospital, Texas University Medical Center, Houston, Texas.

Arrows	=	Highly echogenic regions in a mucinous adenocarcinoma of the colon
B	=	Urinary bladder
Ca	=	Calcification within the mass
F	=	Foot
FC	=	Foley catheter
H	=	Head
L	=	Left
M	=	Solid pelvic masses
P	=	Level of the symphysis pubis
R	=	Right
Sh	=	Shadowing behind the calcification
U	=	Umbilical level

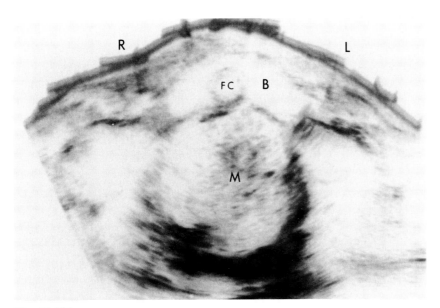

Fig. 11.128

Unusual Pelvic Tumors: Malignant Melanoma and Liposarcoma

Figure 11.129 is a transverse scan of a 49-year-old man who was admitted for re-staging and treatment of his malignant melanoma. The primary lesion had been on his left foot and had been widely excised 4 years earlier. On the present admission, he was noted to have a left pelvic mass. Figure 11.129 is a transverse scan of the pelvis with the urinary bladder deviated posteriorly and to the right side by an echogenic mass. The mass is situated anterior to the urinary bladder and on the left side. The soft echoes indicate a solid lesion. It was diagnosed as metastatic malignant melanoma at surgery.

Figures 11.130–11.132 are scans of a middle-aged man with a large pelvic and abdominal mass. At surgery, this was found to be liposarcoma. The mass (figs. 11.130 and 11.131) has an echogenic ultrasonic appearance. Figure 11.132 is a CAT scan which shows the mass to be situated in the pelvis, displacing the rectum and sigmoid colon posteriorly and to the left side.

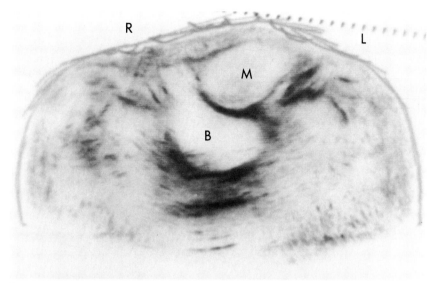

Fig. 11.129

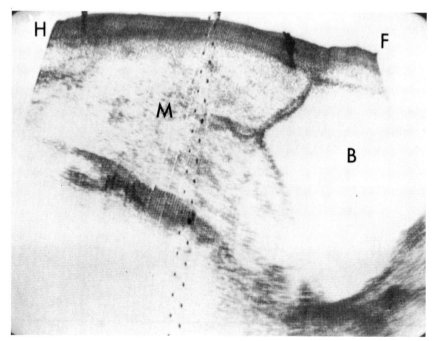

Fig. 11.130

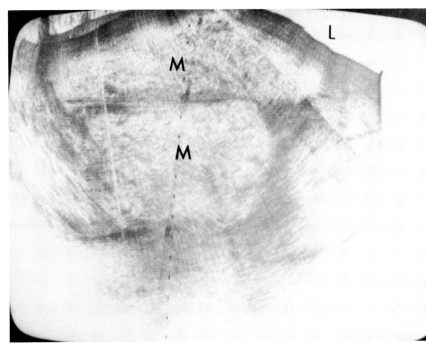

Fig. 11.131

SOURCE: The case in figure 11.129 is provided through the courtesy of Dr. B. Green, M. D. Anderson Hospital, Texas University Medical Center, Houston, Texas.

B	=	Urinary bladder
F	=	Foot
H	=	Head
IP	=	Iliopsoas muscle
L	=	Left
M	=	Soft-tissue masses in the pelvis
R	=	Right
Re	=	Rectum
Si	=	Sigmoid colon

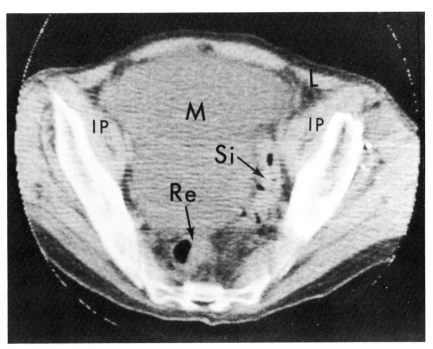

Fig. 11.132

Bladder Duplication Artifacts: Foley Catheter; Blood Clot, and Vaginal Carcinoma

Figure 11.133 is an excellent example of a bladder duplication artifact. It has already been mentioned that a bladder can often present as a sonolucent mass in the pelvis, secondary to a duplication artifact. In this instance, we have a complete duplication artifact of the bladder that is situated posterior to the urinary bladder. What makes this scan so interesting is the duplication artifact of the vagina. The vaginal duplication artifact is situated posterior to the duplication artifact of the bladder. The artifact arises from the strong echo off the posterior urinary bladder wall hitting the transducer-skin interface and making a second trip. This yields a duplication artifact of the urinary bladder and the vagina. Duplication artifacts are discussed in greater detail in chapter 1.

Figure 11.134 illustrates a mass secondary to a Foley Catheter within the urinary bladder. This is quite easy to detect once it is recognized. The distal portion of the tube extending from the water-filled portion of the Foley catheter also is seen.

Figure 11.135 is a transverse scan of the urinary bladder with an echogenic mass on the posterior wall. Although this could represent a bladder tumor, it is a blood clot which presented as an echogenic mass within the urinary bladder.

Figure 11.136 is a longitudinal scan of a patient who had a hysterectomy 15 years previously. She was found to have a mass posterior to the urinary bladder on ultrasound examination. The lucent anterior portion of the vagina is seen directly posterior to the urinary bladder. Deep to this, however, is an echogenic mass which turned out to be a vaginal tumor. This vaginal carcinoma would be somewhat difficult to separate from the rectum as far as ultrasound is concerned. We see the lucent anterior muscularis of the vagina, however, separated from the vaginal tumor by a strong echogenic interface. The strong echogenic interface represents the vaginal mucosa. This unusual case

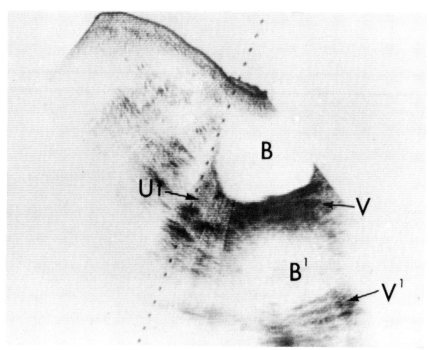

Fig. 11.133

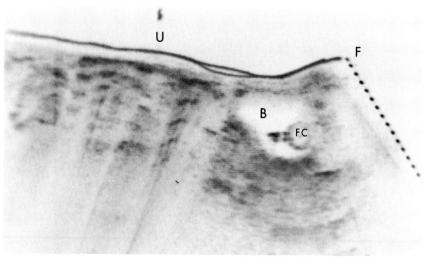

Fig. 11.134

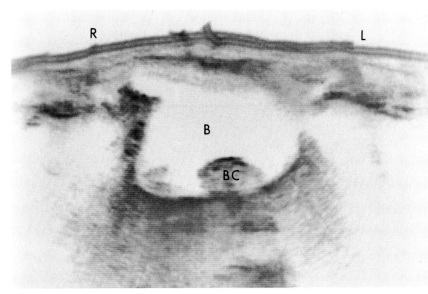

Fig. 11.135

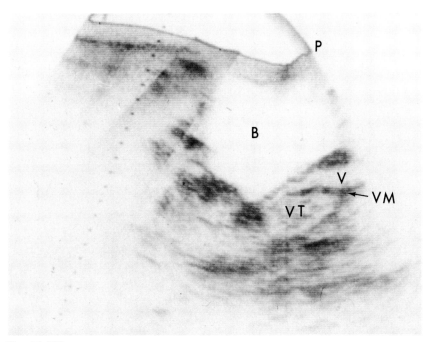

Fig. 11.136

demonstrates the marked thickening of the muscularis region of the posterior aspect of the vagina as compared to the relatively normal thickness for the anterior vaginal muscular area.

SOURCE: Figures 11.134 and 11.135 are provided through the courtesy of Dr. B. Green, M. D. Anderson Hospital, Texas Medical Center, Houston, Texas.

B	=	Urinary bladder
BC	=	Blood clot
B¹	=	Bladder duplication artifact
F	=	Foot
FC	=	Foley catheter
L	=	Left
P	=	Level of the symphysis pubis
R	=	Right
T	=	Vaginal tumor
U	=	Umbilical level
Ut	=	Uterus
V	=	Normal vaginal region anteriorly
V	=	Vagina
V¹	=	Vaginal duplication artifact
Vm	=	Vaginal mucosa
VT	=	Vaginal tumor

Bladder Tumors

Figures 11.137 and 11.138 are pelvic scans of a 42-year-old woman who had some difficulty on urination. The longitudinal scan (fig. 11.137) demonstrates bladder wall thickening (arrows) on the posterior aspect. The bladder wall is approximately 1–1.5 cm in thickness, directly anterior to the vagina. Figure 11.138 is a transverse scan of the bladder wall thickening (arrows) on the posterior aspect of the bladder. The soft echoes, with no evidence of shadowing, indicate a soft-tissue tumor. This could represent either a blood clot or debris in the bladder. With the suggestion of wall thickening, however, a bladder tumor is most likely. At surgery, the patient was found to have urinary bladder carcinoma on the posterior left aspect of the bladder wall.

Another example of a urinary bladder wall carcinoma is seen in figures 11.139 and 11.140. The bladder tumor is approximately 2 cm in thickness. We see a marked irregular surface to the bladder wall which is in contact with urine (arrows). Also noted on the transverse scan in figure 11.139 is a circular structure secondary to a Foley catheter. When a soft tissue density is noted within the urinary bladder or urinary bladder wall, the possibility of a urinary bladder carcinoma should be considered.

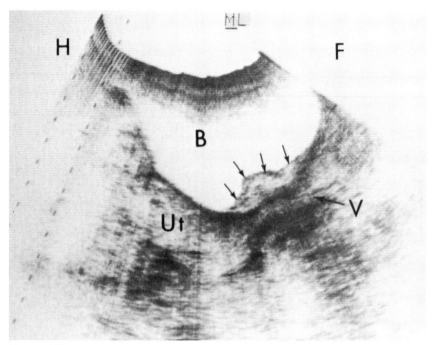

Fig. 11.137

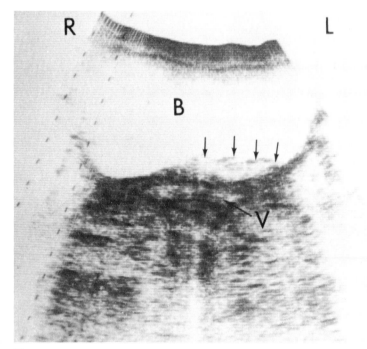

Fig. 11.138

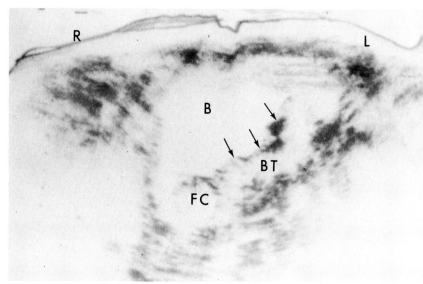

Fig. 11.139

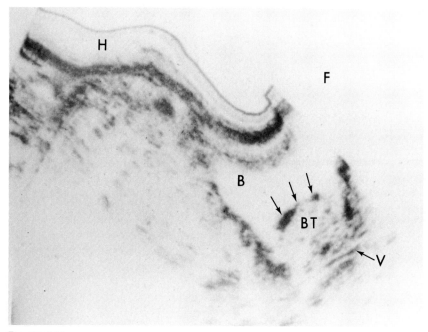

Fig. 11.140

Arrows	=	Urinary bladder wall carcinoma
B	=	Urinary bladder
BT	=	Urinary bladder wall tumor
F	=	Foot
FC	=	Foley catheter
H	=	Head
L	=	Left
R	=	Right
Ut	=	Uterus
V	=	Vagina

Urinary Bladder Diverticulum

Figure 11.141 is a longitudinal scan of the pelvis with a sonolucent mass posterior to the urinary bladder. This may be considered an ovarian cyst or other fluid-filled structure. The possibility of a bladder diverticulum, however, should be considered. In figure 11.141 the communication between the urinary bladder and the bladder diverticulum is not demonstrated. Figures 11.142 and 11.143 of the same patient do, however, demonstrate communication in the longitudinal and transverse planes. We see an opening, approximately 6–7 mm in diameter, indicating the communication between the bladder and the bladder diverticulum. If this communication can be seen, the diagnosis and explanation of the sonolucent mass can be determined.

Figure 11.144 is another example of a bladder diverticulum in the right pelvis, lateral to the urinary bladder.

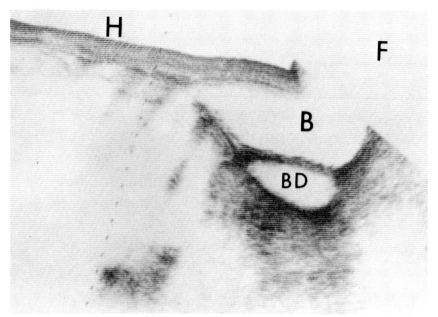

Fig. 11.141

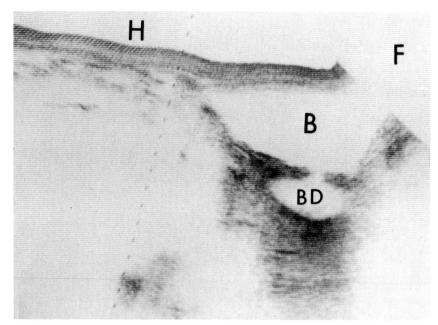

Fig. 11.142

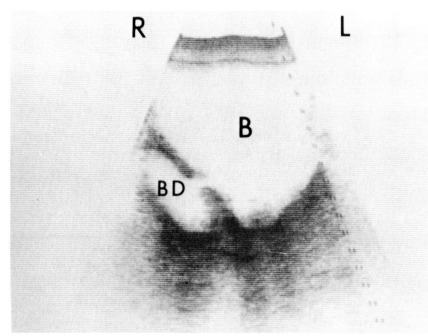

Fig. 11.143

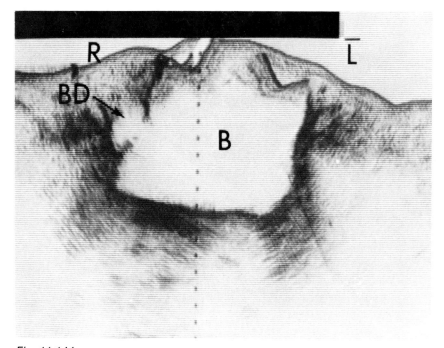

Fig. 11.144

B = Urinary bladder
BD = Bladder diverticulum
F = Foot
H = Head
L = Left
R = Right

Normal Prepubescent Pelvis

When examining the prepubescent pelvis, it is important to visualize the uterus in its long axis. Normally, the cervical region of the prepubescent uterus is larger than the fundal region.

Figures 11.145 and 11.146 are longitudinal scans of a female child approximately 4 years of age (fig. 11.145) and a female infant, 6 months of age (fig. 11.146). The cervical region is as large or larger than the fundal region in both cases. Following puberty and hormonal stimulation, a reversal will occur, and the fundus of the uterus will become larger and more bulbus than the cervical region. Examination of the newborn and the pediatric pelvis can be quite difficult because the patients move about quite markedly during the course of a study. It is important, however, to attempt to visualize the uterus. Real-time examination can often facilitate the study and yield more rapid examination.

Finding the ovaries in a prepubescent child is also difficult. They are usually quite small, 1 cm or less. Again, the study can be quite difficult but usually does not require anesthesia.

Figure 11.147 is a transverse scan demonstrating the ovaries bilaterally. The right ovary is approximately 1 cm in diameter; and the left ovary is less than 1 cm in diameter. Here we visualize the ovaries cephalad to the uterus. The rectum is seen between the ovaries.

Figure 11.148 is a longitudinal scan of the right ovary. It appears as a relatively sonolucent oval-shaped structure in the adnexa. The marked difficulty encountered in visualizing the ovaries is due to their small size and poor patient cooperation.

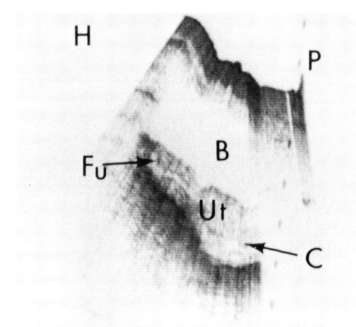

Fig. 11.145

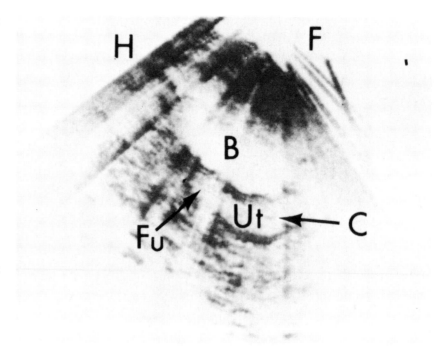

Fig. 11.146

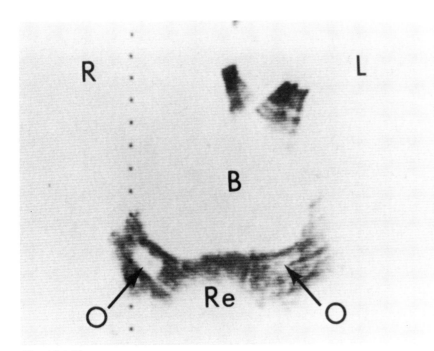

B = Urinary bladder
C = Cervix
Fu = Fundus of the uterus
H = Head
L = Left
O = Ovaries
P = Level of the symphysis pubis
R = Right
Re = Rectum
Ut = Uterus

Fig. 11.147

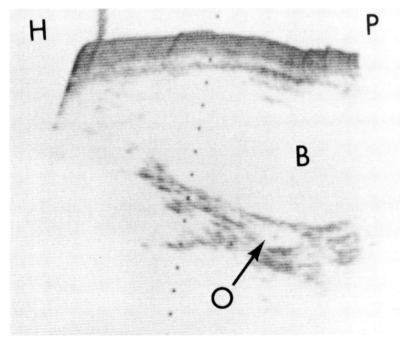

Fig. 11.148

Precocious Puberty; Testicular Feminization

Figures 11.149–11.151 are scans of a 6-year-old child with precocious puberty. In precocious puberty, hormonal stimulation leads to changes in the uterus. The fundal size of the uterus is increased and becomes larger than the cervix. In a transverse scan (fig. 11.149) the uterus is visualized slightly to the left of midline. This uterus is much larger than normal in a 6-year old. The ovaries are also quite large, measuring approximately 2 cm or greater in diameter in the transverse plane. Figure 11.150 is a longitudinal scan with a configuration of the uterus that is more characteristic of the adult, or poststimulated, uterus. The fundus has a more bulky or bulbous appearance than the cervical region. Usually, in the unstimulated uterus the fundus is much smaller than the cervical region. In this 6-year-old with precocious puberty, however, the fundus was large compared with the cervical region. Figure 11.151 is a longitudinal scan of the right ovary. Again, the ovary appears much larger than expected in a 6-year-old. Normally, this should be 1 cm or less in diameter. This ovary is at least 2 cm in diameter and is impinging on the posterior aspect of the urinary bladder.

Figure 11.152 is a transverse scan of a 16-year-old who entered the hospital for an evaluation of primary amenorrhea. No pelvic organs can be seen. The uterus was not identified. Various pelvic musculature, such as the iliopsoas muscle, the obturator internus muscle, and the piriform muscles can be seen, but we were never able to identify the ovaries during the course of the examination. The patient also underwent a pelvic examination, and her vagina was found to end in a blind pouch. The cervix was not identified. The findings are consistent with testicular feminization. For this entity, a pelvic ultrasound can be quite helpful. We were looking for a normal prepubescent uterus and ovaries but were unable to identify any such structures during the course of pelvic sonography.

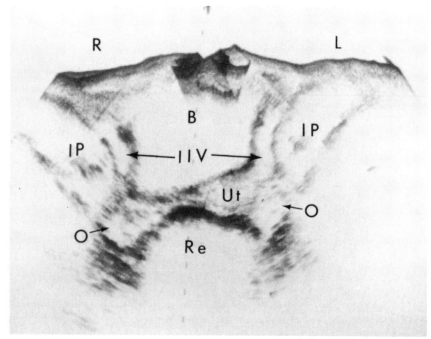

Fig. 11.149

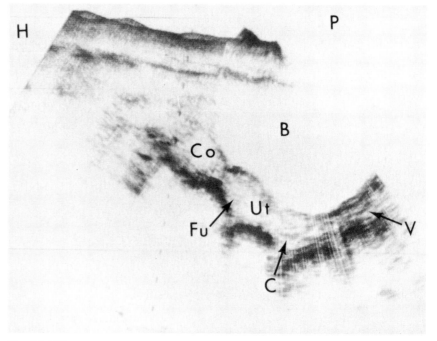

Fig. 11.150

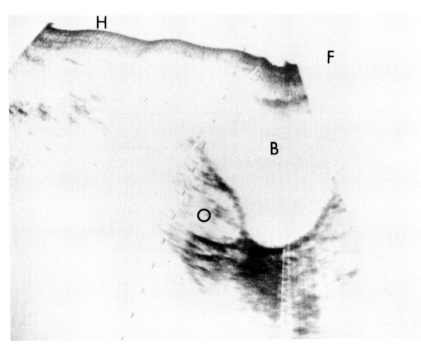

Fig. 11.151

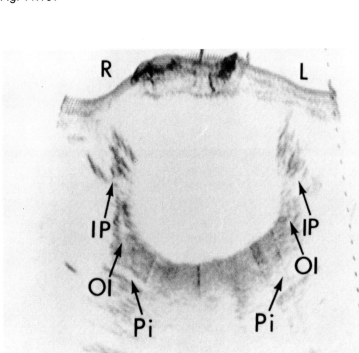

Fig. 11.152

B	=	Urinary bladder
C	=	Cervix
Co	=	Colon
F	=	Foot
Fu	=	Fundus of the uterus
H	=	Head
IIV	=	Internal iliac vessels
IP	=	Iliopsoas muscles
L	=	Left
O	=	Ovaries
OI	=	Obturator internus muscle
P	=	Level of the symphysis pubis
Pi	=	Piriform muscle
R	=	Right
Re	=	Rectum
Ut	=	Uterus
V	=	Vagina

Normal Prostate; Benign Prostatic Hypertrophy

When examining the prostate with ultrasound, it is necessary to fill the urinary bladder. The transducer, however, must be angled more caudally in both the longitudinal and transverse scans. The prostate is situated quite caudally, and if the transducer beam is perpendicular to the tabletop or slightly cephalad in angulation, the prostate gland cannot be visualized.

Figure 11.153 is a longitudinal scan with the prostate noted as a soft echogenic region posterior to the urinary bladder and caudal to the seminal vesicles. Examination in the longitudinal planes best visualizes the prostate when the transducer beam is angled markedly caudally as in this case.

Figure 11.154 is a transverse scan with caudal angulation with the prostate indenting the posterior aspect of the urinary bladder. In the center of the prostate gland, a strong central echo represents the urethra and periurethral glands within the prostate.

Benign prostatic hypertrophy is suggested when a markedly enlarged prostate without disruption of the prostatic capsule is present on ultrasound (figs. 11.155 and 11.156). In Figure 11.155 we see marked indentation of the posteroinferior urinary bladder wall caused by the enlarged prostate. The circular appearance to the prostate in the longitudinal scan is indicative of prostatic enlargement. The transverse scan (fig. 11.156) demonstrates a nodularity to the prostate with two prominent curvilinear indentations on the posterior aspect of the bladder wall. A rectal ultrasonic probe gives excellent visualization of the prostate. B-scan evaluation of the prostate does not determine volume quite as easily as the rectal probe scanner.

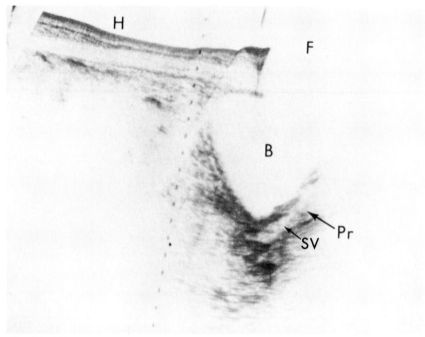

Fig. 11.153

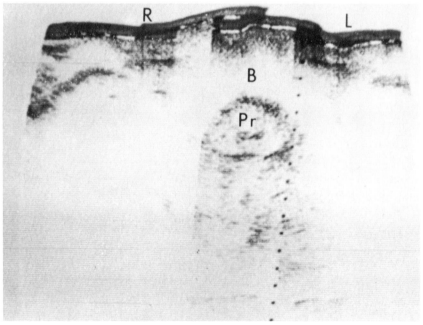

Fig. 11.154

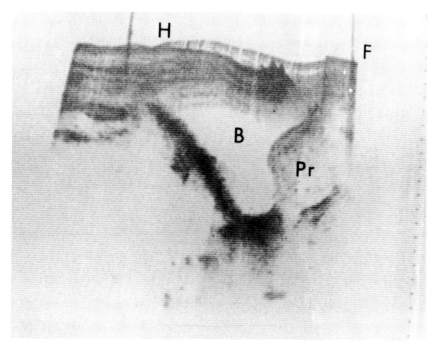

Fig. 11.155

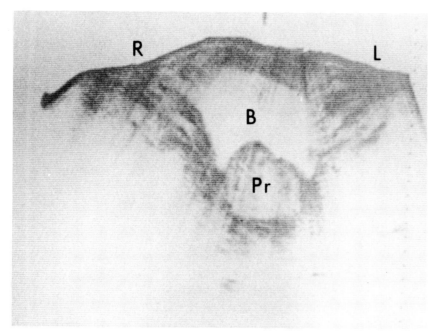

Fig. 11.156

B	=	Urinary bladder
F	=	Foot
H	=	Head
L	=	Left
Pr	=	Prostate
R	=	Right
SV	=	Seminal vesicles

Prostatic Carcinoma; Prostatitis

Figures 11.157 and 11.158 are of a patient with prostatic carcinoma. The prostate is markedly enlarged and indenting the posterior aspect of the urinary bladder. It has a rather uneven echo pattern compared with that of the normal prostate. The irregular echogenicity is also accompanied by a somewhat irregular margin to the prostate wall. The interface between the urinary bladder and prostate is not as sharply seen as in a normal examination. The patient was found to have prostatic carcinoma. An uneven echo pattern and an irregular wall to the prostate is highly suspicious for prostatic carcinoma.

Figures 11.159 and 11.160 are scans of a patient with prostatitis. In figure 11.159, the prostate has a fairly even echo pattern. The seminal vesicles, however, are seen to be much more lucent than usual. The transverse scan (fig. 11.160) demonstrates fairly large seminal vesicles. They are not only more lucent, but they are increased in size, as compared with the normal findings.

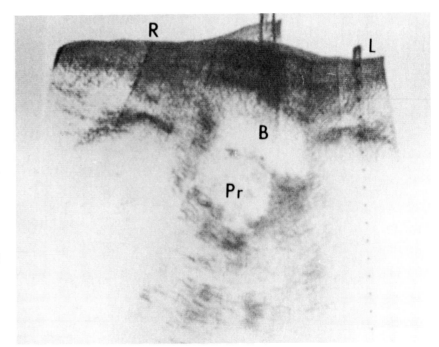

Fig. 11.157

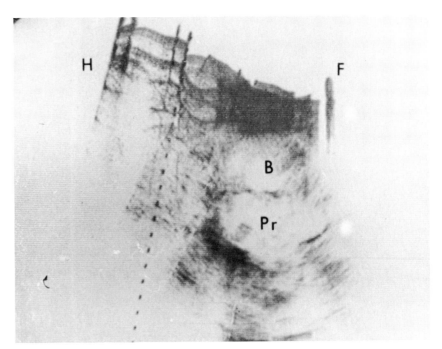

Fig. 11.158

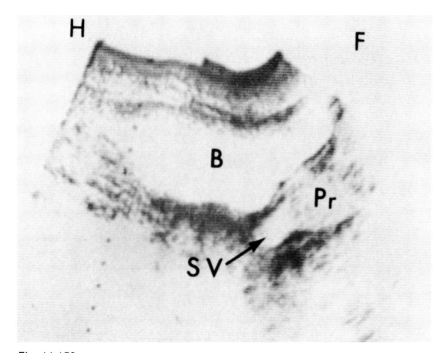

Fig. 11.159

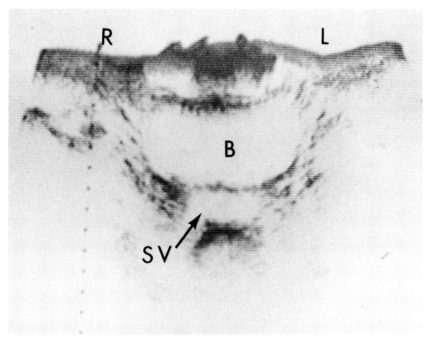

Fig. 11.160

12.
Obstetrical Ultrasonography

Michael S. Shaub, M.D.
Dennis A. Sarti, M.D.

Historically, the examination of the female pelvis with diagnostic ultrasound was one of the earlier applications of this burgeoning area of medical imaging (Donald, MacVicar, and Brown 1958; Donald and Brown 1961; MacVicar and Donald 1963; Taylor et al. 1964). The safety, speed, and information obtained from the examination of the gravid uterus has made it one of the most rewarding and useful of all ultrasound examinations. Many improvements have taken place since the days of the first experiments performed by Dr. Ian Donald in Scotland (Donald, MacVicar, and Brown 1958). Examinations may now be performed by a skilled operator with relative ease and speed; most procedures require less than 20 minutes from start to finish.

Technique for Examination

The examination consists of a series of longitudinal and transverse scans, obtained with the patient in the supine position. The final images are used by the examiner to develop a three-dimensional image of the contents of the gravid uterus. No attempt will be made here to discuss the various types of equipment and transducers available, but current state-of-the-art scanning requires use of gray scale ultrasound equipment with either a 3.5- or 2.25-MHz transducer.

Preparation of the patient for the study is minimal; only a full urinary bladder is required. The importance of a full bladder cannot be overemphasized. When the urinary bladder is empty or poorly filled, the normal uterus is oriented in an anteroposterior direction, facing the anterior abdominal wall. Examination in this position will cause distortion and the resultant scans will be through the long axis of the uterus. As the bladder distends, the fundus rotates cephaladly and dorsally, and the subsequent scans will be accurate longitudinal and transverse depictions of the uterus. The full urinary bladder also will push any bowel interfering with the image superiorly and provide an excellent "window" through which to view the pelvic organs. The distended bladder also provides a known cystic reference, if needed. Thus, when examining the early, slightly enlarged, gravid uterus, the amount of distention of the bladder can determine the accuracy of the diagnostic examination obtained. In later pregnancy, the full bladder allows visualization of the lower uterine segment, which is necessary to determine the lower placental margin. Throughout the pregnancy, the adnexal areas can be evaluated best with a full bladder.

Prior to the actual examination, the procedure is explained to the patient with stress on the fact that no ionizing radiation is involved and that she will experience absolutely no discomfort. She is then placed in a supine position on the examination table, usually with her head to the examiner's left. The examiner is usually in a position, either sitting or standing, along the patient's right side. The skin is coated with a suitable acoustic-coupling agent in order to conduct the high-frequency, low-energy sound into and out of the body. Mineral oil is most commonly used as the coupling agent, but many other suitable agents are commercially available. The water-soluble agents are less desirable because of their tendency to dry out. Normally, the examination is begun with a longitudinal scan in the midline in order to identify the major landmarks and to adjust the various controls for gain, image size, and the location on the monitor. After this, a systematic series of longitudinal sections should be obtained both to the right and left of the midline. At the completion of the longitudinal scans, the examiner should have a good understanding of the anatomy present within the gravid uterus, including the position and number of fetuses present and the location of the placenta.

Systematic transverse scans are then obtained to confirm the findings seen on the longitudinal images and for measurement of the biparietal diameter, defined as the widest distance between the fetal temporal bones when the fetal head is scanned at right angles to the midline. The scans obtained for each examination should encompass the entire length and width of the uterus and should also include the adnexal areas. If additional abnormalities are seen in the abdomen or pelvis, scans should be obtained of these areas as well. Surface landmarks on the patient's skin may be designated by a vertical movement of the transducer over such points as the symphysis pubis, umbilicus, midline, drain site, point of maximal tenderness, and palpable mass. The conditions for each examination will dictate what points are required for later identification. The range markers should, for measurement purposes, also be on every scan obtained during the examination so that any structure can be measured accurately. On occasion, the significance of a finding will not be initially appreciated; but on a subsequent scan, it will become apparent. If no range markers are on the appropriate image on the initial scan, no size comparison between the two scans can be made.

After the biparietal diameter is measured (this will be discussed more fully later in this chapter), fetal viability is determined. This is most commonly done by Doppler examination. The location of the fetal heart can easily be determined from the completed longitudinal and transverse scans, and the Doppler transducer is pointed to this area to detect the characteristic fetal heart tones. If a Doppler unit is not available, the B-scan transducer can be pointed to the same area, and fetal heart activity can be observed on the A-mode display, or the unit can be switched to M-mode with subsequent visualization of fetal heart movement on the monitor. A fetal echocardiogram can also be obtained. Several investigators are currently doing routine fetal intrauterine echocardiograms in high-risk mothers, such as those with previous children with congenital heart disease, exposure to toxins, or German measles. When the examination is performed with the real-time unit, the actual beating fetal heart is readily visible.

Gestational Age

The usual clinical reason for requesting ultrasound is to confirm gestational age, and this is usually done later in pregnancy. Unfortunately, the biparietal diameter grows at approximately 1–2 mm per week during the last trimester. This represents a small change in anatomical structure and a high degree of patient variability. More accurate dating of pregnancy can be obtained if the ultrasound exam is performed within the first 10 weeks after the last menstrual period. During this period of early pregnancy, there is rapid change and growth of anatomical structures and little patient variability, all of which permit fairly precise dating of pregnancy.

Before delving into the ultrasonic findings of early pregnancy, discussion of the pertinent anatomy is in order. Several ovarian follicles begin to mature and ripen at the same time with usually only one rupturing and entering the distal fallopian tube. The remaining, less ripened follicles undergo atresia. The ovum is transported down the tube via ciliary action and muscular contraction. It takes approximately 3–4 days to traverse the tube and enter the uterus. If fertilization fails to occur, the corpus luteum begins to decrease in size approximately 9 days after ovulation. This decreases the progesterone level and eventually causes menstrual bleeding 14 days after ovulation (Langman 1969). Without fertilization, the oocyte becomes nonviable within 1–2 days.

Fertilization usually occurs in the ampullary end of the fallopian tube. The corpus luteum increases in size and remains functionally active through the first half of pregnancy; it secretes progesterone, so menstruation does not occur. During the 3–4 days needed to traverse the tube, the fertilized ovum increases to the 8- to 16-cell stage. It has a mulberry appearance and is called a morula. As the morula enters the uterine cavity, fluid begins to accumulate centrally, and a blastocyst is formed. This floats within the uterine cavity until it finally attaches to the endometrium around the sixth day after fertilization. Trophoblastic cells begin to penetrate the epithelial cells of the uterine mucosa due to the production of proteolytic enzymes by the trophoblast. By the eleventh to twelfth day, the blastocyst is completely embedded within the endometrial stroma. The decidua is fairly even over the entire blastocyst along with the developing villous system. The decidua basalis is that area in contact with the chorion frondosum which eventually develops into the placenta. This area has an excellent blood supply and gives rise to high-level echoes on ultrasound. The decidua capsularis is in contact with the chorion laeve, which is also highly echogenic early in pregnancy.

As gestation advances, and the blastocyst enlarges, however, the blood supply of the expanding decidua capsularis decreases, and the villous system, which is the chorion laeve, atrophies and disappears. The chorion frondosum maintains abundant blood supply, proliferates, and develops into a placenta. It is this stage, at approximately 10–11 menstrual weeks, that the gestation sac "disappears" due to the decreasing blood supply of the stretched and enlarging decidua capsularis and the eventual atrophy of the chorion laeve.

While the gestational sac is primarily fluid-filled, the embryo is growing rapidly. The following table (Langman 1969) indicates the crown–rump length compared to the weeks since fertilization.

Weeks since fertilization	Crown–rump length
5	5–8 mm
6	10–14 mm
7	17–22 mm
8	28–30 mm

At the fifth week after fertilization or the seventh week after menstruation, the embryo finally obtains a size large enough to be detected by ultrasound. Prior to this, only the highly echogenic chorionic villi of the gestation sac can be visualized.

Normal Gestational Sac

Ultrasonic visualization of the gestational sac first occurs around the fourth to fifth menstrual week. By this time, the blastocyst has implanted itself in the endometrium and is completely surrounded by highly echogenic, vascular chorionic villi. The blastocyst enlarges to 5 or 10 mm and is finally detected by B-scan. A gestational sac has a circular to oval shape, and its borders are intact. The size of the gestational sac increases rapidly from the fourth to the tenth menstrual week, enlarging from one to approximately 6 cm in mean gestational sac diameter (Gottesfeld 1970). This rapid growth rate gives rise to the accurate dating of pregnancy (Garrett, Grunwald, and Robinson 1970; Gottesfeld 1970). Follow-up examination 7–10 days after an initial study will normally demonstrate a measurable increase in the gestational sac of approximately 7–10 mm. A repeat examination showing appropriate growth is the most accurate and reliable means of determining a viable pregnancy. The majority of gestational sacs are situated in the fundal or mid uterine segments. A small percentage have a low implantation site, which can be normal or may lead to placenta previa or abortion (Donald 1969; Garrett, Grunwald, and Robinson 1970; Horger, Kreutner, and Underwood 1974).

Since highly vascular chorionic villi initially surround the sac in its entirety, a high-level echo arises from the gestational sac which is two to three shades of gray darker than surrounding myometrium. This high-level echogenicity is extremely important in evaluating viability, since it documents a healthy surrounding vascular supply. By the tenth menstrual week, the echoes from chorionic villi in contact with the decidua capsularis begin to weaken due to atrophy of the vascular supply, and the gestational sac "disappears." Echoes arising from the embryo within the gestational sac can be seen about the seventh menstrual week when the embryo is approximately 5 mm in size. Fetal cardiac activity can also be detected at this time (Robinson 1972).

Single as well as multiple gestational sacs may be detected in utero. Recent reports have indicated a much higher incidence of twins conceived than are delivered (Robinson and Caines 1977). Multiple gestational sacs, however, may also indicate an impending abortion and follow-up studies are necessary.

Abnormal Gestational Sac

Several signs have been described which indicate possible abnormality of the gestational sac. These include: (1) pointed segment; (2) single break or fragmentation; (3) lack of growth; (4) weak surrounding echoes; (5) lack of fetal echoes by the seventh to eighth week; (6) low implantation; and (7) double sac. Several of the above findings are indicative of a nonviable pregnancy while others are only suggestive. As mentioned earlier, the shape of a gestational sac is usually circular to oval. A pointed segment often signals difficulty with the pregnancy if no adjacent masses are present. Distortion of a gestational sac may be caused by uterine myomas or other masses. If the sac has a sharply pointed segment with no identifiable adjacent mass, however, fragmentation or a single break often follows (Donald, Morley, and Barnett 1972; Donald 1969; Hellman et al. 1969). Before diagnosing a break or fragmentation, care must be taken to rule out technical artifacts. If an artifact is not present, these findings are then indicative of a nonviable pregnancy.

The third and probably most important finding of an abnormal gestational sac is lack of adequate growth. If there is any question as to the viability of a pregnancy, the patient should be reexamined in 1 week to 10 days. In this period of time, the sac should enlarge approximately 1 cm in diameter. Lack of growth or decrease in size confirms a nonviable pregnancy (Donald, Morley, and Barnett 1972; Donald 1969; Hellman et al. 1969; Robinson and Caines 1977).

High-level echoes arising from the vascularity of the chorionic villi are evidence of a healthy blood supply to the developing embryo and sac. Therefore, weak surrounding sac echoes, which may be the only sign, are extremely important in diagnosing a nonviable pregnancy. Echoes surrounding the gestational sac are of a higher amplitude than the adjacent myometrium. Normally, there is a decrease in echogenicity of the chorionic villi in contact with the decidua capsularis at approximately the tenth or eleventh menstrual week. This is due to atrophy of the chorionic villi as they outgrow their blood supply. The chorion frondosum, which becomes placenta, maintains its high-level echogenicity. Therefore, a pregnancy that is in difficulty and has its blood supply interrupted or decreased will manifest weak surrounding echoes. This finding is most easily detected from the fifth to ninth menstrual week when the surrounding echoes are normally uniform in thickness and amplitude. However, by the tenth or eleventh menstrual week, the gestational sac has "disappeared" secondary to normal vascular atrophy. This normal event should not be misinterpreted as evidence of a nonviable pregnancy.

As noted in the previous discussion of normal anatomy, the embryo attains a size of 5 mm by the seventh mentrual week. By the seventh to eighth menstrual week, echoes arising from the embryo should be noted within the gestational sac. Cardiac activity can also be detected by A- or M-mode and Doppler. An anembryonic pregnancy should be detected by the eighth or ninth menstrual week, when a definite diagnosis of a nonviable pregnancy can be reached.

The last two signs of possible gestational sac abnormality, low implantation and double sac, are only suggestive of abnormality and must be reevaluated by a later ultrasound examination. There are conflicting reports as to the implication of a low implantation site. The usual implantation site is fundal or mid uterine. Several investigators have reported an increased incidence of abortion (Donald, Morley, and Barnett 1972; Donald 1969; Hellman et al. 1969). Others have found no increased incidence of abortion unless bleeding is clinically evident (Garrett, Grunwald, and Robinson 1970; Kohorn and Kaufman 1974). The safest course to follow with a low implantation pregnancy is a repeat examination one to two weeks later to evaluate the progression of the pregnancy. A low implantation is felt by some investigators to lead to placenta previa (Horger, Kreutner, and Underwood 1974), but this is disputed by others and further studies are necessary to answer the question (Kohorn and Kaufman 1974). Double gestational sac is the final sign which can be indicative of an impending abortion (Garrett, Grunwald, and Robinson 1970; Hellman et al. 1969; Robinson and Caines 1977). Doubling of the gestation sac may indicate a twin gestation, but it may also indicate an abnormal pregnancy and a follow-up examination in 7–10 days is indicated.

From the thirteenth week on, the fetal biparietal diameter is usually measurable for accurate gestational age determinations. But, before discussing biparietal diameter measurements, it is worthwhile to discuss the so-called "blind time" in gestational age determinations (Hellman, et al. 1969). This problem arose because between the eleventh and thirteenth weeks of gestation, before visualization of the fetal head, the decidua parietalis and decidua capsularis begin to fuse with subsequent dissolution of the gestational sac. Not only was it felt that the gestational age could not be accurately determined at this stage of pregnancy, but it was occasionally difficult to differentiate a normally developing pregnancy from a hydatidiform mole and impending abortion with a degenerated fetus, or even from degenerating fibroids. This "blind time" was really a product of the bistable ultrasound equipment in use at that time. With the current gray scale units available, there are no longer any "blind times" in the developing pregnancy. The fetal parts are now identifiable from approximately the seventh week on, and the gestational sac can be identified and measured throughout the first trimester of pregnancy (Ghorashi and Gottesfeld 1977).

By the thirteenth week of pregnancy, the fetal skull is ultrasonically visible in 75% of cases; by the end of the fourteenth week, it is visible in 95% of cases (Leopold and Asher 1975). With visualization of the fetal skull, the fetal biparietal diameter may be measured (Sanders and Conrad 1975). During the remainder of the pregnancy, this is by far the most accurate way to assess the gestational age. Unlike radiographs, the ultrasonic biparietal diameter measurement does not suffer the distortion or magnification that can be present in a radiograph with different locations of the fetal head relative to the radiographic film. Numerous studies have been reported to document the accuracy of the ultrasonic measurement of the fetal biparietal diameter (Campbell 1969; Flamme 1972; Levi 1971; Poll 1976; Thompson et al. 1965). There are some slight differences among the various reported biparietal diameter-gestational age graphs. These appear to be due to the various patient populations studied, for example, black versus white, and sea level versus high altitude. It is recommended that each examiner develop his or her own chart using a particular patient population, or that examiners use a chart that has been developed with a similar patient population.

The actual mechanics of measuring the fetal biparietal diameter are not difficult and can easily be learned. In the early stages of pregnancy, the fetal head has a more rounded appearance, but later it develops the more classical oval or ellipsoidal shape. In either case, when the transducer is angled through the appropriate

widest diameter of the skull, a strong linear midline echo will be present. If this echo runs the entire length of the skull, its origin is either from the falx cerebri or the interhemispheric fissure. Scans should be obtained just caudal to this level, which should be at the level of the third ventricle and thalamus. This measurement is through the widest portion of the fetal skull and should measure slightly larger than the sections through the falx. When scanning at the level of the third ventricle, the strong linear midline echo will still be present, but it will be shorter than the falx echo which extends the entire length of the skull (Brown 1975). When incorrect sections are obtained, the fetal head will have a distorted or asymmetrical appearance, and the midline echo will be absent or off center. Experience will teach the examiner which changes in scan obliquity and/or angulation are necessary to obtain the correct biparietal diameter.

When the fetus is in a cephalad position, the usually slight dorsal flexion of the head is easily appreciated on the longitudinal scans. Deviation of the long axis of the fetal head from the vertical plane is the angle of asynclitism and the amount of angular deviation dictates how much cranial transducer angulation is required in order to be perpendicular to the fetal skull (Brown 1975). When doing the transverse scans for the biparietal diameter determination, the transducer is normally angled in a slightly cephalad direction to insure that it is directed through the two parietal eminences and is perpendicular to the midline. The amount of angulation is determined by the degree of dorsal flexion of the fetal head (angle of asynclitism). Some examiners measure the exact angle, but with experience we can easily estimate the degree of transducer angulation necessary to insure that the transducer axis is perpendicular to the fetal midline. On occasion, a good biparietal diameter will be obtained on the initial longitudinal sections, but in the vast majority of cases, it can only be obtained with transverse sections. When an apparently good biparietal diameter has been obtained, several additional sections should be taken slightly above and below this level to insure that the largest is measured. Rarely, the position and orientation of the fetal skull is such that an accurate biparietal diameter cannot be obtained. If the fetal skull is low in the pelvis, various maneuvers may be tried, such as putting the patient in the Trendelenberg position or applying gentle manual pressure to elevate the fetal head. If these are unsuccessful, repeat examination on another day will often show a change in the position of the fetal head, which will allow an adequate biparietal diameter to be obtained. It should be noted, however, that a cross-section of the fetal abdomen, at the level of the umbilical vein within the liver, usually can be obtained, even when the fetal head is in an unfavorable position. This diameter can be used as a rough guide to estimate the fetal gestational age because, in a normal pregnancy, this abdominal diameter is approximately the same as the biparietal diameter.

From the sixteenth to approximately the thirtieth week, the fetal biparietal diameter increases 3 mm per week. During the remainder of the pregnancy, it increases at approximately 1.8 mm per week (Gottesfeld 1975). Thus, the biparietal diameter-gestational age assessment and incremental growth assessment are most accurate from the sixteenth to approximately the thirtieth week of gestation. Furthermore, if we are trying to differentiate the dysmature fetus (intrauterine-growth retardation or "IUGR") from the normal but small fetus, serial determinations, at no closer than 2-week intervals, should be obtained from the twentieth to the thirtieth week. The dysmature infant will show abnormal incremental biparietal diameter growth, and the normal small fetus will have a normal incremental growth rate (Sanders and Conrad 1975). Determination of the growth-retarded fetus later in pregnancy, when the incremental biparietal diameter increase is only approximately 1.8 mm per week, is much more difficult. When a patient is referred near term for a single examination with a diagnosis of "rule out IUGR," the ultrasound examination has very little to offer. Recently, total intrauterine volume has proved more beneficial in detecting IUGR. Numerous studies have been performed to estimate the fetal weight in utero (Gottesfeld 1975; Kurjak and Breyer 1976; Lunt and Chard 1976; Morrison and McLinnan 1976; Sanders and Conrad 1975; Stocker et al. 1975; Thompson and Makowski 1971). The different methods show varying degrees of accuracy. Although several of the techniques are quite tedious, they can be very helpful in selected cases.

A great deal of controversy surrounds the choice of method for recording the fetal biparietal diameter (i.e., bistable, gray scale, or real time). Most laboratories currently record and measure it using the bistable display, because it is felt to be easier to measure with the fetal calvarial echoes when they are thinner and sharper. The measurement is usually from the outer edge of the proximal table to the inner edge of the distal table, which is similar to the "leading edge" measurement with A-mode. With gray scale, the fetal skull echoes are often quite thick and secondary to skin, hair, and subcuta-

neous tissue, and it is difficult to be certain where to place the calipers for measurement. It should be noted, however, that a recent study has shown little difference between the biparietal diameter values obtained using bistable, gray scale, or real-time images (Cooperberg et al. 1976). Thus, the best method is probably the method with which the examiner is most familiar. No matter which method is used, the image on the screen should be as large as possible to decrease measurement errors. The image should also be positioned in the center of the screen to decrease image distortion and subsequent measurement errors due to its curvature. It is also advantageous to place the range markers through the biparietal diameter to decrease errors in measurements.

It should be remembered, then, that the gestational age of the developing fetus may be estimated by measuring the distance between the two fetal parietal eminences, known as the fetal biparietal diameter. With experience, and sometimes with considerable frustration, we can become adept at obtaining the exact plane of this measurement. It cannot be overemphasized that even when the biparietal diameter can be measured to a tolerance of 1 mm, the gestational age remains an estimate of fetal maturity to an accuracy of ± 7–10 days. If this contradicts the marvels of modern electronics, we should think of the numerous biological variables that are simultaneously at work. If we were to construct a chart relating the fetal beparietal diameter to gestational age by working backward from a known delivery date, we would immediately encounter the problem of determining the exact age of a single, term, healthy infant. The acceptable ages, provided the fetus is neurologically mature and weighs more than 2500 g, range from 37 to 41 weeks! This is already a spread of 4 weeks, and this difference of opinion is incorporated into the error on the graph. We dwell upon this seemingly minor point only because it invariably becomes a major problem in communicating with the clinician.

Normal Placental Findings

From the first description of the ultrasonic placental localization in 1966, ultrasonic placentography has advanced greatly (Gottesfeld, Thompson, Holmes, and Taylor 1966). With currently used high-resolution gray scale equipment, there often is a suggestion of the exact site of early placental development at nine weeks of pregnancy.

This is seen as a thickening of the gestational sac along one or more sides of the uterus (Ghorashi and Gottesfeld 1976). At 11 weeks of gestation, the decidua parietalis and decidua capsularis start to fuse, and the site of the developing placenta can be recognized as a dense area bordered on one side by a chorionic plate attached to the uterine wall. By 13 weeks of gestation, the gestational sac has disappeared, leaving the placental implantation site recognizable. The placenta continues to increase in size, and in the early stages of pregnancy, it can occupy 50–75% of the volume of the uterus. The uterus, however, enlarges faster than the placenta; and in later pregnancy the placenta occupies only approximately 25–30% of the uterine cavity (Sanders and Conrad 1975). The placenta may also appear to change position during pregnancy ("placental migration").

The placenta can be accurately located in approximately 97–98% of cases, which makes ultrasound placental localization the procedure of choice (Gottesfeld, Thompson, Holmes, and Taylor 1966; Sanders and Conrad 1975). Multiple studies have shown ultrasonic placental localization to be of greater accuracy than the other previously used methods, such as soft-tissue radiography and radioisotopic localization (Cohen et al. 1972; King 1973). Furthermore, the ultrasound examination does not employ ionizing radiation and, therefore, can be repeated as often as necessary without risk to the fetus or mother.

Ultrasonic display of the placenta allows the examiner to evaluate not only the placental location, but also its size, margins, internal structures, and surfaces. The fetal surface (chorionic plate) of the placenta is typically displayed as a strong linear echo on its inner surface. This is best seen when the transducer is perpendicular to its surface and can be difficult to image in fundal or laterally located placentas where the chorionic plate is oriented parallel to the ultrasound beam. Short segments of the chorionic plate may not be imaged when a portion of the fetus is in contact with it. In both of these situations, however, there is usually no difficulty in identifying the placental mass itself. Between the chorionic plate and uterine myometrium lies the actual mass of the placenta. Placental tissue gives a speckled appearance due to the multiple placental villi in complex interfaces, collagen and fibrous tissue, and occasional calcification present within the tissue.

When the placenta is located anteriorly, the chorionic plate and speckled appearing placenta are usually easily identifiable. In posteriorly located placentas, the placenta and chorionic plate will be visualized where amniotic fluid is located anterior to it. In areas located behind the fetus, the placenta may appear clear due to "acoustic shadowing" by the fetus. A complete ultrasound examination, however, consists of a series of longitudinal and transverse scans encompassing the entire uterus. Therefore, several images usually show a portion of the posteriorly located placenta. When oligohydramnios is present, with decreased amounts of amniotic fluid, the natural intrauterine contrast between the amniotic fluid and solid structures is lost. In this situation, the placenta is frequently much more difficult to identify. With experience, this problem can usually be overcome; but the resultant ultrasound images frequently will not be as definitive. A recent observation in the normal "mature" placenta is the presence of multiple sonolucencies within the placental mass secondary to placental infarction. This is a normal finding and indicates that the pregnancy is near term (Winsberg 1973). This finding in itself, however, should not replace the gestational age determination by biparietal diameter measurement.

In most laboratories, common indications for ultrasound placentography are (1) evaluation of vaginal bleeding to exclude a placenta previa or abruptio placenta, (2) abnormal fetal lie to ascertain whether the fetus is being displaced by a low-lying placenta, and (3) examination prior to amniocentesis to assure that the aspiration needle does not pass through the placenta or the fetus.

Abnormal Placental Findings

The patient with painless vaginal bleeding during the third trimester presents an enormous dilemma to her physician. How should the management of this patient proceed? Is this a benign manifestation of the pregnancy or does it foretell of something more ominous, such as placenta previa or abruptio placenta? Elimination of the latter two possibilities certainly would change the complexion of the problem. It would obviate the need for complete bed rest in the hospital, expensive medications, or termination of the pregnancy. With ultrasound examination of this type, we are usually able to locate accurately the placenta, its margins, the cervix, lower uterine segment, and fetal position. Accuracy and reliability should approach 97%, which is considerably more efficacious for the patient. The small percentage that may remain in a nondiagnostic category must still be treated conservatively in a high risk manner, but the number of patients in this group is considerably reduced.

The ultrasound examination for placenta previa must be performed with a full, distended urinary bladder, which allows adequate visualization of the cervix and lower uterine segment. A distended urinary bladder also will help to displace the fetal head superiorly and allow better visualization of these structures. Determination should be made as to whether the placenta is low-lying, involves the margin of the internal cervical os (marginal placenta previa), or completely covers the internal cervical os (complete previa). When the placenta is anterior its lower margin is usually quite easy to define. With a posteriorly located placenta and a breech or transverse position of the fetus, amniotic fluid is usually adjacent to the lower uterine segment, and the lower placental margin can be well visualized. Diagnostic difficulties can arise with the posteriorly situated placenta and a fetus which is in a cephalad position with the head low in the pelvis. In this situation, the lower placental margin may be difficult to identify with certainty, due to the overlying fetus and subsequent acoustic shadowing beneath the fetal skull. The patient may be put into a Trendelenberg position, and an attempt made to gently elevate the fetal head by manual palpation. The maternal bladder may also be slightly overdistended to elevate the head. On occasion, none of these maneuvers will elevate the fetus, and the distance between the fetal calvarium and the anterior margin of the maternal sacrum will be of paramount importance. When this separation is greater than 15 mm, it may indicate extension of the lower placental margin over the sacral promontory onto the lower uterine segment (King 1973). Closer scrutiny of the lower uterine segment is required. If the separation is less than 15 mm, a low-lying placenta is usually excluded because the distance between the maternal sacrum and fetal skull is not sufficient for extension of the placenta. The examiner should communicate to the clinician the diagnostic limitations of the examination, and the referring physician must treat the patient based on the clinical evaluation. One last comment should be made in regard to the erroneous evaluation of the maternal sacrum-fetal skull distance. This distance may appear falsely large if the fetal skull is off center, or if a fetal extremity is located posterior to the skull. Furthermore, if the cervix is identified other than in the midline, it

may be shown to have no placental extension, even with a widened maternal sacrum-fetal skull distance.

Several interesting phenomena related to apparent change in the location of a placenta recently have been reported. First, a rare and interesting phenomenon is that on serial ultrasound examinations, the placenta will appear to have changed locations within the uterus— for example, anterior to posterior or right side to left side. This is brought about by the fact that the gravid uterus can rotate about its long axis, and thus, the placental location can apparently shift. This is especially true when urinary bladder filling is varied. Second, early in pregnancy, the placenta can appear to be in two separate areas on one examination and only in one area on later examination. At this time, this is felt to be due either to uterine contractions with subsequent transient myometrial thickening or to unsoftened portions in the uterus. Third, the last area of apparent change in placental location is so-called "placental migration." This was first described by King in 1973 and is now recognized as a commonly occurring entity (King 1973). Prior to King's article, all ultrasonographers were confronted with the perplexing problem of cases reported as having a placenta previa early in pregnancy, which subsequently cannot be determined from ultrasound examination.

King demonstrated that the position of the placenta can change during pregnancy, with "migration" away from the cervix with uterine growth, and thus, an apparent low implantation can change to a high implantation. The etiology of this "migration" is felt to be due to differential growth rate of the lower uterine segment compared with the remainder of the uterus.

An analogy that is helpful in understanding this compares the uterus to a lettered balloon frequently given to children at the shoe store. For discussion purposes, the hole where one blows up the balloon is the cervix and the letters on the balloon are the placenta. Initially, the letters are located in close proximity to the balloon orifice. When the balloon is inflated, the fixed letters are located a great distance away from the orifice. This is because of differential expansion or growth rate of different segments of the balloon. Thus, we can see how a fixed and implanted low-lying placenta can "migrate" away from the cervix during the growth and development of the gravid uterus. It is doubtful that a complete previa, implanted on both sides of the internal os, can ever be converted, although even this may also resolve with time. The important point to be gained from this discussion is that whenever the placenta is low-lying early in pregnancy, a repeat examination should be obtained near delivery to reevaluate the lower placental margin at that time.

The ultrasonic diagnosis of abruptio placenta is frequently difficult, and the diagnostic accuracy does not approach that in the ultrasonic diagnosis of placenta previa. The most common finding seen with ultrasound is separation of the placenta from the myometrial surface by an interposed fluid collection (hemorrhage). In normal pregnancy, an apparent separation of a portion of the placenta can be due to scanning a segment of the placenta obliquely. In this case, the apparently separated placental segment appears to be free within the uterine cavity. Review of all the longitudinal and transverse scans will usually make the etiology of this apparently separated area obvious. On occasion, large venous structures at the placenta-myometrium junction can be confused with an area of abruption. Thus, we should correlate the diagnosis of abruptio placenta with appropriate clinical findings. An abruptio placenta may rarely appear as a thickened placenta. If blood clots have formed in the area of abruption, the site of abruption may not appear sufficiently different from adjacent placental tissue, and the ultrasound appearance will be that of a thickened placenta. Another rare presentation of an abruption can be seen if the area of hemorrhage is into the placental tissue itself. When this occurs, hemorrhage in the placenta may act ultrasonically different from the remainder of the placenta, having either increased or decreased echo formation. Care must be taken, however, not to misinterpret as an abruption the sonolucent areas, which are usually multiple, that can be normally seen in a mature placenta (Winsberg 1973). Furthermore, with the better resolution now obtainable, the normal placental-myometrial interface can be seen and should not be confused with an abruption. In a patient with posttraumatic vaginal bleeding, placental abruption will look the same as the nontraumatic variety of abruption. We rarely can identify intrauterine or extrauterine posttraumatic hematomas which should resolve on serial scans.

As previously noted, the placenta early in pregnancy is larger and occupies a much larger volume in the uterus (50–75%) than later in pregnancy (25–30%). This is important to be aware of because an enlarged or thickened placenta usually indicates an abnormality in the pregnancy. To date, no large studies of the upper limits of placental thickness have been conducted, but a placental thickness of 5.5–6.0 cm usually is considered the

upper limit of the normal range. As with most things in ultrasound, care must be taken when evaluating the placental thickness, and it can only be measured where there is a good placental cross-section and with the transducer oriented perpendicular to the chorionic plate. Oblique or tangential sections of the placenta will cause it to be artifactually thick.

The most common etiologies of an abnormally large placenta are diabetes mellitus and Rh incompatibility (Ghorashi and Gottesfeld 1976; Gottesfeld 1975; Shaub and Wilson 1976). In the pregnant diabetic patient, everything is enlarged including the fetus (macrosomia) and the placenta. In Rh incompatibility, the placenta also may be markedly enlarged. In the fetuses affected, the ultrasound examination may disclose evidence of fetal ascites or skin edema. Demonstration of these fetal abnormalities is very significant in the management of the pregnancy. With severe involvement of the fetus, intrauterine fetal transfusions are no longer of any value (Shaub and Wilson 1976). A rarer cause of placental thickening is transplacental syphilis. With transplacental syphilis, the placenta may be markedly enlarged, and fetal ascites may be seen. An additional cause of increased placental thickening, which has previously been discussed, is abruptio placenta. Lastly, an extremely rare cause of total or partial placental thickening is the existence of a normal intrauterine pregnancy with a hydatidiform mole (Beisher 1961).

Intrauterine pregnancies manifesting a thickened placenta are usually referred for ultrasound examination from a high-risk obstetrical clinic where they are being followed. The ultrasound information obtained in these cases may be invaluable in the management of the pregnancy and may dictate whether an intrauterine fetal transfusion, placental localization for amniocentesis, early delivery of the abnormal fetus, or other course of action must be undertaken. Other cases manifesting a thickened placenta will be discovered during a routine ultrasound examination or during an examination ordered for some other unrelated problem. In these cases, the abnormally thickened placenta will necessitate appropriate laboratory tests to exclude diabetes mellitus, Rh isoimmunization, or syphilis.

Maternal Uterine Size Larger Than Expected for Dates

A common referring diagnosis for ultrasound examination during pregnancy is that the patient is larger than she should be according to her menstrual dates. The most common finding in this clinical setting is that her gestational age dating is inaccurate. Some patients are not sure of their last menstrual period, and others may have had slight menstrual bleeding after becoming pregnant. In either case, the biparietal diameter measurement will disclose that the fetus is more mature than was indicated by the patient's apparent menstrual history and that the problem of the discrepancy in uterine size is easily solved.

Another frequent cause of the patient being larger than her gestational date is multiple gestation. Twins can usually be suspected by about the sixth to seventh week of gestation with the visualization of two gestational sacs. Multiple gestation has been diagnosed as early as 5 weeks (menstrual age). A case of quintuplets was diagnosed at 9 weeks, and Gottesfeld has examined sextuplets at 18 weeks gestation (Campbell and Dewhurst 1970; Gottesfeld, Sundgren, and Chavez 1974; Levi 1976). Despite these and many other reports of the early diagnosis of multiple gestation, extra care must be taken in the first trimester of pregnancy. Recent reports have shown a greater number of multiple gestational sacs identified during ultrasound examination in early pregnancy than observed at delivery (Hellman, Kobayashi, and Cromb 1973; Levi 1976). In a study of 6690 pregnant patients reported by Levi, a greater rate of multiple pregnancies than that observed at delivery was found. Seventy-one percent of twin gestations diagnosed before 10 weeks turned out to be single fetuses at delivery (Levi 1976). All cases of multiple gestation diagnosed after 15 weeks' gestation were correct, with more than one fetus delivered. These results indicate that all cases of multiple gestation diagnosed in the first trimester must be reconfirmed after 15 weeks, at which time the fetal skulls are visible.

The diagnosis of multiple gestation is relatively simple and requires visualization of more than one fetus. The biparietal diameter determination may be difficult because of the not infrequent unusual position of one or both fetal heads. If there is difficulty in obtaining the biparietal diameter measurement, a repeat examination at another time frequently shows a change in fetal position, allowing an adequate determination to be made. In the cases studied at Los Angeles County University of Southern California Medical Center, a significant difference in the biparietal diameter measurements of single versus multiple gestations was not found, and only one biparietal diameter chart was used for both single and multiple gestations. A recently reported study by Scheer has confirmed this, with his finding that the measurement for each twin is usually the same as in a single pregnancy of the same gestational maturity (1974). Two potential sources of error in the diagnosis of twins are triplets and excessive fetal activity. We must take care not to diagnose triplets as twins. This is easier to do than it seems, especially if the twins are active and moving within the uterus during the examination. It should also be borne in mind that the fetus can be very active and it is not unusual for a single active fetus, in the third trimester, to switch position during the course of a single examination. Before diagnosing the number of fetuses in a multiple gestation, we should try to image all the fetal heads on a single picture.

Polyhydramnios can also result in uterine enlargement. The diagnosis of excessive amounts of amniotic fluid is actually a subjective judgement with no good figures for measurements available to guide in the computation. With minimal experience, however, it is not a difficult diagnosis to make. Most polyhydramnios is benign and will resolve spontaneously. This may be due to the "lazy baby syndrome" with a fetus that is slow in learning to swallow. Polyhydramnios, however, does have a high incidence of occurrence in anencephaly, high fetal gastrointestinal obstructions, maternal problems such as diabetes mellitus, and the "transfusion syndrome" with twins (Benirschke and Driscoll 1967; Gottesfeld 1975; Sanders and Conrad 1975). When polyhydramnios is identified and no evidence of fetal or maternal abnormalities is apparent clinically or on ultrasound examination, this information is very important to the delivering obstetrician and will alert the attending pediatrician to evaluate the infant carefully after delivery.

A patient with a molar pregnancy will also frequently present with a "large-for-dates" history and commonly will have increased blood pressure, hyperemesis, and vaginal bleeding. The ultrasound diagnosis of this condition is usually simple, accurate, and has nearly replaced the older diagnostic methods of amniography or angiography. Ultrasound examination of a molar pregnancy discloses an enlarged uterus completely filled with placental (trophoblastic) tissue (Leopold 1971; Sanders and Conrad 1975; Thompson 1973). There will be no evidence of a developing fetus, and multiple larger sonolucent areas may be seen within the molar tissue, representing areas of degeneration or internal hemorrhage. Theca-lutein cysts frequently are found in association with molar pregnancies and are seen as adnexal cysts. They can achieve a very large size and may grow larger than the uterus itself. Their occurrence is due to the elevated human chorionic gonadotrophin levels that are routinely identified in patients with molar pregnancies. On occasion, the ultrasound picture of a molar pregnancy may be simulated by a degenerating leiomyoma, missed abortion with retained products of conception, or a chronic ectopic pregnancy in the midline (Leopold 1971; Morrison and McLinnan 1976; Sanders and Conrad 1975; Thompson 1973). Clinical history will aid in the differential diagnosis, and human chorionic gonadotrophin levels will not be elevated to the degree seen with a hydatidiform mole. Treatment for a molar pregnancy is complete evacuation of the uterine contents. Approximately 2–8% of cases prove to be choriocarcinoma, the malignant counterpart of the benign hydatidiform mole (Eastman and Hellman 1966). They cannot be differentiated with ultrasound, and the clinical history, evidence of metastatic disease, and tissue pathological examination will differentiate these two conditions.

A normal intrauterine pregnancy with an associated tumor can be yet another cause for a patient referred with a large-for-dates history. This can either be a uterine tumor such as a leiomyoma and/or an adnexal mass. The most frequent mass found in association with an intrauterine pregnancy is uterine leiomyomata. They frequently demonstrate the same characteristics as when they are found in the nongravid uterus. They can manifest a variable ultrasonic picture with some appearing as solid tumors with a diffuse echo pattern, others as a "mixed" mass with solid and cystic areas due to cystic degeneration and/or hemorrhage, and still others as a primarily cystic mass due to almost complete cystic degeneration. Although their ultrasonic appearance can be variable, their continuity with, and deformity of, the uterus allows the diagnosis to be made. If the myoma is on a thin pedicle, the diagnosis will be more difficult because its attachment to the uterus may not be apparent. The size of the myoma may change with the pregnancy, and those located in the lower portion of the uterus may not allow a normal vaginal delivery. The size and number of the myomata can be variable and can rarely cause massive uterine enlargement. Rare uterine anomalies such as a bicornuate or double uterus can also present with the picture of excessive uterine enlargement on clinical examination.

Adnexal masses adjacent to the uterus may give the clinical impression that the uterus is larger than it should be for the patient's menstrual age. In this situation, the ultrasound examination is invaluable in clarifying the situation. The most frequently associated pelvic mass is a simple ovarian cyst. These can achieve a large size, but are completely cystic or occasionally can show evidence of septations. The dimensions of the cyst are important, because a cyst larger than 5–7 cm in size frequently requires exploratory surgery to exclude malignancy. These cysts should not be confused with corpus luteum cysts which can occur normally during the first trimester of pregnancy. They rarely are larger than 4–5 cm and will disappear after the first trimester of pregnancy. Cystic teratomas, or dermoid tumors, can also be found in association with a normal intrauterine pregnancy. If a layering of echogenic material is present in the mass, or if strong echoes secondary to calcification are present, this diagnosis should be suggested. Other less common adnexal masses that can be found in association with a normal intrauterine pregnancy include: ovarian malignant tumors, pelvic kidneys, tubal ovarian abscesses, and hematomas.

Ectopic Pregnancy

A brief explanation of the pathological changes with ectopic pregnancy is important in understanding its ultrasonic presentation (Rogers, Shaub, and Wilson 1977). Ectopic pregnancy is similar to a normal pregnancy with hormonal stimulation causing uterine hypertrophy and the development of a decidua. Endometrial changes appear almost identical to a normal pregnancy except for the absence of chorionic villi. The conditions for trophoblastic growth in the wall of the tube are different in comparison to growth in a normal intrauterine pregnancy. The paucity of decidual development augments vascular penetration and invasion of the muscularis. Hematomas often result after rupture into adjacent structures. An "acute" ectopic pregnancy usually denotes a combination of abrupt pain, syncope, or shock from massive hemorrhage. In a "chronic" ectopic pregnancy, the process persists and becomes walled off with organization. Chronic ectopic pregnancies often have a history of irregular, recurrent vaginal bleeding, fever, and palpable masses.

The classical ultrasonic description of an ectopic pregnancy finds a slightly enlarged uterus, with uniform internal echoes and no evidence of intrauterine pregnancy, combined with an extrauterine cystic or semi-cystic mass, gestational sac, fetal structures, or fluid in the cul-de-sac (Kobayashi, Hellman, and Cromb 1972; Rogers, Shaub, and Wilson 1977). The ultrasonic picture of an "empty" (nongravid) uterus with an adjacent adnexal mass is certainly not diagnostic for an ectopic pregnancy, because this pattern can be seen in numerous other entities, including tubal ovarian abscesses, simple ovarian cysts, neoplasms, endometriosis, teratomas, or fluid in the bowel loops. The clinical history, including the pregnancy test, is vitally important in allowing the diagnosis of an ectopic pregnancy to be made ultrasonically. If free fluid is present within the abdomen or pelvis, as in the cul-de-sac region, a ruptured ectopic pregnancy is suggested. Another identified pattern of ectopic pregnancy is a slightly enlarged or normal uterus with no visualization of an adjacent adnexal mass or free fluid. In other words, the ultrasound examination is essentially normal. If the patient is known to be at approximately 5–6 weeks gestation, at which time the gestational sac will definitely be ultrasonically visible, an intrauterine pregnancy can be excluded. In this situation, the area of the ectopic pregnancy cannot be located for the clinician, but it can be determined that it definitely is not within the uterus. If there is a possibility that the patient may have just converted her pregnancy test and is only at 4 weeks gestation, a repeat scan in 2 weeks will clarify whether the first examination was performed before the intrauterine gestational sac was ultrasonically visible, or if, in fact, it lies outside of the uterus. In all four cases with the preceding findings which we studied, the findings at exploratory surgery disclosed very small (1–2 cm) unruptured tubal ectopic pregnancies that were too small to be discernible with ultrasound.

Chronic ectopic pregnancies usually present an entirely different ultrasonic picture than acute ectopic pregnancies (Rogers, Shaub, and Wilson 1977). There can be a variable ultrasonic appearance, but the most frequent appearance is that of a midline mass in the expected location of the uterus. The mass frequently is "uterine" in shape and may appear primarily solid in nature, or present a complex pattern with solid and cystic components. The contour of the mass frequently is very irregular, but it can appear fairly well circumscribed. Unfortunately, the ultrasonic appearance of chronic ectopic pregnancies is not specific and strongly resembles an enlarged myomatous uterus with areas of cystic de-

generation, or occasionally, a large pelvic abscess. If a separate uterus could be identified, the diagnosis would be much simpler; this, however, is rarely the case. It is not surprising, though, when the pathology of the lesion is considered. At surgery, the large midline mass has incorporated the uterus within it and the associated inflammatory reaction has obliterated the normal tissue planes, making the uterus unidentifiable as a separate structure on ultrasound. Thus, when a midline solid or complex pelvic mass is present in the expected location of the uterus, a chronic ectopic pregnancy should be included in the differential diagnosis and correlation with the laboratory and clinical data should assist in making the diagnosis in appropriate cases.

Incompetent Cervix

Incompetent cervix presents in the second trimester as a painless, bloodless abortion with minimal warning. It is frequently secondary to previous trauma such as a difficult delivery or previous D and C. Other etiologies such as emotional factors or a weakness of the cervical muscle ring have been entertained.

Ultrasound examination of the lower uterine segment and endocervical canal now can confirm the clinical impression of an incompetent cervix. Most often, these patients present with two or three previous abortions in the second trimester. If such a patient is encountered, an ultrasound examination of the endocervical canal should be undertaken.

The technique for examination of the endocervical canal is extremely important. Transverse scans should initially be obtained perpendicular to the long axis of the cervix. The right and left borders of the cervix should be marked on the patient's skin. The transducer arm should then be realigned parallel to the long axis of the cervix for the longitudinal scans. Often, this is a midline scan; occasionally, however, the cervix is oriented obliquely to the right or left. The initial transverse scans will delineate the oblique angle of the cervix. The longitudinal scan should then begin to the right or the left and proceed at half centimeter intervals through the entire cervix. The majority of the scans will demonstrate the echogenic muscle of the cervix, but when the mid portion of the cervix is approached, a strong linear echo arising from the endocervical canal will be noted within the muscle tissues of the cervix. This strong linear echo should be visualized in its entirety, from the external to the internal os. If an incompetent cervix is present, sonolucency due to amniotic fluid will be noted in the endocervical canal. This may extend nearly the entire length of the endocervical canal. It is extremely important that adequate bladder distension be present to ensure adequate visualization of the lower uterine segment and cervix. It should also be noted that overdistension of the urinary bladder can lead to collapse of the cervix from the increased pressure in the urinary bladder. Therefore, if on initial examination the urinary bladder appears overly distended, the patient should partially void and then be reexamined to determine if the lower uterine segment distends and fluid is noted in the endocervical canal.

It is extremely difficult and unusual to visualize an incompetent cervix with ultrasound prior to the fourteenth or fifteenth week. At this early stage of pregnancy, the volume of the fluid and fetus within the uterus is not adequate to cause distension of the lower uterine segment and cervix. By the seventeenth or eighteenth week of pregnancy, however, an incompetent cervix can be visualized with ultrasound.

In any patient clinically suspected of having an incompetent cervix, an ultrasound examination of the lower uterine area should be performed serially at 2 or 3-week intervals until about the twenty-fourth week. By this stage of pregnancy, if fluid is not identified in the endocervical canal by ultrasound, it is extremely unlikely an incompetent cervix is present.

Fetal Death

The verification of fetal death is vastly simplified by the use of an ultrasound examination. In most ultrasound laboratories, a common indication for ultrasound examination is "no FHTs, rule out fetal death." These patients usually arrive for ultrasound examination from the obstetrical clinic where the clinician was unable to detect fetal heart tones on auscultation. On occasion, the ultrasound examination will discover a molar pregnancy, but in the vast majority of cases, a viable pregnancy will be present. The advantage that the ultrasonographer has over the clinician, who has blindly attempted to detect fetal heart tones, is that the ultrasound examination will disclose the location of the fetal heart within the thorax, and a Doppler transducer can then be directed at the

known location of the fetal heart. The absence of fetal heart tones on Doppler examination performed in this manner is pathognomonic of fetal death. If the examination is performed with a real-time unit, lack of visualization of a beating fetal heart is also indicative of fetal death.

The B-scan findings in fetal death can show various abnormalities. The findings in early gestation have previously been discussed; thus, this discussion will be limited to the findings of fetal death in later pregnancy. Within hours of fetal death, amniotic fluid penetrates rapidly into the skin of the fetus and results in increased fluffiness and coarsening of the fetal outline (Gottesfeld 1970; Leopold and Asher 1975; Sanders and Conrad 1975). As the fetal scalp is separated from the calvarium by the edema fluid, a double outline of the skull (halo sign) can be identified; less commonly, the edema fluid will create a double outline of the fetal body as well. The double contour is not pathognomonic of fetal death in that it can be seen in edematous hydropic fetuses secondary to Rh incompatibility, in infants of diabetic mothers, or in those affected with sickle cell disease. A partial double contour can be seen if the fetus moves during the scanning procedure. This double contour will not be completely circumferential and will intersect the calvarium at some point, because it is really a composite of two fetal skull outlines. Furthermore, it will not be a consistent finding on repeated scans. Other scan findings in fetal death include deformity of the fetus itself with later collapse of the fetal skull (Spaulding's sign), fetal body, and spine. There will be lack of fetal and uterine growth on serial examinations. When the examination is performed with a real-time unit, similar fetal structural abnormalities can be identified. In addition, there will be an absence of identifiable fetal movement, and the fetal heart will show no evidence of contraction (Levine and Filly 1977).

Normal Fetal Anatomy

The advent of recent refinements in gray scale imaging has allowed visualization of normal fetal structures to a degree unmatched by any other noninvasive diagnostic modality. Intracranial detail, including midline structures of the falx and third ventricle, are routinely imaged. Kossoff (1974) has identified the lateral ventricles and mid brain. The fetal heart and lungs can be identified within the thorax, and a fetal echocardiogram can be obtained in most cases (Garrett, Kossoff, and Lawrence 1975; Kossoff, Garrett, and Radavonovich 1974). In the abdomen, the liver, umbilical vein, gallbladder, kidneys, urinary bladder, and bowel loops are routinely identified (Flanigan and Butiny 1977; Lee and Blake 1977). The fetal extremities are easily imaged, and frequently even small fetal digits can be seen. Finally, male genitalia can occasionally be identified (Flanigan and Butiny 1977).

Abnormal Fetal Anatomy

With the improved intrauterine visualization of normal fetal anatomy has come the expected identification of more and more abnormal fetal anatomy. The following is a discussion of fetal anomalies described to date.

Anencephaly is the most common and one of the most easily detected anomalies diagnosed by ultrasound examination. It is the most frequent fetal malformation affecting the central nervous system, and its overall incidence is 1/1000 possible deliveries (Cecuk and Breyer 1976; Cunningham and Walls 1976; Warkany 1971). The recurrence rate is 1 in 25 and after two successively affected fetuses, the risk rises to 1 in 10 (Warkany 1971). Ultrasonic diagnosis is made when a normal cephalic outline is absent. The anencephalic fetus is usually very well seen because of the presence of polyhydramnios in 30 to 50% of cases (Warkany 1971). The fetal body appears normal, and there usually is a dense cluster of echoes in the expected location of the fetal skull. Many cases will be discovered late in pregnancy when being scanned for a "large-for-dates" history due to polyhydramnios. Because of the high recurrence rate in anencephaly and other neural tube defects (meningomyeloceles, etc.), all patients with a previous infant delivered with a neural tube defect should have a screening ultrasound examination at 14–15 weeks, at which time the fetal skull should be visible. If there is no evidence of a fetal skull at this time, a repeat examination should be performed in 2–3 weeks to confirm the diagnosis, so that the pregnancy can be terminated. Amniocentesis will also result in elevated alpha-fetoprotein in anencephaly, as well as other open neural tube defects.

Microcephaly can also be easily diagnosed with ultrasound. Unlike the anencephalic fetus, the microcephalic has a diminutive skull. The diagnosis of microcephaly can be made when there is a large discrepancy between the fetal body and fetal head size, and the body is greater than head. This, of course, presumes that the fetal body is normal and is not enlarged due to ascites or tumor.

At the opposite end of the spectrum is the hydrocephalic fetus. This has been diagnosed prior to 20 weeks of gestation due to a large head-body discrepancy, so that the head is greater than the body, and accelerated growth of the biparietal diameter on serial examinations (Freeman et al. 1977). Typically, however, the patient is first examined near term, and the biparietal diameter will be noted to be excessive. Most laboratories consider a measurement greater than 10.7 or 10.8 cm to be indicative of hydrocephalus (Sanders and Conrad 1975). The fetal skull will frequently act ultrasonically cystic, due to the excessive amount of cerebral spinal fluid present, and the enlarged ventricles themselves may be identified. In diabetic patients, the upper limit of 10.8 cm should be used with caution. Infants of diabetic mothers do not show the decrease in the biparietal diameter growth rate near term that is noted in normal pregnancies. Macrosomic infants of diabetic mothers demonstrate both a large body-chest size and a large biparietal diameter. Thus, the hydrocephalic discrepancy in the body-head diameters will not be present in these infants. In order to diagnose hydrocephalus in the fetus of a diabetic patient, the fetal measurement must be disproportionately increased in comparison with the large fetal body.

Fetal ascites is easily demonstrable whether it is due to Rh incompatibility, syphilis, urinary tract obstruction, or, as in a recently reported case, due to a fetal lung tumor (Garrett, Kossoff, and Lawrence 1975; Ghorashi and Gottesfeld 1976; Leopold and Asher 1975; Shaub and Wilson 1976). Clinical history is of paramount importance in determining the etiology, but associated ultrasonic findings of fetal scalp edema, body edema, or marked placental enlargement can be helpful in suggesting the diagnosis of Rh incompatibility or possibly transplacental syphilis. With newer high-resolution gray scale units, the normal fetal kidneys can be seen, and findings due to congenital hydronephrosis or multicystic kidney can be identified (Flanigan and Butiny 1977; Garrett, Grunwald, and Robinson 1970; Lee and Blake 1977; Santos-Ramos and Duenhoelter 1975). Renal anomalies, especially obstructive urinary tract disease, are also frequently associated with fetal urinary ascites

(Leopold and Asher 1975). Masses or tumors projecting from the fetus also can be identified, and the intrauterine detection of fetal meningocele, meningomylecele, cystic lymphangioma, oomphalocele, and cystic hygroma have all recently been reported (Herzog 1975; Mitchell and Bradley-Watson 1973; Morgan et al. 1975; Shaub, Wilson, and Collea 1976). Conjoined twins have rarely been diagnosed prior to the onset of labor, but several reports of antepartum diagnosis recently have appeared in the world literature (Fagan 1977; Wilson, Shaub, and Cetrulo 1977).

With multiple gestation pregnancies, intrauterine-growth retardation of one of the fetuses can be detected when there is a repeatedly significant difference in fetal biparietal diameters (Dorros 1976). Ultrasound examination of a twin gestation also may disclose evidence of the so-called "transfusion syndrome," where evidence of fetal ascites or polyhydramnios can be seen (Benirschke and Driscoll 1967). In this situation, there are vascular anomalies and vascular connections within the placentas and one fetus receives a larger amount of the placental blood flow. The ascites develops secondary to high-output cardiac failure in one fetus (hypervolemic) or hypovolemic failure in the other. If one fetus does not survive, the abnormal hemodynamic conditions disappear, and the ascites resolves in the surviving fetus.

Amniocentesis

Transabdominal amniocentesis following placental and amniotic fluid localization has become one of the most commonly requested obstetrical ultrasonic procedures. It is most frequently used in the diagnosis of genetic diseases where the aspirated amniotic fluid is used in tissue-cell culture analysis to detect biochemical defects or aberrations in the number or structure of chromosomes. This allows genetic counseling to be based on in utero diagnosis, and not on probability of risk (Arger et al. 1976; Milunsky et al. 1970; Nadler and Gerbie 1970). Amniocentesis also is commonly done to determine the amniotic fluid lecithin/sphingomyelin (L/S) ratio to predict fetal pulmonary maturity. Furthermore, in cases of suspected or known Rh isoimmunization, the determination of the amniotic fluid delta-450 bilirubin peak is an indicator of fetal Rh involvement. Intrauterine fetal transfusions with ultrasonic localization and guid-

ance can also be performed when the fetus is affected. The amniocentesis procedure itself is an invasive procedure with a low morbidity rate of approximately 1% (Schwartz 1975).

Amniocentesis usually is performed at 14–18 weeks gestation for genetic counseling and in the third trimester of pregnancy for detection of the lecithin/sphingomyelin ratio or delta-450 bilirubin peak (Arger et al. 1976). The actual procedure and the preceding ultrasound examination are the same in either case. A routine obstetrical ultrasound scan is done with transverse and longitudinal sections obtained for placental localization and biparietal diameter measurement. The best aspiration site is then determined. If possible, this site should avoid penetration of the placenta or fetus and be in an area of amniotic fluid accumulation. If the placenta is in an anterior location, a "clear" area must be found where the placental tissue is absent. On occasion, the accessible area will be quite small, and rarely will there be an area completely free of placental tissue. When this is the case, the clinical necessity for the amniocentesis must be weighed against the fact that the aspiration needle will knowingly pass through the placenta with the slightly higher attendant risks. Use of a 22-gauge needle is recommended when the amniocentesis is to be performed through placental tissue.

When the placenta is located posteriorly, almost any area can be used for percutaneous puncture. In early pregnancy, however, the posterior placenta is frequently quite large and bulky and may approach contact with the anterior wall of the uterine cavity. In this situation, the distance from the skin to the placenta may be measured from the ultrasound scan, and the aspiration needle may be marked with a flange or sterile piece of tape to preclude penetration into the bulky posterior placenta. When the amniocentesis is to be performed at a later time, outside the ultrasound laboratory, selection of the best aspiration site may be a problem. This arises from the fact that the ultrasound-descriptive landmarks used (symphysis pubis, umbilicus) are fixed, and the uterus itself is mobile. Thus, if the degree of bladder distension is significantly different at the time of the amniocentesis versus the time of the ultrasound examination, a surface skin landmark may no longer be close to the selected uterine tap site. The problem can be overcome if the patient voids completely after the ultrasound examination and is then rescanned with the skin marked over the selected aspiration site. Then, as long as the amniocentesis is performed with an empty urinary bladder, the surface skin mark will still correctly localize the selected uterine tap site.

Real-time Ultrasonography

Real-time ultrasound in obstetrics is becoming increasingly popular because of the speed and ease of examination. Most commercially available units are small and portable and can be taken to the patient's bedside or to the labor area. Several commercial manufacturers have also recently made real-time units available as an option on their standard contact B-scan unit at a nominal additional cost.

Most of the real-time units employ either a linear array of multiple transducer elements or a sector scanner accomplished either mechanically or electrically. This is done quite rapidly with frame rates of around 40 B-scan images per second (Levine and Filly 1977). This is slightly above the flicker rate of the human eye, which is 16–18 frames per second. The examiner perceives a continuum of motion (i.e., a "fluoroscopic" image of the fetus).

An analogy to better understand this difference between contact B-scanning and real-time would be as follows. If we were to take rapid still photographs (contact B-scan pictures) of an object passing by a window and then developed and viewed them, the resultant pictures would each individually show different positions and locations of the object, but no perception of actual motion would be apparent. On the other hand, if a motion picture of the same object were obtained, the resultant viewed images would show apparent actual motion. The motion pictures, however, are actually only multiple individual pictures (like the still photographs), but they are viewed at a rapid rate that is above the flicker rate of the human eye. The viewer, thus, appears to see actual motion. Therefore, the contact B-scan images are similar to the still photographs, the real-time images are similar to motion picture images which appear to show actual motion. Actually, they are only multiple separate B-scans projected at the rapid rate.

Real-time examination is performed after coating the skin with an appropriate acoustic coupling agent (e.g., mineral oil). The transducers most commonly employed are either 2.25- or 3.5-MHz. In smaller patients, a 5.0-MHz transducer is sufficient. The actual transducers are small, handheld, and easily guided over the skin and/or angled to quickly obtain the required images. With experience in doing this type of examination, the complete procedure can be done in one-half to one-fourth the time required for a contact B-scan study. Furthermore, the operation of a real-time unit can be learned much more quickly. Polaroid images are usually taken of important findings (placental localization, fetal position, biparietal diameter, etc.), and the entire examination is usually recorded and stored on videotape. The real-time examination allows complete visualization of all the appropriate intrauterine anatomy but also allows the examiner to visualize fetal movement and the actual beating fetal heart.

After the preceding glowing review of real-time ultrasound, we may wonder why all obstetrical ultrasound examinations are not done with real-time units. It is generally felt that in the near future, this will be the case, with real-time ultrasound becoming the examination of choice in obstetrics. In addition, because of the cheaper cost of the portable real-time units (approximately one-fourth to one-third that of contact B-scan units) and the speed in performing the examination, the cost of the examination can be decreased to an amount which makes it financially reasonable to perform the study routinely on all pregnant patients. Articles have recently appeared in the literature advocating exactly this (Scheer 1977). Only time and future refinement and development of the real-time ultrasound units will show whether this comes to pass.

References

Arger, P. H. et al. Ultrasound assisted amniocentesis in prenatal genetic counseling. *Radiology* 120:155, 1976.

Barone, C. M. Ultrasonic diagnosis in hydatidiform mole with a coexistant fetus, *Radiology* 124:798, 1977.

Beisher, N. A. Hydatidiform mole with coexistant fetus. *Br. J. Obstet. Gynaecol.* 68:231, 1961.

Benirschke, K. E., and Driscoll, S. G. *The pathology of the human placenta*. New York: Springer-Verlag, 1967.

Brown, R. E. *Ultrasonography. Basic principles and clinical applications,* St. Louis: Warren H. Green, Inc., 1975.

Campbell, S. The prediction of fetal maturity by ultrasonic measurement of the biparietal diameter. *Br. J. Obstet. Gynaecol.* 76:603, 1969.

Campbell, S., and Dewhurst, C. J. Quintuplet pregnancy diagnosed and assessed by ultrasonic compound scanning. *Lancet* 1:101, 1970.

Cecuk, A. K., and Breyer, B. Prediction of maturity in first trimester of pregnancy by ultrasonic measurement of fetal crown-rump length. *J. Clin. Ultrasound* 4:83, 1976.

Cohen, W. N. et al. Correlation of ultrasound and radioisotope placentography. *Am. J. Roentgenol.* 116:843, 1972.

Cooperberg, P. L.; Chow, T.; Kite, V.; and Austin, S. Biparietal diameter: a comparison of real time and conventional B-Scan techniques. *J. Clin. Ultrasound* 4:421, 1976.

Cunningham, M. E., and Walls, W. J. Ultrasound in the evaluation of anencephaly. *Radiology* 118:165, 1976.

Donald, I.; MacVicar, J.; and Brown, T. G. Investigation of abdominal masses by pulsed ultrasound, *Lancet* 1:1188, 1958.

Donald, I., and Brown, T. G. Demonstration of tissue interfaces within the body by ultrasonic echo sounding. *Brit. J. Radiol.* 34:539, 1961.

Donald, I.; Morley, P.; and Barnett, E. The diagnosis of blighted ovum by sonar. *Br. J. Obstet. Gynaecol.* 79:304, 1972.

Donald, I. Sonar as a method of studying prenatal development. *J. Pediatr.* 75:326, 1969.

Dorros, G. The prenatal diagnosis of intrauterine growth retardation in one fetus of a twin gestation. *Obstet. Gynecol.* 48:475, 1976.

Eastman, N. J., and Hellman, L. M. *Obstetrics.* New York: Appleton-Century-Crofts, 1966.

Fagan, C. J. Antepartum diagnosis of conjoined twins by ultrasonography. *Am. J. Roentgenol.* 129:921, 1977.

Flamme, P. Ultrasonic fetal cephalometry: percentile curve. *Br. Med. J.*, 3:384, 1972.

Flanigan, D. J., and Butiny, J. H. Ultrasonic imaging of normal intrauterine anatomy. *J. Clin. Ultrasound* 5:334, 1977.

Freeman, R. T. et al. The diagnosis of fetal hydrocephalus before viability. *Obstet. Gynecol.* 49:109, 1977.

Garrett, W. J.; Kossoff, G.; and Lawrence, R. Grey scale echography in the diagnosis of hydrops due to fetal lung tumors. *J. Clin. Ultrasound* 3:45, 1975.

Garrett, W. J.; Grunwald, G.; and Robinson, D. E. Pre-

natal diagnosis of fetal polycystic kidney by ultrasound. *Aust. N. Z. J. Obstet. Gynaecol.* 10:7, 1970.

Ghorashi, B., and Gottesfeld, K. R. The grey scale appearance of the normal pregnancy from 14 to 16 weeks of gestation. *J. Clin. Ultrasound* 15:195, 1977.

Ghorashi, B., and Gottesfeld, F. R. Recognition of the hydropic fetus by grey scale ultrasound. *J. Clin. Ultrasound* 4:193, 1976.

Gottesfeld, K. The ultrasonic diagnosis of intrauterine fetal death. *Am. J. Obstet. Gynecol.* 108:623, 1970.

Gottesfeld, K. R.; Sundgren, C.; and Chavez, F. The diagnosis of sextuplets by ultrasound—a case report. *J. Clin. Ultrasound* 2:291, 1974.

Gottesfeld, K. R. Ultrasound in obstetrics & gynecology. *Semin. Roentgenol.* 10:305, 1975.

Gottesfeld, K. R.; Thompson, H. E.; Holmes, J. H.; and Taylor, E. S. Ultrasonic placentography—a new method for placental localization. *Am. J. Obstet. Gynecol.* 96:538, 1966.

Hellman, L. M. et al. Growth and development of the human fetus prior to the twentieth week of gestation. *Am. J. Obstet. Gynecol.* 103:789, 1969.

Hellman, L. M.; Kobayashi, M.; and Cromb, E. Ultrasonic diagnosis of embryonic malformations. *Am. J. Obstet. Gynecol.* 115:615, 1973.

Herzog, K. A. The detection of fetal meningocele & meningoencephalocele by B-scan ultrasound: a case report. *J. Clin. Ultrasound* 3:307, 1975.

Horger, E. D.; Kreutner, A. K.; Underwood, P. B. Ultrasonic diagnosis of low implantation preceding placenta previa. *Am. J. Obstet. Gynecol.* 120:1119, 1974.

King, D. L. Placental ultrasonography. *J. Clin. Ultrasound* 1:21, 1973.

Kobayashi, M.; Hellman, L. M.; and Cromb, E. *Atlas of Ultrasonography in obstetrics and gynecology.* New York: Appleton-Century-Crofts, 1972.

Kohorn, E. I., and Kaufman, M. Sonar in the first trimester of pregnancy. *Obstet. Gynecol.* 44:473, 1974.

Kohorn, E. I.; Morrison, J.; Ashford, C.; and Blackwell, R. J. Ultrasonic scanning in obstetrics and gynecology. *Obstet. Gynecol.* 34:515, 1969.

Kossoff, G.; Garrett, W. J.; and Radavonovich, G. Grey scale echography in obstetrics and gynecology. *Australas. Radiol.* 18:62, 1974.

Kurjak, A., and Breyer, B. Estimation of fetal weight by ultrasonic abdomenometry. *Am. J. Obstet. Gynecol.* 125:962, 1976.

Langman, J. *Medical Embryology.* Baltimore: The Williams & Wilkins Co., 1969.

Lee, T. G., and Blake, S. Prenatal fetal abdominal ultra-sonography and diagnosis. *Radiology* 124:475, 1977.

Leopold, G. R., and Asher, W. M. *Fundamentals of abdominal and pelvic ultrasonography.* Philadelphia: W. B. Saunders Co., 1975.

Leopold, G. R. Diagnostic ultrasound in the detection of molar pregnancy. *Radiology* 98:171, 1971.

Levi, S. The use of ultrasonic biparietal diameter mea-surement of the fetus in assessing gestational age. *Acta. Obstet. Gynecol. Scand.* 50:179, 1971.

Levi, S. Diagnostic use of ultrasonics in abortion. A study of 250 patients. *Int. J. Gynaecol. Obstet.* 11:195,1973.

Levi, S. Ultrasonic assessment of the high rate of hu-man multiple pregnancy in the first trimester. *J. Clin. Ultrasound* 4:3, 1976.

Levine, S. C., and Filly, R. A. Accuracy of real-time sonography in the determination of fetal viability. *Obstet. Gynecol.* 49:475, 1977.

Lunt, R., and Chard, T. A new method for estimation of fetal weight in late pregnancy by ultrasonic scanning. *Br. J. Obstet. Gynaecol.* 83:1, 1976.

MacVicar, J., and Donald, I. Sonar in the diagnosis of early pregnancy and its complications. *Br. J. Obstet. Gynaecol.* 70:387, 1963.

Milunsky, A. et al. Prenatal genetic diagnosis. *N. Engl. J. Med.* 283:1498, 1970.

Mitchell, R. C., and Bradley-Watson, P. J. The detection of fetal meningocele by ultrasound B-scan. *Br. J. Obstet. Gynaecol.* 80:1100, 1973.

Morgan, C. L. et al. Antenatal detection of fetal struc-tural defects with ultrasound. *J. Clin. Ultrasound* 3:287, 1975.

Morrison, J., and McLinnan, M. J. The theory, feasibility, and accuracy of an ultrasonic method of estimating fetal weight. *Brit. J. Obstet. Gynaecol.* 83:833, 1976.

Nadler, H. L., and Gerbie, A. B. Role of amniocentesis in the intrauterine detection of genetic disorders. *N. Engl. J. Med.* 282:596, 1970.

Poll, V. Precision of ultrasonic fetal cephalometry. *Br. J. Obstet. Gynaecol.* 83:217, 1976.

Robinson, H. Detection of fetal heart movement in first trimester of pregnancy using pulsed ultrasound. *Br. Med. J.* 4:466, 1972.

Robinson, H. P., and Caines, J. S. Sonar evidence of early pregnancy failure in patients with twin concep-tions. *Br. J. Obstet. Gynaecol.* 84:22, 1977.

Rogers, W. F.; Shaub, M. S.; and Wilson, R. Chronic

ectopic pregnancy: ultrasonic diagnosis. *J. Clin. Ultrasound* 5:257, 1977.

Sanders, R. C., and Conrad, M. R. Sonography in obstetrics. *Radiol. Clin. N. Am.* 13:435, 1975.

Sanders, R. C.; Curtin, M. J.; and Tapper, A. J. Ultra-sound in the management of elective abortion. *Am. J. Roentgenol.* 125:469, 1975.

Santos-Ramos, R., and Duenhoelter, J. H. Diagnosis of congenital fetal abnormalities by sonography. *Obstet. Gynecol.* 45:279, 1975.

Scheer, K. Ultrasound in twin gestation. *J. Clin. Ultra-sound* 2:197, 1974.

Scheer, K. Sonography as a routine obstetrical diagnos-tic procedure. *J. Clin. Ultrasound* 5:101, 1977.

Schwartz, R. N. Amniocentesis. *Clin. Obstet. Gynecol.* 18:1, 1975.

Shaub, M., and Wilson, R. Erythobastosis fetalis: ultra-sonic diagnosis. *J. Clin. Ultrasound* 4:19, 1976.

Shaub, M.; Wilson, R.; and Collea, J. Fetal cystic lymph-angioma (cystic hygioma): prepartum ultrasonic findings. *Radiology.* 121:449, 1976.

Stocker, J.; Mawad, R.; Deleon, A.; and Desjardins, P. Ultrasonic cephalometry—its use in estimating fetal weight. *Obstet. Gynecol.* 45:275, 1975.

Taylor, E. S.; Holmes, J. H.; Thompson, H. E.; and Gottesfeld, K. R. Ultrasound diagnostic techniques in obstetrics and gynecology, *Am. J. Obstet. Gyne-col.* 90:655, 1964.

Thompson, H.; Holmes, J.; Gottesfeld, K.; and Taylor, E. Fetal development as determined by ultrasonic pulse echo technique. *Am. J. Obstet. Gynecol.* 92:44, 1965.

Thompson, H. E., and Makowski, E. L. Estimation of birth weight and gestational age. *Obstet. Gynecol.* 37:44, 1971.

Thompson, H. E. Ultrasonic diagnostic procedures in obstetrics and gynecology. *J. Clin. Ultrasound* 1:160, 1973.

Warkany, J. Congenital malformations. Chicago: Year Book, 1971.

Williams, P. L.; Wendell-Smith, C. P.; and Treadgold, S. Basic human embryology. Philadelphia: J. B. Lippin-cott Co., 1966.

Wilson, R.; Shaub, M.; and Cetrulo, C. The antepartum findings of conjoined twins. *J. Clin. Ultrasound* 5:35, 1977.

Winsberg, F. Echographic changes with placental ag-ing. *J. Clin. Ultrasound* 1:52, 1973.

CASES
Dennis A. Sarti, M.D.
W. Frederick Sample, M.D.

Normal Gestational Sac

Fertilization takes place in the distal third of the fallopian tubes, approximately 2 weeks after menstruation. The fertilized ovum travels down the fallopian tube and reaches the uterus approximately 2–3 days after fertilization. The blastocyst then floats in the uterine cavity and finally embeds in the uterine mucosa after about 3 or 4 more days. Therefore, approximately 7 days after fertilization, the blastocyst has finally embedded itself within the uterine mucosa. The blastocyst cannot be visualized at this time because of its small size. At about two weeks after fertilization, however, ultrasound can visualize the first evidence of a beginning gestational sac.

Figure 12.1 is a longitudinal scan of the uterus with a strong central echo in the fundal region; this is the beginning gestational sac. This is approximately 2–2½ weeks after fertilization, which would correspond to 4–4½ weeks after the last menstruation. This is the earliest visualization of the gestational sac. We do not see any central fluid at this time. The gestational sac continues to enlarge. In figure 12.2 the gestational sac is seen at approximately 5 menstrual weeks. A central sonlucency within the gestational sac represents the amniotic fluid. This is a more typical appearance of the gestational sac with the strong surrounding echoes of the chorionic villi and the decidual reaction. The surrounding echoes are very important, for they give an impression of the normal vascularity to the gestational sac. The high-amplitude echoes are a good sign of prominent chorionic villi developing within the uterus.

Figure 12.3 is another longitudinal scan at approximately 5–6 menstrual weeks. Again, the strong surrounding echoes of the chorionic villi are seen. The central portion of the gestational sac is fluid-filled. The embryo is not visualized at this time, since it is too

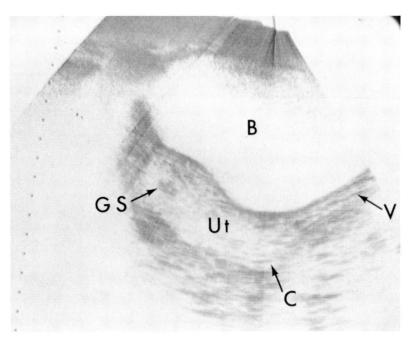

Fig. 12.1

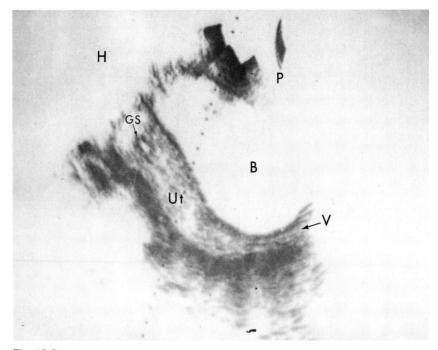

Fig. 12.2

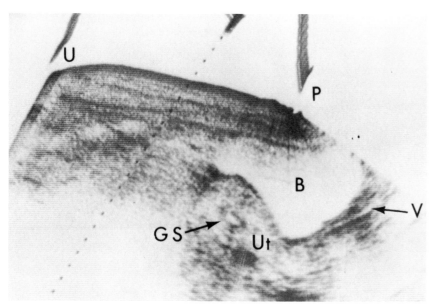

Fig. 12.3

small to be detected with ultrasound. The important finding is the strong surrounding echoes of the gestational sac, which indicate a normal adequate blood supply.

Figure 12.4 is a transverse scan of the pregnant uterus at approximately 6 menstrual weeks. Again we see the strong surrounding echoes of the chorionic villi in the gestational sac. Fluid is noted centrally without evidence of an embryo at this time. An ovarian cyst is on the right side, consistent with a corpus luteum cyst of pregnancy.

B	=	Urinary bladder
C	=	Cervix
GS	=	Gestational sac
H	=	Head
L	=	Left
O	=	Ovary
OC	=	Ovarian cyst
P	=	Level of the symphysis pubis
Pi	=	Piriformis muscles
R	=	Right
U	=	Umbilical level
Ut	=	Uterus
V	=	Vagina

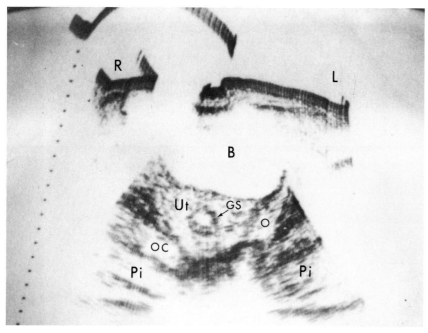

Fig. 12.4

Normal Gestational Sac

The gestational sac continues to grow in size during the first 10 weeks. It grows at approximately 1 cm per week in mean diameter. Therefore, normal growth is easy to measure in serial examinations. The embryo can be seen at approximately the seventh menstrual week, when it attains a size large enough for ultrasonic detection. Figure 12.5 is a longitudinal scan in which we see a gestational sac situated in the fundus of the uterus. It is approximately 2–3 cm in diameter. Strong surrounding echoes indicate good vascular supply to the chorionic villi. A small echo (arrow) is noted in the central portion of the gestational sac. This is the early detection of the embryo by ultrasound. The embryo is approximately 5 mm in size by the seventh menstrual week.

Figure 12.6 is a longitudinal scan of the pregnant uterus at approximately 8 weeks gestation. The fetus has enlarged to approximately 1 cm in diameter. It is easily recognizable within the amniotic fluid of the gestational sac. The gestational sac is now strongly surrounded by echoes that are thicker on one side in the region that will eventually become the placenta. The thicker portion of the gestational sac will become the placenta, while the thinner portion will eventually atrophy and completely disappear. That portion of the gestational sac that is away from the implantation site eventually outgrows its blood supply and atrophies completely. This leads to the disappearance of the gestational sac.

Occasionally, two fluid-filled areas are seen within the uterus separated by a curvilinear septum (figs. 12.7 and 12.8). This is an indication of a twin pregnancy. In figure 12.7, we see two fluid-filled sacs separated by a curvilinear septum. In one sac the internal echoes indicate a fetus. The other sac is completely clear. This could represent an anembryonic pregnancy on one side. Close examination of the gestational sac, however, is necessary, since we may not be passing the transducer beam over the site of the fetus. Figure 12.8 is the same patient. A fetus is visualized in both sides of the gestational sac. This is a

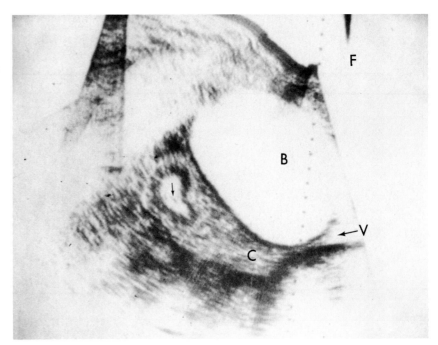

Fig. 12.5

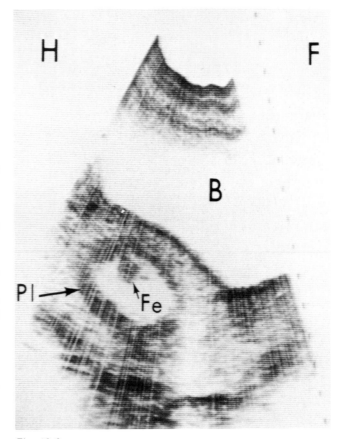

Fig. 12.6

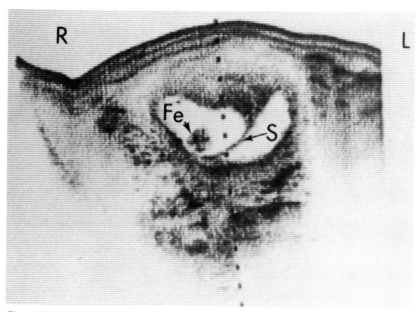

Fig. 12.7

normal twin pregnancy with separate amniotic cavities.

Arrows = Early embryo
B = Urinary bladder
C = Cervix
F = Foot
Fe = Fetus
H = Head
L = Left
Pl = Placenta
R = Right
S = Septum separating a twin pregnancy
V = Vagina

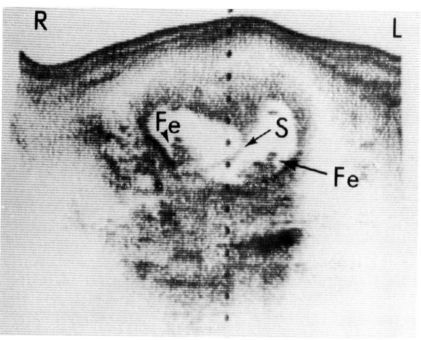

Fig. 12.8

Normal Gestational Sac

As the gestational sac continues to enlarge, the region of the placenta becomes thicker. The area that will no longer be the placenta continues to thin out and eventually disappears. Figure 12.9 is a longitudinal scan of the gestational sac at approximately 9 weeks gestation. Here we see a thickened placenta situated posteriorly. The anterior portion of the gestational sac is less echogenic and much thinner; this indicates normal atrophy. The myometrium situated posterior to the placenta has a lighter echo pattern to it than the highly echogenic placenta. A corpus luteum cyst is seen in the region of the cul-de-sac.

Figure 12.10 is a longitudinal scan at approximately 9–10 weeks gestation. Again we see a thickened echogenic region posteriorly; this represents the placental site. Thinning and decreasing echogenicity to the surrounding gestational sac, secondary to normal vascular atrophy, is seen in the anterior portion (arrows).

Figure 12.11 is a transverse scan with a thick posterior placenta. Again, the anterior portion of the gestational sac is much thinner. This normal disappearance of vascular supply is very important to appreciate. It can become very difficult to diagnose an impending abortion around 10 weeks of pregnancy because of the normal atrophic appearance to the gestational sac. If decreased echogenicity is seen at 6, 7, or 8 weeks, the diagnosis of an impending abortion is more likely.

Figure 12.12 is a pregnancy at approximately 11 weeks. This is a time in which the gestational sac has disappeared. The placenta is situated posteriorly. It is quite thick and has a high echogenicity which indicates good vascular supply. It is important, however, to notice the surrounding portion of the gestational sac. We no longer see the thick surrounding echoes (arrows). Instead, amniotic fluid in contact with myometrial echoes is visualized. It is around the eleventh to twelfth week that the gestional sac disappears, and only placental tissue is evident.

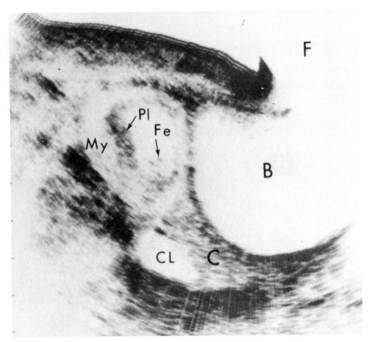

Fig. 12.9

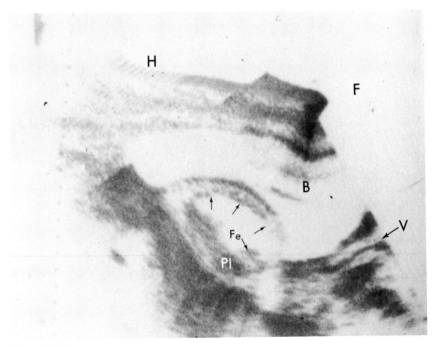

Fig. 12.10

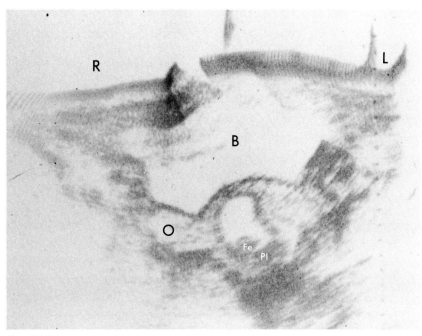

Fig. 12.11

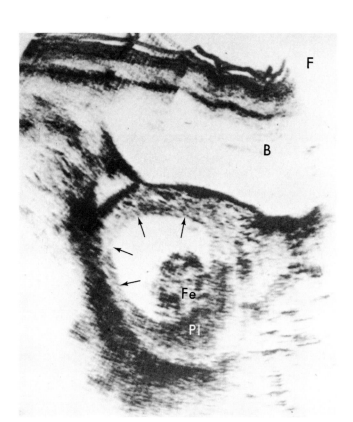

Fig. 12.12

Abnormal Gestational Sac

Numerous ultrasonic signs can indicate an abnormal gestational sac. In figure 12.13 a longitudinal scan demonstrates a gestational sac without the usual round or oval appearance. In the caudal portion of the gestational sac we see a pointed segment. A pointed segment is a strong indication that an abnormal sac is present. The same patient was scanned in the transverse plane (fig. 12.14). Here we see an uneven thickness and echogenicity to the surrounding echoes of the gestational sac. Areas of thinner echogenicity (arrows) present on the anterior and posterior segments of the gestational sac (fig. 12.14). This is compatible with decreased vascular supply to an abnormal sac. The vascularity of a gestational sac can be visualized by the thickness and strength of the surrounding echoes. Here we have evidence of an abnormal vascular supply.

The patient was brought back 10 days later (figs. 12.15 and 12.16). Figure 12.15 is a longitudinal scan indicating marked decrease in the surrounding echoes (arrows). A transverse scan confirms the decreased echogenicity. Also of extreme importance is the fact that the gestational sac did not increase in size. If there is any question as to an abnormal sac, the patient should be studied 7–10 days later. In this time period, the mean diameter of the sac should increase at least 1 cm. The main findings of this case are the pointed segment and decreased echogenicity indicating an abnormal gestational sac.

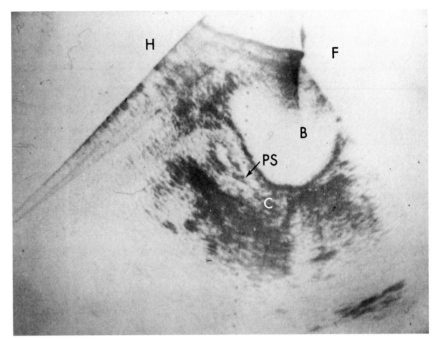

Fig. 12.13

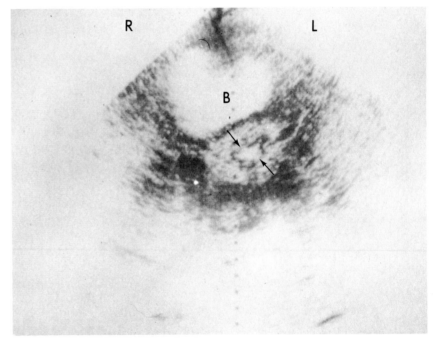

Fig. 12.14

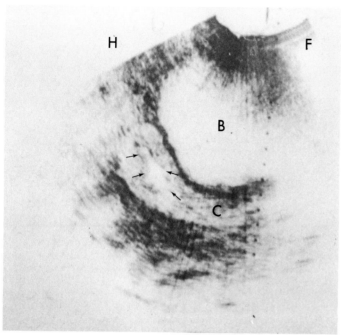

Fig. 12.15

Arrows = Decreased vascular supply to the
gestational sac
B = Urinary bladder
C = Cervix
F = Foot
H = Head
L = Left
PS = Pointed segment
R = Right

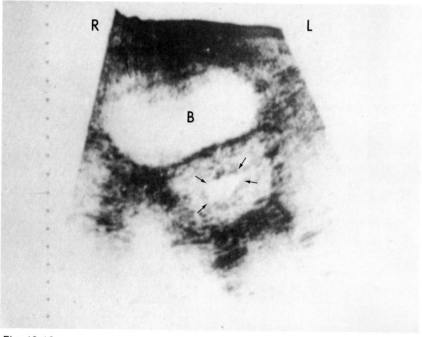

Fig. 12.16

Abnormal Gestational Sac

Figure 12.17 is an example of an abnormal gestational sac with evidence not only of a pointed segment but also an actual break in the gestational sac. The caudal portion of the gestational sac is markedly abnormal compared with the previous normals.

Often, a double gestational sac is present. This may represent a normal twin gestation, but the possibility of an abnormal pregnancy should also be considered. Figure 12.18 is a longitudinal scan with two gestational sacs (numbers 1 and 2) in the mid portion of the uterus. It is important to notice that a small fluid collection is present above the two gestational sacs. This patient went on to have a complete abortion approximately 1 week later.

The implantation site of a normal gestational sac is usually fundal or mid-uterine in location. Occasionally, a low implantation site is seen (fig. 12.19). The gestational sac is located in the cervical region of the uterus. The patient was examined 1 week later, and a complete abortion occurred (fig. 12.20). Here we see no evidence of the gestational sac. Low implantation may indicate an impending abortion. These cases should be followed carefully.

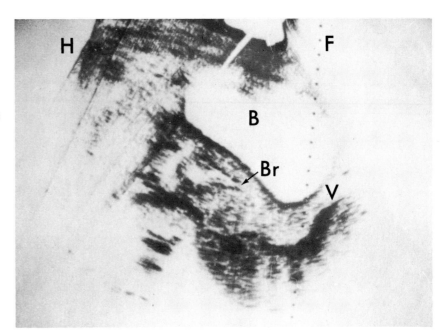

Fig. 12.17

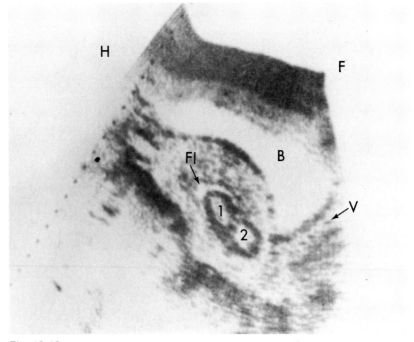

Fig. 12.18

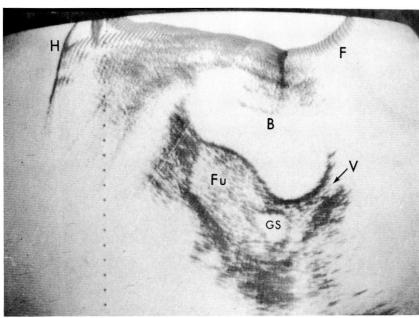

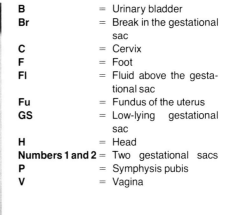

B = Urinary bladder
Br = Break in the gestational sac
C = Cervix
F = Foot
Fl = Fluid above the gestational sac
Fu = Fundus of the uterus
GS = Low-lying gestational sac
H = Head
Numbers 1 and 2 = Two gestational sacs
P = Symphysis pubis
V = Vagina

Fig. 12.19

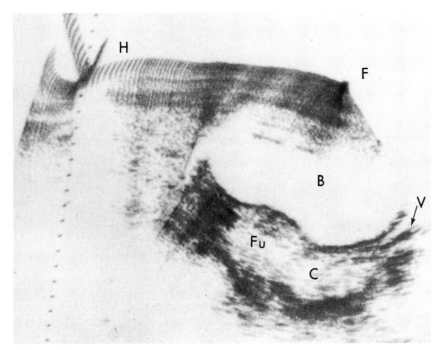

Fig. 12.20

Abnormal Gestational Sac

Frequently a large amount of fluid is seen in the gestational sac, but without evidence of any fetal echoes. This has been termed an anembryonic pregnancy or a blighted ovum. A longitudinal scan of the uterus (fig. 12.21) demonstrates a large amount of fluid in the gestational sac. The surrounding echoes however, are quite thin and weak, indicating an abnormal pregnancy. A break in the gestational sac with some fragmentation of the surrounding echoes supports this. Figure 12.22 is a transverse scan of an anembryonic pregnancy with markedly weak surrounding echoes (arrows). This indicates a poor vascular supply to the gestational sac. We do not find evidence of any fetal echoes within this rather large gestational sac. Once a gestational sac reaches a size of approximately 2–3 cm, it should demonstrate fetal echoes. If fetal echoes are not present on a close and meticulous examination, then an anembryonic pregnancy can be diagnosed.

Figures 12.23 and 12.24 are longitudinal and transverse scans of a patient with an anembryonic pregnancy. Here we see an empty gestational sac. Weak, thin surrounding echoes (arrows) indicate poor vascular supply to this pregnancy. When there is no evidence of a placental site with a gestational sac of this size, an anembryonic pregnancy can be diagnosed. This gestational sac is approximately 7–8 cm. By this time a markedly thick portion which will eventually be the placental site is seen. The fetus should also be quite large by this time.

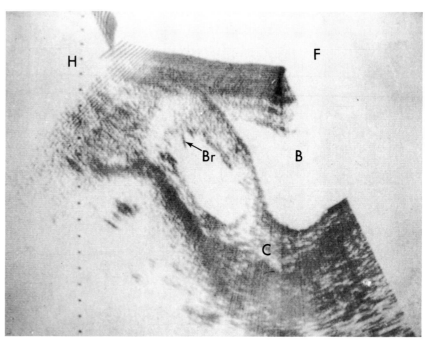

Fig. 12.21

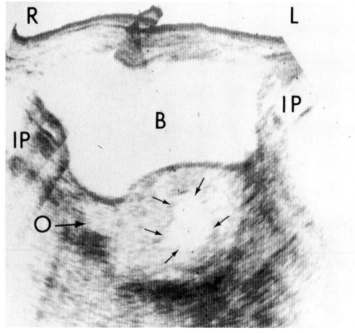

Fig. 12.22

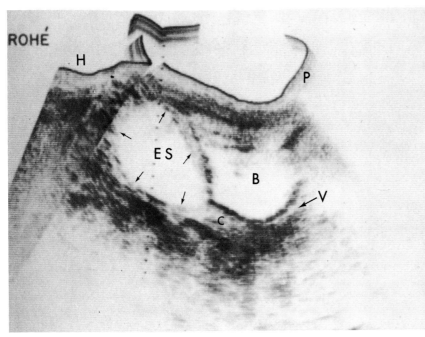

Fig. 12.23

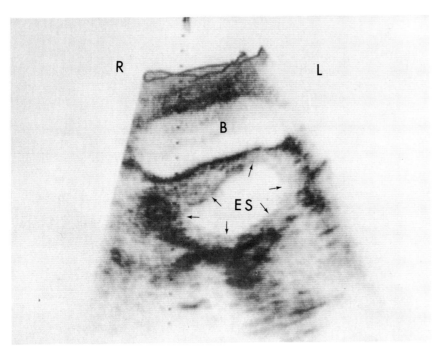

Fig. 12.24

Arrows = Weak and thin surrounding echoes indicating an abnormal gestational sac
B = Urinary bladder
Br = Break in the gestational sac indicating fragmentation
C = Cervix
ES = Empty gestational sac
F = Foot
H = Head
IP = Iliopsoas muscle
L = Left
O = Right Ovary
R = Right

Incomplete Abortion

Often, a patient is sent for an ultrasound examination to determine whether or not she has aborted completely. Clinically, she will be having some spotting and pain. It is not felt that the pregnancy is viable, but it must be determined whether or not the uterus has completely emptied itself.

Figures 12.25 and 12.26 are typical of a patient who has had an incomplete abortion. Strong echoes (arrows) are seen in the endometrial cavity which is somewhat thicker than we usually see with normal menstruation. In the right clinical setting, however, the findings are compatible with an incomplete abortion. The patient can be followed for several weeks to see whether or not the uterus empties itself completely. If central echoes are still present over a prolonged period of time, a D and C should be performed.

Figures 12.27 and 12.28 are of an incomplete abortion which has gone on for longer than 3 years. The patient had an abortion 3 years previously without complete emptying of the uterus. Strong central echoes (arrows) are seen within the mid portion of the uterus. In this instance, shadowing is distal to the echoes indicating calcification within the mid portion of the uterus. The retained products of conception actually contained bony structures from the fetus.

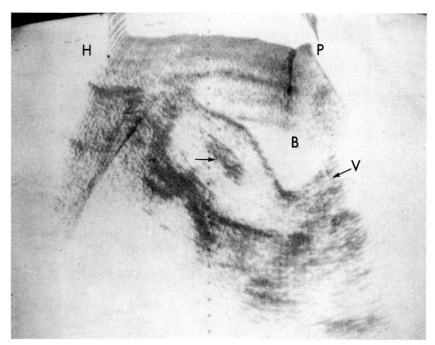

Fig. 12.25

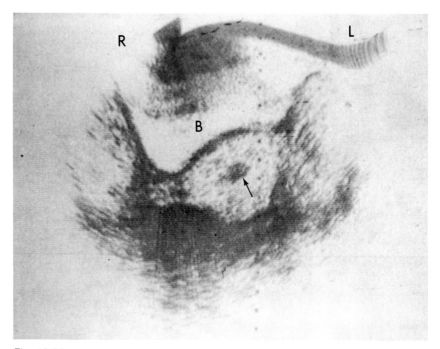

Fig. 12.26

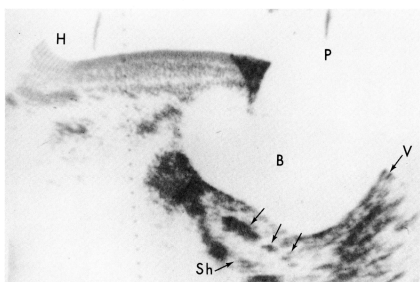

Arrows = Strong central echoes indicating
         an incomplete abortion
B   = Urinary bladder
FT = Left fallopian tube
H   = Head
L   = Left
P   = Level of the symphysis pubis
R   = Right
Sh = Shadowing behind retained fetal
         products
V   = Vagina

Fig. 12.27

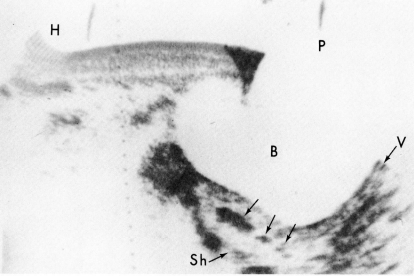

Fig. 12.28

Incomplete Abortion

Figure 12.29 is another example of retained products (arrows) within the central portion of the uterus. It almost appears to be an incomplete sac. The uterus had, however, been almost twice as large approximately 2 weeks earlier. Not only did the uterus contract down, but also the central echoes of the uterus became smaller. These findings are compatible with incomplete, inevitable abortion.

Occasionally, the uterus will reach a fairly large size. If an abortion is present, degeneration of the fetus and placenta will occur. Often, this may be difficult to distinguish from a molar pregnancy. Figure 12.30 is a transverse scan of a patient with an incomplete abortion. The uterus is markedly enlarged. Diffuse, irregular echoes within it could be confused with a molar pregnancy. We can often distinguish an incomplete abortion from a molar pregnancy by the strong echoes present in an incomplete abortion.

Figure 12.31 is a longitudinal scan on the same patient demonstrating numerous strong echoes (arrows) within the uterus. This uneven echo pattern is highly suggestive of an inevitable abortion, rather than a molar pregnancy. Figure 12.32 further confirms this diagnosis, since calcification is noted within the uterus. That this is a calcific density is confirmed by the shadow distal to it. If such strong calcific echoes can be identified, the diagnosis of an inevitable abortion, as opposed to a molar pregnancy, can be made.

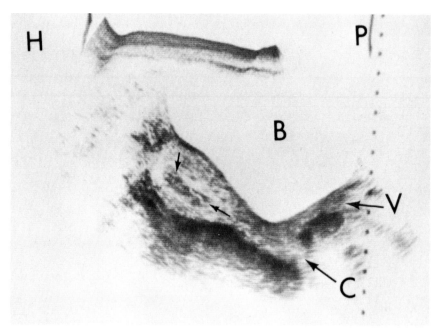

Fig. 12.29

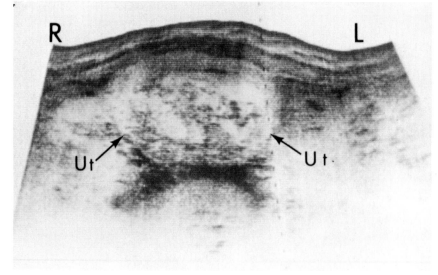

Fig. 12.30

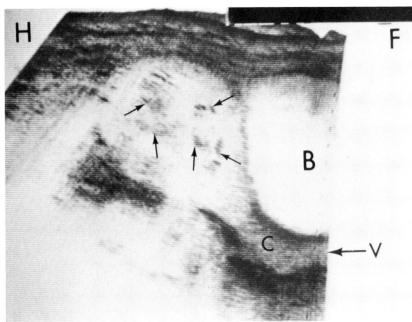

Arrows = Retained products of conception
B   = Urinary bladder
C   = Cervix
Ca   = Calcification
H   = Head
L   = Left
P   = Level of the symphysis pubis
R   = Right
Sh   = Shadowing
Ut   = Uterus
V   = Vagina

Fig. 12.31

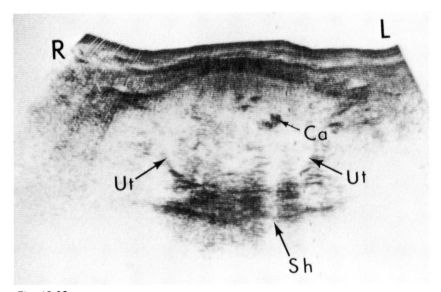

Fig. 12.32

Gestational Age

During the course of a pregnancy, several anatomic structures can be measured, all of which will give a fairly accurate assessment of gestational age. In the first 10 weeks of pregnancy, the gestational sac is used to measure the length of pregnancy. A mean gestational diameter is used by taking height, width, and length measurements and dividing these by three. Figure 12.33 is a longitudinal scan with the gestational sac seen in the central portion of the uterus. We can obtain a length and a height of the gestational sac, corresponding to the dark lines seen in figure 12.33. By obtaining a transverse scan and measuring the width, we can then determine the mean gestational sac diameter. This can be used from the fifth to the tenth menstrual week.

After the disappearance of the gestational sac, it is difficult to visualize the biparietal diameter for several weeks. During this period of time, the crown–rump length can be used to determine the gestational age. Crown rump length is often used from the seventh to the fifteenth or sixteenth menstrual week. Figure 12.34 is an example of the crown rump length measured from the top of the fetal skull (number 1) to the sacral region (number 2).

The biparietal diameter is used to estimate gestational age from the fifteenth week of gestation to term. This diameter can occasionally be seen as early as the eleventh or twelfth week of gestation. By the fifteenth or sixteenth week, we should be able to obtain a biparietal diameter in 100% of cases. Figure 12.35 is a transverse scan of the fetal skull with a strong central linear echo which arises from the falx cerebri. On each side of the falx cerebri are some lucent areas arising from the lateral ventricles. When visualizing the lateral ventricles, we are too cephalad to obtain an accurate biparietal diameter. The biparietal diameter should be measured at the widest diameter of the fetal skull, which is at the level of the thalami.

Dr. Michael Johnson of the University of Colorado, Denver, Colorado, has recently developed newer concepts in understanding the anatomy of the fetal

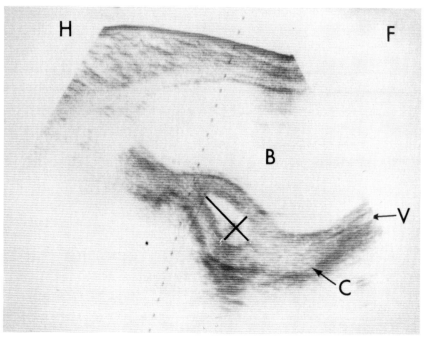

Fig. 12.33

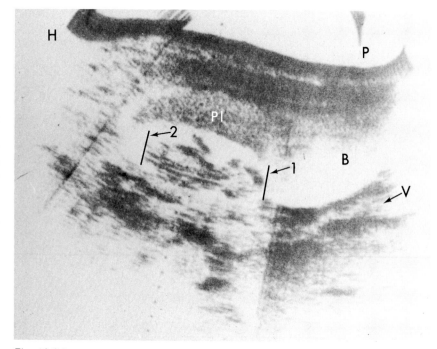

Fig. 12.34

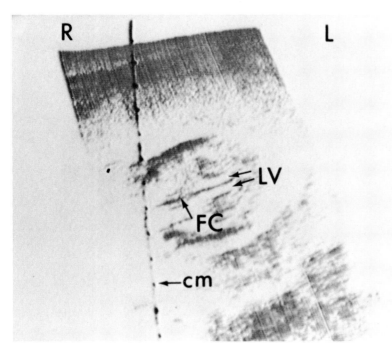

Fig. 12.35

skull. He has determined that the most accurate measurements for biparietal diameters are obtained at the level of the thalami. Figure 12.36 is a transverse scan of the fetal skull with the sonolucencies of the thalami situated near the central portion of the brain. The strong central echo between the thalami is arising from the third ventricle (number 3V). The continuation of the linear echo of the third ventricle arises from the septum pellucidum. A break is seen in the midline structures as the corpus callosum crosses the midline. The linear echoes then continue anteriorly formed by the falx cerebri. The biparietal diameter can then be obtained when visualizing the thalamic level. The biparietal diameters are measured from the near fetal skull to the far fetal skull.

B	=	Urinary bladder
C	=	Cervix
CC	=	Corpus callosum
cm	=	centimeter markers
F	=	Foot
FC	=	Falx cerebri
FS	=	Fetal skull
H	=	Head
L	=	Left
LV	=	Lateral ventricles
Numbers		
1 and 2	=	Crown-rump length (fig. 12.34)
Number		
3V	=	Third ventricle
P	=	Symphysis pubis
Perpendic-		
ular lines	=	Length and height of the gestational sac (fig. 12.33)
PL	=	Placenta
R	=	Right
SP	=	Septum pellucidum
T	=	Thalami
V	=	Vagina

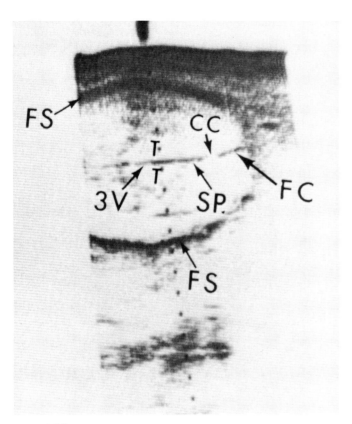

Fig. 12.36

Normal Placenta

Placental tissue will present either as an echogenic area or as a sonolucent area, depending upon its position in relationship to the fetus and to the transducer. If an anterior placenta is present in which there are only the uterine and abdominal walls between the placenta and the transducer, it will present as an evenly speckled, echogenic mass. Figure 12.37 is an example of an anterior placenta with an even, soft echogenic appearance to it. A strong linear echo is between the placenta and the amniotic fluid which is arising from the chorionic plate. Since the chorionic plate is a specular reflector, we must be close to the perpendicular in order to visualize the chorionic plate. It is not unusual to scan over an anterior placenta and, because of this physical limitation, be unable to visualize the chorionic plate. Figure 12.38 is another midline longitudinal scan with a homogeneous echo pattern arising from the anterior placenta. The placenta has an even texture with no masses evident within it. Mature placentas later on in pregnancy will tend to give an uneven coarser echo appearance.

Figures 12.39 and 12.40 are placentas with some small sonolucencies situated just beneath the chorionic plate. These are secondary to choriol cysts. They are a normal anatomic variant and of no clinical significance. Their usual location is directly beneath the chorionic plate.

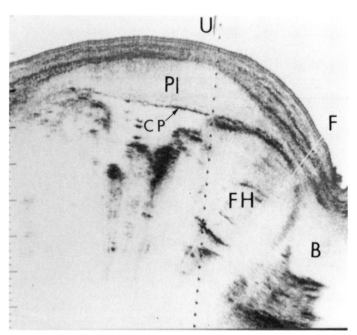

Fig. 12.37

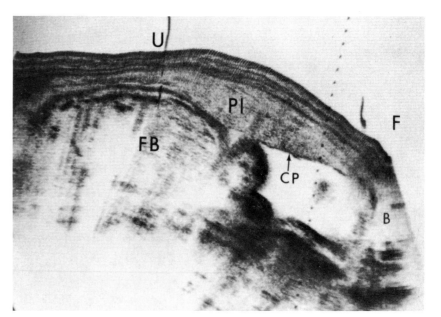

Fig. 12.38

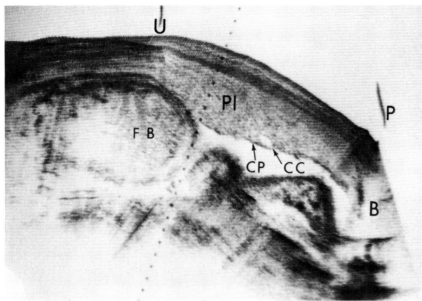

Fig. 12.39

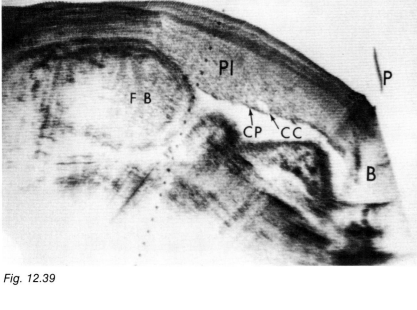

Fig. 12.40

B	=	Urinary bladder
CC	=	Choriol cysts
CP	=	Chorionic plate
F	=	Foot
FB	=	Fetal body
FH	=	Fetal head
P	=	Symphysis pubis
PI	=	Placenta
U	=	Umbilical level

Normal Placenta

When the placenta is situated posteriorly, it can give a variety of echogenic appearances. If it is situated behind the fetus, it will appear as a sonolucent mass. The reason for this is that the echoes arising from the placenta are too weak to pass through the markedly attenuating oseous structures of the fetus. Therefore, the echoes are not registered on the transducer during their return from the placental interfaces. Figure 12.41 is an example of a longitudinal scan in which we have a posterior fundal placenta. Placental tissue in the fundal region deep to amniotic fluid is speckling in, much as the anterior placentas did on the previous scans. The intervening amniotic fluid does not attenuate the placental tissue. The placenta, however, is also situated deep to the fetal extremities and the fetal head. Placental tissue in this location appears as a sonolucent mass because of the attenuation from the fetus.

Figure 12.42 is another example of echogenic placental tissue deep to amniotic fluid. Areas of placental shadowing, however, are noted when the placenta is scanned deep to the fetal extremities. There is a small region of through transmission as we scan between the fetal extremities. This is an extremely important technical concept to understand, because the limits of a posterior placenta are often quite difficult to detect.

Figure 12.43 is a transverse scan of a posterior lateral placenta with shadowing deep to the fetal body and fetal extremities. The left lateral portion of the placenta is seen. Here we have excellent visualization of the placental myometrial interface (arrows). The placental tissue is higher in amplitude and has a much finer echo appearance than the surrounding myometrium.

Figure 12.44 is a transverse scan of a posterior placenta. The placental tissue echoes normally when it is deep to the amniotic fluid on the left side. However, echogenicity from the placenta on the right side is also visualized when it is deep to the fetal body. The placenta was actually scanned from the right lateral aspect of the maternal abdomen. There-

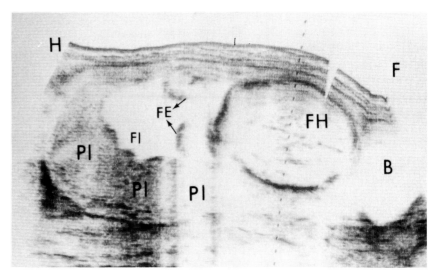

Fig. 12.41

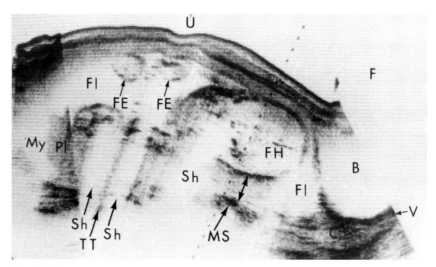

Fig. 12.42

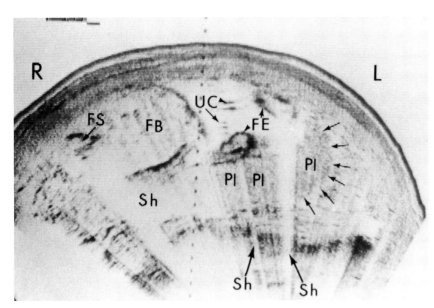

Fig. 12.43

fore, we did not pass the sound beam through the fetal body in order to speckle in the placenta on the right side. If we had scanned this patient from the anterior right abdomen, the placenta would have appeared sonolucent because of fetal body attenuation. The difference in echogenicity between the myometrium and placenta can be noted.

Arrows	=	Placental myometrial interface (fig. 12.43)
B	=	Urinary bladder
Ce	=	Cervix
F	=	Foot
FB	=	Fetal body
FE	=	Fetal extremity
FH	=	Fetal head
FI	=	Amniotic fluid
FS	=	Fetal spine
H	=	Head
L	=	Left
MS	=	Maternal sacrum
My	=	Myometrium
PI	=	Placenta
R	=	Right
Sh	=	Shadowing
TT	=	Through transmission
U	=	Umbilical cord
UC	=	Umbilical cord
V	=	Vagina

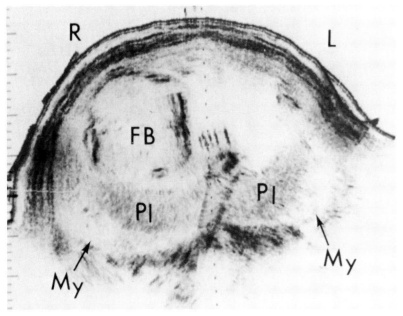

Fig. 12.44

Normal Placenta

A fundal placenta usually yields echogenicity similar to an anterior placenta when no fetus is situated between the placenta and the transducer. Figure 12.45 is an example of the fundal posterior placenta. The echogenic portion of the placenta is visualized in the fundal region. The sonolucent myometrium is noted cephalad to the placental tissue. When we are scanning over the fetal body, however, the placenta, situated deep to the fetus, appears as a sonolucent mass. A transverse scan through a fundal placenta (fig. 12.46) demonstrates an even echo pattern to the placental tissue surrounded by the relatively more lucent myometrium. If we were to scan the entire uterus and this picture were obtained, a hydatidiform mole would be considered. Scanning a placenta tangentally, however, can give an appearance similar to figure 12.46.

There has been much discussion about placental migration and the disappearance of a placenta previa with time. This has been attributed by many to the fact that the myometrium grows at a differential rate compared to placental tissue. Another important point that must be understood, however, is that the uterus undergoes contractions during the course of many ultrasonic examinations. Figures 12.47 and 12.48 are excellent examples of uterine contraction apparently changing the placental location.

Figure 12.47 is a midline scan with an anterior placenta which is somewhat low-lying. The difference in echogenicity between the placenta and myometrium is noted. The arrows in figure 12.47 represent the placental myometrial interface. The patient was then scanned approximately 5 minutes later after slight emptying of the bladder. The following scan (fig. 12.48) indicates the anterior placenta to be no longer low-lying. The myometrium in figure 12.47 is also much thicker in the anterior lower uterine segment than that in figure 12.48. This represents a uterine contraction drawing the placenta closer to the endocervical canal in figure 12.47. With relaxation of the contraction (fig. 12.48), the placenta moves much more cephalad.

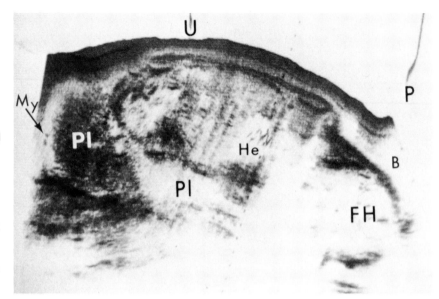

Fig. 12.45

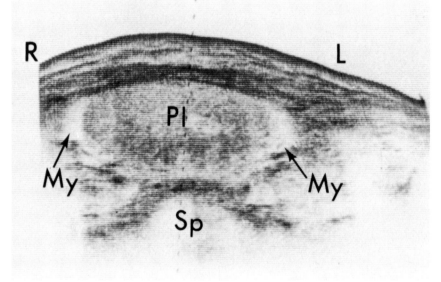

Fig. 12.46

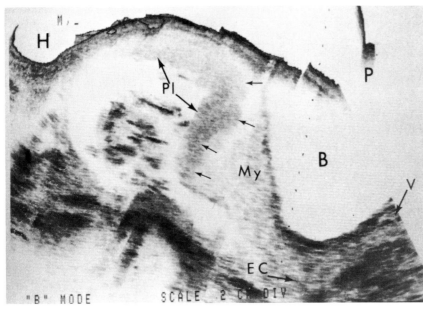

Fig. 12.47

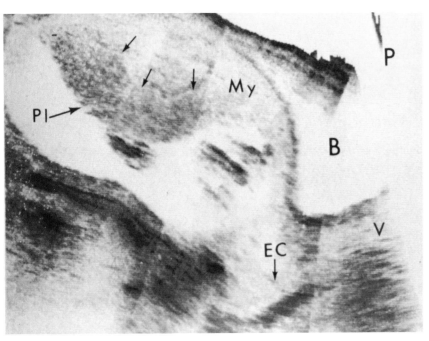

Fig. 12.48

Placental Myometrial Interface; Mature Placenta

When examining the placenta in a longitudinal or transverse plane, numerous tubular sonolucencies are often seen situated deep to it. In reality, this represents the myometrium with its rich vascular bed supplying the placenta. Figures 12.49 and 12.50 are longitudinal and transverse scans in which we see a markedly lucent and tubular myometrium deep to the placental tissues. This is not always a constant finding. In many individuals the myometrial-placental interface is not as dramatic as in these cases. When these marked tubular structures are present, however, they represent a normal variant with venous lakes within the myometrium standing out more prominently than usual. This should not be misdiagnosed as an abnormality or myometrial bleed. It does not represent an abruptio placenta, but rather a normal variant. Numerous parallel lines which represent the umbilical cord are also noted in figure 12.49. This is a normal finding on obstetrical examinations.

After the thirty-third or thirty-fourth week of pregnancy, many placentas will have an echogenic pattern different from the usual, even parenchymagram noted earlier in pregnancy. The appearance of the placenta will be much coarser and irregular. This is secondary to placental infarction which is a normal occurrence later on in pregnancy. Figure 12.51 is a longitudinal scan with a placenta with an even echo pattern in certain areas. Other areas, however, have very strong curvilinear echoes (arrows) that even cast a shadow. This is secondary to placental infarction and may eventually lead to placental calcification. Figure 12.52 is another longitudinal scan through the placenta. Multiple circular sonolucent areas represent the cotyledons of the placenta. These are surrounded by strong, highly echogenic rims (arrows) that represent areas of fibrosis and calcification. If we see this type of pattern earlier in pregnancy, around 27 weeks, we should be concerned about premature placental maturation.

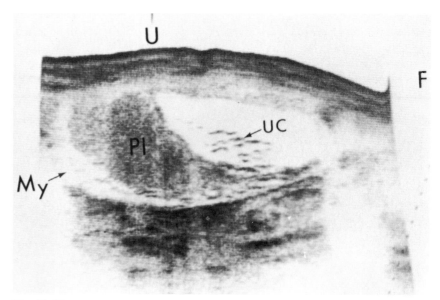

Fig. 12.49

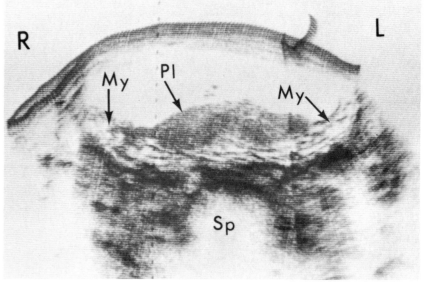

Fig. 12.50

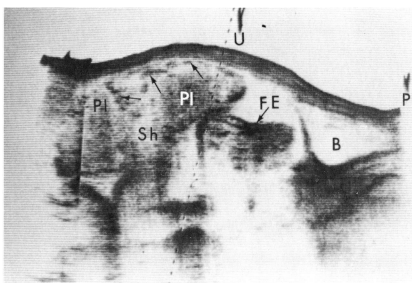

Fig. 12.51

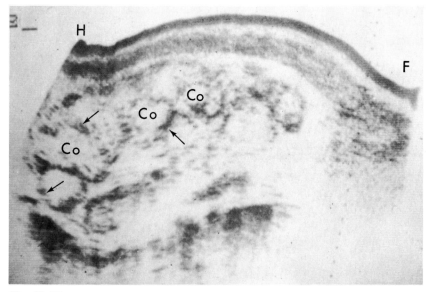

Fig. 12.52

Arrows	=	Areas of placental fibrosis and calcification
B	=	Urinary bladder
Co	=	Placental cotyledons
F	=	Foot
FE	=	Fetal extremity
H	=	Head
L	=	Left
My	=	Myometrium
P	=	Level of the symphysis pubis
Pl	=	Placenta
R	=	Right
Sh	=	Shadowing
Sp	=	Spine
U	=	Umbilical level
UC	=	Umbilical cord

Placenta Previa

In examining a third-trimester bleeder for placenta previa, it is extremely important to visualize not only the cervix but also the endocervical canal. Figure 12.53 is a longitudinal scan with the strong linear echo of the endocervical canal seen within the myometrial echoes of the cervix. Since the cervix is quite wide, we can scan over a 4-cm area and just visualize the cervical myometrium without visualizing the endocervical canal. An important measurement in ruling out a posterior placenta previa is visualization of the distance between the fetal head and the maternal sacrum. In figure 12.53 the distance between the fetal head and maternal sacrum (small arrows) is only about 1 cm. This is within normal limits, since anything less than 1.6–2 cm is considered within normal limits. Figure 12.54 is another longitudinal scan with a normal distance between the fetal head and maternal sacrum. Again, it is extremely important to visualize the linear echo of the endocervical canal, which is well seen in figure 12.54.

Figure 12.55 is an example of an increased distance between the fetal head and maternal sacrum. In this instance it is approximately 3 cm. When the fetal head is elevated above the maternal sacrum, the possibility of a posterior previa should be considered. Other causes for the elevation of the fetal head include an extremity interposed between the fetal head and the maternal sacrum, or a fetal head that is off center, causing us to scan a lateral aspect that will appear to be elevated off the maternal sacrum. Whenever there is any question, it is important to have the patient continue filling her bladder and to make strong efforts to visualize the endocervical canal.

Figure 12.56 is an example of a bladder filled adequately enough to allow visualization of the endocervical canal. The placenta extends completely over the cervix on this scan. The placental-myometrial interface (arrows) is well seen on this study. When attempting to diagnose a posterior placenta previa, it is extremely important to visualize not only the cervix but also the endocervical

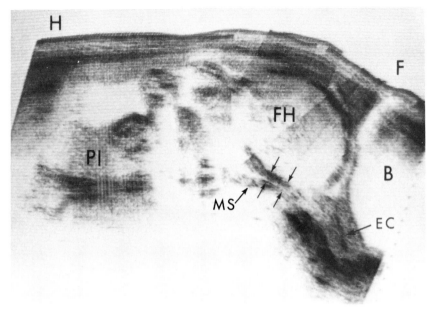

Fig. 12.53

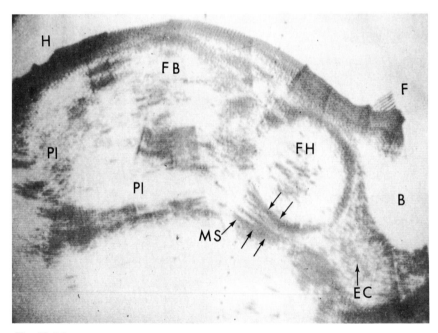

Fig. 12.54

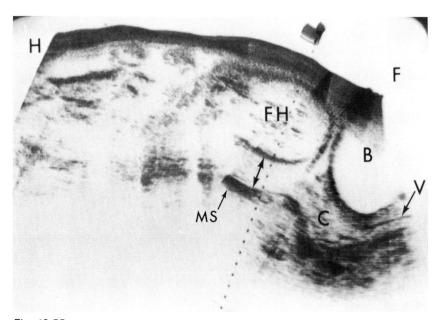

Fig. 12.55

canal and the placental myometrial interface, as is seen in figure 12.56. If this placental-myometrial interface can be seen extending over the entire cervix, the diagnosis of posterior placenta previa can be made.

Arrows = Fetal head-maternal sacral distance
Arrows = Placental-myometrial interface (fig. 12.56)
B = Urinary bladder
C = Cervix
EC = Endocervical canal
F = Foot
FB = Fetal body
FH = Fetal head
H = Head
MS = Maternal sacrum
PI = Placenta
V = Vagina

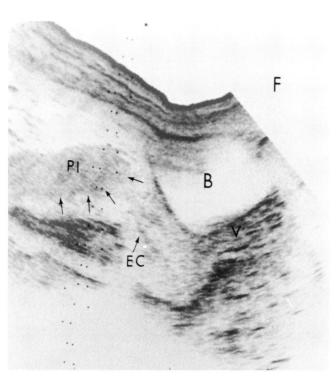

Fig. 12.56

Placenta Previa

A central previa exists when the placenta is situated over the mid portion of the cervix with an equal component over the anterior myometrium and an equal component over the posterior myometrium. We are near the midline, since we are able to visualize the cervix on this scan (fig. 12.57). The placental-myometrial interface (arrows) is well visualized as a relatively lucent band caudal to the placenta itself. This is consistent with a central placenta previa.

Figure 12.58 is a longitudinal scan with a central previa with a large anterior component. Again we see the placental tissue situated over the endocervical canal. This is a complete previa, since placental tissue is situated both anterior and posterior to the cervix. When we see this much placenta over the endocervical canal, we should have no difficulty in diagnosing a placenta previa.

Figures 12.59 and 12.60 are examples of placenta previa with sonolucent areas also visualized within the placenta. In figure 12.59 we see a sonolucent area secondary to hemorrhage situated just beneath the chorionic plate of the placenta. This is a complete posterior previa, since placental tissue is seen over the cervix and endocervical canal. In figure 12.60 longitudinal scan demonstrates not only a posterior placenta previa, but also hemorrhage slightly separating the placenta from the cervix. This is a posterior previa with a sonolucent area situated between the placenta and cervix, corresponding to the area of hemorrhage.

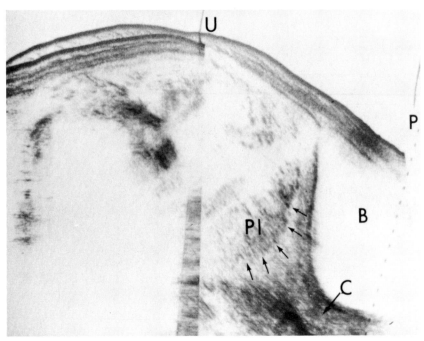

Fig. 12.57

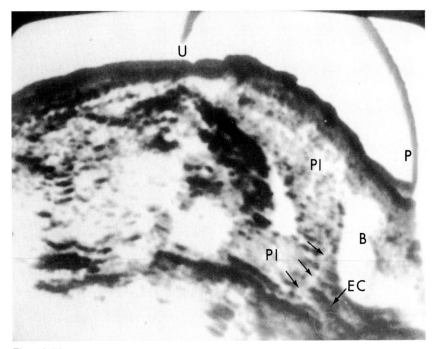

Fig. 12.58

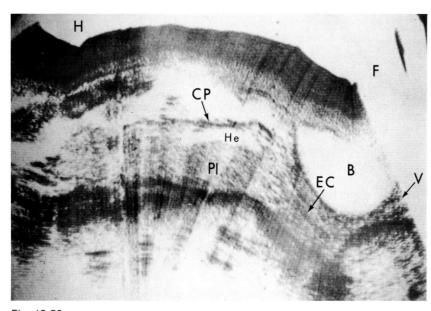

Fig. 12.59

SOURCE: The case in figure 12.58 is provided through the courtesy of Dr. M. Shaub, Centinela Valley Hospital, Los Angeles, California.

Arrows	=	Placental myometrial interface
B	=	Urinary bladder
C	=	Cervix
CP	=	Chrionic plate
Ec	=	Endocervical canal
F	=	Foot
Fe	=	Fetus
H	=	Head
He	=	Area of hemorrhage
P	=	Level of symphysis pubis
Pl	=	Placenta
U	=	Umbilical level
V	=	Vagina

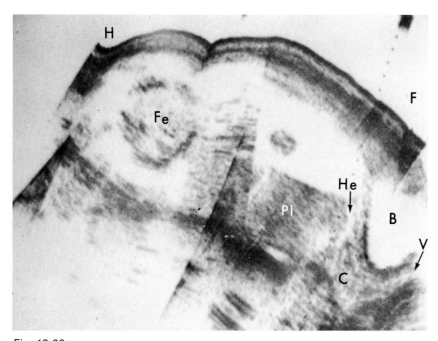

Fig. 12.60

Thick Placenta; Uterine Hematoma

Five centimeters is considered the upper limits for normal placental thickness. Several clinical entities can cause an increase in placental volume and thickness. The most common is Rh sensitization. Increase in placental thickness, however, can also be seen in diabetes and syphilis.

Figures 12.61 and 12.62 demonstrate examples of extreme placental thickness in a patient who had Rh sensitization with placental and fetal findings. Here we see marked thickness to the placenta, which is taking up the majority of the volume of the uterus. Figure 12.61 is a longitudinal scan in which only a portion of the fetal head is visualized, while the remainder of the uterine volume is filled with the placenta. Figure 12.62 is a transverse scan showing not only a thickened placenta but also ascites within the fetal abdomen. The fetal bowel is displaced away from the fetal abdominal wall. Only a small amount of amniotic fluid is present on this scan. This was true throughout the rest of this study. Practically the entire uterus is placenta-filled. Not only is the placenta markedly thickened in Rh sensitization, but it also has a high amplitude echogenicity.

Figures 12.63 and 12.64 are scans of an unusual patient with an area of hemorrhage in the cervical region of the uterus. Figure 12.63 is a longitudinal scan obtained on the patient on the same day that she suffered injuries in an auto accident. A sonolucent mass over the cervical region was suspected to be a uterine hematoma. The patient was followed for several weeks, and figure 12.64 is a study performed approximately 3–4 weeks after the previous examination. The uterine hematoma has completely resolved, and no sonolucent mass is evident in the lower uterine segment. This is an example of hemorrhage within the myometrium with complete resolution.

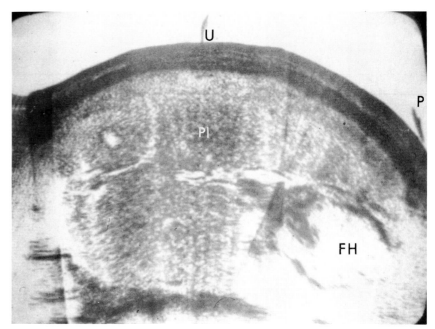

Fig. 12.61

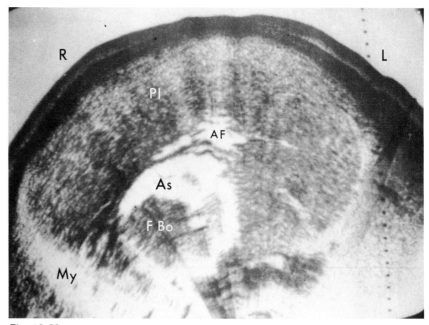

Fig. 12.62

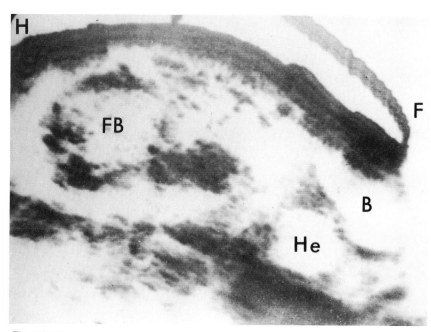

Fig. 12.63

SOURCE: The case in figures 12.63 and 12.64 was provided through the courtesy of Dr. M. Shaub, Centinela Valley Hospital, Los Angeles, California.

AF	=	Amniotic fluid
As	=	Fetal ascites
B	=	Bladder
F	=	Foot
FB	=	Fetal body
FBo	=	Fetal bowel
FH	=	Fetal head
H	=	Head
He	=	Uterine hematoma
L	=	Left
My	=	Myometrium
P	=	Level of the symphysis pubis
Pl	=	Placenta
R	=	Right
U	=	Umbilical level

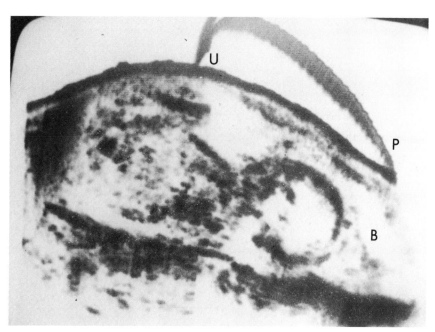

Fig. 12.64

Placental Implantation on a Uterine Septum

Occasionally during the course of an ultrasound examination we come across a placenta that has an unusual configuration. Figure 12.65 is an example of a 23-year-old woman with a confusing routine obstetrical ultrasound examination. On closer scrutiny of the study, however, a placental implantation on a uterine septum was diagnosed (fig. 12.65). In the center of figure 12.65 is a drawing which represents the findings at cesarian section. The fetus is in the breech position with the placenta implanted on a uterine septum. The fetal head is noted left of the placenta with the left arm situated on the right side of the uterine septum.

Part A of figure 12.65 is a transverse scan, quite cephalad with the fetal head on the left side of the uterus, to the left of the placenta. The placenta is situated against the lateral uterine wall on the right side. A transverse scan at part B shows that the placenta is now displaced away from the lateral uterine wall in which we see a sonolucent area of fluid. More caudally in part C of figure 12.65, we see the fetal extremity situated to the right lateral aspect of the placenta. The fetal body is situated to the left side. Part D is most important, for we are able to actually see the tip of the placenta as it extends into the amniotic fluid. The fetal extremity is visualized underneath the placenta with the fetal body to the left side.

Longitudinal scans corresponding to parts F, G, H, and I confirm the finding of a placental septum with the fetal extremity situated below the placenta and the fetal head and body situated on the left side. Cesarian section was performed on the patient and the findings corresponded to the initial ultrasonic interpretation.

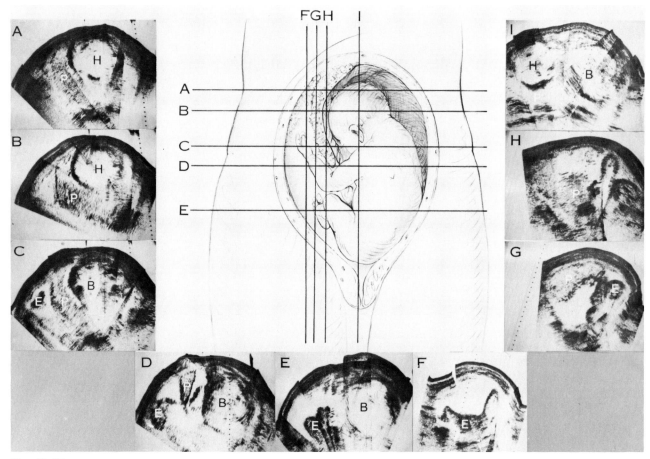

Fig. 12.65

B   = Fetal body
E   = Fetal extremity
H   = Fetal head
P   = Placenta

Multiple Gestation

One of the more common referral diagnoses for obstetrical ultrasound is that the patient is too "large for dates." Most often the reason for this discrepancy between size and dates is the fact that the patient is unsure of her last menstrual period. Another cause, however, is multiple gestation. In the first 10 weeks of pregnancy, we may actually be able to visualize two gestational sacs (fig. 12.66). This transverse scan demonstrates a septum (arrow) between the two gestational sacs (numbers 1 and 2). Later on in pregnancy, when attempting to diagnose a multiple gestation, it is important to visualize the two fetal heads. Figure 12.67 is an example of two fetuses in the vertex presentation. Both fetal heads are seen.

In figure 12.68 we are able to visualize one fetal head and two areas of amniotic fluid (numbers 1 and 2). Between the two areas of fluid is a linear echo representing the septum between the two amniotic fluid cavities. Figure 12.69 is another example with the linear echo (arrow) separating the fetal body on one side and the fetal pelvis on the other.

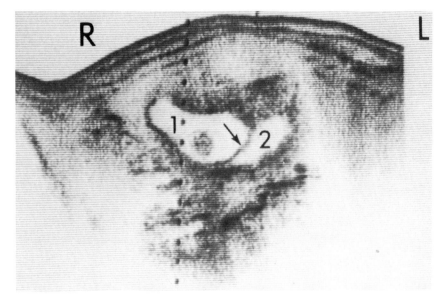

Fig. 12.66

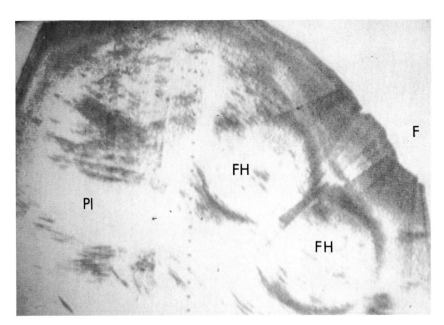

Fig. 12.67

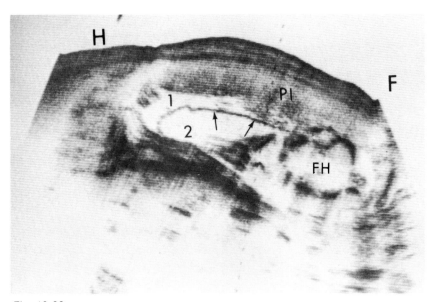
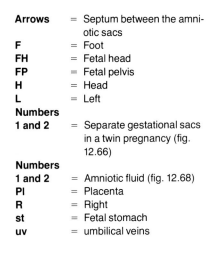

Fig. 12.68

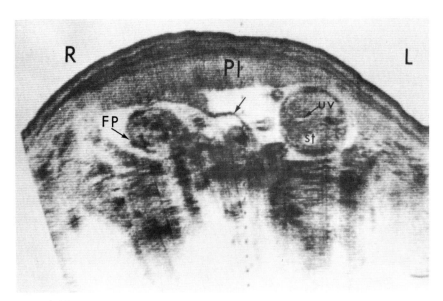

Fig. 12.69

Arrows = Septum between the amni-
otic sacs
F = Foot
FH = Fetal head
FP = Fetal pelvis
H = Head
L = Left
Numbers
1 and 2 = Separate gestational sacs
in a twin pregnancy (fig.
12.66)

Numbers
1 and 2 = Amniotic fluid (fig. 12.68)
Pl = Placenta
R = Right
st = Fetal stomach
uv = umbilical veins

Multiple Gestation

If several heads or bodies are present on ultrasound examination, the possibility of triplets should be considered. Most often, when several fetal heads are seen, the diagnosis of twins is made quite easily. An effort should be made, however, to map out the position of the fetuses on the patient's abdomen with a marking pencil. If carefully done, the diagnosis of triplets will not be missed. If we casually make the diagnosis of twins without attempting to determine the position of the fetus, however, we may miss triplets or quadruplets.

Figure 12.70 is a longitudinal scan with three fetal heads and one fetal body. When doing an examination on a patient who has a multiple gestation, it is extremely helpful to line up the fetal heads on one scan to confirm the number of fetuses present. On this scan, three of the fetal heads are aligned with one of the fetal bodies. Figure 12.71 demonstrates triplets with two fetal heads and one fetal body. We know, however, that the fetal body is separate from the two fetal heads because of the septum (arrows) separating the one fetal body from the two visualized fetal heads. The third fetal head was present much more caudally than this transverse cut.

Figures 12.72 and 12.73 are scans of another patient obtained several months apart. The initial scan was performed when the patient was at approximately 15–16 weeks' gestation. In figure 12.72 the transverse scan demonstrates a fetal head situated quite anteriorly. Suggestion of a second fetal head was noted in the posterior aspect of the uterus. This was approximately the same size as the first fetal head, and the possibility of twins was raised. The questionable fetal head, however, is situated posterior to the placenta and

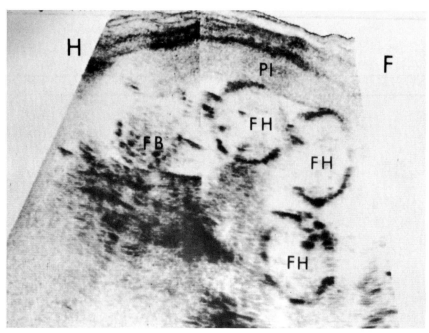

Fig. 12.70

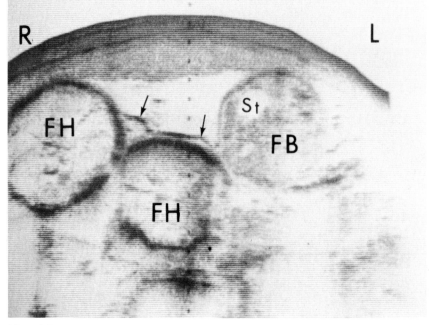

Fig. 12.71

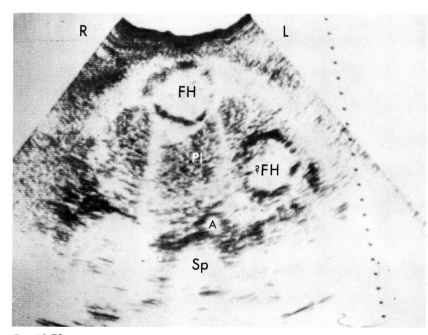

Fig. 12.72

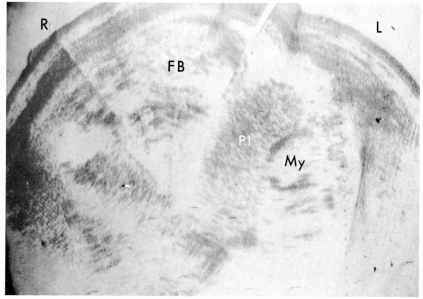

Fig. 12.73

actually in the myometrium. It was felt that this was a calcified myoma which happened to be approximately the same size as the fetal head at 16 weeks' gestation. The patient was re-examined approximately 2 months later after adequate growth of fetal head and body. Figure 12.73 is a transverse scan in which a much larger fetal body is seen anterior to the placenta. The myoma is now visualized in the myometrium of the uterus posterior to the placenta. Therefore, the finding in figure 12.72 was a calcified myoma in the myometrium that just happened to have the appearance of a fetal head.

A	=	Aorta
Arrows	=	Septum separating the amniotic cavities
F	=	Foot
FB	=	Fetal body
FH	=	Fetal head
H	=	Head
L	=	Left
My	=	Calcified myoma
Pl	=	Placenta
R	=	Right
Sp	=	Spine
St	=	Stomach

Polyhydramnios

Another cause for the patient being "large for dates" is polyhydramnios. This is commonly caused by a slight imbalance between the mother and fetus, with no definite etiology arising from the fetus. Other causes which can be diagnosed by ultrasound are anencephaly and a high gastrointestinal obstruction in the fetus. When making the diagnosis of polyhydramnios, it is important to scan the entire uterus. We often can have one or two transverse scans or one longitudinal scan demonstrating a large amount of fluid; when the entire uterus is scanned, however, it will be realized that a normal amount of fluid is present. In the case of polyhydramnios, practically all scans demonstrate a large quantity of fluid.

Figures 12.74–12.77 are transverse and longitudinal scans of a patient with an anencephalic fetus. In every scan we see an inordinate amount of fluid. The amniotic fluid is markedly increased in quantity compared to the amount of fetal echoes visualized. The placenta is quite thin, due to pressure from the polyhydramnios. Only the fetal body can be visualized in this study. During the course of the entire examination, the fetal head was never identified. One sign of polyhydramnios is that fetal extremities are seen to be floating in the amniotic fluid on numerous scans. The amount of amniotic fluid is difficult to quantitate presently. Consequently, diagnosing polyhydramnios is still a subjective procedure. In the future we hope to be able to quantitate the amount of fluid present in the uterus.

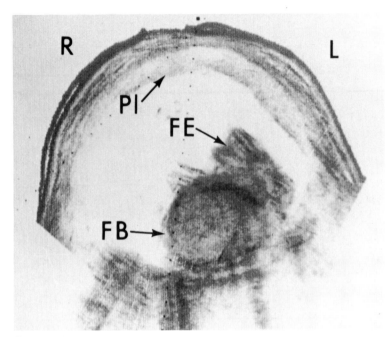

Fig. 12.74

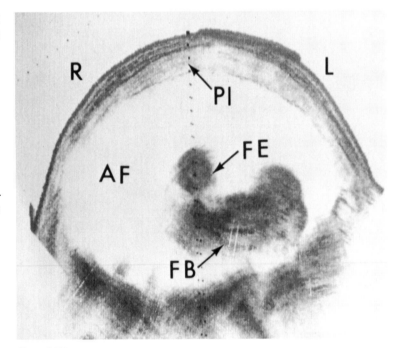

Fig. 12.75

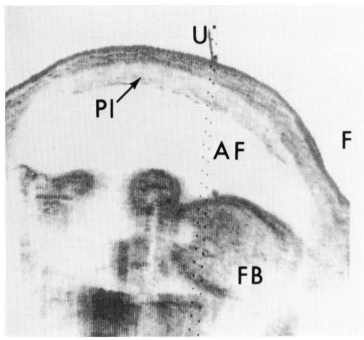

Fig. 12.76

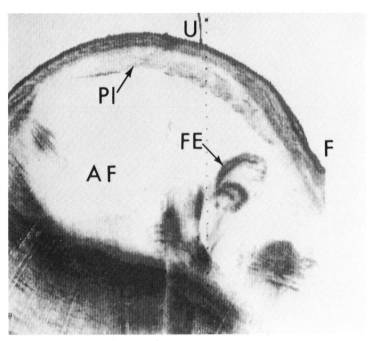

Fig. 12.77

AF = Amniotic fluid
F = Foot
FB = Fetal body
FE = Fetal extremity
L = Left
Pl = Placenta
R = Right
U = Umbilicus

Mass Associated With Pregnancy

Another reason for a patient referred to ultrasound as "large for dates" is a pelvic mass found in addition to a pregnancy. Often, a pelvic mass will elevate the uterus out of the pelvis, and clinically, the patient will appear to be "large for dates." One common mass seen during pregnancy is a corpus luteum cyst which supports the pregnancy for the first 4–5 months. Figure 12.78 is a longitudinal scan with a corpus luteum cyst situated in the cul-de-sac, elevating the fundus of the uterus to a higher position than is normally expected for the time of gestation. A gestational sac is situated in the fundus of the uterus.

Figure 12.79 is a longitudinal scan of a patient with an ovarian cyst above the fundus of the uterus. The ovarian cyst was actually palpated as the fundus of the uterus, and the patient was felt to be 6–8 weeks further along than she actually was. A gestational sac of approximately 7–8 weeks' gestation is seen. The top of the ovarian cyst, however, is approximately at the umbilical level, which would place this pregnancy at 16 weeks.

Figures 12.80 and 12.81 are transverse and longitudinal scans of a patient with a sonolucent mass in the right adnexal region. The pregnancy is situated in the midline and to the left of midline with the large sonolucent mass on the right side. The sonolucent mass has a strong linear echo in its posterior aspect indicating that this is not a simple cyst. It turned out to be a multilocular ovarian cyst that was quite large and also led to a "large-for-dates" discrepancy early on in the pregnancy.

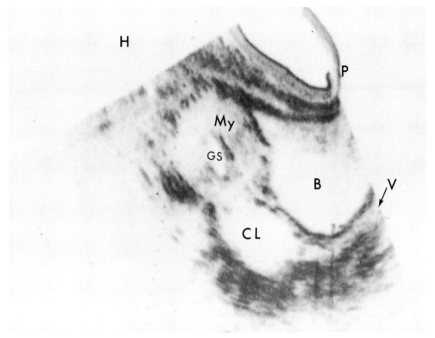

Fig. 12.78

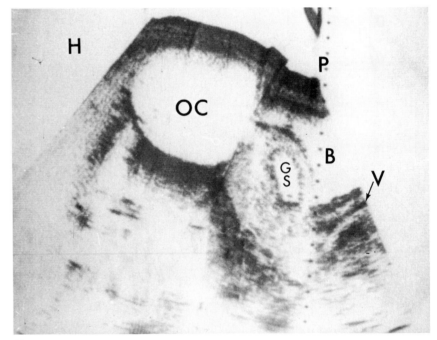

Fig. 12.79

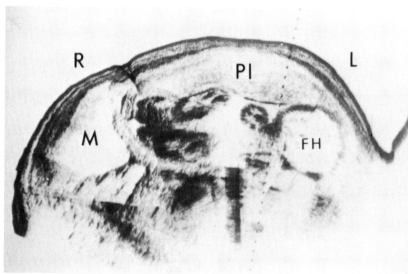

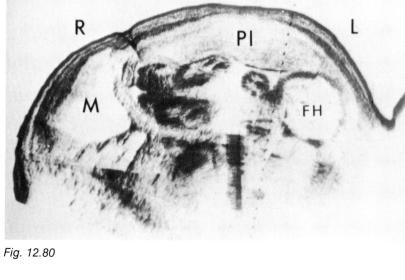

B = Urinary bladder
CL = Corpus luteum cyst
F = Foot
FH = Fetal head
GS = Gestational sac
H = Head
L = Left
M = Multiloculated ovarian cyst
My = Myometrium of the fundus of the uterus
OC = Ovarian cyst
P = Level of the symphysis pubis
PI = Placenta
R = Right
U = Umbilical level
V = Vagina

Fig. 12.80

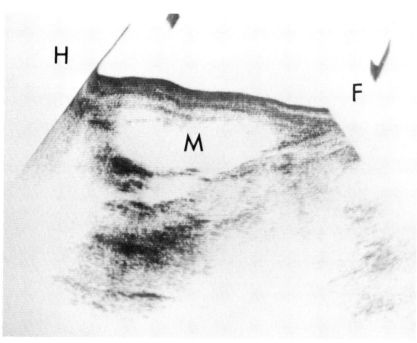

Fig. 12.81

Masses Associated with Pregnancy

Figure 12.82 is a longitudinal scan of a patient who also was considered to be "large for dates." We see a large sonolucent mass situated in the lower pelvis posterior to the cervix. The cervix is elevated anteriorly. This was not the urinary bladder. The urinary bladder was completely empty on this longitudinal scan. At surgery, it was found to be a cystic teratoma situated in the cul-de-sac and markedly elevating the lower uterine segment anteriorly and cephaladly. The large size of the mass indicates that the fundus of the uterus would be elevated 6–8 cm higher than it normally would.

Frequently, the uterus itself may have a mass which causes it to be enlarged. Figure 12.83 demonstrates a small myoma in the posterior aspect of the uterus. A gestational sac is situated in the normal fundal position. Through transmission is posterior to the gestational sac, as the myometrium has increased echoes. The myoma elevates the uterus slightly and could give a mistaken diagnosis of an enlarged uterus.

Figure 12.84 is of another myomatous uterus with the fundal region of the uterus markedly more cephalad than it would be under normal circumstances. Here we see a gestational sac situated in the fundal region of the uterus. It is approximately 4 cm in diameter which would place it at 9–10 weeks. The myoma, however, is approximately 10–12 cm in diameter. This places the fundus of the uterus at approximately 24 weeks' gestation, rather than the expected 8 weeks according to the size of the gestational sac. This would yield a clinical diagnosis of a "large-for-dates" patient. The myoma has a thoroughly characteristic echo pattern with attenuation seen posteriorly.

Figure 12.85 is a transverse scan of an interesting patient with approximately 7 weeks' gestation, as demonstrated by the size of the gestational sac. A strong echogenic mass is situated anterior to the uterus. A cleavage plane is between the mass and the uterus. This turned out to be an ovarian neoplasm which gave the patient a "large-

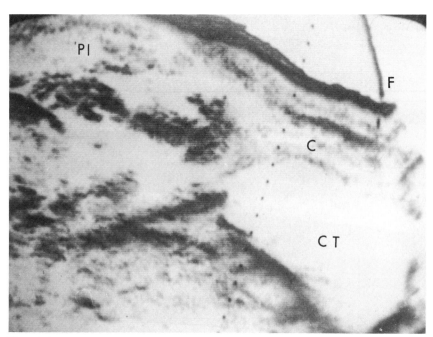

Fig. 12.82

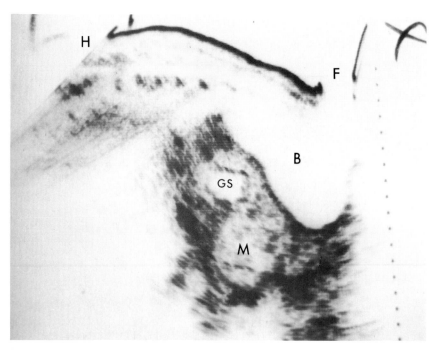

Fig. 12.83

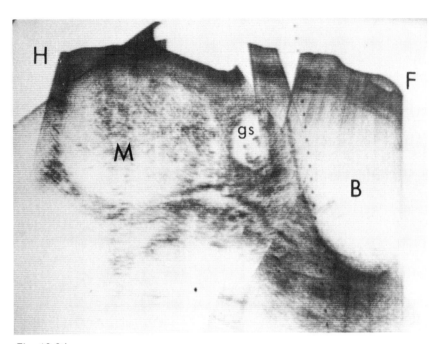

Fig. 12.84

for-dates" diagnosis. Also present in the left adnexal region is a small amount of fluid. Fluid in the pelvis is not unusual and very often is secondary to the rupture of functional cysts.

SOURCE: Figures 12.82 and 12.83 are provided through the courtesy of Dr. M. Shaub, Centinela Valley Hospital, Los Angeles, California.

B	=	Urinary bladder
C	=	Cervix
CT	=	Cystic teratoma
F	=	Foot
FI	=	Fluid
GS	=	Gestational sac
gs	=	gestational sac
H	=	Head
L	=	Left
M	=	Neoplasm (fig. 12.84)
M	=	Myoma
PI	=	Placenta
R	=	Right

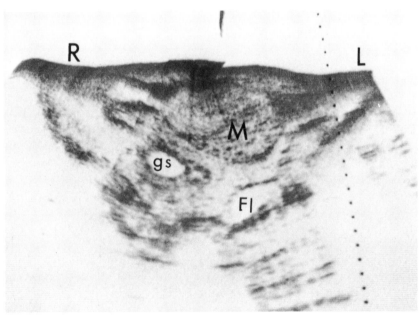

Fig. 12.85

Pelvic Kidney; Renal Transplant

Another cause for a "large-for-dates" referral, along with various masses in the pelvis, are ectopic kidneys or renal transplants. Figures 12.86 and 12.87 are scans of a pregnant woman with a pelvic kidney. The longitudinal scan (fig. 12.86) shows the kidney to be posterior to the fundal region of the uterus. The fetus is situated in the amniotic fluid with an anterior placenta. A transverse scan of the same patient is present in figure 12.87 with the kidney again seen posterior to the uterus.

Figures 12.88 and 12.89 are scans of a patient with a renal transplant in the right iliac fossa. Figure 12.88 is a transverse scan with a kidney situated in the right lateral abdomen lateral to the fetal head. A small amount of fluid is present within the kidney, secondary to mild hydronephrosis. Figure 12.89 is a longitudinal scan of the right lateral abdomen with the kidney situated in the lower right abdomen. Cephalad to the kidney, we see a relatively lucent echogenic region scanned tangentially through the myometrium of the uterus.

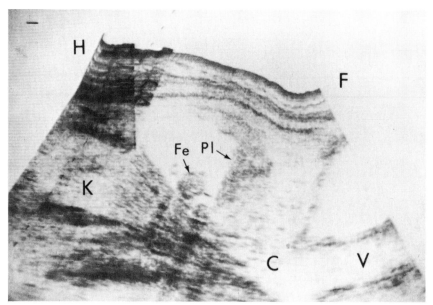

Fig. 12.86

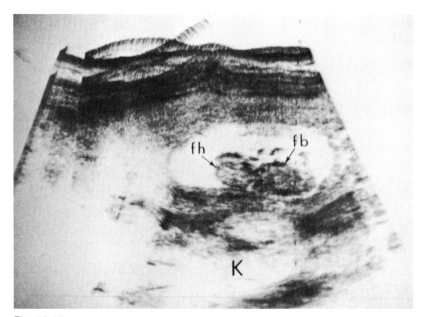

Fig. 12.87

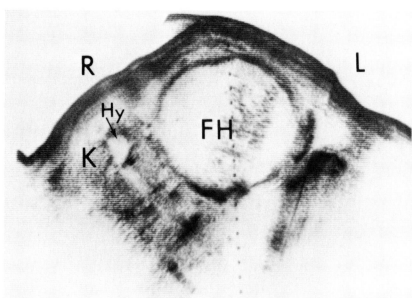

Fig. 12.88

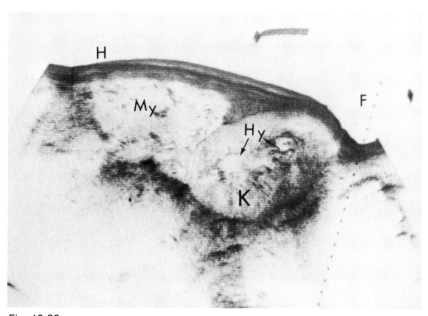

Fig. 12.89

Hydatidiform Mole

Yet another cause for a "large-for-dates" referral is a hydatidiform mole. In this instance, the fetus is felt to be at 16 or 18 weeks gestation, and no fetal heart tones are present. Usually, the clinician will request an ultrasound study to rule out fetal death. A hydatidiform mole gives a fairly characteristic echo pattern on ultrasound. Figures 12.90 and 12.91 are longitudinal and transverse scans of a patient with a molar pregnancy. Here we see a fairly even echo pattern throughout the uterus. The mole looks like placental tissue throughout. If, when scanning the uterus we find echogenicity of placental tissue throughout, the diagnosis of a molar pregnancy can be made.

Figures 12.92 and 12.93 are of another molar pregnancy within the confines of the uterus. Here we see some lucent structures indicating the larger grapelike structures within a hydatidiform mole. This type of molar pregnancy can be confused with a degenerated placenta and fetus. Even when scanning the uterus in its entirety, however, we do not find any calcific echoes or shadows when dealing with a molar pregnancy.

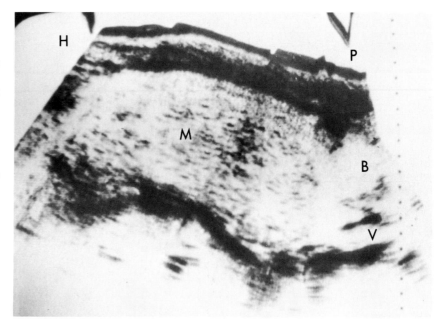

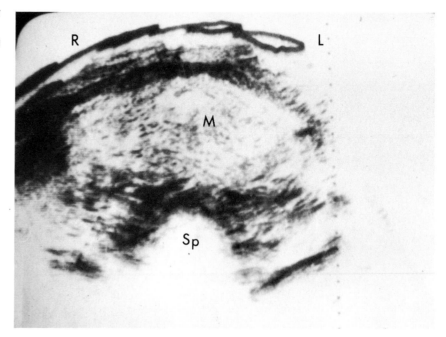

Fig. 12.91

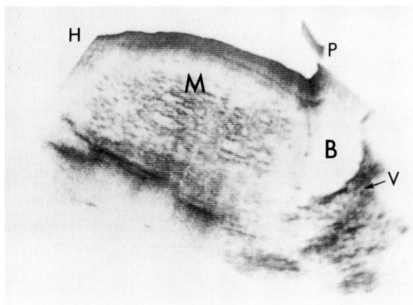

B = Urinary bladder
H = Head
L = Left
M = Hydatidiform mole
P = Level of the symphysis pubis
R = Right
Sp = Spine
V = Vagina

Fig. 12.92

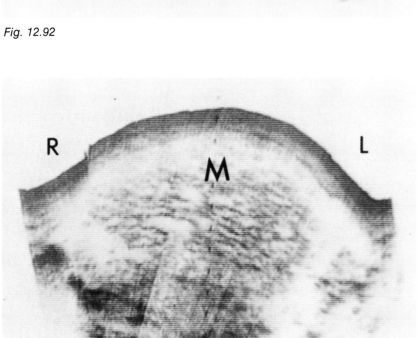

Fig. 12.93

Degenerating Placenta and Fetus

A hydatidiform mole can easily be confused for a degenerating pregnancy. Figures 12.94 and 12.95 are examples of early degeneration of the placenta (arrows). Numerous sonolucent structures are seen within the placental tissue. This is highly suggestive of a hydatidiform mole. In figure 12.94, however, we have enough amniotic fluid present, so there is no difficulty in distinguishing this as a pregnancy rather than a molar pregnancy. Figure 12.95 is a transverse scan with some remaining fetal echoes. When severe placental and fetal degeneration occurs, this picture can often be confused with a hydatidiform mole.

Figures 12.96 and 12.97 are of a degenerating pregnancy with some confusion as to whether or not we are dealing with a molar pregnancy. The longitudinal scan (fig. 12.96) demonstrates numerous strong echoes (arrows) throughout the uterus. A molar pregnancy usually has a fairly even echo pattern to it, more consistent with placental tissue. A degenerating pregnancy, as in this case, tends to have a coarser echogenic appearance. Figure 12.97 is the same case. Several sonolucent areas (arrows) are dispersed throughout the uterus. We are usually able to determine a degenerating pregnancy because of the coarseness and unevenness of the echo pattern. A molar pregnancy has a rather even speckled appearance to it. Because of the spectrum, however, overlap of the two entities is possible. In some instances, distinguishing between the two can be quite difficult.

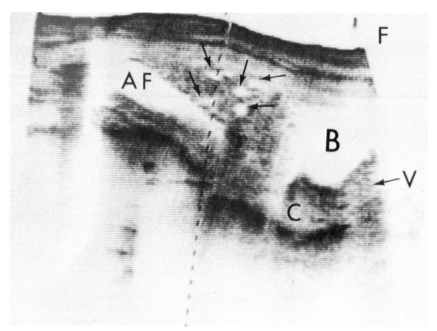

Fig. 12.94

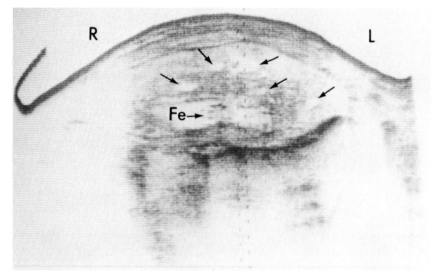

Fig. 12.95

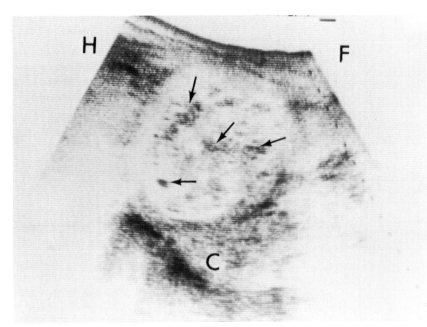

Fig. 12.96

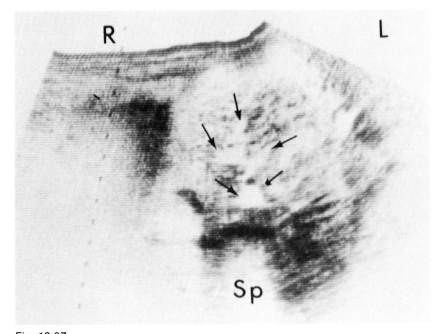

Fig. 12.97

Arrows = Degenerating placenta
AF = Amniotic fluid
B = Urinary bladder
C = Cervix
F = Foot
Fe = Fetus
H = Head
L = Left
R = Right
Sp = Spine
V = Vagina

Normal Fetal Anatomy

When examining the obstetrical patient, it is important to pay particular attention to the anatomy of the fetus. While doing a routine obstetrical study, a great deal can be discovered about the normal anatomy. This becomes extremely important when examining the fetus for various congenital anomalies. Figure 12.98 is an example of a fetal head with fluid-filled lateral ventricles. Recognizing the normal lateral ventricles is extremely important when ruling out hydrocephalus. The lateral ventricles are much more easily visualized on real-time examination.

Frequently, an evaluation of the fetal spine for such entities as spina bifida or meningomyelocele is requested. Figure 12.99 is a longitudinal scan in which we see the tubular structure of the fetal spine. Shadowing is seen also over the thoracic region secondary to the fetal ribs.

Figure 12.100 is another of the fetal spine. In the region of the cervical spine, the fetal head and upper fetal spine are seen quite well. Posterior to the fetal spine is amniotic fluid. To rule out a meningocele or a meningomyelocele, close scrutiny of this cervical region would be ncessary. In following the fetal spine in a cephalad portion, a mass in the posterior cervical region can be ruled out. We can also scan the fetal spine in the lower sacral area to rule out any masses in this region. Figure 12.101 is a longitudinal scan in which the step-like echoes of the vertebral bodies are actually seen. The vertebral bodies yield this characteristic echo which can identify the fetal spinal column quite easily.

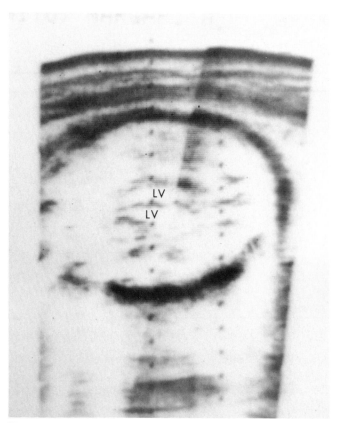

Fig. 12.98

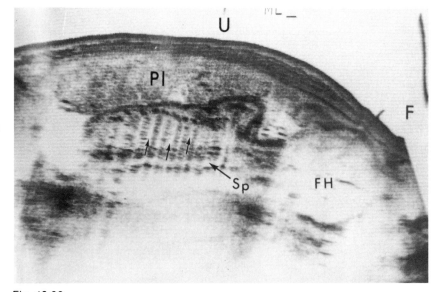

Fig. 12.99

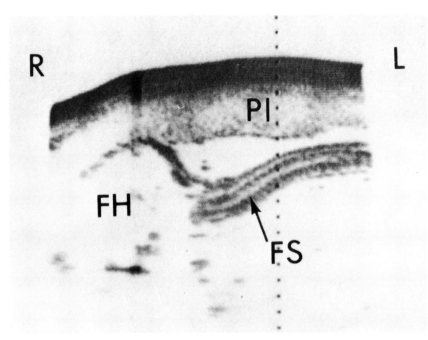

AF = Amniotic fluid
Arrows = Shadowing from the ribs
F = Foot
FH = Fetal head
FS = Fetal spine
H = Head
L = Left
LV = Lateral ventricles
PI = Placenta
R = Right
Sp = Fetal spine
U = Umbilical level
Ve = Vertebral bodies

Fig. 12.100

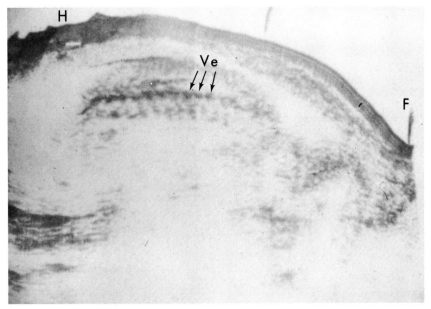

Fig. 12.101

Normal Fetal Anatomy

Figure 12.102 is a transverse section of a fetus in the thoracic region. Here we see the fetal spine in a transverse plane. It appears as a circular echogenic region in the posterior aspect of the fetus. If a severe spina bifida were present, a defect would appear in the posterior aspect of the spine. A sonolucency is noted in the anterior half of the fetal thorax on this scan; this represents the fetal heart. By scanning slowly over the fetal cardiac region in either a transverse or longitudinal plane, fetal cardiac activity can be documented by B-scan. If there is any question at all, either Doppler or real time can be used to document fetal cardiac activity.

Figure 12.103 is a transverse scan over the fetal abdomen. Again we see the fetal spine in the posterior aspect of the fetal abdomen. A sonolucent area is present in the left upper quadrant; this is secondary to fluid in the fetal stomach. We can document fetal swallowing as fluid is recognized routinely in the fetal stomach. The linear tubular structure in the anterior half of the fetal abdomen is secondary to the umbilical vessels coursing through the fetal abdomen. This is an important landmark when attempting to measure the abdominal circumference of the fetus. Figure 12.104 is another transverse scan through the fetal abdomen with the fetal spine situated posteriorly. The left kidney is recognized posterior to the fetal stomach. Looking for renal abnormalities in utero, we can easily identify the fetal kidneys in the mid and third trimester.

Another transverse scan (fig. 12.105) allows both kidneys to be visualized this time. The left kidney is situated posterior to the fluid-filled fetal stomach again. In this instance, the fetal spleen is recognized lateral to the left kidney and fetal stomach. The paraspinous muscles are posterior to the kidneys.

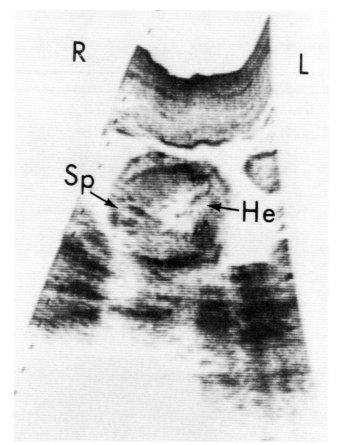

Fig. 12.102

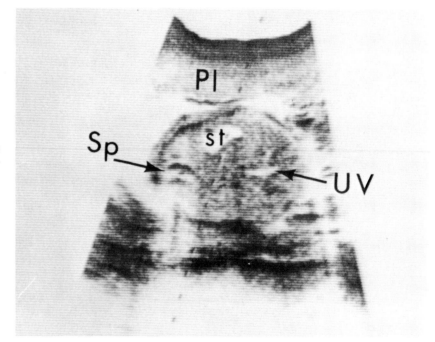

Fig. 12.103

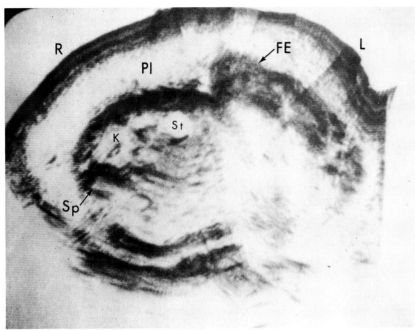

Fig. 12.104

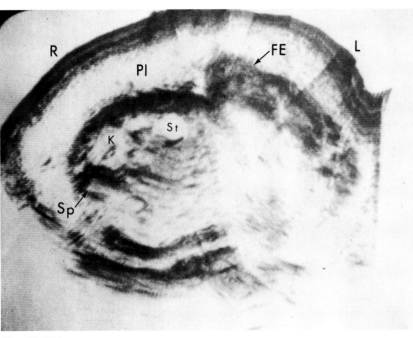

Fig. 12.105

FE = Fetal extremity
He = Fetal heart
K = Fetal kidneys
L = Left
Pl = Placenta
PM = Paraspinous muscles
R = Right
S = Spleen
Sp = Fetal spine
St = Fetal stomach
st = Stomach
UV = Umbilical vessels

Normal Fetal Anatomy

Figure 12.106 is a coronal section of the fetus with the fetal heart in the thorax of the fetus. Just caudal to the fetal heart is the sonolucency of the stomach. This scan is an unusual one; the left kidney is visualized in the coronal plane. Figure 12.107 is another coronal section with the descending aorta just below the fetal heart. In this scan we are able to visualize both the right and left kidneys in a coronal section.

In figure 12.108 the thoracic and abdominal aorta is seen. The aorta in longitudinal scans presents as a small tubular structure. When scanning over the aorta at a rather slow rate, cardiac pulsations can actually be detected in the walls. The small size of the aorta in this scan is noted. The lumen is approximately 2 mm in diameter which demonstrates some of the resolution presently available with the various equipment. The mother often asks to know the sex of the baby. If the scan is successful, and the sex is evident, the scrotum may be detected. Figure 12.109 is a scan through the pelvis of the fetus; the urine-filled fetal bladder is seen. The scrotum is recognized in the amniotic fluid. Fetal urine production can be followed by measuring the volume of the fetal bladder at various intervals.

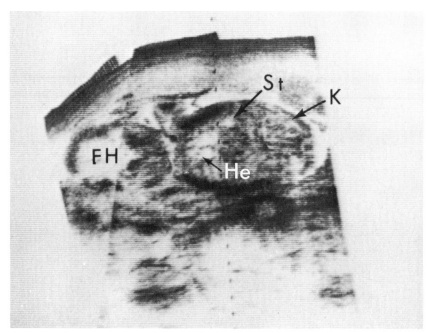

Fig. 12.106

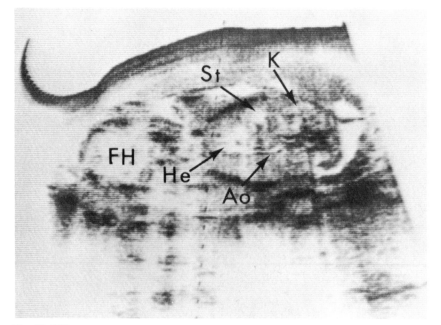

Fig. 12.107

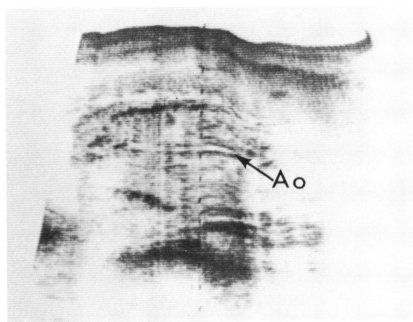

Ao = Aorta
FB = Fetal bladder
FH = Fetal head
He = Heart
K = Kidney
L = Left
R = Right
Sc = Scrotum
St = Stomach

Fig. 12.108

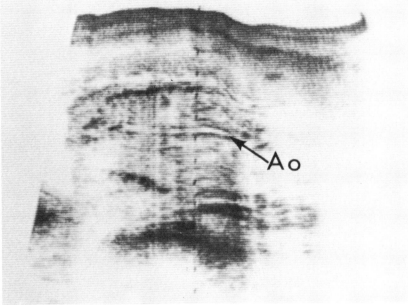

Fig. 12.109

Normal Fetal Anatomy

Figure 12.110 is a longitudinal scan over the lateral uterus with the characteristic echoes of a fetal extremity cut transversely. The fetal extremities yield a strong central echo arising from the osseous structure surrounded by the soft echoes of the muscle. Numerous parallel lines are noted on this scan. These are characteristic echoes arising from the umbilical cord. Figure 12.111 is a scan of the lower extremity of the fetus. The femur is situated in the thigh. Caudal to this, the tibia is visualized in the calf. The diagnosis of dwarfism may be possible with ultrasound when the osseous structures can be seen in such detail. Figure 12.112 is an excellent example of visualization of the upper extremity. The arm can be seen situated lateral to the fetal trunk. The strong echoes arising from the humerus are seen between the shoulder and fetal elbow. The forearm and digits of the hand can be seen quite well. Figure 12.113 is a well-known slide provided by Dr. Peter Cooperberg. It expresses most aptly the feeling of the majority of fetuses to ultrasonic probing.

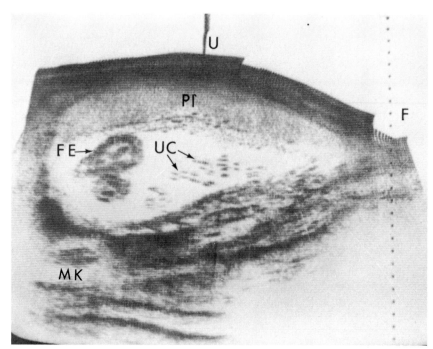

Fig. 12.110

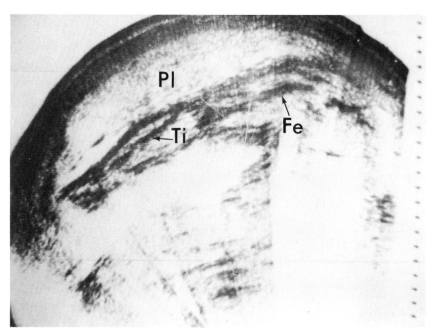

Fig. 12.111

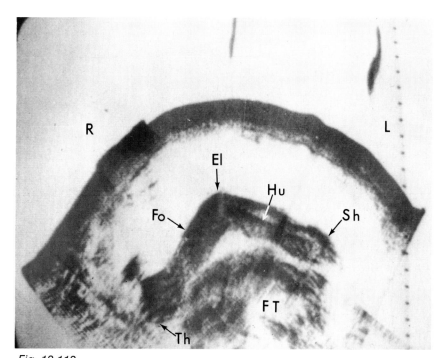

Fig. 12.112

SOURCE: Figure 12.113 is provided through the courtesy of Dr. P. Cooperberg, University of British Columbia, Vancouver, British Columbia, Canada.

El	=	Elbow
F	=	Foot
FE	=	Fetal extremity
Fe	=	Femur
Figure 12.113	=	Bowel loops in ascites
Fo	=	Forearm
FT	=	Fetal trunk
Hu	=	Humerus
L	=	Left
MK	=	Maternal kidney
Pl	=	Placenta
R	=	Right
Sh	=	Shoulder
Th	=	Thumb
Ti	=	Tibia
U	=	Umbilical level
UC	=	Umbilical cord

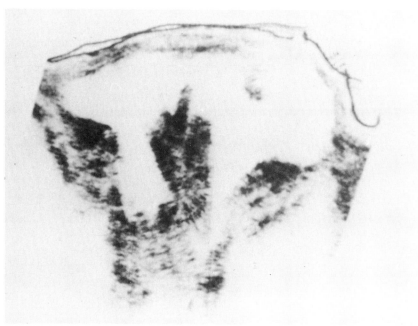

Fig. 12.113

Anencephaly; Hydrocephaly

An elevated alpha fetoprotein in the amniotic fluid very often indicates a neural tube defect. One of the commoner reasons for elevation of the alpha fetoprotein is anencephaly. Figures 12.114 and 12.115 are examples of an ultrasound examination on anencephalic fetuses. It is extremely important to attempt to line up the fetal body with the supposed site of the fetal head when trying to detect an anencephalic fetus. If the fetal body can be lined up correctly, a cluster of echoes can be visualized in the region of the fetal head. This cluster of echoes is fairly characteristic for an anencephalic fetus.

Figure 12.114 demonstrates numerous ill-defined echoes in the region of the fetal head. These are not the characteristic echoes of a biparietal diameter. The discrepancy in size between the fetal head and the fetal body is noted. This is usually present in an anencephalic. Figure 12.115 is another example with a cluster of echoes in the region of the fetal head. Again, the diameter and size of the fetal head is smaller than expected for the size of the fetal body.

Figures 12.116 and 12.117 are examples of a hydrocephalic fetus. In this instance, the opposite size discrepancy is true. The head size is much larger than expected for the fetal body. In figure 12.116 the head is one-and-a-half times as large as expected for the size of the fetal body. In figure 12.117 the head size is not only large, but fairly sonolucent for its size. Hydrocephalus often is most easily diagnosed by real-time examination. In real-time studies the ventricles stand out more easily than on a B-scan examination.

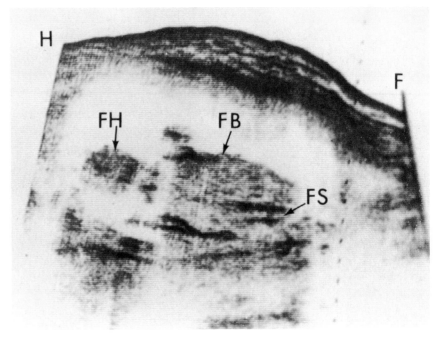

Fig. 12.114

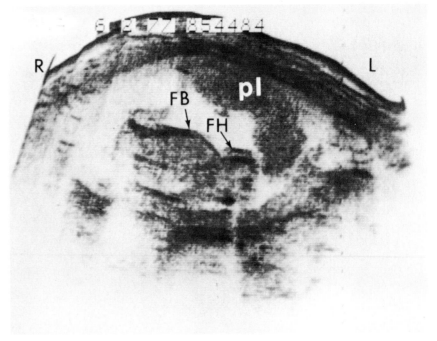

Fig. 12.115

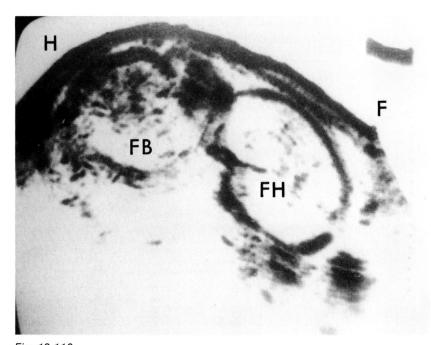

Fig. 12.116

SOURCE: Figures 12.116 and 12.117 are provided through the courtesy of Dr. M. Shaub, Centinela Valley Hospital, Los Angeles, California.

B	=	Urinary bladder
F	=	Foot
FB	=	Fetal body
FH	=	Fetal head
FS	=	Fetal spine
H	=	Head
L	=	Left
Pl	=	Placenta
R	=	Right

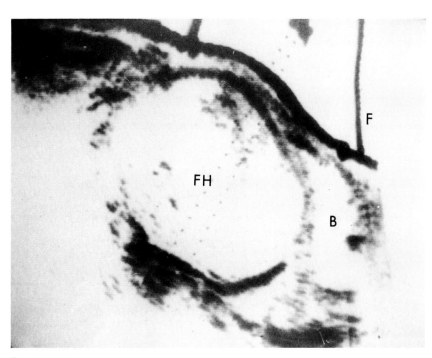

Fig. 12.117

Dandy-Walker Syndrome; Single Ventricle; IUGR; Triploidy

When examining the fetus during the course of an obstetrical study, we may find a discrepancy between the size of the fetal head and body. It then becomes necessary to determine whether or not the head, the body, or one of the two is inordinately "small for dates." In this instance, it is important to have an adequate menstrual history in an effort to determine the abnormality. Figure 12.118 is a scan of a fetus with a markedly enlarged fetal head. There are no echoes noted within the head, indicating that it is a fluid-filled structure. The size of the head is markedly enlarged compared with the size of the fetal body. This was an extremely unusual case of an abnormally dilated fourth ventricle in the Dandy-Walker syndrome. Not only is the head size abnormal, but its sonolucent appearance indicates that the abnormality is in the head and not in the fetal body.

Figure 12.119 is another example of a markedly enlarged and sonolucent head in comparison to the fetal body. As in figure 12.118, the fetal head is relatively sonolucent, indicating that it is a fluid-filled structure. This case turned out to be a single ventricle in which the brain substance was markedly compressed, secondary to the ventricular fluid.

Occasionally, however, we encounter a fetus in which the fetal body is actually small compared to a normally sized head. One of the more common reasons for this is intrauterine-growth retardation. Often, the fetus will spare the fetal brain at the expense of the fetal body in the entity of intrauterine growth retardation.

Figure 12.120 is an example of such a case. There is a normally sized fetal head and an abnormally small fetal body. This actually represents fetal wasting, secondary to growth retardation. Total intrauterine volume has been used to diagnose intrauterine-growth retardation earlier than has been previously possible. This severe degree of growth retardation, with the fetal body smaller than the fetal head, usually is an ominous sign.

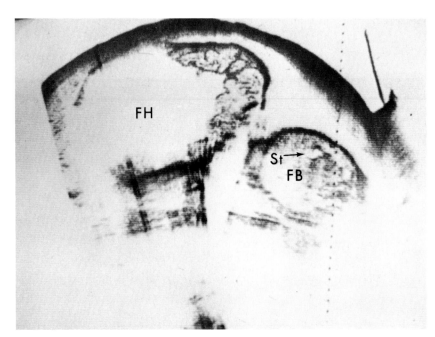

Fig. 12.118

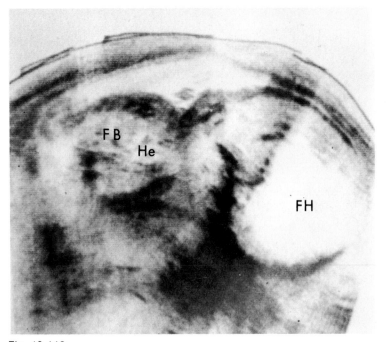

Fig. 12.119

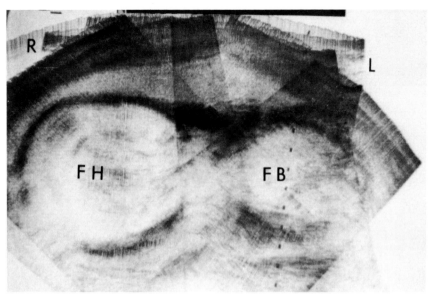

Fig. 12.120

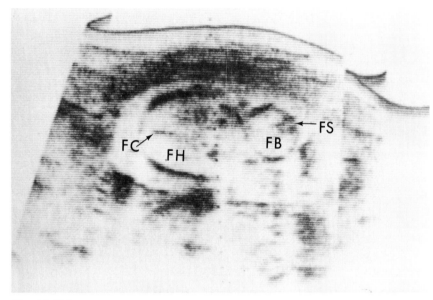

Fig. 12.121

Figure 12.121 is a case of an abnormally small fetal body in early pregnancy at approximately 20 weeks. In this instance, the fetal head was of normal size and growing at a normal rate. The fetal body, however, not only was abnormally small, but its growth rate was decreased over the normal range. Because of the ultrasonic findings, the patient underwent an elective abortion. She was found to have a triploidy (69 chromosomes) in which the fetal head was within normal size, and the fetal body was abnormally small.

SOURCE: The case for figure 12.119 is provided through the courtesy of Dr. R. Filly, University of California, San Francisco, California.

FB	=	Fetal body
FC	=	Falx cerebri
FH	=	Fetal head
FS	=	Fetal spine
He	=	Heart
L	=	Left
R	=	Right
St	=	Stomach

Cystic Lymphangioma

During the course of an ultrasound examination, an inordinate amount of fluid may be found and the diagnosis of polyhydramnios made. We should, however, look closely at the fluid to make sure that is free within the uterine cavity. Very rarely, a fluid-filled mass contained within a curvilinear echo will be seen.

Figures 12.122–12.125 represent two separate cases with large fluid-filled masses contained within a structure that appears to be attached to the fetus. The possibility of a meningocele or meningomyelocele was strongly considered. Both of these cases are examples of cystic lymphangiomas arising from the fetal neck and base of the skull. Figures 12.122 and 12.123 show the large fluid-filled mass contained within a structure which appears to be separate from the amniotic fluid. In figure 12.123, the mass is situated in close proximity to the fetal head.

Figures 12.124 and 12.125 are another case, again with a large sonolucent mass. Figure 12.125 is the more important scan in that the curvilinear echo demonstrates that the fluid-filled mass is not amniotic fluid. If it were secondary to amniotic fluid, the fetus would be seen floating more freely in the uterine cavity. In most of these cases, the fetus is situated on one side of the uterine cavity, because it is displaced by the large cystic mass.

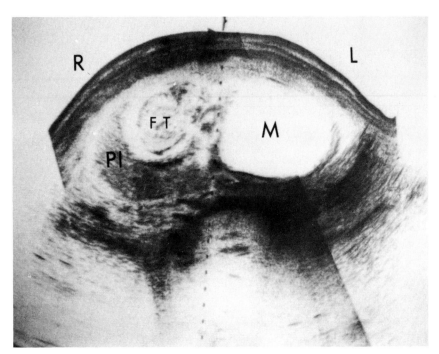

Fig. 12.122

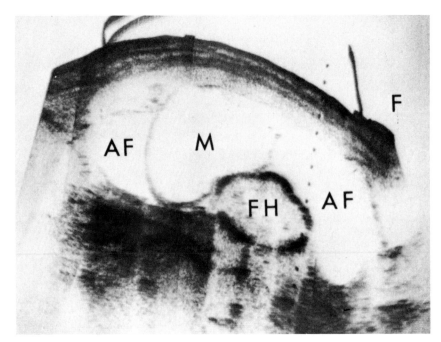

Fig. 12.123

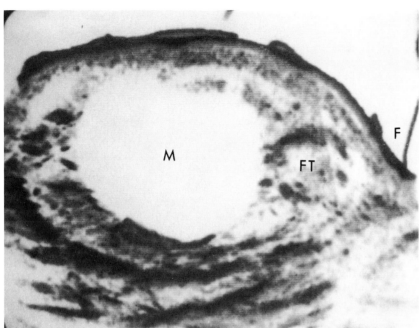

Fig. 12.124

SOURCE: Figures 12.124 and 12.125 are provided through the courtesy of Dr. M. Shaub, Centinela Valley Hospital, Los Angeles, California.

AF = Amniotic fluid
F = Foot
FH = Fetal head
FT = Fetal trunk
L = Left
M = Cystic lymphangioma
Pl = Placenta
R = Right

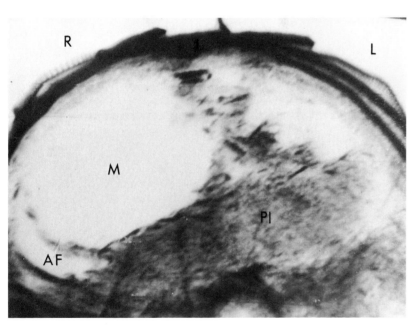

Fig. 12.125

Siamese Twins; Fetal Death of One Twin

During the course of an ultrasound examination of fetal twins, often a normal biparietal diameter is obtained for one twin, but there is difficulty with the biparietal diameter of the second, usually because of its position. It is important to be meticulous in the examination of twins because of the possibility of fetal abnormalities to either one or both. Figures 12.126–12.128 are examples of an unusual case in which the diagnosis of Siamese twins was made by ultrasound examination. In the transverse scan of the abdomen (fig. 12.126) the fetal heads of the twins are seen. At this level, the twins are definitely separate, and there is no difficulty in detecting the fact that a twin pregnancy is present. Continuing down the maternal abdomen, however, we begin to see evidence of fusion of the fetal trunks (fig. 12.127). Even though there is suggestion of a separation, the twins could not be completely separated at this point. Figure 12.128 is a transverse scan of the maternal abdomen, slightly more caudal than figure 12.127. It is at this juncture that separation of the fetal abdomen is completely impossible. Complete fusion of the fetal bodies, with no discernible septum, is seen. Because of the ultrasonic findings, the diagnosis of Siamese twins was suggested. This was confirmed at cesarian section.

When examining twins, we may find marked abnormality of one of the fetuses. Figure 12.129 is an example of a twin pregnancy with a normal fetal head seen near the lower uterine segment. A large amount of amniotic fluid is present. The linear septum, which indicates a twin pregnancy, is visualized, but in the fundal region of the uterus is a cluster of echoes representing the second fetus. It was difficult to make out any normal anatomy within this fetus. A biparietal diameter was not obtainable. Echoes about the fetal body were also difficult to visualize. Because of this finding, the possibility of fetal anomaly or fetal death was considered.

The patient delivered approximately 4 days after the ultrasound examination. The viable fetus died of respiratory dis-

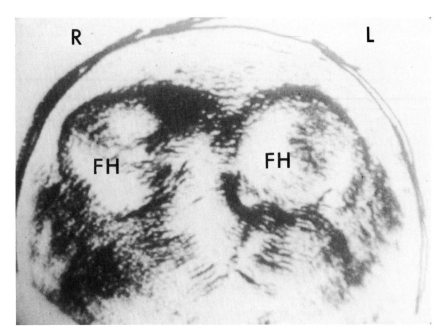

Fig. 12.126

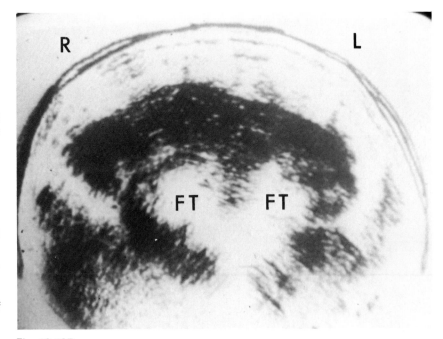

Fig. 12.127

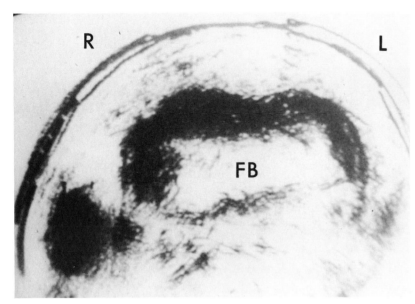

Fig. 12.128

tress syndrome 36 hours after delivery. The second fetus had undergone marked degeneration and decomposition from a fetal death in utero. Because of the marked distortion of the fetus, secondary to death, the ultrasound picture was quite confusing.

SOURCE: The case for figures 12.126–12.128 is provided through the courtesy of Dr. M. Shaub, Centinela Valley Hospital, Los Angeles, California.

B = Urinary bladder
FB = Fetal body
Fe = Fetal demise
FH = Fetal head
FT = Fetal trunk
L = Left
P = Level of the symphysis pubis
PI = Placenta
R = Right
S = Septation separating the twin pregnancy
U = Umbilicus

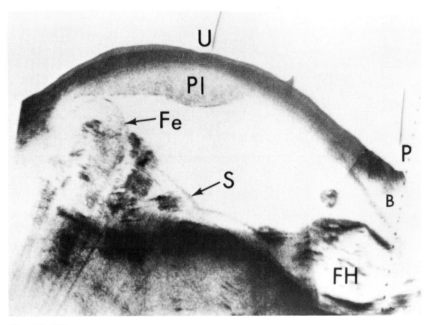

Fig. 12.129

Jejunal Atresia; Prune-belly Syndrome; Omphalocele

We normally can see fluid in the fetal stomach during a fetal examination. The urinary bladder of the fetus may also be fluid-filled. Very rarely, a few small lucencies in the abdomen will be noted secondary to normal filling of the small bowel with amniotic fluid. If there is an inordinate amount of bowel loops or sonolucent masses present in the abdomen, it is necessary to scrutinize the fetus in closer detail. Figure 12.130 demonstrates numerous sonolucent structures which remained fairly well fixed in position in the fetal abdomen during the course of an ultrasound examination. Three large sonolucent circular structures, which represent fluid-filled bowel, are seen. This fetus was eventually diagnosed as having jejeunal atresia. Very often, a high gastrointestinal obstruction in the fetus can lead to polyhydramnios. When fluid-filled structures within the fetus, which do not change position, are seen the possibility of a gastrointestinal obstruction should be considered.

Figures 12.131 and 12.132 are another example of a fetus with numerous large circular and tubular fluid-filled structures. In this instance, however, the fluid-filled structures were secondary to the genitourinary tract. This was found to be hydroureter and hydronephrosis, secondary to prune-belly syndrome. We see the large fluid-filled ureters filling the entire abdomen and causing marked distention of the fetal abdomen. Because of the large abdomen, a cesarian section had to be performed in order to deliver the fetus.

Figure 12.133 is an unusual case with the fetal abdominal contents visualized outside the fetal body. This is a case of an omphalocele. Fetal omphalocele will elevate the alpha fetal proteins as will neural tube defects. When examining a fetus with an elevated alpha fetal protein, not only should the cervical and sacral regions be studied for meningoceles, but also the anterior abdomen should be inspected to rule out an omphalocele.

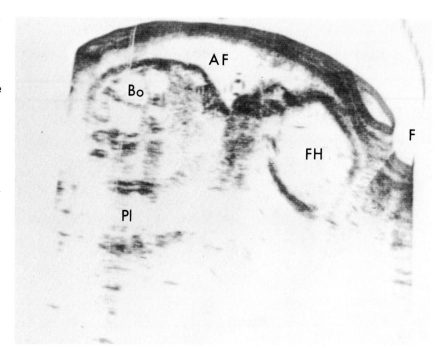

Fig. 12.130

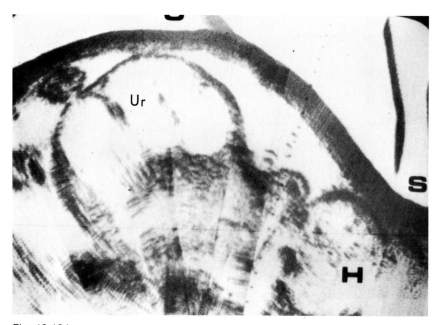

Fig. 12.131

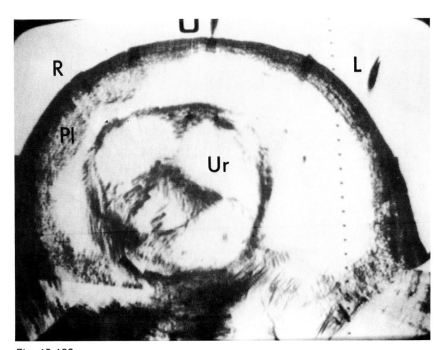

Fig. 12.132

Source: Figure 12.130 is provided through the courtesy of Dr. R. Hoffman, Torrance Memorial Hospital, Torrance, California.

Figure 12.133 is provided through the courtesy of Dr. D. McQuown, Long Beach Memorial Hospital, Long Beach, California.

Ab	=	Abdominal contents outside the fetal body secondary to an omphalocele
AF	=	Amniotic fluid
Bo	=	Dilated bowel secondary to jejeunal atresia
F	=	Foot
FB	=	Fetal body
FH	=	Fetal head
H	=	Fetal head
L	=	Left
Pl	=	Placenta
S	=	Level of the symphysis pubis
R	=	Right
U	=	Level of the umbilicus
Ur	=	Dilated ureter secondary to prune-belly

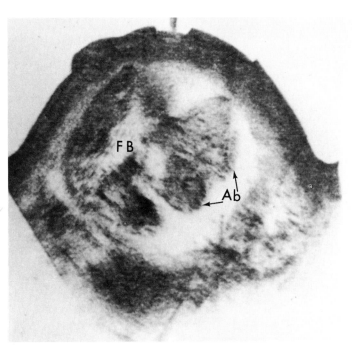

Fig. 12.133

Fetal Ascites

Fetal ascites presents ultrasonic findings similar to those seen in the adult. Fetal ascites can occur in a patient with Rh sensitization. When the fetus is severely affected with Rh incompatibility, marked ascites can develop. Figure 12.134 is a longitudinal scan of the fetus with a large amount of ascitic fluid. The abdomen is somewhat enlarged, secondary to the amount of ascitic fluid. Cephalad to the ascitic fluid, the highly echogenic liver is seen. Figure 12.135 is a transverse scan of the upper abdomen with the characteristic findings of ascites similar to that found in the adult. The ascitic fluid is situated between the abdominal wall and the liver, which is floating away from the abdominal wall. The circular structure in the liver is secondary to a dilated umbilical vein. Figure 12.136 is an interesting transverse scan of the fetus. The umbilical cord, as it enters the fetal abdomen, actually can be seen. It divides in the ascitic fluid as it enters the fetal abdomen.

Ultrasound can be used to assist in fetal transfusions. Used in conjunction with fluoroscopy, the fluoroscopy time can be decreased markedly. Figure 12.137 is a scan performed on the lateral aspect of the mother while a fetal transfusion was being performed. Here we see the needle as it enters the fetal abdomen. It is easily detected because of the surrounding ascitic fluid.

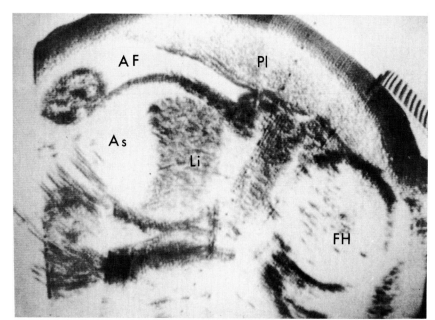

Fig. 12.134

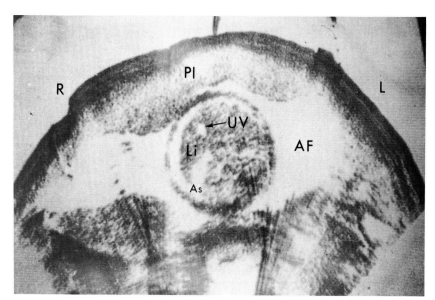

Fig. 12.135

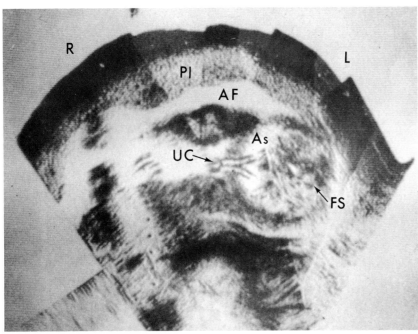

AF = Amniotic fluid
As = Ascitic fluid
FH = Fetal head
FS = Fetal spine
L = Left
Li = Liver
N = Transfusion needle
PI = Placenta
R = Right
UC = Umbilical cord
UV = Umbilical vein

Fig. 12.136

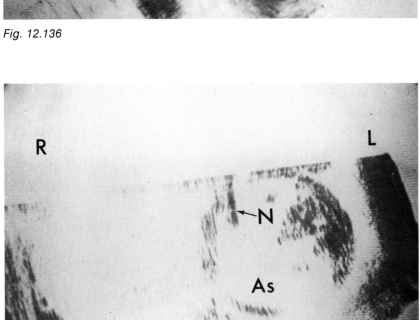

Fig. 12.137

Maternal Anatomy

Often, when scanning the pregnant uterus, sonolucent structures are visualized posterior to the uterus. Very often, this represents the maternal aorta and inferior vena cava if it is near the midline. We will, however, occasionally see a sonolucent structure posterior to the lateral aspect of the uterus. Figure 12.138 is a transverse scan with a circular structure posterior to the uterus on the right side. This represents a dilated right ureter. Of course, this is a common finding in pregnancy, since right hydroureter and hydronephrosis is often seen. Figure 12.139 is a longitudinal scan which attempts to delineate further the right ureter. The dilated tubular ureter is seen on top of the right iliopsoas muscle. The placenta and amniotic fluid are anterior to the right ureter.

Figure 12.140 is a longitudinal scan of the right kidney in the supine position. There is evidence of mild hydronephrosis secondary to the right hydroureter. Occasionally, when examining the lower uterine segment, a sonolucent structure is seen posterior to the vagina. Figure 12.141 is an example of such a case; fluid is actually seen in the rectum. This may be seen following enemas or in cases where the mother is suffering from gastrointestinal problems.

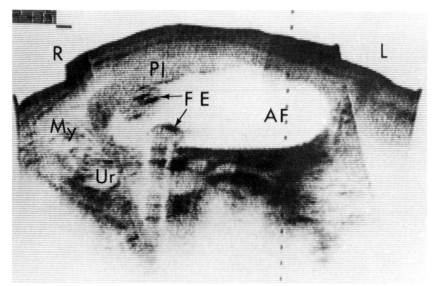

Fig. 12.138

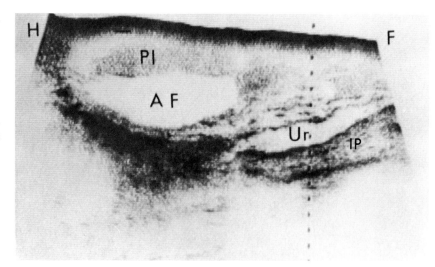

Fig. 12.139

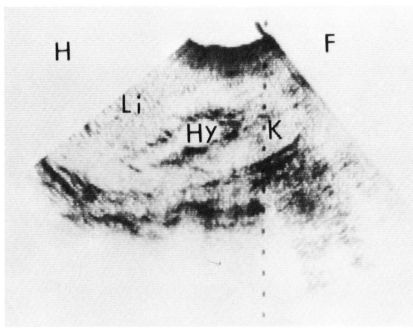

Fig. 12.140

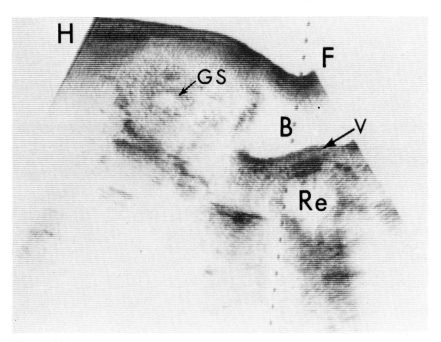

Fig. 12.141

AF = Amniotic fluid
B = Urinary bladder
F = Foot
FE = Fetal extremities
GS = Gestational sac
H = Head
Hy = Mild hydronephrosis
IP = Iliopsoas muscle
K = Kidney
L = Left
Li = Liver
My = Myometrium
Pl = Placenta
R = Right
Re = Fluid-filled rectum
Ur = Dilated right ureter
V = Vagina

Fetal Death

If there is any question as to fetal viability, it is important to do a Doppler or real-time examination in an effort to detect fetal cardiac activity. Several signs, however, give evidence of fetal death on a routine B-scan examination. The most common sign is finding fetal edema about the head or the body. Although this is not automatically consistent with fetal death, it is highly suspicious. Fetal edema and congestive heart failure may be seen in the fetus. Figures 12.142 and 12.143 are examples of fetal edema registering as a double ring sign around the fetal head. Edema is usually seen entirely around the fetal head. Mistakes can be made when the fetus is in close contact to the urinary bladder which will give a false double ring sign.

Another sign of fetal death is evidence of collapse of the normal contour of the fetal head. Figure 12.144 is an example of distortion of the fetal head. Marked straightening (arrows) of the fetal contour which is markedly abnormal is noted. When we see abnormality of the fetal skull, a Doppler or real-time examination should be performed. Figure 11.145 is an example of the overlapping of the skull bones which is another sign of fetal death. Ultrasonic visualization of overlapping of the fetal skull has the same significance as the X-ray finding of an overlapping skull. Both indicate fetal death.

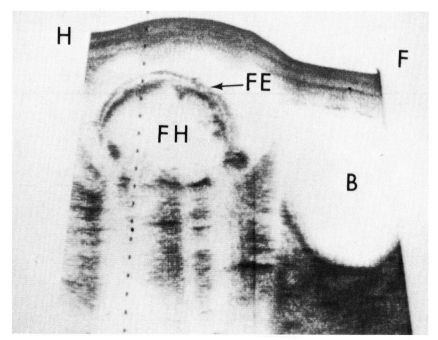

Fig. 12.142

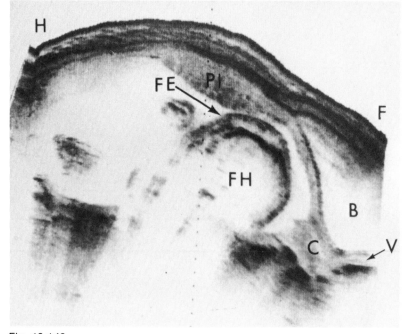

Fig. 12.143

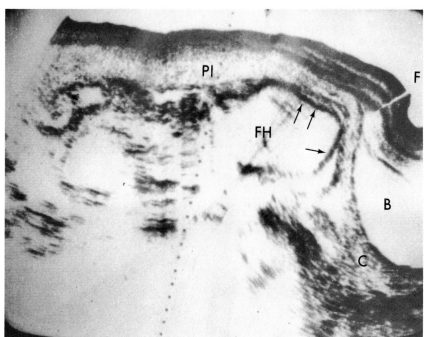

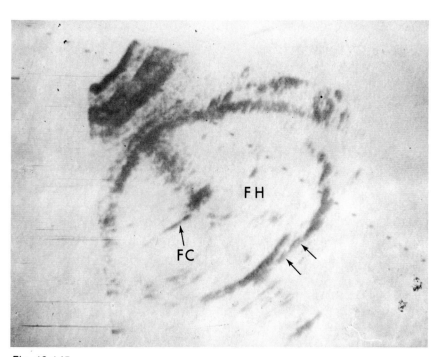

Arrows = Distortion of fetal skull (fig. 12.144)
Arrows = Overlapping skull echoes (fig. 12.145)
B = Urinary bladder
C = Cervix
F = Foot
FC = Falx cerebri
FE = Fetal edema
FH = Fetal head
H = Head
Pl = Placenta
V = Vagina

Fig. 12.144

Fig. 12.145

Fetal Death

Another indication of fetal death is the empty fetal thorax sign. When the fetal thorax is markedly distorted, this should be considered. Figures 12.146 and 12.147 are of a twin pregnancy. One of the twins is no longer viable. Here we see the empty-thorax sign. The normal echo pattern of the fetal thorax is not seen. Instead, the thorax appears more lucent with coarser echoes within it. There is a marked distortion of the contour of the fetal thorax compared with normal fetal body seen in figure 12.147. The normal circular-to-oval structure of the fetal thorax is lost. We are seeing evidence of degeneration of the fetus with collapse of the fetal thorax, similar to collapse of the fetal skull.

Figure 12.148 is an example of distortion of the fetal spine (arrows). Normally the fetal spine is fairly straight on longitudinal scan. Marked distortion and angulation of the fetal spine, however, are present. This ultrasonic finding corresponds to the marked angulation in fetal death on X-ray. We again see evidence of fetal degeneration when this marked anatomic distortion takes place. Figure 12.149 is an example of collapse of the fetal head and the fetal body. We see severe oligohydramnios along with marked difficulty in visualizing the normal fetal structures.

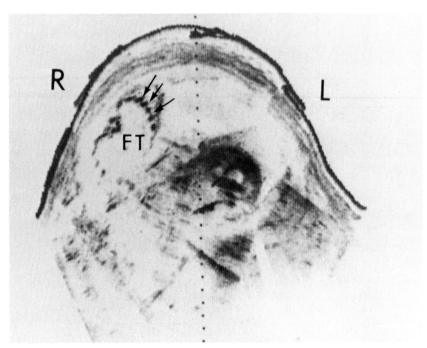

Fig. 12.146

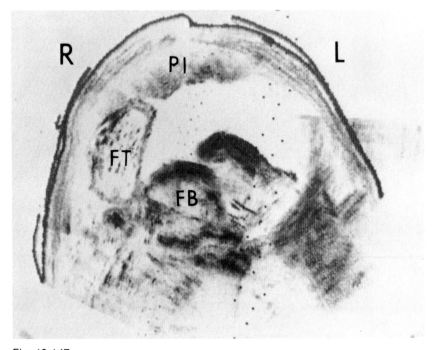

Fig. 12.147

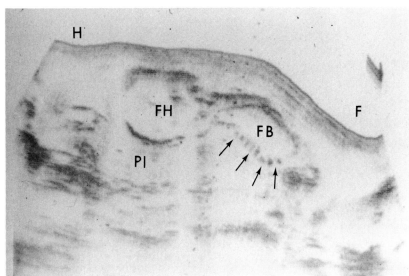

Fig. 12.148

Arrows = Ribs (fig. 12.146)
Arrows = Collapse and marked angulation
of the fetal spine (fig. 12.148)
B = Urinary bladder
F = Foot
FB = Fetal body of the normal twin
FH = Fetal head
FT = Collapsed fetal thorax
H = Head
L = Left
PI = Placenta
R = Right

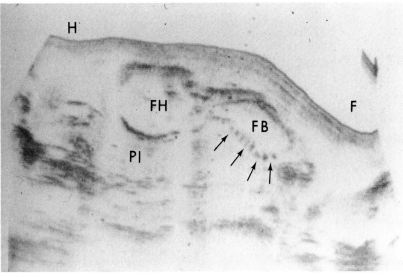

Fig. 12.149

Fetal Death

Separation of the amnion from the chorion may be visualized in fetal death. During early pregnancy, the amnion and chorion are not in contact. Chorionic fluid is found between the amnion and chorion. By approximately the eighteenth to twentieth week of pregnancy, the amnion and chorion come into contact, with no evidence of any space between them. In some instances of fetal demise, however, fluid may collect between the amnion and chorion, separating the amnion away from the placenta and the surrounding uterine cavity. The case in figures 12.150–12.153 is an example of separation of the amnion (arrows) from the chorion. The potential space of the chorionic cavity is now filled with fluid. Sometimes, this finding can be confused for a fetal abnormality such as a meningomyelocele or other fluid collection attached to the fetus. When examining the fetus closely, however, we often find that this curvilinear echo is completely surrounding the fetus. It actually represents separation of the amnionic membrane from the lining of the uterine cavity.

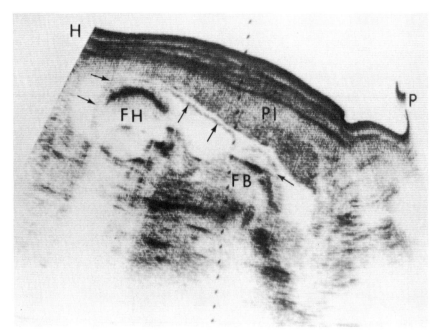

Fig. 12.150

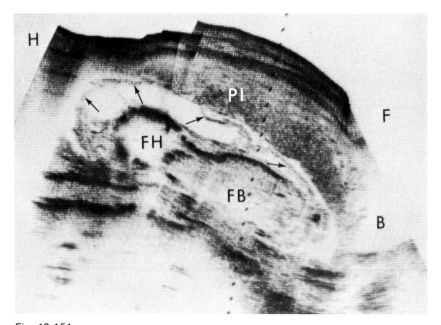

Fig. 12.151

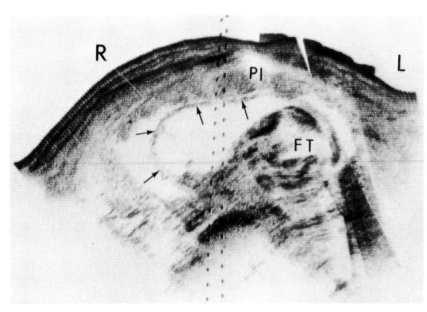

Fig. 12.152

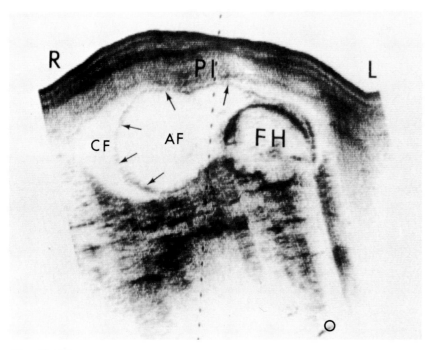

Fig. 12.153

Arrows	=	Amnionic membrane
AF	=	Amniotic fluid
B	=	Urinary bladder
CF	=	Chorionic fluid
F	=	Foot
FB	=	Fetal body
FH	=	Fetal head
FT	=	Fetal thorax
H	=	Head
L	=	Left
P	=	Level of the symphysis pubis
PI	=	Placenta
R	=	Right

Incompetent Cervix

The incompetent cervix is clinically described as a painless, bloodless, dilatation of the endocervical canal usually occurring during the second trimester of pregnancy. Ultrasound can easily visualize fluid in the endocervical canal and therefore confirm the diagnosis of incompetent cervix. Figure 12.154 is a longitudinal examination demonstrating the normal appearance of the endocervical canal. The endocervical canal appears as a strong linear echo in the mid portion of the myometrial echoes of the cervix. The normal length of the endocervical canal varies from approximately 2.5–6 cm. There should be no evidence of fluid in the endocervical canal during the course of a normal pregnancy. When examining a patient for incompetent cervix, it is important to have the bladder well filled. Overdistention of the bladder, however, may actually lead to collapse of an incompetent cervix.

Figure 12.155 is an example of a longitudinal scan in a patient with incompetent cervix and an overdistended bladder. The urinary bladder is markedly distended and actually compressing the cervix. The patient was asked to partially void to relieve bladder pressure. Figure 12.156 is a scan of the same patient following partial bladder emptying. Now the fluid in the endocervical canal confirms the diagnosis of an incompetent cervix.

We now routinely examine a patient suspected of having an incompetent cervix with a full urinary bladder and partial bladder emptying. If the bladder is markedly overdistended, it may cause closure of an incompetent cervix. Figure 12.157 is a transverse scan through an incompetent cervix with fluid in the endocervical canal.

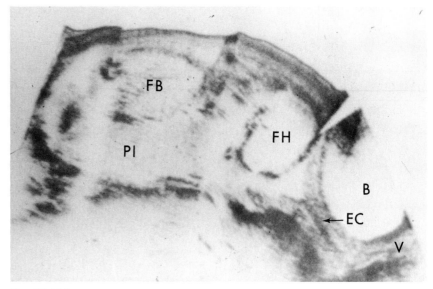

Fig. 12.154

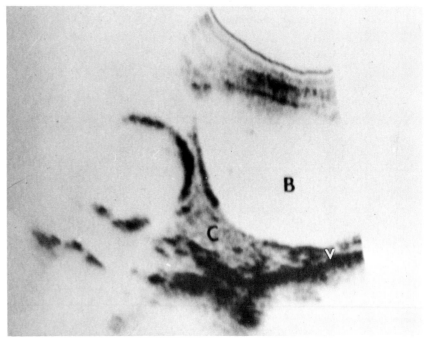

Fig. 12.155

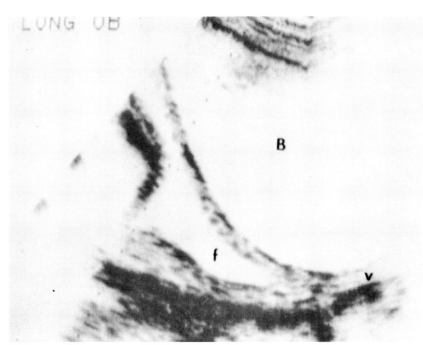

B	= Urinary bladder
C	= Cervix
EC	= Normal endocervical canal
f	= Fluid in the endocervical canal, secondary to incompetent cervix
FB	= Fetal body
FH	= Fetal head
Pl	= Placenta
V	= Vagina
v	= Vagina

Fig. 12.156

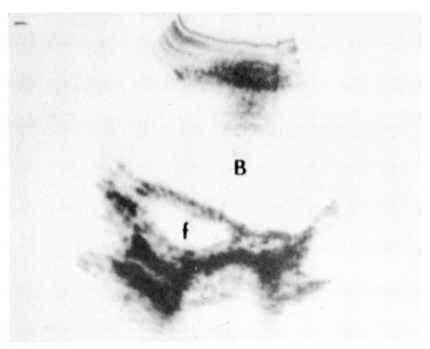

Fig. 12.157

Incompetent Cervix

Figure 12.158 is another example of incompetent cervix with amniotic fluid in the endocervical canal. The amniotic fluid is visualized almost to the external os. When examining a patient for incompetent cervix, it is important to align the transducer parallel to the long axis of the endocervical canal. This is best determined on the transverse scans by marking the right and left border of the cervix on the patient's skin. Longitudinal scans are then begun parallel to the long axis of the cervix.

Figure 12.159 is an example of incompetent cervix in a twin pregnancy. A cephalic fetus with the fetal head near the internal os is seen. Amniotic fluid is noted in the endocervical canal, again nearly completely to the external os. A second fetus is noted in the breech position in the fundal region of the uterus.

Figures 12.160 and 12.161 are examples of another case of incompetent cervix. There is markedly severe dilatation of the endocervical canal by amniotic fluid. This patient had marked bulging membranes; this is easily visualized on the ultrasound examination. Amniotic fluid is seen actually bulging into the proximal vagina.

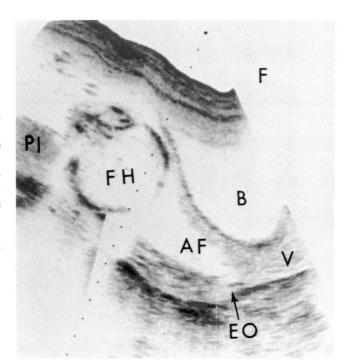

Fig. 12.158

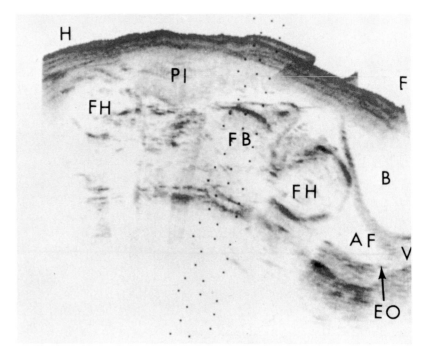

Fig. 12.159

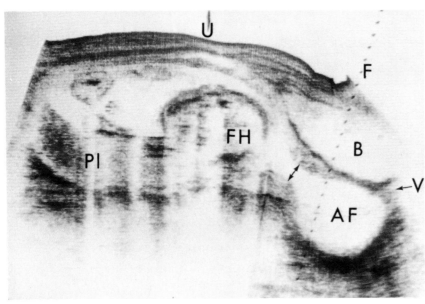

Fig. 12.160

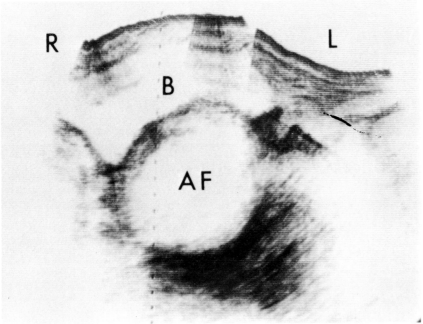

Fig. 12.161

AF = Amniotic fluid
B = Urinary bladder
EO = External os
F = Foot
FB = Fetal body
FH = Fetal head
H = Head
L = Left
PI = Placenta
R = Right
U = Umbilical level
V = Vagina

Ectopic Pregnancy

Patients are often sent for ultrasound examination to rule out ectopic pregnancy. Often, they have a positive pregnancy test and pelvic or lower abdominal pain. The ultrasound examination initially centers on visualizing the uterus to determine whether or not a gestational sac is present. If we visualize a normal gestational sac, ectopic pregnancy can be ruled out. If the uterus is empty, however, the study then concentrates on visualizing the adnexal regions to determine whether or not a mass is present. Figure 12.162 is an example of an ectopic pregnancy with the gestational sac within the tube on the right side. Here we see strong surrounding echoes, indicating decidual reaction. Even some internal echoes arise from the fetus within the gestational sac in the right adnexa. Strong linear echoes are present in the uterus, secondary to a Lippe's loop as seen in figure 12.163. The intrauterine device has the characteristic steplike pattern of a Lippe's loop. Figure 12.164 is a longitudinal scan of the same patient with the gestational sac situated in the right tube. Most ectopic pregnancies are not quite this classic. If we see a classic gestational sac within the tube, the diagnosis is quite easy.

Figure 12.165 is another example of an ectopic pregnancy on the right side. Fetal echoes inside the fluid-filled gestational sac are seen. Also noted in the pelvis are areas of hemorrhage behind the uterus and right adnexa. This is a common occurrence with some pelvic fluid secondary to hemorrhage associated with the ectopic pregnancy.

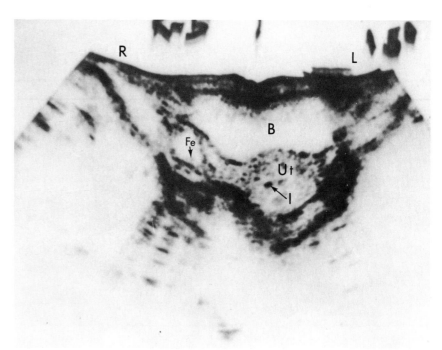

Fig. 12.162

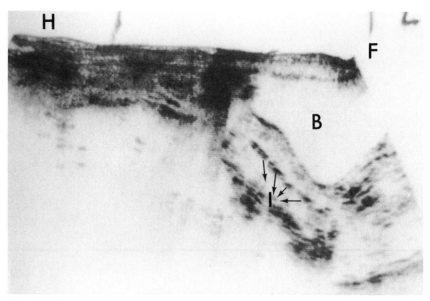

Fig. 12.163

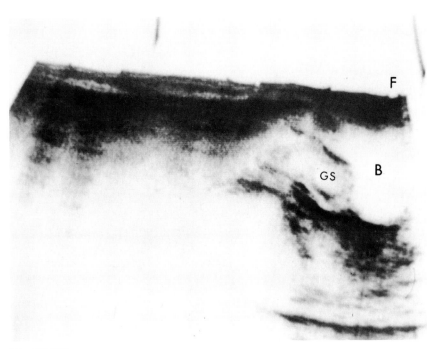

Fig. 12.164

SOURCE: The case in figures 12.162–12.164 is provided through the courtesy of Dr. M. Shaub, Centinela Valley Hospital, Los Angeles, California.

B	=	Urinary bladder
F	=	Foot
Fe	=	Fetal echoes
GS	=	Gestational sacs
H	=	Head
He	=	Hemorrhage
I and arrows	=	Intrauterine device
L	=	Left
R	=	Right
Ut	=	Uterus

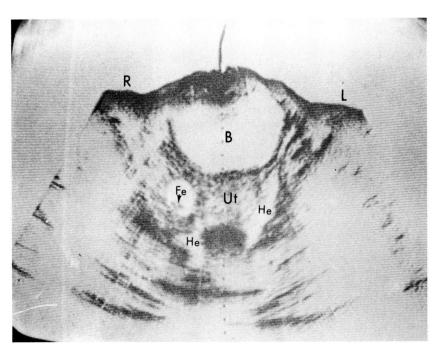

Fig. 12.165

Ectopic Pregnancy

The usual ultrasonic finding in ectopic pregnancy is an ill-defined adnexal mass rather than a clearly defined gestational sac, as noted previously. Figures 12.166 and 12.167 are scans of a patient with an ectopic pregnancy in the right adnexal region. The transverse scan in figure 12.166 demonstrates a solid-appearing echogenic mass that is larger than the normally sized left ovary. No gestational sac is clearly discernible. This is a more characteristic appearance of an ectopic pregnancy. A small central echo (arrow) is noted within the uterus. Often in an ectopic pregnancy, endometrial proliferation will be noted within the uterine cavity. This is the normal uterine response to the pregnant state, even though the pregnancy is outside the uterus.

The case in figures 12.168 and 12.169 is another characteristic ultrasonic appearance to an ectopic pregnancy. Figure 12.168 is a longitudinal scan of the right adnexal region with a mixed echogenic mass in the right adnexa. This fluid- and solid-containing mass was secondary to an ectopic pregnancy. Also noted in this patient was fluid situated in the cul-de-sac posterior to the uterus. This is seen in figure 12.169, and the fluid was secondary to hemorrhage from the ectopic pregnancy.

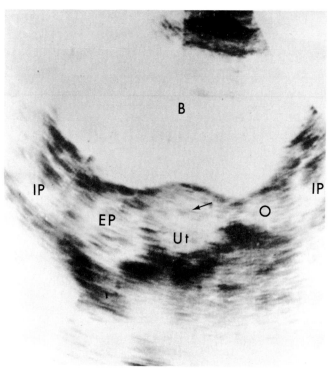

Fig. 12.166

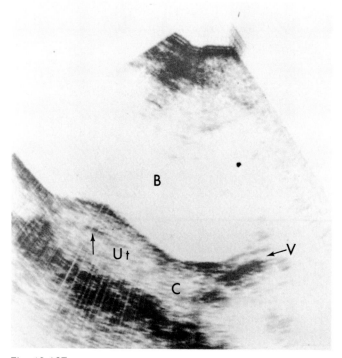

Fig. 12.167

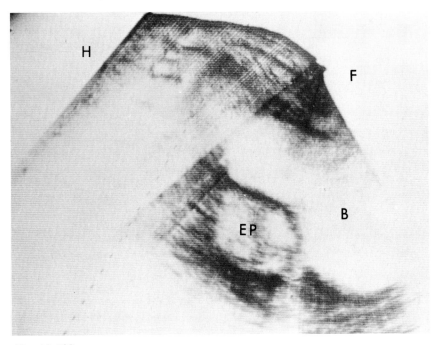

Arrow	=	Endometrial proliferation
B	=	Urinary bladder
C	=	Cervix
EP	=	Ectopic pregnancy
F	=	Foot
FI	=	Fluid in the cul-de-sac
H	=	Head
IP	=	Iliopsoas muscles
O	=	Normal left ovary
Ut	=	Uterus
V	=	Vagina

Fig. 12.168

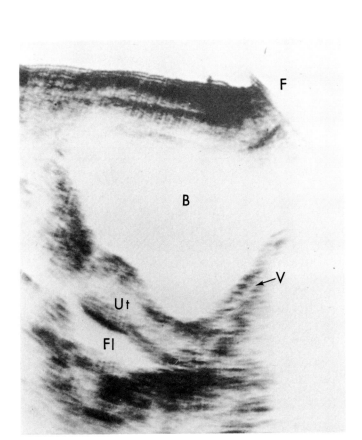

Fig. 12.169

Ectopic Pregnancy

Frequently, an ectopic pregnancy yields a large ill-defined mass in the pelvis very adherent to the uterus. When the borders between the uterus and the mass are lost, the findings can be similar to chronic pelvic inflammatory disease or endometriosis. The case in figures 12.170–12.172 is such an instance in which a chronic ectopic pregnancy is quite similar to chronic pelvic inflammatory disease. In figure 12.170 the ectopic pregnancy is present on the right side with a gestational sac surrounded by echogenic material. It is difficult to distinguish the border between the chronic ectopic pregnancy and the uterus. Within the uterus is a central echo consistent with endometrial proliferation. Posterior to the uterus is fluid in the cul-de-sac. Figure 12.171 is a longitudinal scan in the midline, again with endometrial proliferation within the uterus. Posterior to the uterus is the fluid in the cul-de-sac. Scanning to the right side of the patient, we see the gestational sac in figure 12.172 on a longitudinal scan. The highly echogenic material surrounding the gestational sac, which is secondary to hemorrhage and debris, is visualized.

Occasionally, a chronic ectopic pregnancy can reach a fairly large size. Figure 12.173 is a longitudinal scan in the midline with a chronic ectopic pregnancy which could be confused for a myomatous uterus. There is a loss of the tissue planes between the uterus and the chronic ectopic pregnancy, so that we cannot visualize the uterine borders.

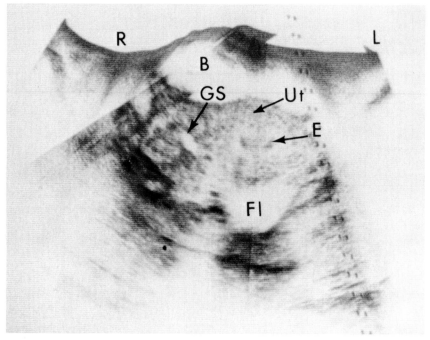

Fig. 12.170

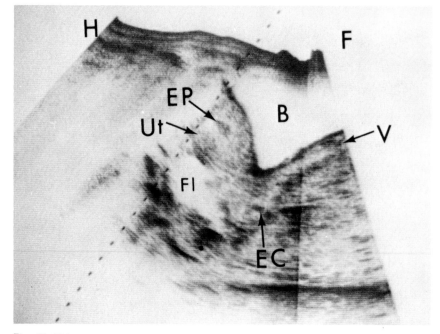

Fig. 12.171

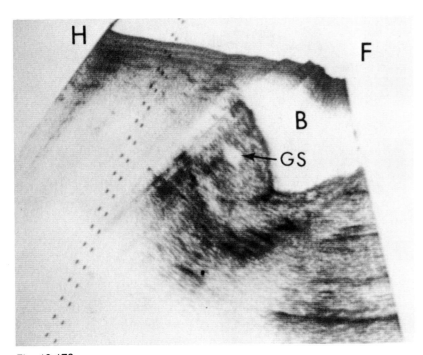

Fig. 12.172

SOURCE: Figure 12.173 is provided through the courtesy of Dr. M. Shaub, Centinela Valley Hospital, Los Angeles, California.

B	= Urinary bladder
C	= Chronic ectopic pregnancy
E	= Endometrial cavity
EC	= Endocervical canal
EP	= Endometrial proliferation
F	= Foot
FI	= Fluid in the cul-de-sac
GS	= Gestational sac
H	= Head
L	= Left
R	= Right
Ut	= Uterus
V	= Vagina

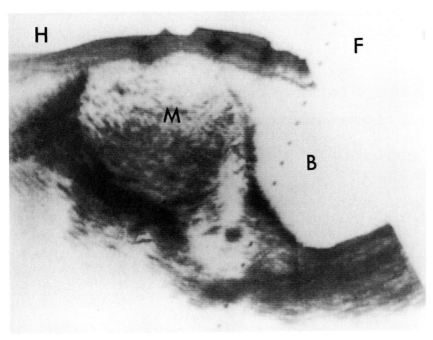

Fig. 12.173

Intrauterine Devices Associated with Pregnancy

Ultrasound examination is often requested to locate an intrauterine device. If this request occurs during the first 10 weeks of pregnancy, the exam can be successful. During this time period, the intrauterine device will stand out as a strong echo adjacent to the gestational sac. If it is after the tenth or eleventh week of pregnancy, however, numerous fetal echoes are present within the uterine cavity. The strong echoes arising from the fetus will make distinguishing the fetus from the intrauterine device difficult.

The gestational sac is seen as a fluid-filled structure in the mid portion of the uterus in figure 12.174. A strong circular echo is noted in the myometrium on the right side of the uterus. This is secondary to a Copper 7 intrauterine device. Figure 12.175 is a longitudinal scan through the mid portion of the uterus, demonstrating the gestational sac with fetal echoes within it. Figure 12.176 is the same patient; the right side of the uterus is being scanned. The strong echo of the intrauterine device is seen. The intrauterine device can be visualized at this time in the pregnancy, because the echoes arising from the fetus are not numerous enough to give any difficulty. Figure 12.177 is another example of a gestational sac present in conjunction with an intrauterine device. Here we see the gestational sac on the right side of the uterus. The strong circular echo is the characteristic echo arising from a Copper 7 intrauterine device on the left half of the uterus.

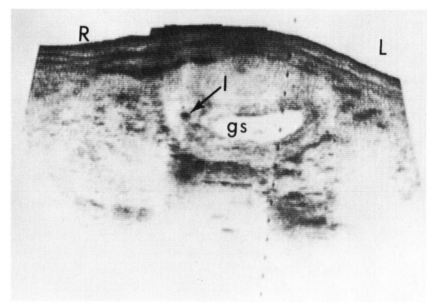

Fig. 12.174

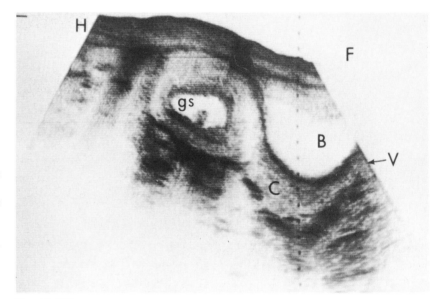

Fig. 12.175

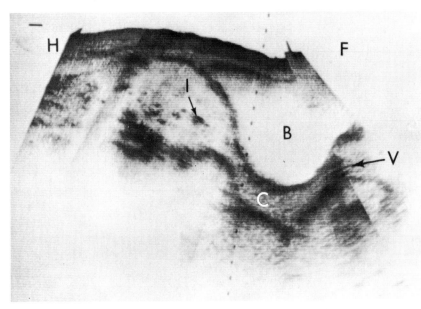

B = Urinary bladder
C = Cervix
F = Foot
gs = Gestational sac
H = Head
I = Intrauterine device
L = Left
R = Right
V = Vagina

Fig. 12.176

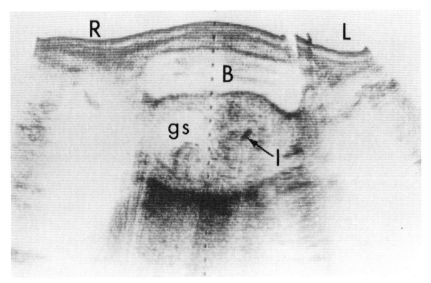

Fig. 12.177

Bicornuate Uterus

Occasionally, we will encounter a pregnancy in a bicornuate uterus, with a gestational sac on one side and myometrial echoes on the other side. The case in figures 12.178–12.180 is from a patient who requested a therapeutic abortion. Following a D and C, no gestational products were removed. Consequently, the patient underwent ultrasound examination. Figure 12.178 is a transverse scan following the attempted therapeutic abortion. We find evidence of a gestational sac with fetal echoes on the right side of the uterus. On the left side of the uterus there is a mixed echo pattern consistent with hemorrhage. Myometrium is present between the gestational sac and hemorrhage. Because of this finding, the diagnosis of a bicornuate uterus was made. We then lined up the gestational sac with the cervix and obtained an oblique longitudinal scan in figure 12.179. Here we see the pregnant cornua with a gestational sac in the fundal region of the uterus. A second oblique longitudinal scan was obtained, lining up the area of hemorrhage with the cervix. This is shown in figure 12.180. The other cornua with hemorrhage is visualized and lined up with the cervix and vagina. This is evidence of a pregnancy in a bicornuate uterus. The therapeutic abortion was not successful because the nonpregnant cornua was entered.

Figure 12.181 is another example of a pregnancy in a bicornuate uterus. The gestational sac is seen on the right side. In the left cornua we see strong high-amplitude echoes, indicating endometrial proliferation in the nonpregnant cornua.

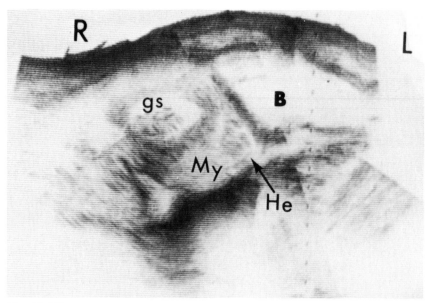

Fig. 12.178

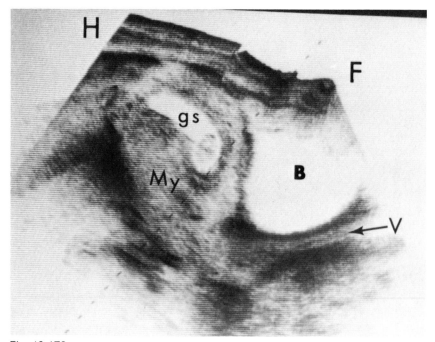

Fig. 12.179

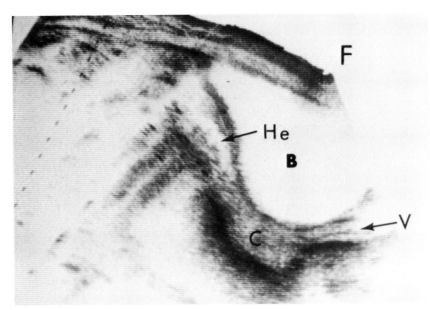

B	= Urinary bladder
C	= Cervix
EP	= Endometrial proliferation
F	= Foot
GS	= Gestational sac
gs	= Gestational sac
H	= Head
He	= Hemorrhage
L	= Left
My	= Myometrium
R	= Right
V	= Vagina

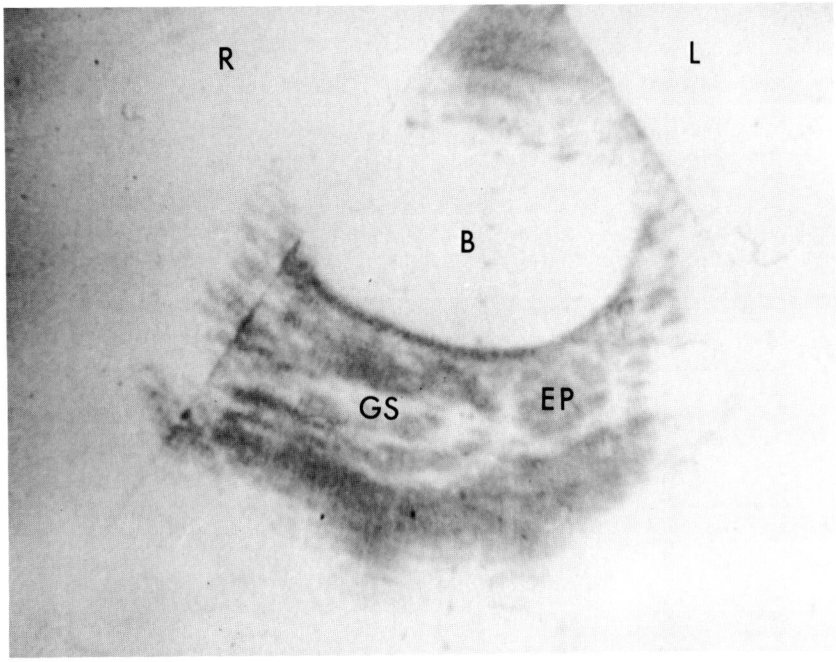

Fig. 12.180

Fig. 12.181

Index

The following figures have been reproduced in this text with the permission of the editors and publishers of their respective journals:

Figure 1.41 11.19 Sample, W. F. Normal anatomy of the female pelvis: computed tomography and ultrasonography. *Clinics in Diagnostic Ultrasound 2* (in press).
11.14 11.21
11.15 11.22
11.16 11.24
11.18 11.53

Figure 1.53 Sample, W. F. The unsoftened portion of the uterus: a pitfall in gray scale ultrasound studies during midtrimester pregnancy. *Radiology* 126:227–230, January 1978.
1.54
1.55

Figure 3.19 Sample, W. F. Diagnostic value and limitations in digestive disorders. Chapter 10 in *Developments in digestive diseases: clinical relevance* J. E. Berk, ed. Lea & Febiger, Philadelphia, 1977.
3.24
3.58
3.74

Figure 3.8 4.15 Sample, W. F. Normal abdominal anatomy defined by gray scale ultrasound. *Radiol. Clin. North Am.* 17:3–11, April 1979.
3.67 4.17
3.72 4.25
4.7 7.111
4.9 11.20
4.13

Figure 3.75 Sample, W. F.; Sarti, D. A.; Goldstein, L. I.; Weiner, M.; and Kadell, B. M. Gray scale ultrasonography of the jaundiced patient. *Radiology* 128:719–725, September 1978.
3.76

Figure 4.79 Carroll, B., and Sample, W. F. Pancreatic cystadenocarcinoma: CT body scan and gray scale ultrasound appearance. *Am. J. Roentgenol.* 131:339–341, August 1978.
4.80

Figure 4.10 Sample, W. F., and Sarti, D. A. Computed body tomography and gray scale ultrasonography: anatomic correlations and pitfalls in the upper abdomen. *Gastrointest. Radiol.* 3:243–249, 1978.
4.11
4.26

Figure 4.49 4.55 Sarti, D. A. Rapid development and spontaneous regression of pancreatic pseudocysts documented by ultrasound. *Radiology* 125:789–793, December 1977.
4.50 4.56
4.51 4.57
4.52 4.58
4.53 4.59
4.54 4.60

Figure 4.16 Sample, W. F., and Sarti, D. A. Computed tomography and gray scale ultrasonography of the adrenal gland: a comparative study. *Radiology* 128:377–383, August 1978.
7.137
7.147
7.169

Figure 7.110 Callen, P. W.; Filly, R. A.; Sarti, D. A.; and Sample, W. F. Ultrasonography of the diaphragmatic crura. *Radiology* 130:721–724, March 1979.
7.116
7.134

Figure 7.105 Cahill, P. J.; Cochran, S.; and Sample, W. F. Conventional radiographic and ultrasonic imaging in renal transplantation. *Urology* (Supplement) 10:33–42, July 1977.
7.108

Figure 7.112 7.146 Sample, W. F. Adrenal ultrasonography. *Radiology* 127:461–466, May 1978.
7.114 7.150
7.119 7.154
7.135 7.156

Figure 7.117 7.125 Sample, W. F. A new technique for the evaluation of the adrenal gland with gray scale ultrasonography. *Radiology* 124:463–469, August 1977.
7.118 7.143
7.123 7.144
7.124

Figure 7.227 7.256 Sample, W. F.; Gottesman, J. E.; Skinner, D. G.; and Ehrlich, R. M. Gray scale ultrasound of the scrotum. *Radiology* 127:225–228, April 1978.
7.248 7.259
7.252 7.263

Figure 10.9 Sarti, D. A.; Louie, J. S.; Lindstrom, R. R.; Nies, K.; and London, J. Ultrasonic diagnosis of a popliteal artery aneurysm. *Radiology* 121:707–708, December 1976.
10.10